Performance-Enhancing Substances in Sport and Exercise

Michael S. Bahrke, PhD
Human Kinetics

Charles E. Yesalis, MPH, ScD
Pennsylvania State University

Editors

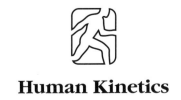

Human Kinetics

Library of Congress Cataloging in Publication Data

Bahrke, Michael S., 1949-
    Performance-enhancing substances in sport and exercise / Michael S. Bahrke, Charles
E. Yesalis.
       p. cm.
    Includes bibliographical references and index.
    ISBN 0-7360-3679-2
      1. Doping in sports. I. Yesalis, Charles. II. Title.

    RC1230 .B347 2002
    362.29'088'796--dc21

                          2002017199

ISBN-10: 0-7360-3679-2
ISBN-13: 978-0-7360-3679-5

The Web addresses cited in this text were current as of February 20, 2002, unless otherwise noted.

Acquisitions Editor: Loarn D. Robertson, PhD; **Developmental Editor:** Renee T. Thomas; **Assistant Editor:** Amanda S. Ewing; **Copyeditor:** Joyce Sexton; **Proofreader:** Red Inc.; **Indexer:** Susan Danzi Hernandez; **Permission Manager:** Dalene Reeder; **Graphic Designer:** Nancy Rasmus; **Graphic Artist:** Denise Lowry; **Cover Designer:** Jack W. Davis; **Art Manager:** Carl D. Johnson; **Illustrator:** Brian McElwain; **Printer:** Sheridan Books Inc.

Printed in the United States of America   10   9   8   7   6   5

Human Kinetics
Web site: www.HumanKinetics.com

United States: Human Kinetics, P.O. Box 5076, Champaign, IL 61825-5076
800-747-4457
e-mail: humank@hkusa.com

Canada: Human Kinetics, 475 Devonshire Road, Unit 100, Windsor, ON N8Y 2L5
800-465-7301 (in Canada only)
e-mail: info@hkcanada.com

Europe: Human Kinetics, 107 Bradford Road, Stanningley
Leeds LS28 6AT, United Kingdom
+44 (0) 113 255 5665
e-mail: hk@hkeurope.com

Australia: Human Kinetics, 57A Price Avenue, Lower Mitcham, South Australia 5062
08 8372 0999
e-mail: info@hkaustralia.com

New Zealand: Human Kinetics, Division of Sports Distributors NZ Ltd.
P.O. Box 300 226 Albany, North Shore City, Auckland
0064 9 448 1207
e-mail: info@humankinetics.co.nz

Contents

Foreword

The word competition is derived from the Latin "come together" and has taken on the English meaning of a "trial of skill or ability; a contest." Rules in sport define the field and mode of play—the essence of the trial of skill. There is no mystical meaning behind the arbitrary determination that a basketball rim is 10 feet above the court or that only 14 clubs are allowed in a golf bag during a round. The essence of sport, of a fair trial, is that the competitors abide by the rules of fair play.

In their trials of skill, all competitors look for an advantage in their pursuit of superiority. The advantage may be sought in the form of an equipment advance—such as a new golf club or ball, a clap skate, or a full-body swimsuit that reduces drag. It may also be sought in the form of improved training. And when the training becomes more than the athlete can endure, chemical and pharmacological means of gaining an advantage may be used. Chemical and pharmacological methods may also be viewed as the easy way to achieve an end.

Sport has a responsibility to maintain a level playing field for the trial of skill. The use of chemical and pharmacological agents is cheating—just like using a corked baseball bat. But unlike the broken corked bat lying on the field for all to see, doping is shrouded in mystery. There are a number of reasons for the difficulty in understanding doping. First, the athletes and their advisors, in an effort to find an advantage, continually seek to exploit "gray areas" surrounding the rules of sport. If something is not explicitly forbidden, then it must be permitted. If training at altitude to enhance the oxygenation of muscle is allowed, then wouldn't the use of an altitude (or nitrogen) tent be permitted? And if the nitrogen tent is permissible, then why not the use of recombinant erythropoietin? This slippery slope of rationalization, once embarked upon, is at once treacherous and appealing to a player or team seeking the glory and financial reward of modern sport.

One of the concerns of those responsible for the oversight of sport is the potential for unethical human experimentation, particularly under the pressure to succeed. The government-sanctioned doping system that formed the foundation of the East German success in athletics in the 1970s and 1980s is a frightening example.

Anabolic-androgenic steroids were administered to adolescent female athletes when the long-term outcome of such administrations was unknown. In addition to relying on the siren's song of Olympic glory, the athletes were coerced into taking the drugs by the threat of being dismissed from the governmental sports program and losing associated benefits.

While the potential for such programs still exists, the Internet provides a more insidious method of coercion. Undocumented, unreviewed testimonials and articles about new compounds abound. Such testimonials rave about success in adding muscle and weight and in some cases the use of excessive dosages and unusual routes of administration, such as snorting anabolic steroid powders up the nose with a straw. Without appropriate knowledge, these testimonials might be appealing. If a substance is natural, it must be okay to use, right? Wrong. Strychnine, hemlock, and many other poisons are natural too.

In toxicology, it is widely known that the dose makes the poison. A further impediment to providing reliable information is that the medical community is bound by the rules of medical ethics. Thus even investigating the long term effects of some of these compounds at the dosages used by athletes would not be allowed due to the possibility of harm to those participating in the study. In addition, studies may be carried out under one set of conditions, when in fact the athletes use the drug in much different dosages and in combination with other agents. An example would be androstenedione, which was shown to be converted to estrogen. However, combination with a substance that would prevent this conversion could result in increases in testosterone that were not found in the study. When studies are undertaken, the design of the study itself may not allow the investigators to draw the conclusion they desire. A recent study of the impact of creatine on kidney function made use of a medical test that is insensitive to small changes in kidney function, then concluded that there was no risk. Clearly any changes that might have occurred would have been small, but the limitations of the study made it through the scientific peer review process and into print. In the end, concern for the health of the athletes must result in erring on the side of safety.

The second reason for the difficulty in understanding doping is that information presented to the public about doping tends to be sensational and incomplete. People want to believe the deathbed revelations of Lyle Alzado whose use of steroids and other drugs to enhance his sports career resulted in the cancer that led to his death. To the scientific community, this revelation is simply an unproven hypothesis—one of many possible explanations for his illness. Many athletes are taking numerous substances to supplement their diet, making clear identification of a problematic compound extremely difficult.

Third, doping exists at the confluence of science and the law. It is important to uphold athletes' rights, and thus an athlete having a positive drug test is entitled to a hearing. Occasionally an athlete will admit breaking the rules, but more frequently the athlete retains an attorney in an attempt to avoid a sanction. Frequently the defense will make its case in the press, while the sports organization and the laboratory remain silent lest their responses be construed as creating bias in the case. As one example, a linkage between supplement use, exercise, and a positive drug test was reported in the press. The fact that the supplements were later found to be contaminated with the drug was not reported in the press. The net result is that some continue to believe there is a linkage between exercise, supplement use, and positive drug findings. In many scientific studies, the purpose of the study is to look for the common element among the participants. In the hearing room, the possibility that the athlete is an exception is always raised. In almost all cases, detailed scientific issues are presented to a legal panel who must weigh their merits against the rules of sport and arrive at a reasoned opinion. Sometimes the case turns on a technicality or a weakness in the prosecution of the case. For the uninformed, this can appear to be a flaw in the doping control system.

An additional problem arises when experts extend themselves beyond their area of expertise and begin to mix opinion and personal bias with their scientific expertise. Usually, a cross-examination at a hearing can clarify these issues. On the Internet, however, a number of individuals have published pages purporting to be critics of testing procedures or the inclusion of substances on the prohibited classes of compounds. It is frequently not clear to the reader where the authors obtained the information (since it is not referenced) or what credentials the authors have that allow them to critically analyze the information. The same is true when scientific studies are intermingled with quotes from newspapers, which give the latter an air of truth to which they are frequently not entitled. Thus, a complex area is made more difficult by the dissemination of misinformation.

Finally, there is the issue of ethics. When confronted with a new substance for which there is no test but there is potential for harm of the athlete, it could be argued that sport has a responsibility to act. The violation of any rule of sport is cheating. In the report of the Taskforce appointed by the Finnish Ministry of Education to investigate the widespread use of plasma expander infusions by the Finnish cross-country ski teams at the 2001 World Nordic Championships in Lahti, Finland, one of the most disappointing statements was that the coaches, physicians, and some skiers on the Finnish cross-country team knew that plasma expanders were prohibited and discussed whether or not HemoHES would show in the doping test. The athletes must have responsibility in the fight against drugs. This in turn requires that they have confidence that other athletes are not able to cheat and go undetected. The recent investment in anti-doping research by both the World Anti-Doping Agency and the United States Anti-Doping Agency is an important start in building this confidence.

It is apparent that there is a need for increased education both among athletes and among the public with respect to the issues surrounding the use of doping substances and methods in sports. Dr. Bahrke, Dr. Yesalis, and the numerous contributors to this book have successfully illuminated many of these issues in a scholarly and unbiased way. *Performance-Enhancing Substances in Sport and Exercise* is a strong contribution to the international fight against doping.

Frank Shorter
Chairman
Board of Directors
United States Anti-Doping Agency
Colorado Springs, Colorado

Larry D. Bowers, PhD
Senior Managing Director
Technical/Information Resources
United States Anti-Doping Agency
Colorado Springs, Colorado

Preface

The use of drugs and supplements by athletes to enhance performance and appearance is not new. The Berserkers of Norse mythology used bufotein for stimulating effects (Prokop, 1970). West Africans used *Cola acuminita* and *Cola nitida* for running competitions (Strauss & Curry, 1987). The ancient Greeks ate hallucinogenic mushrooms and sesame seeds to enhance performance (Wadler & Hainline, 1989). Roman gladiators used stimulants to overcome fatigue and injury (Wadler & Hainline, 1989). South American natives have chewed coca leaves for centuries to increase endurance (Boje, 1939; Karpovich, 1941). In the 1800s, performance-enhancing drug use among athletes was commonplace (Boje, 1939; Hoberman, 1992; Prokop, 1970), and it was during this time that the word *dop* first appeared in an English dictionary. At this time (1889) dop was defined as a narcotic mixture of opium used for racehorses (Voy and Deeter, 1991).

During the early 20th century the term *doping* was used to describe certain methods designed to augment the functional efficiency of athletes by means of highly active drugs (Boje, 1939). In the mid-20th century, people began to use the term in a general sense to describe any method of improving athletic performance temporarily, either during training or in conjunction with competitive meets (Boje, 1939). However, as the list of potential performance-enhancing substances (PES) grew longer during the last decade of the 20th century, the definition of doping became even broader and more confusing. As International Olympic Committee (IOC) Vice President Richard Pound admitted, "We still have no clearly stated definition of what doping is" (Lucas, 1992). Prohibiting and limiting substances such as ephedrine and caffeine, while permitting the use of others including creatine monohydrate, melatonin, ginseng, and asthma medications (e.g., salbutamol), exemplify the confusion around defining doping in sport that exists currently (Wilson, 2000).

Today, according to the IOC, doping is considered to contravene the ethics of both sport and medical science (IOC, 2000). It consists of the administration of substances belonging to prohibited classes of pharmacological agents and/or the use of various prohibited methods. Prohibited classes of substances used to enhance performance include stimulants (e.g., amphetamines), narcotics (e.g., morphine), anabolic agents (e.g., nandrolone), diuretics (e.g., furosimide), peptide hormones, mimetics, and analogs (e.g., growth hormone). Prohibited methods include blood doping and pharmacological, chemical, and physical manipulation. In addition, there are classes of drugs subject to certain restrictions; these include alcohol, cannabinoids (e.g., marijuana), local anesthetics (e.g., lidocaine), corticosteroids, and beta blockers (IOC, 2000).

Interestingly, while doping is banned in sport, some athletes, coaches, physicians, and others defend their use of various substances because they view these substances more as "performance enablers," "engenderers," or "restoratives" (e.g., pseudoephedrine for colds, beta blockers to reduce anxiety, and anti-inflammatories) that permit athletes to compete rather than as "performance enhancers" or "assistive additives" employed to improve their performance (e.g., anabolic steroids). This was the argument put forward by East German physicians and coaches who claimed they were only returning training-depressed testosterone levels to the normal range in their athletes, thus permitting their athletes to perform at previous levels—the levels they would have performed at had testosterone not been depressed as the result of intense training regimes. As French cycling star Richard Virenque (charged with various offenses related to encouraging and facilitating the use of illegal drugs in sporting competitions in connection with the 1998 Tour de France) stated, "We don't say doping. We say we're preparing for the race. To take drugs is to cheat. As long as the person doesn't test positive, they're not taking drugs." Virenque told the court he took certain products that "for me were vitamins, fortifiers" without being drugs. "My hope was not to fall ill, not to test positive" (Lille, France, Associated Press, October 24, 2000).

Later, Virenque tried to explain how he was led to indulge in doping. "Bike riding requires permanent sacrifice. It means training 11 months out of 12 and 110 days of racing in whatever the weather conditions. Early in life I realized I did not have the intellectual potential so I dedicated myself to cycling. As a teenager I did not smoke, I did not go out to discos like 95 per cent of youngsters do. After a while, suffering becomes harder. Your heartbeats swing from 140 to 180 a minute for long hours. It's not just like walking up stairs, you can only overcome pain with treatment (doping in cycling's slang) and fan's support" (Lille, France, electronicTelegraph, October 28, 2000).

Another example of the use of performance enablers is the case of Olympic all-round women's gymnastics gold medalist Andreea Raducan of Romania, who tested positive for a substance (two cold pills containing the banned stimulant pseudoephedrine prescribed by her team's physician) banned by the IOC during the 2000 Sydney Games and was subsequently disqualified (Sydney, Australia, Reuters, September 25, 2000). Many sports medicine specialists later agreed that the drug and the dose taken would not result in improved gymnastics performance and perhaps may have hindered her performance.

Athletes continue to use a wide variety of drugs and substances to enhance performance and appearance, including, among others, caffeine; amphetamines; human growth hormone; erythropoietin; clenbuterol; androstenedione; diuretics; gamma hydroxybutyric acid; creatine; anabolic-androgenic steroids; recreational drugs such as marijuana; and various vitamins, minerals, and herbals.

Although the vast majority of the athletic community accepts that many of these substances enhance performance and appearance, the extent to which this occurs and the factors influencing such effects remain incompletely understood and documented. While the short-term health effects of PES have been increasingly studied and reviewed, the long-term effects are generally unknown. Numerous adverse effects related to the use of PES include those to the cardiovascular, hepatic, and reproductive systems.

Unfortunately, much of our knowledge concerning the efficacy and adverse effects of PES is anecdotal. Also, much of the research examining the effectiveness and adverse effects of PES is fraught with methodological problems such as poor research design (e.g., small sample size; lack of blinded, placebo-controlled studies), use of a variety of substances (whose purity and content are often suspect), inconsistent dosages, concurrent use of several drugs by subjects (polypharmacy), and so on. In addition, the clinical application of these substances may have been hampered by the media's concern over the abuse of these substances in sport. Significant positive clinical benefits resulting from these drugs (e.g., testosterone) also may not have been fully examined. Moreover, it is quite possible that the lack of accurate and balanced reporting by the media on the performance effects of these substances has hindered efforts to prevent and reduce their use, especially at the elite level. Despite

enactment of legislation to restrict the use of PES, a diverse population continues to use these substances to promote improved health, performance, and physical appearance. A scholarly, heavily referenced book that thoroughly and effectively summarizes the research behind PES is needed. The purpose of this book is to examine the scientific evidence documenting the efficacy and safety of PES.

We have brought together many of the leading experts in the field of PES to provide exercise scientists, sports medicine specialists, sport administrators, coaches, and athletes with the latest and most comprehensive review of each PES. While it is beyond the scope of this book to include every substance thought to enhance performance, what we have done is include substances that are known or believed to have performance-enhancing properties, many of which are prohibited by the various sport governing organizations.

The history of the use of PES is discussed in part I, as are the methodological issues related to various aspects of the products: development (lack of clinical trials); manufacturing and production (purity, content, improper and inaccurate labeling); marketing and advertising (false, unsubstantiated, and improper claims); and legal, legislative, and enforcement aspects (scheduling, warnings, recalls).

Part II ("Anabolics") includes four chapters devoted to several very different anabolic drugs (anabolic-androgenic steroids, β2-agonists, human growth hormone and insulin-like growth factor, and testosterone precursors such as androstenedione). Anabolic-androgenic steroids are synthetic derivatives of testosterone, the natural male hormone responsible for the masculinizing (androgenic) and tissue-building (anabolic) effects noted during male adolescence and adulthood. Anabolic-androgenic steroids are used by athletes to increase muscle mass and strength, to reduce recovery time between training sessions, and, at times, for their aggression-increasing properties. Beta-2 agonists, such as clenbuterol, are classified as stimulants and are used to treat asthma in Europe and other countries. Although β2-agonists are not anabolic-androgenic steroids, they have been found to possess anabolic properties, that is, to increase lean muscle mass and reduce body fat in animals. Human growth hormone is secreted by the anterior pituitary gland. It stimulates bone growth and affects the metabolism of protein, carbohydrate, and fat. Synthetic (recombinant human growth hormone) forms are available and are used by athletes to increase muscle mass, decrease body fat, and speed recovery following training. Testosterone precursors such as androstenedione have become popular because of their use by athletes like Mark McGwire in his successful quest to break professional baseball's single-season home run record. Human chorionic gonadotropin, the topic of the fifth chapter in part II, is not an anabolic steroid; but it is used by athletes to stimulate endogenous testosterone production following long-term anabolic steroid use.

Erythropoietin, secreted by the kidneys, stimulates the formation of red blood cells in the bone marrow. Synthetic erythropoietin (recombinant erythropoietin), used by endurance athletes to increase the number of red blood cells—thus improving the oxygen-carrying capacity of the blood and ultimately the athlete's endurance performance—is the basis for part III ("Blood Doping"). Heterologous and autologous transfusions are also discussed in part III.

Diuretics such as Lasix and furosemide, prescribed therapeutically to increase the secretion of urine and to eliminate excess body water, are often used by athletes in weight-restricted sports such as wrestling and weightlifting and by bodybuilders to enhance muscle definition. Diuretics are also used by athletes to dilute urine for the purpose of circumventing drug testing. These drugs are discussed in part IV.

Part V covers narcotic and non-narcotic analgesics, used to suppress pain, and depressants such as hypnotics, tranquilizers, and β-adrenergic antagonists often used to reduce anxiety levels. The use of narcotic analgesics may permit athletes to perform beyond their normal pain limits. Depressants may reduce anxiety levels and result in improved performance in fine-motor skill sports. Non-narcotic analgesics, such as nonsteroidal anti-inflammatories and corticosteroids, are used for the pain and disability associated with muscle injuries or strains, muscle contusions, and delayed-onset muscle soreness. Narcotic and non-narcotic analgesics may also allow athletes to perform at their usual, normal performance levels.

Four chapters (on macronutrients and metabolic intermediates, creatine, sodium bicarbonate, and herbals) make up part VI ("Nutritional Ergogenic Aids"). These substances are used by athletes to increase muscle mass, supply energy to working muscles, and increase the rate of energy production in the muscle.

Part VII ("Social/Recreational Drugs") consists of two chapters, on alcohol and marijuana. Although alcohol is a recreational drug and classified as a depressant, it is sometimes used by athletes to reduce elevated levels of anxiety that can hamper the fine-motor skills required in sports such as marksmanship. Marijuana, another recreational drug, is often used by athletes for its relaxation effect and as an appetite stimulant (weight lifters).

Part VIII ("Stimulants") includes four chapters (on amphetamine, caffeine, cocaine, and ephedrine) that address the question "Do stimulants enhance performance?" Amphetamines may improve reaction time and increase muscular strength and endurance.

Caffeine stimulates the central nervous system, increasing arousal and fat utilization. Cocaine, used as a stimulant, may help athletes by reducing fatigue and enhancing endurance performance. Increase in physical power and suppression of appetite for weight control are two uses of ephedrine by athletes.

Part IX ("Miscellaneous Substances") includes information on gamma hydroxybutyric acid, designer drugs, and other substances used to enhance performance and improve appearance. Also included is a chapter on future performance-enhancing drugs and substances.

Two chapters (on masking agents and legal aspects) make up part X ("Drug Testing"). Masking agents such as Probenicid have been used by athletes to dilute the urine and avoid positive drug tests. Drug trafficking and enforcement efforts, drug testing, privacy issues and due process, and the legal consequences of drug abuse are a few of the topics discussed in the chapter on the legal aspects of drug use and abuse in sport and exercise.

Conclusions and future directions are included in part XI ("Conclusion"). Virtually all organizations overseeing athletic competitions oppose the use of performance-enhancing drugs. The drug policies, programs, regulations, and position stands and papers of various sport governing and sports medicine associations can be found at the Web sites included in the appendix.

References

Boje, O. (1939). Doping. *Bulletin of the Health Organization of the League of Nations, 8*, 439-469.

Hoberman, J. (1992). The early development of sports medicine in Germany. In J. Berryman & R. Park (Eds.), *Sport and exercise science: Essays in the history of sports medicine.* Champaign, IL: University of Illinois Press.

International Olympic Committee. (2000). *International Olympic committee medical code.* Lausanne, Switzerland: International Olympic Committee.

Karpovich, P.V. (1941). Ergogenic aids in work and sports. *Research Quarterly, 12*(Suppl.), 432-450.

Lucas, J.A. (1992). *Future of the Olympic Games.* Champaign, IL: Human Kinetics.

Prokop, L. (1970). The struggle against doping and its history. *Journal of Sports Medicine and Physical Fitness, 10*(1), 45-48.

Strauss, R.H., & Curry, T.J. (1987). Magic, science and drugs. In R.H. Strauss (Ed.), *Drugs and performance in sports* (pp. 3-9). Philadelphia: Saunders.

Voy, R., & Deeter, K.D. (1991). *Drugs, sport, and politics.* Champaign, IL: Human Kinetics.

Wadler, G., & Hainline, B. (1989). *Drugs and the athlete.* Philadelphia: Davis.

Wilson, S. (2000). Concerns over medication, athletes. *Associated Press,* November 15.

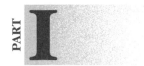

PART I

Introduction

CHAPTER 1

History of Doping in Sport

Charles E. Yesalis, MPH, ScD

Michael S. Bahrke, PhD

"I feel sorry for Ben Johnson. All sportsmen—not all, but maybe 90%, including our own—use drugs."

Anonymous Soviet coach
The New York Times, October 1988
1988 Seoul Olympics

"Americans like to think the U.S. leads the 'Sports without Drugs Crusade,' but 'the reality is that the U.S. is viewed as one of the dirtiest nations in the world,' says John Ruger, past chair of the United States Olympic Committee Athletes' Advisory Council."

"Mass Deception: Today's Athlete Is Getting Bigger, Stronger, Faster . . . Unnaturally"
Sport, August 1998

When humans compete against one another—either in war, in business, or in sport—the competitors, by definition, seek to achieve an advantage over their opponent. Frequently they use drugs and other substances to gain the upper hand. Furthermore, there have always been individuals who in the pursuit of victory have transcended social norms. In sport such conduct is termed cheating, and it has existed as long as sport has existed. Today, stone pedestals line the entranceway to the Olympic stadium in Olympia, Greece, site of the ancient Games (776 B.C.-394 A.D.). During the ancient Games these pedestals supported zanes, bronze life-size statues of Zeus (Pausanias, 1959). Zanes were placed there not to honor the great athletes of the time, but rather to punish, in perpetuity, athletes who violated Olympic rules. These cheaters were banished for life from competing in the Games. Inscribed on each stone pedestal is the offending athlete's name, his transgression

(e.g., bribing an opponent), and the names of family members. The statues also served as a warning to athletes of the day who had to pass them on their way into the stadium to compete before 40,000 spectators.

Interestingly, while the violation of Olympic rules was dealt with harshly in the ancient Games, it does not appear that the use of drugs and other substances to improve athletic performance was considered cheating. Nor does it appear that any culture in early history made any effort to discourage the use of ergogenic substances. In fact, after doping in sport blossomed during the latter part of the 19th century, it was viewed as a standard practice—out in the open—until after World War I (Hoberman, 1992b). Not until the 1920s was there any widespread attempt to admonish against doping in sport, much less designate it as a formal violation of rules or as cheating (Hoberman, 1992b). In 1933 Dr. Otto Rieser, in his prophetic work "Doping and Doping Substances," discussed the prevalence of doping as well as the culpability of medical professionals.

> The use of artificial means [*to improve performance*] has long been considered wholly incompatible with the spirit of sport and has therefore been condemned. Nevertheless, we all know that this rule is continually being broken, and that sportive competitions are often more a matter of doping than of training. It is highly regrettable that those who are in charge of supervising sport seem to lack the energy for the campaign against this evil, and that a lax, and fateful, attitude is spreading. Nor are the physicians without blame for this state of affairs, in part on account of their ignorance, and in part

because they are prescribing strong drugs for the purpose of doping which are not available to athletes without prescriptions (Hoberman, 1992b).

By 1933 the word *doping* had become a normal part of the English language (Prokop, 1970). While Rieser and others continued to speak out against doping, it was not until 1967 that the International Olympic Committee (IOC) voted to adopt a drug-testing policy banning the use of specific drugs (Todd & Todd, 2001). However, even in 1969 an investigative report by *Sports Illustrated* concluded that "not a single major U.S. sporting organization, amateur or professional . . . has specific anti-doping regulations with an enforcement apparatus" (Gilbert, 1969c). In 1982 the National Football League finally began drug testing players, although the NFL did not test for anabolic steroids until 1987 (Ferstle, 2000). The National Collegiate Athletic Association (NCAA) did not initiate a drug-testing program until 1986. In 1998 baseball slugger Mark McGwire acknowledged that he used androstenedione, an anabolic steroid that is banned specifically by the IOC, the NCAA, and the NFL. Professional baseball has not banned this or any other steroid and has no drug-testing program in place for performance-enhancing drugs (Ferstle, 2000). Today professional sports in the United States that do test for drugs have programs that, on average, are substantially less rigorous than the IOC program (Ferstle, 2000). Interestingly, while doping was outlawed in horse racing as early as 1903 (Donohoe & Johnson, 1986), it was not until at least the latter third of the 20th century that major sport organizations began to proscribe doping—formally designating it as a form of cheating. In 1939 in his paper titled "Doping," Boje commented on this apparent irony:

In sports in which animals took part, the use of stimulants was so widespread that several countries introduced legislation to forbid it on the grounds of its cruelty to the animals. Equal attention ought also to be paid to human beings participating in sports.

Early History

The use of drugs to enhance physical performance has been a feature of human competition since the beginning of recorded history (Prokop, 1970; Strauss & Curry, 1987). The goal of the user most often was to increase strength or overcome fatigue. Today we classify such drugs as anabolics and stimulants.

It has been argued that the first instance of doping occurred in the Garden of Eden when Adam and Eve ate the forbidden fruit to gain godlike powers (Csaky, 1972). The ancients learned empirically of the anabolic and androgenic function of the testes by observing the effects of castration on domesticated animals (Newerla, 1943). Furthermore, the ancients as well as people of the medieval

period indulged in organotherapy (the eating of the organs of animals and humans) to cure disease and to improve vitality and other aspects of performance (Newerla, 1943). As early as 1400 B.C., the Susruta of India advocated the ingestion of testis tissue to cure impotence. Likewise, the ancient Egyptians accorded medicinal powers to the testicles (Hoberman & Yesalis, 1995). A heart may have been eaten to promote bravery, and the brain to improve intelligence. Testicular extract was prescribed by Johannes Mesue the Elder (777-837 A.D.) as an aphrodisiac (Rolleston, 1936).

The works of Aretaeus (1854) the Cappadocean (ca. 150 A.D.) portend the endocrine function of the testis, in particular the anabolic and androgenic effects of testosterone: "For it is the semen, when possessed of vitality, which makes us to be men, hot, well braced in limbs, well voiced, spirited, strong to think and act. . . . But if any man be continent in the emission of semen, he is bold, daring, and strong as wild beasts as is proved from such of the athletae as are continent. . . . Vital semen, then, contributes to health, strength, courage, and generation."

In the ancient Games, many of the "athletes tried, persistently . . . to improve their performance not only by studying the techniques of their particular sport but also by . . . experimenting with their diet among other things . . ." (Finley & Plecket, 1976). Charmis, the Spartan winner of the *stade* race (~200 yd [183 m]) in the Olympic Games of 668 B.C., purportedly used a special diet of dried figs. Other athletes ate wet cheese and wheat meal. On the other hand, Dromeus from Stymphalos, who won the *dolichos* race (1-3 miles [1.6-4.8 km]) twice at Olympia, twice at Delphi, three times at Isthmia, and five times at Nemea, ate a meat diet (Pausanias, 1959).

The use of stimulants also dates to ancient times. The Greeks drank various brandy and wine concoctions (Voy, 1991) and ate hallucinogenic mushrooms and sesame seeds to enhance performance. Likewise, the gladiators in the Roman Colosseum used unspecified stimulants to overcome fatigue and injury (Wadler & Hainline, 1989). Medieval knights also reportedly used unnamed stimulants to improve their stamina in battle (Donohoe & Johnson, 1986).

Many of the early stimulants were of plant origin. The legendary Berserkers of Norse mythology used bufotein to "increase their fighting strength twelve fold" (Prokop, 1970). This drug came from fly-agaric *(Amanita muscaria)*, a mushroom containing muscarine (a deadly alkaloid) (Boje, 1939). The Samoyeds used the same stimulant to induce a heightened state of combativeness. The African plant *Catha edulis* contains norpseudo-ephedrine, a psychomotor stimulant that has been used by the people of the region to increase strength and delay the onset of fatigue (Ivy, 1983). From ancient times West

Africans used *Cola acuminita* and *Cola nitida* for running competitions (Boje, 1939). For centuries Andean Indians of Peru have chewed coca leaves or drunk coca tea to increase endurance and protect against mountain sickness (Jokl, 1968). The Tarahumara Indians of northern Mexico used peyote (which has strychnine effects) in their multiday runs that were among the requirements of a fertility ritual (Hoberman, 1992b). The Australian aborigines ate the pituri plant for its stimulant effect (Boje, 1939; Karpovich, 1941; Williams, 1974). In Styria and Tyrol in Austria, lumberjacks ingested large amounts of arsenic to increase their endurance (Csaky, 1972).

Nineteenth Century

The last half of the 19th century saw the beginnings of modern medicine and, not coincidentally, a significant growth in the use of drugs and other substances to improve performance. While the primary emphasis was on stimulants as ergogenic aids, this period also marked the birth of scientific experimentation with the anabolic effects of hormones.

Stimulants

The stimulant effect of coffee (caffeine) has long been recognized. According to Catton (1951) in *The Army of the Potomac,* during the Civil War "the coffee ration was what kept the *(Union)* army going." The ration was "ample for three or four pints of strong black coffee daily. . . . Stragglers would often fall out, build a fire, boil coffee, drink it, and then plod on to overtake their regiments at nightfall." The use of coffee by foot soldiers also serves as an early example that such ergogenic practices were not universally embraced: "cavalry and artillery referred to infantry, somewhat contemptuously, as 'coffee boilers'" (Catton, 1951).

Coffee was also "the drug of choice for any number of literati, scientists, and artists" of that period whose work necessitated a well-functioning brain (Hoberman, 1992b). Liquors too were considered artificial stimulants to be used by "soldiers and laborers working in stressful conditions" (Hoberman, 1992b).

In the last third of the 19th century, the use of stimulants among athletes was commonplace, and moreover, there was no attempt to conceal drug use with the possible exception of some trainers who guarded the proprietary interest in their own special "doping recipes." Swimmers, distance runners, sprinters, and cyclists used a wide assortment of drugs to gain an edge over their opponents (Boje, 1939; Hoberman, 1992b; Prokop, 1970). As early as 1865, a doping episode involving canal swimmers of Amsterdam was reported (Prokop, 1970). Boxers of the day used strychnine tablets and mixtures of brandy and cocaine (Prokop, 1970).

In 1879, "Six Day" bicycle races began, each race proceeding continuously, day and night, for 144 hours. It is not surprising that stimulants and a variety of doping strategies were employed in these grueling contests of prolonged athletic exertion.

"French racers preferred mixtures on caffeine bases, the Belgians preferred sugar cubes dipped in ether, and others used alcohol-containing cordials, while the sprinters specialized in the use of nitroglycerine" (Prokop, 1970).

The cyclists of the day also used coffee "spiked" with caffeine; and as the race progressed, they would add increasing doses of cocaine and strychnine (Donohoe & Johnson, 1986). (Note: Strychnine when taken at low doses has a stimulant effect, while at higher doses it is poisonous.) As trainers continued their experiments with a variety of powerful drugs and poisons, it is little wonder that someone died. The first fatality attributed to doping was reported in 1886: Arthur Linton, an English cyclist, is said by some to have overdosed on "tri-methyl" (probably a compound containing either caffeine or ether) during a 600-km (373-mile) race between Bordeaux and Paris (Prokop, 1970). Others have argued that in fact Linton won the race in question and did not die until 10 years later, in 1896, of typhoid fever (Donohoe & Johnson, 1986). Whatever the case, given the potency of many of the doping substances being used at that time, it is clear that the health of the athlete was at risk.

Another popular sport during that period in both the United States and England was the professional sport of pedestrianism (or ultramarathoning). These "go-as-you-please" walking and/or running marathon races usually lasted six days and six nights (Lucas, 1968). The contestant who had covered the most miles at the end of the six days was declared the winner. During some of the more famous ultramarathons, several of the contestants in one race each completed over 500 miles (805 km), and in 1884 George Haezel of England became the first man to cover 600 miles (966 km) in the six-day period (Lucas, 1968)! By their very nature, stimulants lent themselves to use in this sport. Trainers employed a variety of concoctions to keep their man going. These included milk-punch champagne and brandy, as well as belladonna, strychnine, and "morphine in hot drops" (Osler & Dodd, 1979).

Anabolics

The age of scientific organotherapy began on June 1, 1889, when the 72-year-old Charles Edouard Brown-Sequard, a prominent physiologist and neurologist, addressed the Society of Biology in Paris. In his talk (and a paper published shortly after), Brown-Sequard reported how over a three-week period he had self-administered 10 subcutaneous injections that contained "first, blood of the testicular veins; secondly, semen; and thirdly, juice extracted from a testicle . . . from a dog or guinea pig" (Brown-Sequard, 1889). He enthusiastically described "radical" changes in his health including significant improvements in physical and mental energy. One month after the last injection he "experienced almost a complete return of the state of weakness. . . ." While today most experts believe that the "rejuvenation" experienced by Brown-Sequard was the result of the placebo effect, he was correct, not only in his rudimentary understanding of testicular function, but also about the potential value of hormonal replacement or supplementation therapy. Because of this he is considered the father of modern endocrinology.

Brown-Sequard offered free samples of his *liquide testiculaire* to physicians willing to test them. In addition, various laboratories, including some in the United States such as the New York Pasteur Institute, began preparing the extract for use (Borell, 1976). This began a swell of experiments not only in France but throughout the Western world employing testicular extracts to rejuvenate as well as treat a wide variety of diseases (Hoberman & Yesalis, 1995). The "Fountain of Youth" had been found—once again—and a cultlike following arose (Herman, 1982). Numerous similar accounts of rejuvenation soon followed and continued until the early 1920s. Ironically, these uncontrolled studies and bold claims also stimulated important research in clinical endocrinology.

The "athleticizing" of testicular extracts came quickly after Brown-Sequard's initial report. In 1894 Oskar Zoth and Fritz Pregl assessed the effects of the extracts on muscular strength (Hoberman, 1992b). Although Zoth concluded that these "orchitic" extracts improved muscular strength, it is highly unlikely they had any therapeutic or ergogenic effect beyond the power of suggestion (Hoberman & Yesalis, 1995). Nevertheless, Zoth in a 1896 paper provides a chilling prophecy of the use of anabolic hormones in sport in the 20th century when he states in the final sentence: "The training of athletes offers an opportunity for further research in this area and for a practical assessment of our experimental results" (Hoberman & Yesalis, 1995).

Twentieth Century

Looking at elite sport in the 20th century, an unstable picture emerges of a doping pandemic. This section discusses the use of anabolics and stimulants during the 20th century; the current use of PES by Olympic, professional, collegiate, and adolescent athletes; and the response of organized sport to this problem.

Anabolics

In 1912, another form of glandular therapy debuted with the transplantation of animal and human testicular material into patients with testicular dysfunction (Hamilton, 1986, Hoberman & Yesalis, 1995). As with the injection of

extracts, the purposes of these transplants were curative and restorative. The practitioners of these procedures believed, incorrectly, that these testicular transplants would survive in the recipient and would function. Many respected surgeons around the world performed these transplants through the 1920s and published case reports of favorable findings in well-respected medical journals, including *Endocrinology* and the *Journal of the American Medical Association* (Lespinasse, 1913; Stanley, 1922). However, in the mid-1920s, serious concern arose in the medical community regarding these overt claims of rejuvenation (Fishbein, 1925). As a result an international committee was appointed to evaluate these claims and concluded that they were unfounded (Parkes, 1985, 1988). The practice disappeared by 1935 when scientists isolated, chemically characterized, and synthesized the hormone testosterone and elucidated the basic nature of its anabolic effects (Butenandt & Hanisch, 1935; David, Dingemanse, Freud, & Laqueur, 1935; Kochakian & Murlin, 1935). Shortly thereafter, both oral and injectable preparations of testosterone were available to the medical community. While there is no record of systematic use of testicular transplants or the injection of testicular extracts by athletes, these procedures likely helped lay the foundation for the subsequent use of testosterone as an ergogenic aid.

It has been rumored that some German athletes were given testosterone in preparation for the 1936 Berlin Olympics (Francis, 1990). Although the effects of other drugs on the physiology of human performance are well documented in the German medical literature, no mention of the use of testosterone as an ergogenic aid has been noted during that period (Hoberman, 1992a & 1992b). Moreover, Hoberman contends:

> It is likely that public anti-doping sentiment after 1933 was related to Nazi strictures against the self-serving, individualistic, record-breaking athlete and the abstract ideal of performance. It is also consistent with Nazi rhetoric about sportsmanship, e.g., the importance of the "noble contest" and the "chivalric" attitude of the German athlete.

Wade (1972) has alleged that during World War II, German soldiers took steroids before battle to enhance aggressiveness. This assertion, although often cited, has yet to be documented, in spite of efforts in this regard. Furthermore, the Nazis were opposed to organism-altering drugs in general (Hoberman, 1992a & b). There was a concerted campaign against the "poisons" alcohol and tobacco, and the Nazis "were not particularly interested in the popular gland transplant techniques of that period, since their idea of race improvement was genetic" (Hoberman, 1992a & b).

Boje, writing in the *Bulletin of the Health Organization of the League of Nations* in 1939, appears to have been the first to suggest that sex hormones, based on their physiologic actions, might enhance physical performance. At the same time, the anabolic effects of anabolic steroids were being confirmed in eunuchs and in normal men and women (Kenyon, Knowlton, Sandiford, Koch, & Lotwin, 1940; Kenyon, Sandiford, Bryan, Knowlton, & Koch, 1938). Uncontrolled studies also demonstrated improvements in strength and dynamic work capacity in eugonadal males (Simonson, Kearns, & Enzer, 1941) and otherwise healthy older males complaining of fatigue (Simonson, Kearns, & Enzer, 1944).

The first recorded case of an "athlete" using testosterone was a gelding trotter named Holloway (Kearns, Harkness, Hobson, & Smith, 1942). Prior to the implantation of testosterone pellets, this 18-year-old horse had "declined to a marked degree in his staying power and during February of 1941 in several attempts at ice racing, failed to show any of his old speed or willingness" (Kearns et al., 1942, p. 199). After the administration of testosterone and several months of training, Holloway won or placed in a number of races and established a trotting record at age 19.

In *The Male Hormone*, de Kruif (1945) further raised hopes and expectations for the newly synthesized anabolic steroids. He argued that these hormones had the potential to rejuvenate individuals and improve their productivity, and he assuredly reported that testosterone "caused the human body to synthesize protein [and] . . . to be able to build the very stuff of its own life" (p. 130). De Kruif went on:

> I'll be faithful and remember to take my twenty to thirty milligrams a day of testosterone. I'm not ashamed that it's no longer made to its old degree by my own aging body. It's chemical crutches. It's borrowed manhood. It's borrowed time. But just the same, it's what makes bulls bulls. (p. 226)

With regard to athletes, de Kruif commented,

> We know how both the St. Louis Cardinals and the St. Louis Browns have won championships supercharged by vitamins. It would be interesting to watch the productive power of an industry or a professional group (of athletes) that would try a systematic supercharge with testosterone. (p. 223)

De Kruif's writings were not without effect. When these were combined with the significant positive observations reported from clinical studies in professional journals, it was a relatively easy extrapolation for some in the physical culture of bodybuilding to expect that additional anabolic-androgenic hormones, at that time universally assumed to exert no adverse effects when taken in therapeutic dosages, would allow development of greater-than-"normal" body size and strength. According to several interview reports,

experimental use of the new testosterone preparations began among West Coast bodybuilders in the early 1950s (Wright et al., 1998 unpublished). Also suggestive of anabolic steroid use are physique photos of this time showing highly significant changes over relatively short periods in the muscle mass of established elite bodybuilders. Since then, bodybuilding has been and continues to be strongly and consistently linked to steroid use (Duchaine, 1982, 1989; Fussell, 1990; Klein, 1986, 1993; Nack, 1998; Phillips, 1990; Wright, 1978), as has the sport's most well-known participant, Arnold Schwarzenegger (Johnston, 1974; Leigh, 1990). The elite bodybuilding community has maintained its position at the "cutting edge" of experimentation with performance-enhancing drugs. By the early 1980s and beyond, the use of human growth hormone (hGH) was well established on that community's drug menu (Duchaine, 1982, 1989; Fahey, 2001). In 1982 Fred Hatfield in his controversial book, *Anabolic Steroids: What Kind and How Many,* stated that hGH had "become 'the state of the art' strength and size drug in the free world."

The initiation of systematic use of anabolic steroids in sport has been attributed to reports of their use by successful Soviet weightlifting teams in the early 1950s. Statistical analysis of the performance of the Soviet lifters during this period is consistent with this assertion (Fair, 1988).

In 1954, at the world weightlifting championships in Vienna, Dr. John Ziegler, the U.S. team physician, reportedly was told by his Soviet counterpart that the Soviets were taking testosterone (Fair, 1993; Starr, 1981; Todd, 1987). Ziegler returned to the United States and experimented with testosterone on himself and a few weight lifters in the York Barbell Club. Dr. Ziegler was concerned, however, with the androgenic effects of testosterone; and in 1958, when the Ciba Pharmaceutical Company released Dianabol (methandrostenolone), he began experimentation with this new drug. After several of the weight lifters with whom Ziegler was working achieved championship status while using anabolic steroids, news of the efficacy of these drugs apparently spread by word of mouth during the early 1960s to other strength-intensive sports, from field events to football.

Stimulants

Continuing the practices of their 19th-century counterparts, athletes during the first three decades of the 20th century used a variety of substances (alcohol, cocaine, strychnine, caffeine, and nitroglycerine) for their purported "stimulant" effects (Boje, 1939; Prokop, 1970; Jokl, 1968). Noticeably absent from this doping menu is any mention of the use of amphetamines, even though they were first synthesized in 1887 (Hart & Wallace, 1975). In the 1920s and 1930s other derivatives of amphetamines were synthesized. However, it was not until the mid-1930s that amphetamines were identified as a central nervous system stimulant, and in 1937 they became available as a prescription tablet (Ray & Ksir, 1996). In the late 1930s, amphetamines were publicized as "a means of dissipating mental fog" and were thereafter adopted by college students "to ward off sleep and clear their minds" (*Air Surgeon's Bulletin,* 1944).

The first systematic use of amphetamines as an ergogenic aid was seen during World War II, when both Axis and Allied powers used these drugs to combat fatigue and improve endurance. The British army used amphetamines when men "were markedly fatigued physically or mentally and circumstances demanded a particular effort" (Robson, 1999). According to a report in the *Air Surgeon's Bulletin* (1944), ". . . one pill (*Benzedrine*) may be worth a Flying Fortress when the man who is flying it can no longer stay awake." Going beyond staving off fatigue, the Japanese were said to have used heavy doses of amphetamines to arouse or "psych up" their kamikaze pilots in preparation for the suicide missions (Scott, 1971). Similarly Mandell (1981) suggested that amphetamines could be used by soldiers to create a sense of fearlessness.

The use of these "pep pills" by prewar college students, combined with the experiences of servicemen who used them to competitive advantage in armed services football, appears to have laid the foundation for introduction of amphetamines to professional and collegiate sport at the end of the World War II (Mandell, 1978). The spread of amphetamine use must have proceeded rather quickly, because by 1969 Gilbert (1969b) concluded:

> On good evidence—which includes voluntary admissions by physicians, trainers, coaches, athletes, testimony given in court or before athletic regulatory bodies, and autopsy reports— amphetamines have been used in auto racing, basketball, baseball (at all levels down to children's leagues), boxing, canoeing, cycling, football, golf, mountain climbing, Roller Derby, rodeo, Rugby, skating, skiing, soccer, squash, swimming, tennis (both lawn and table), track and field, weight lifting and wrestling.

Cycling

Cycling plays a central role in the explosion of stimulant use in sport after World War II. Prokop (1970) describes cycling competitions of that era as "special hotbeds of doping." Of 25 urine samples taken from riders in a 1955 race, five were positive for stimulants. In the 1960 Rome Olympic Games, Knut Jensen, a 23-year-old Danish cyclist, collapsed during competition and died. Autopsy results revealed the presence of amphetamines (Donohoe

& Johnson, 1986). During the 13th leg of the 1967 Tour de France, English cyclist Tom Simpson, 29, collapsed and died. His autopsy showed high levels of methamphetamine, "a vial of which had been found in his pocket at the time of his death" (Gilbert, 1969b). The impact of Simpson's death was extensive, in part because "this was the first doping death to be televised" (Donohoe & Johnson, 1986). His death substantially added to the mounting pressure on the IOC and member federations to establish doping control programs, which they did at the end of 1967 (Ferstle, 2000). One year later another cyclist, Yves Mottin, died from "excessive amphetamine use" two days after winning a race (Todd & Todd, 2001).

Tests conducted on Belgian cyclists in 1965 showed that 37% of professionals and 23% of amateurs were using amphetamines, while reports from Italy showed that 46% of professional cyclists tested positive for doping (Donohoe & Johnson, 1986). In 1967 Jacques Anquetil, a five-time winner of the Tour de France, stated:

> For 50 years bike racers have been taking stimulants. Obviously we can do without them in a race, but then we will pedal 15 miles an hour [*instead of 25*]. Since we are constantly asked to go faster and to make even greater efforts, we are obliged to take stimulants (Gilbert, 1969).

Longtime team masseur for professional cycling, Willy Voet, summarized the past 40 years of doping in cycling by describing the three drug eras of the sport: amphetamines in the 1960s and 1970s, anabolic steroids and cortisone in the 1980s, and, thereafter, hGH and erythropoietin (EPO) (Swift, 1999). In fact, there is strong speculation that more than a dozen deaths of elite cyclists that took place the late 1980s were the result of the use of EPO (Ramotar, 1990; Fisher, 1991).

The breadth and depth of the level of doping in the cycling world were exposed to full public view in 1998 when Voet was arrested by French customs police for transporting performance-enhancing drugs. Voet began detailing the use of drugs in cycling, and a large-scale investigation by both French and Italian authorities, as well as by a number of journalists, ensued. The results of these investigations implicated many of the top teams and riders in the sport as part of a highly organized, sophisticated, and long-lived doping scheme (*USA Today,* 1998d; Swift, 1999). Just hours before the 2000 Tour de France was to begin, three cyclists failed a mandatory EPO test and were expelled from competition (King5.com, 2000). Perhaps the magnitude of this problem in cycling is best summarized by Daniel Delegove, the presiding judge of the doping trial of France's cycling superstar Richard Virenque. After hearing compelling evidence of widespread doping, Judge

Delegove said, "These are not racers, they are pedaling test tubes" (Ford, 2000).

Modern Olympic Sports

Thomas Hicks, the winner of the marathon in the 1904 St. Louis Olympic Games, was administered strychnine and brandy several times during the race. Dr. Charles Lucas, a physician who attended to Hicks, commented that "the Marathon race, from a medical standpoint, demonstrated that drugs are of much benefit to athletes" (Dyreson, 1998). Likewise, the "winner" of the 1908 Olympic marathon was suspected of taking strychnine, although he was later disqualified because spectators assisted him the last few feet of the race (Donohoe & Johnson, 1986). Wilhelm Knoll, a Swiss physician, administered a stimulant, Coramin, to skiers at the St. Moritz Olympic Games in 1928 (Hoberman, 1992b).

In the 1932 Los Angeles Olympic Games, the victories of Japanese swimmers were rumored to be the result of their being "pumped full of oxygen" (Boje, 1939; Hoberman, 1992b). There were accusations of strychnine use at the 1956 Melbourne Games, while some of the urine samples taken from cyclists after the races during the Tokyo Games "were actually *blue* in colour due to the use of various drugs" (Donohoe & Johnson, 1986).

Anabolic steroid use was apparently not a major problem at the 1960 Olympic Games in that it was probably limited to Soviet strength athletes and a few American weight lifters. By 1964, however, the secret behind the startling progress of a number of strength athletes began to leak out, and as a result steroids were soon being used extensively by athletes in all the strength sports (Connolly, 1973; Gilbert, 1969a, b, & c; Payne, 1975; Starr, 1981; Todd, 1987).

Weight lifters themselves were quickly convinced that steroids made them bigger and stronger, and they began to tout the drugs. In track and field, the throwers were early converts. By the mid-1960s most of the top-ranking throwers began using anabolic steroids, including Randy Matson, the 1968 Olympic champion and world-record holder in the shot put; Dallas Long, the 1964 Olympic shot put champion; Harold Connolly, the 1956 Olympic champion in the hammer throw; and Russ Hodge, a world-record holder in the decathlon (Gilbert, 1969a, b, & c).

By 1968, according to H. Connolly (1973) and Francis (1990), athletes in a number of track and field events, including sprinters, hurdlers, and middle-distance runners, were using anabolic steroids. Dr. Tom Waddell, a U.S. decathlete, estimated that one-third of the entire U.S. track and field team (not just strength and field-event athletes) had used steroids at the 1968 pre-Olympic training camp (Todd, 1987). Dr. H. Kay Dooley, a team physician for the U.S. weight lifters, stated, "I don't think it is possible for a weight man to compete internationally without using anabolic steroids. . . . All the weight men on the Olympic team had to take steroids. Otherwise they would not have been in the running" (Gilbert, 1969a). This was a time when steroid use was not banned and had become much less secretive than previously. It was also the year after the IOC established a medical committee and banned certain drugs.

During the 1968 Olympic Games in Mexico City, athletes and coaches did not debate the morality or propriety of taking drugs; the only debate was over which drugs were more effective. Bill Toomey, gold medalist in the decathlon at the 1968 Olympics and winner of the Amateur Athletic Union's prestigious Sullivan Award, admitted he used drugs to aid his performance at the Mexico City Olympics (Scott, 1971).

Dosages of anabolic steroids used by strength athletes had increased by the late 1960s to two to five times therapeutic recommendations (for replacement therapy); and the variety of steroids used had increased as well, although it was not until this time that use of multiple drugs (stacking) and the simultaneous use of oral and injectable anabolic steroids began. From the time substances marketed as anabolic steroids were introduced, some athletes preferred them to the more androgenic preparations (such as the oral and injectable testosterones and fluoxymesterone), primarily because the anabolic steroids were marketed for their "anabolic" effects but also because of concern over what athletes considered undesirable androgenic effects (including aggression). However, steroid users who wished to maximize muscle mass and strength continued to use the more "androgenic" preparations.

By 1969, the cat was completely out of the bag. Users were praising the effects of anabolic steroids on performance (Brown & Tait, 1973), and Jon Hendershott (1969), then editor of *Track and Field News,* was nonfacetiously categorizing anabolic steroids as the "breakfast of champions." That same year a mainstream sport magazine published a three-part expose of drug use in sport, indicating on the basis of numerous interviews and observations that "athletes were popping more pills for more purposes than were dreamt of in anybody's philosophy—or pharmacy" (Gilbert, 1969c, p. 30).

After the 1968 Olympic Games, a U.S. weight lifter "admitted most of his colleagues took a few amphetamines before competing to get that extra little lift" (Gilbert, 1969a). In 1970 at the Weightlifting World Championships, 9 of the first 12 medalists tested positive for amphetamines (Scott, 1971). After winning the 1971 Pan Am games in Cali, Colombia, weight lifter Ken Patera relished meeting Russian superheavyweight Vasily Alexeyev in the 1972 Olympics in Munich. Patera was quoted in the *Los Angeles Times:*

> Last year the only difference between me and him was I couldn't afford his drug bill. Now I can.

When I hit Munich I'll weigh in at about 340, or maybe 350. Then we'll see which are better, his steroids or mine. (Scott, 1971)

Since 1971, blood doping (i.e., the reinfusion of an athlete's own concentrated oxygen-carrying red blood cells or those of a typed-matched donor, shortly before competition) has been alleged to have been used for several years by European distance runners, cyclists, cross-country skiers, and biathletes (Williams, 1980). However, it was brought to the attention of the lay public during the 1976 Summer Olympic Games when several TV commentators suggested that Finnish distance runner Lasse Viren, gold medalist in the 5000- and 10,000-m (5468 and 10,936 yd) races, used blood doping (Zorpette, 2000).

After the 1980 Moscow Olympics, a new assay for exogenous testosterone, developed by Dr. Manfred Donike, was retroactively applied to all urine samples. Twenty percent of all athletes (males and females) would have tested positive. This group included 16 gold medalists (Todd & Todd, 2001).

Before the 1984 Olympics, a newspaper article alleged that shot-putters and throwers of the discus, javelin, and hammer had been given information by the coordinator of a U.S. Olympic Committee's instructional program, within the year before the Olympics, to help them circumvent tests for anabolic steroids (*Tampa Bay Tribune,* 1984). Others have argued that this program was merely an educational effort to familiarize the athletes with the adverse consequences of anabolic steroid use and had nothing to do with evading drug tests.

Human growth hormone was described by a well-known sport physician as the "fad anabolic drug" of the Los Angeles Olympic Games (Todd & Todd, 2001). Interestingly, 12 years later the Atlanta Olympic Games were jokingly referred to as the "Growth Hormone Games" by some athletes (Bamberger & Yaeger, 1997). Tests at the 1984 Games also revealed that most of the competitors in the modern pentathlon had used beta blockers (i.e., for their anti-tremor and anti-anxiety effects), although these drugs were not on the banned list at that time (Todd & Todd, 2001). After the Games, 24 members of the U.S. men's cycling team admitted to blood doping prior to competition (Cramer, 1985; Zorpette, 2000).

In the 1988 Seoul Games, two gold medalist weight lifters tested positive for diuretics. However, the big story of the Seoul Games concerned the fact that Ben Johnson, winner of the 100-m (109 yd) dash, tested positive for an anabolic steroid (Todd & Todd, 2001). A subsequent investigation by the *New York Times* concluded that "at least half of the athletes who competed at the Olympics in Seoul used anabolic steroids to enhance their performances . . ." (Janofsky, 1988).

During the 1990s, not only were weight lifting and the field events still enmeshed in performance-enhancing drug use (Noden, 1993; *USA Today,* 1995, 1997a, 1998b), but also the use of anabolic steroids, hGH, and EPO was present in other Olympic sports, including hockey, swimming, cycling, skiing, volleyball, wrestling, handball, pentathlon, bobsledding, and soccer (Dubin, 1990; Todd & Todd, 2001; *USA Today,* 1997b).

After a lengthy investigation of drug use in Olympic sports, Bamberger & Yaeger (1997) concluded,

. . . three distinct classes of top-level athletes have emerged in many Olympic sports. One is a small group of athletes who are not using any banned performance enhancers. The second is a large, burgeoning group whose drug use goes undetected; these athletes either take drugs that aren't tested for, use tested-for drugs in amounts below the generous levels permitted by the IOC or take substances that mask the presence of the drugs in their system at testing time. The third group comprises the smattering of athletes who use banned performance enhancers and are actually caught.

The Sydney Olympic Games did little to dispel this grim conclusion. They were scarred as the "Dirty Games" as tens of dozens of news articles were published about the Sydney Games that dealt with the ongoing epidemic of drug use in Olympic sport and the IOC's continued inability (or insincerity) to effectively deal with it (Abrahamson & Wharton, 2000; Longman, 2000a; Begley & Clifton, 2000; Cazeneuve & Layden, 2000; Fish, 2000; Harvey, 2000; Humphries, 2000; Reid, 2000; Sullivan & Song, 2000). In one of these articles Dr. Don Catlin, director of one of the IOC drug-testing laboratories, observed, "There's probably a lot more drugs out there in sport than the general public would think. They'd be fairly horrified" (Humphries, 2000). In another, Frank Shorter, 1972 Olympic marathon champion and chairman of the U.S. Anti-Doping Agency, not only recognized the magnitude of the problem but also saw that doping has consequences that reach far beyond the Olympic Games (Longman, 2000). He stated,

Every 14-year-old kid knows that to be in strength and endurance sports, if he wants to go on with his career, 'I have to go on these drugs.'

An intensive two-year investigation of doping in Olympic sport conducted for the U.S. Office of National Drug Control Policy concluded that while estimates of the magnitude of the doping epidemic vary widely (from 10% to 90% of athletes), there exists an atmosphere in our society that fosters drug use by athletes (National Center on Addiction and Substance Abuse, 2000):

. . . the high financial stakes for Olympic athletes, corporate sponsors, the TV broadcast and cable industries and sport governing bodies, coupled with the pharmacopoeia of performance-enhancing substances, the athlete's drive to win and the absence of an effective policing mechanism, create an environment that encourages doing anything—including doping—to win.

Female Athletes

It is reasonable to assume that the use of anabolic steroids, stimulants, and blood doping (or EPO) by female athletes followed closely on the heels of adoption of use by male athletes. The use of anabolic steroids by female athletes is of particular interest because these drugs have a significantly more pronounced effect in women than in men. The powerful masculinizing effects of anabolic steroids in females had been established before 1960 (Kochakian, 1976; Kruskemper, 1968). It is likely that the Soviet female track and field athletes of the 1960s, or perhaps even the 1950s, were the first women athletes to use these drugs.

The masculine appearances of a number of female track and field athletes from the Eastern bloc countries in the mid-1960s led to speculation that they were either hermaphrodites or men disguised as women. In response, a chromosome test was initiated in 1967 at the European Cup (Todd, 1987). Although several athletes did indeed fail the screening over the years and several others mysteriously retired from competition before being tested, one might wonder if many of the women who initially were suspected were neither genetic "rarities" nor charlatans but simply had been administered testosterone and other anabolic steroids.

The spread of steroid use among female athletes probably followed a pattern similar to that of males, with the strength athletes the first among women to adopt the drugs. Evidence of steroid use among female throwers from Eastern bloc countries goes back at least to the 1968 Olympic Games at Mexico City (Fikotova-Connolly, personal communication, 1991; Franke & Berendonk, 1997). By the 1972 Munich Games, it was alleged that several U.S. women participating in the field events had used anabolic steroids (Connolly, 1989). While anabolic steroids continue to be used by female athletes in strength sports (Franke & Berendonk, 1997; Patrick, 1997), based on government records, testimonials, and the results of drug tests, by the late 1970s steroid use had spread to sprinters and middle-distance runners, swimmers, rowers, and athletes in various winter sporting events as well (Franke & Berendonk, 1997; Dubin, 1990; Williams, 1989). The 1976 Montreal Olympics foreshadowed the doping problem among elite female athletes. The Games saw the first female athlete to test positive for anabolic steroids and the emergence of East German women as a dominant force internationally. In particular, suspicions (now confirmed; see later) were raised by the masculine appearance and overpowering performance of the German Democratic Republic (GDR) female swimmers. When an East German coach was asked about rumored steroid use and observations about the deep voices of his female athletes, he allegedly answered, "We have come here to swim, not to sing" (Todd & Todd, 2001).

As with men, women's steroid use has diffused beyond Olympic sport and has now been reported at the collegiate level in sports including basketball, volleyball, soccer, field hockey, swimming, gymnastics, lacrosse, and softball (Anderson, Albrecht, McKeag, Hough, & McGrew, 1991; *NCAA News,* 1997; Yesalis, Anderson, Buckley, & Wright, 1990; see chapter 3 in this text). In 1995 a 14-year-old female long jumper and sprinter from South Africa became the world's youngest athlete to test positive for anabolic steroid use (*New York Times,* 1995). The 1980s and 1990s saw numerous doping scandals throughout the world involving female athletes; and this argues that, at least at the elite level, there is little or no difference in the prevalence of doping between the sexes.

National Doping Programs

Although the existence of well-organized, nationwide sport doping programs has been rumored for decades, solid evidence has now come to light to document their reality. National doping programs transcend the all-too-common informal collusion of elite athletes, coaches, and rogue physicians and sport scientists to use performance-enhancing drugs. Indeed they are constituted under the direction or strong support of government and sport federation officials, as well as with the active collaboration of mainstream physicians and scientists.

Thanks to the courage and persistence of Werner Franke and Brigitte Berendonk (1997), we now have detailed information on the heinous activities of the GDR sport doping system.

Top-secret doctoral theses, scientific reports, progress reports of grants, proceedings of symposiums of experts, and reports of physicians and scientists who served as unofficial collaborators for the Ministry of State Security ("Stasi") reveal that from 1966 on, hundreds of physicians and scientists, including top-ranking professors, performed doping research and administered prescription drugs as well as unapproved experimental drug preparations. Several thousand athletes were treated with androgens every year, including minors of each sex. Special emphasis was placed on administering androgens to women and adolescent girls because the practice proved to be particularly effective for sport performance.

This Communist state-sponsored program was not only a highly organized assault on the rules of sport; more importantly, it also flagrantly violated scientific and medical ethics. Girls and boys 14 years of age or younger were given anabolic steroids and other drugs—and often they or their parents were not so informed. Successful criminal prosecutions of some of these coaches and physicians has been completed in Germany (*Des Moines Sunday Register,* 1997; *USA Today,* 1998c). Interestingly, the IOC has been denounced for hesitating to aggressively investigate the East German scandal. John Leonard of the World Swimming Coaches Association couched his criticism in terms of the IOC fixation on its image and money:

> The reason the IOC needs to be cautious about this [i.e., *the East German program*] is because this has nothing whatsoever to do with sports. It has everything to do with the IOC's business relationships with its sponsors . . . once you start to pull on the thread of this, the entire garment of the Olympic fabric begins to come apart. . . . And what you begin to realize is the IOC itself has nothing to do with sport. It has to do with raising money and putting money in the IOC's coffers and the relationships it has with its major sponsors.
>
> The evidence has been there since 1989. . . . The IOC doesn't want to act on this because they don't want the full extent of doping activities revealed. (ABC News, 1998)

In addition, it is reasonable to conclude that similar organized sport doping programs existed in the Soviet Union and other Soviet bloc countries (Gilmour, 1998; Hoberman, 1992b; Rosellini, 1992; Voy, 1991). From as early as 1945, there is evidence from a Soviet government document that there were formal discussions regarding the viability of doping in sport (i.e., the use of stimulants) (Gilmour, 1998). The document shows a significant range of opinions on the matter, both pro and con. The conclusions reached in these discussions were that stimulants were already being used in sport, that athletic trainers and coaches were involved, that more research was needed to assess the effects, and that variations in reaction to the drugs did not justify the risks *at that time* (Gilmour, 1998). This latter judgment may well have been reassessed when in 1948 Soviet sport established a goal of meeting or exceeding all world records. Whatever the case, it appears that by 1954 the Soviets employed systematic use of testosterone with their weight lifters and that thereafter use spread to other sports (Starr, 1981; Todd, 1983, 1987). While Edelman (1993) stated that the Soviet program probably was never as well organized or systematic as in the GDR, he nevertheless concluded as follows:

Officials, team doctors, and pharmacologists made drugs available to coaches who were under enormous pressure from the Party to produce winners. Facilities and assistance, especially pre-emptive testing, were provided to insure athletes could escape both detection and death. (Kidd, Edelman, & Brownell, 1998)

After the fall of Communism in Europe, many East German coaches sought employment elsewhere, and a number of these coaches began working in Communist China's sport programs (Fish, 1994; Hersh, 1993b; Whitten, 1994). The Chinese even established the National Research Institute, a high-performance sport science laboratory that appears to eerily parallel the GDR's Research Institute for Physical Culture and Sports in Leipzig (Hoberman & Todd, 1992). Shortly thereafter, Chinese female athletes moved from a position of relative obscurity to world dominance, especially in swimming, track and field, and weight lifting. Almost immediately accusations of doping and comparisons with the GDR spewed forth (Fish, 1993; Hersh, 1993a & b; Montville, 1994; Moore, 1993; Patrick, 1993; *USA Today,* 1994; Whitten, 1994). These accusations were supported in part by the large number of positive drug tests the Chinese athletes experienced during the 1990s, including 29 track and field athletes and 19 swimmers (Allen, 1998). At this time there is no absolute evidence of a centrally controlled system of drug use in China as was the case with the GDR (Kidd et al., 1998). However, it is quite implausible to attribute the numerous documented cases of doping in the totalitarian society that is Communist China to random episodes of "cowboy chemistry." Thus, there is little doubt that highly organized, systematic sport doping has taken place, at the very least, at the provincial level.

Professional Football

The history of drug use in professional football spans at least six decades and comprises primarily the use of stimulants (amphetamines and cocaine), anabolics (anabolic steroids and growth hormone), and painkillers (narcotic analgesics and codeine).

Amphetamine use appeared in the NFL immediately after World War II. An investigative report of drug use in sport published by *Sports Illustrated* in 1969 (Gilbert, 1969b) noted that "among major American sports, amphetamine usage may be the highest in football. . . ." Amphetamines are used in a violent contact sport such as football not to mask fatigue as much as to overcome pain and get "psyched up." Dr. Arnold Mandell (1976), an eminent psychiatrist and team physician to the San Diego Chargers from 1972 to 1974, illustrates this with a quote from a veteran player, "Doc, I'm not about to go out there one on one against a guy who's grunting and drooling and comin' at me with big dilated pupils unless I'm in the same condition!" Mandell goes on to say, "A football player uses amphetamines once a week, like a truck driver takes them to finish a long run or a student takes them to complete a paper or cram for an exam. He usually hates the feeling and looks forward to never having to do it again. It's strictly a way to get the work done."

The first systematic assessment of the incidence of amphetamine use in pro football, conducted in 1972, showed that over half the members of the teams sampled had used amphetamines (Mandell, 1981). George Burman, who played for three teams in the NFL during the 1960s, estimated that approximately one-third of players used the drugs (Padwe, 1973). From 1972 to 1975, Mandell (1981) conducted in-depth interviews with 87 players from 11 NFL teams and found that two-thirds of the players used amphetamines "sometimes" and more than half used them "regularly." Mandell's study also demonstrated position-related dosing to achieve different ends. Players at the skill positions (quarterback, wide receiver, etc.) used relatively low doses to increase energy and enhance "creative performance," whereas defensive linemen used the highest doses to engender a sense of fearlessness or paranoid rage.

Other observers of professional football during that time noted that amphetamine use was particularly high among members of special teams—also referred to as "suicide squads" or "bomb squads"—to help psych themselves up during kickoffs and punt returns when they slam into their opponents at full speed (Scott, 1971). It is very likely that until at least the 1980s, amphetamine use in pro football was relatively open and that for some teams, passing around the cookie jar full of different types of amphetamines was part of the pregame routine (Courson, 1991; Gilbert, 1969b).

Cocaine use has also been a chronic problem among NFL players. Carl Eller, an All-Pro defensive lineman for the Minnesota Vikings during the 1960s, estimated that 40% of professional players were regular cocaine users (Donohoe & Johnson, 1986). Vic Washington, an All-Pro running back with the San Francisco 49ers in the early 1970s, said of cocaine use, "At the time it was viewed as giving the player an edge. . . . We were in a war out there. And using cocaine was seen as a way of getting psyched up to have an edge. I understood it at the time because we were out of reality. Pro football is not reality" (Hewitt, 1993).

Not long after word of the effectiveness of anabolic steroids disseminated among weight lifters and throwers in the early 1960s, football players began to incorporate these drugs into their training regimens. In 1963 the San Diego Chargers hired Alvin Roy, a Baton Rouge gym owner, as the first strength coach in professional football.

Roy, previously an assistant coach for the U.S. Olympic weightlifting team, was probably already familiar with anabolic steroids, and it is alleged that he introduced the San Diego players to Dianabol (Gilbert, 1969a, b, & c; Mix, 1987). Some of the former Chargers say that they were not informed that the "little pink pills" placed next to their plates at the training table were anabolic steroids, and they add that there was a clear implication that players who refused to take the pills would be fined (Scott, 1971). Several years later, Roy left the Chargers to become the strength coach of the Kansas City Chiefs, who were known for their massive offensive and defensive lines during their heyday in the late 1960s. According to the accounts of physicians and players, members of the Kansas City Chiefs, Atlanta Falcons, and Cleveland Browns used anabolic steroids during the 1960s (Gilbert, 1969a, b, & c). It is fair to assume that trades, coaching changes, and word-of-mouth interaction among football players and other strength athletes further facilitated the diffusion of steroid use in the NFL.

From the mid-1970s to the early 1980s, the Pittsburgh Steelers were said to possess one of the most sophisticated strength programs in pro football and one of the most physical styles of play. More importantly, the Steelers were a dominant force in the NFL during this period, as well as in the NFL's Strongest Man competitions (1980 to 1982). Some of the athletes who contributed to this success used anabolic steroids (Courson, 1988, 1991). One cannot easily discount the effect that this might have had on the further spread of steroid use in the league, where strength and power are highly valued.

The testimony of former players supports the apparent escalation of steroid use in the NFL from the late 1970s onward. Pat Donovan, a Dallas Cowboy offensive lineman for nine years who retired in 1983, said, "Anabolic steroids are very, very accepted in the NFL. In my last five or six years it ran as high as 60-70% on the Cowboys on the offensive and defensive lines" (Johnson, 1985, p. 43). In the same article, the Buffalo Bills' Fred Smerlas said he thought that 40% of the players in the NFL used anabolic steroids. "On some teams between 75-90% of all athletes use steroids," said former Los Angeles Raider defensive lineman, Lyle Alzado (p. 43). Other NFL players estimated steroid use as high as 90% (Johnson, 1985).

Joe Klecko, a former New York Jets defensive lineman, said that anabolic steroids were commonplace in the late 1970s. Klecko stated, "I would guess between 65% and 75% were using AS in 1987" (Klecko & Fields, 1989). Klecko added, "I used AS when I wanted to be bear strong for the three NFL (*"Strongest Man in Football"*) contests I entered in the off-season 1979-1981."

In a 1986 article in *Sports Illustrated* (Zimmerman, 1986), Los Angeles Raider defensive end Howie Long estimated the level of steroid use in the NFL: "At least

50% of the big guys. The offensive lines 75%, defensive line 40%, plus 35% of the linebackers. I don't know about the speed positions, but I've heard that they're used there too" (p. 18). From the same article, "Anabolic steroids are the worst problem in the NFL," said Indianapolis linebacker Johnny Cookes (p. 18).

Steve Courson (1988), who played for the Pittsburgh Steelers and Tampa Bay Buccaneers from 1977 to 1985, stated, "My educated guess is that 50% of the linemen use steroids." While testifying before the U.S. Senate Judiciary Committee in 1989, the Atlanta Falcons' All-Pro lineman Bill Fralic described steroid use in the NFL as rampant: "I would say that the guys I play against—that is excluding the quarterbacks, and defensive backs and wide receivers, it is probably about 75%" (Fralic, 1989).

In 1991, prior to his death, NFL All-Pro lineman Lyle Alzado charged that NFL officials had known about players' extensive use of anabolic steroids but had chosen to ignore it. He said that he used drugs during his entire career in the NFL, which spanned nearly two decades. Alzado also said he believed the teams' coaches knew that he and others were taking drugs but "just coached and looked the other way" (Alzado, 1991, p. 27). One of Alzado's coaches admitted that he knew about Alzado's drug use. "When I was coaching him, I was aware that he was using steroids," former Oakland Raiders coach Tom Flores told Steve Kelley of the *Seattle Times* (Kelley, 1991).

The current drug advisor to the NFL, Dr. John Lombardo, has stated, "In the late '70s and the '80s, use of steroids was unbridled, uncontrolled. . . . People felt they had to take them to compete" (Miller, 1996). The precise level of steroid use in the NFL during the 1970s and 1980s probably will never be known, but it appears that steroid use was quite substantial. Unfortunately, the question of performance-enhancing drug use in the NFL persists today. Continued speculation of epidemic levels of drug use has been fueled further by the dramatic increase in the size of NFL players, from quarterbacks to offensive linemen (Keteyian, 1998). In 1987 only 27 NFL players weighed more than 300 lb (136 kg), while in 1997 there were approximately 240 players over 300 lb (Noonan, 1997). Some argue that the size increase is a consequence of high-calorie diets and food supplements such as creatine (Noonan, 1997), while others point their finger at anabolic steroids and hGH as the cause (Bamberger & Yaeger, 1997; Keteyian, 1998).

National Football League officials counter that the NFL's year-round, random drug-testing program has limited steroid use to a few marginal players (Noonan, 1997). However, the very integrity of the NFL drug-testing program has been brought into question. Accusations have been made of covering up positive tests of star players, allowing players to "come back tomorrow" to give their urine sample, or allowing someone else to give "your" sample (Almond, 1993, 1995; *Sports Illustrated,* 1991): if true, all of these actions are flagrant violations of accepted testing policies. Even more disturbing is the revelation of Eric Moore, an offensive lineman for the New York Giants who was arrested in 1993 for possession of anabolic steroids with intent to deliver. During his interrogation by a Drug Enforcement Administration agent (Almond, 1995),

> Moore told the agent that he was usually given advance warning of any test, the centerpiece of the NFL's drug program. Moore said he was allowed to enter the testing room alone and that he kept a clean vial of urine in his jock strap to substitute for his own specimen.

All this is consistent with the comments of Dr. Forrest Tennant, the former NFL drug advisor:

> When I was dealing with cocaine, marijuana, and alcohol, no problem. Everybody supported cleaning that problem up. But when we decided to move into dealing with steroids, that is when you found out how many people around the league knew they worked, knew they wanted to see certain players keep taking them, and you would run into those pockets of resistance. (Burrelle's Information Service, 1992)

The potential problems with the integrity of the testing program, combined with the facts that there is no effective test for hGH and that the tests for testosterone can be circumvented (see chapter 27), argue that performance-enhancing drug use remains a significant and widespread problem in the NFL.

Professional Baseball

In his book, *Pennant Race,* Jim Brosnan (1962), who pitched for the Cincinnati Reds in the early 1960s, admitted using amphetamines as a "pick-me-up." In baseball, amphetamines are not used to increase endurance as in cycling or to heighten aggressiveness as in football, but rather to deal with the monotony and strain of a long season and numerous road trips (Padwe, 1973). The use of amphetamines in major league baseball gained substantial notoriety in 1970 when Jim Bouton, a pitcher for the New York Yankees during the 1960s and author of the highly controversial book, *Ball Four* (1970), admitted using amphetamines and estimated that 40% of other players did as well. However, Bouton argued that the drugs give a false sense of security. "The trouble with them is that they make you feel so great that you think you're really smoking when you're not. . . .

The result is you get gay, throw it down the middle and get clobbered."

As with football, the size and strength of professional baseball players appear to have increased markedly during the past 15 years. As a consequence, suspicions of anabolic steroid use have dramatically escalated during the past half-decade. In 1995 Randy Smith, general manager of the San Diego Padres, stated, "We all know there's steroid use, and it's definitely become more prevalent." Smith estimated the prevalence of use at 10% to 20% of players, while an anonymous American League general manager said, "I wouldn't be surprised if it's closer to 30% . . ." (Nightengale, 1995). Others say 40% (Harvey, 2000; McKinley, 2000). Among power hitters, steroid use is estimated to be as high as 90% (Henderson, 2000). In 1998 (Rosenthal, 1998), an anonymous American League front office executive stated:

> It (*anabolic steroid use*) is absolutely rampant right now. . . . Steroids have completely changed the game. Guys try to cover it up by saying they're using creatine (a muscle enhancer). Or they're just lifting weights now. Come on. It's a completely different look.

Kevin Towers, San Diego Padres general manager, has been outspoken about the prevalence of anabolic steroids in baseball and about baseball's seeming inaction. "I think the stuff is more prevalent in major league clubhouses than alcohol, tobacco or any other drug, but the attitude seems to be, 'Let's not worry about it until someone dies'" (*Denver Post,* 2000).

Perhaps Towers is correct. Major league baseball's response to all these accusations has been interesting. The baseball commissioner has blamed the strong players' union for blocking action on this issue such as instituting drug testing. The players' association, on the other hand, argues that "there's been no hard evidence" that anabolic steroids either improve performance or represent a health or safety hazard (Reilly, 2000a).

College Sports

Given the number of World War II veterans who attended college after being discharged, it is likely that amphetamine use was introduced to college football early on. All-American George Connor (1946-1947) admitted that he took "pep pills" at Notre Dame (Gilbert, 1969b). Rick Sortun, a star football player at the University of Washington in the early 1960s, disclosed that an assistant coach would surreptitiously give players amphetamines before each game (Scott, 1971). Surveys and athlete testimonials in the late 1960s show that amphetamine use was widespread among college football players (Padwe, 1973; Scott, 1971). In a 1997 anonymous survey, 3.1% of the NCAA athletes surveyed acknowledged amphetamine use, and 29% of the users stated that they obtained the drugs from a physician (NCAA Research Staff, 1997).

Although the NCAA outlawed in principle the use of anabolic steroids in 1973, it was not until 1986 that a testing program was initiated—10 years after the IOC began testing for these drugs.

The diffusion of steroid use in college football was undoubtedly delayed by the perceptions of many coaches during the 1950s and 1960s that increased muscle mass and basic strength conditioning did not afford an advantage; some coaches persisted in this thinking even in the early 1970s. Soon after, however, coaches appeared to dismiss the "muscle-bound" theory, and elaborate weight-training facilities and professional strength coaches became an integral part of college football.

Jim Calkins, the cocaptain of the 1969 University of California at Berkeley football team, claimed that he was given anabolic steroids by the team physician in order to gain weight to play tight end (Scott, 1971). Steve Courson (1988), during his playing days at the University of South Carolina, was prescribed Dianabol by the team physician in 1974. During the 1980s, football players at Stanford, the University of Oklahoma, North Dakota State University, Salisbury State, the University of Nevada-Reno, Georgia Southern College, the University of Southern California, the University of Tennessee, Louisiana State University, the University of Pittsburgh, Northwestern University, the University of Texas, the University of Minnesota, and Vanderbilt, among others, were all involved in steroid use (Huffman, 1990; *Tampa Bay Tribune,* 1985; Wadler & Hainline, 1989; Yaeger & Looney, 1993). Furthermore, two of the most famous schools in college football, the University of Nebraska and Notre Dame, have been implicated in widespread steroid use (Keteyian, 1987; Yaeger & Looney, 1993).

The University of Nebraska has been at the cutting edge in strength training at the collegiate or professional level for over three decades. Unfortunately, "no school has a bigger reputation for clandestine steroid involvement than the University of Nebraska" (Yaeger & Looney, 1993). The program placed a great deal of emphasis on strength, speed, and power. "Nebraska at times resembled less of a football team and more of a powerlifting club . . . the powerlifting mind-set that eventually permeated the squad—that led Nebraska players closer and closer to the S-word. Not strength . . . but steroids" (Keteyian, 1987). One of the largest criminal investigations into steroid trafficking in the United States touched Lincoln, Nebraska.

According to the U.S. Attorney's Office in San Diego, where the case was prosecuted, the investigation led to the conviction of Tony Fitton, whom the Feds considered the "kingpin" of steroids in the 1980s. Fitton admitted supplying Nebraska players with steroids. (Yaeger & Looney, 1993)

In another report, a former drug dealer described steroid use at Nebraska as "massive" and estimated use on the 1983 and 1984 teams to be as high as 85% (Keteyian, 1987). Additional evidence of rampant steroid use derives from a number of journalistic investigations implicating such Cornhusker greats as Dean Steinkuhler, Dave Rimington, Danny Noonan, Neil Smith, and Lawrence Pete, all of whom have admitted using steroids while at Nebraska (Keteyian, 1987; Yaeger & Looney, 1993).

Regarding steroid use at Notre Dame, Yaeger & Looney (1993) concluded as follows:

> First Lou Holtz arrived at Notre Dame. Then a lot of steroids did. The connection is inescapable. It also has been devastating. The football team quickly became awash in anabolic steroids, starting in 1986.

On the basis of the results of an anonymous survey of Division I-III athletes, sponsored by the NCAA in 1989, one would expect that on a team with 100 football players, on average 10 (i.e., 10%) would have used steroids in the prior 12 months (Anderson et al., 1991). A more recent survey of NCAA intercollegiate athletes shows that steroid use is on the decline in football (i.e., down to 2%) as well as in other sports (*NCAA News,* 1997). As in the case of pro football, the purported decrease in steroid use among college football players flies in the face of significant increases in the size of players and a drug-testing program fraught with loopholes. Moreover, the validity of anonymous surveys of any group of elite athletes has to be carefully scrutinized because admitting to steroid use poses a potential threat to the athlete's scholarship and future livelihood. In addition, the fear of guilt by association and its potential to adversely affect the athlete's place in sport history may result in a hesitancy to volunteer or be truthful (Yesalis, Kopstein, & Bahrke, 2001).

In addition to football, other collegiate men's sports have been linked to anabolic steroid use. These include track and field, baseball, basketball, gymnastics, lacrosse, swimming, volleyball, wrestling, soccer, and tennis (Anderson et al., 1991; *NCAA News,* 1997; Yesalis et al., 1990).

High School

It is unsettling how quickly the use of performance-enhancing drugs spread to adolescent sport. In the late 1960s, a West Coast athletic trainer described being approached by a track coach for grade school and high school girls to procure amphetamines for his athletes (Gilbert, 1969a). In a letter submitted as testimony to the U.S. Congress in 1973, a mother of two young boys voiced her concern that participants in a local Pop Warner football league (boys 11 to 14 years of age who must weigh less than 140 lb [63.5 kg]) were being given, or encouraged by coaches to take, "drugs, pepper-uppers, speed, pills to keep weight down" (Santos, 1973). In 1969, Gilbert (1969b) described instances of use of amphetamines by high school athletes (basketball and football), with one episode involving a coach supplying the drugs.

Use of anabolic steroids by high school athletes is rumored to have begun as early as 1959 when a physician in Texas allegedly administered Dianabol to a high school football team for an entire season. As part of a clandestine "research" program in the early 1960s, a high school football team was reportedly given steroids by a team physician working in cooperation with a pharmaceutical company (Gilbert, 1969b). In 1965 a physician in Bloomington, California, oversaw a study in which three different commercial brands of anabolic steroids were administered to 10th- and 11th-grade football players (Gilbert, 1969b). Before 1972, some high school coaches in Alabama were rumored to have advised football players to take Dianabol to help them gain weight (Wade, 1972). By the late 1980s anabolic steroid use had been reported in high school baseball, basketball, track and field, and wrestling (Buckley et al., 1988). The spread of steroid use to adolescents likely has involved a variety of paths over the past four decades, including interactions with older athletes, coaches, physicians, and even parents. For further information on the use of anabolic steroids by adolescents, refer to chapter 3.

Other Sports

Because of the competitive nature of our culture and, in some instances, lucrative financial rewards, performance-enhancing drug use has diffused to a variety of other sports and activities. For example, there appears to be an eerie parallel between the spread of anabolic steroids in various types of horse racing and that of their use in human athletics (Cotolo, 1992). As with human athletics, rumors and accusations abound that performance-enhancing drug use is epidemic in horse racing, while others say the problem is overstated; some say drug testing is behind the times and make mention of "designer" drugs, while others argue that testing is working; some critics say a "get tough" policy for cheaters is long overdue, while others propose that drug use should be allowed, but in a controlled fashion; and some veterinarians even argue that anabolic steroids really do not confer a competitive advantage (Cotolo, 1992).

Even golf, a sport with a clean image that is thought by many to be synonymous with integrity, has been under a cloud of doping for over 30 years. In golf there is a constant battle against tension. In 1969, Gilbert (1969b) reported on the use of sedatives and tranquilizers for their "calming" effect by such players as Doug Sanders, Dave Hill, and Al Geiberger. In 2001 the new calming drugs on the golfing menu are beta blockers, which moderate the effects of adrenaline and decrease heart rate (Blauvelt, 2001).

Other sports and activities now under the shadow of doping include rugby, professional wrestling, Paralympics, and even pigeon racing (*Chicago Sun-Times,* 1994b; O'Brien, 1993; Reilly, 2000b; Reuter Information Service, 1995; Struman, 1992; *USA Today,* 1992).

Conclusion

In 1939 Ove Boje appeared to clearly understand the core issues involved in doping:

> There can be no doubt that stimulants are to-day widely used by athletes participating in competitions; the record-breaking craze and the desire to satisfy an exacting public play a more and more prominent role, and take higher rank than the health of the competitors itself.

Looking at elite sport in the 20th century through the eyes of historians and journalists as well as the athletes themselves, an unmistakable picture emerges of a doping pandemic of huge proportions in elite sport. However, sport federation officials most often either have tended to deny that a major doping problem exists or have at least downplayed its magnitude (*Chicago Sun-Times,* 1994a; Donohoe & Johnson, 1986; Gilbert, 1969c; *Milwaukee Sentinel,* 1993; Shipley, 2000; *Sports Medicine Digest,* 1996). In fact, when the Dubin Commission (Dubin, 1990) in Canada investigated the extent of doping in Olympic sport, its report referred to a "conspiracy of silence" and a "pact of ignorance" among those in sport organizations when it comes to discussing the issue of drug use. Ten years later, another investigation of doping in Olympic sport again concluded that in the rush for gold, governments, coaches, or trainers have often turned a blind eye or have actively supported the use of performance-enhancing substances (National Center on Addiction and Substance Abuse, 2000). However, when pushed, some sport officials eventually acknowledge, "we've had problems in the past, but now things are different" (*Champaign News Gazette,* 1995; *Chicago Tribune,* 1992; *USA Today,* 1998a; Yesalis, 1996, 2000).

Although it has taken over a century, there presently appears to be a consensus among various interest groups—including many athletes, physicians, coaches, administrators, and spectators—that performance-enhancing drug use in most sports is a serious and growing problem. Numerous international and national meetings as well as a variety of books and reports have been devoted exclusively to this issue (Dubin, 1990; Lin & Erinoff, 1990; National Center on Addiction and Substance Abuse, 2000; National Steroid Consensus Meeting, 1989; U.S. Drug Enforcement Administration, 1994; Voy, 1991; Yesalis, 1993, 1995; Yesalis & Cowart, 1998).

As with many problems that are long-standing and vexing, society seeks not only solutions but also someone or something to blame. Most if not all the blame to date has been laid at the feet of the athlete by politicians, the press, sport federations, and the medical community. In this regard, when we review the history of performance-enhancing drug use in sport, a number of ironies present themselves. Not only did the medical community develop these drugs, but it also played a role early on in "selling" these potential fountains of youth. It was physicians and trainers who administered powerful "stimulants" to a variety of athletes in the 19th and 20th centuries. It was a physician and some officials and supporters of the U.S. weightlifting team who initiated use of anabolic steroids in the 1950s in this country. It was government scientists and sport federation officials who institutionalized use of performance-enhancing drugs in Eastern bloc countries. It was physicians and/or coaching staffs at the professional, collegiate, or high school level in a number of instances who provided the substances or facilitated or encouraged the use of anabolic steroids and other drugs—the most recent example being the 1998 Tour de France doping scandal. It was physicians who served as the primary source of anabolic steroids for over one-third of the steroid users in this country (Scott, 1971; Yesalis et al., 1990; Green, Uryasz, Petr, & Bray, 2001). It is a number of sport federations that for decades have covered up the doping problem, conveniently looked the other way, or instituted drug-testing programs that were designed to fail (Dubin, 1990; Franke & Berendonk, 1997; Longman, 2000; National Center on Addiction and Substance Abuse, 2000; Voy, 1991; Yesalis & Cowart, 1998). As Boje described over 60 years ago, it was (and is) our society that emphasizes and rewards speed, strength, size, aggression, and, above all, winning. As with other types of drug abuse, doping in sport is primarily a demand-driven problem. In this instance, however, demand encompasses more than the demand for performance-enhancing drugs by athletes and includes the demand by the fan for the high-level performances that doping brings. Arguably, the behavior of athletes and sport officials in the matter of doping is congruent with the desires of their customers. Thus, a key question is, How concerned are sport fans about the doping epidemic? It is likely that the large majority of them really do disapprove of drug use in sport, but the real question is, do they disapprove enough to turn off their televisions?

References

ABC News. (1998, July 6). Cheating at the Olympics: Should history be rewritten? *Nightline.*

Abrahamson, A., & Wharton, D. (2000, August 20). Behind the rings: Inside the Olympic movement. *Los Angeles Times,* 1A.

Air Surgeon's Bulletin. (1944). Benzedrine alert. 1(2), 19-21.

Allen, K. (1998, June 4). China's road to success hits its share of hurdles. *USA Today,* 5E.

Almond, E. (1993, January 29). TV report in 1990 zeroed in on drugs. *Los Angeles Times,* 8C.

Almond, E. (1995, January 23). Drug testing in NFL under a microscope; pro football: Health officials, former players question efforts to detect steroids as athletes continue to get bigger, stronger. *Los Angeles Times,* 1C.

Alzado, L. (1991, July 8). I'm sick and I'm scared. *Sports Illustrated,* 20-27.

Anderson, W.A., Albrecht, M.A., McKeag, D.B., Hough, D.O., & McGrew, C.A. (1991). A national survey of alcohol and drug use by college athletes. *The Physician and Sportsmedicine,* 19(2), 91-104.

Aretaeus. (1854). *The Extant Works of Aretaeus, the Cappodocean.* Edited and translated by F. Adams. London: Sydenbam Society.

Bamberger, M., & Yaeger, D. (1997, April 14). Over the edge. *Sports Illustrated,* 86(15), 60-70.

Begley, S., & Clifton, T. (2000, September 11). The drug charade. *Newsweek,* 42-45.

Blauvelt, H. (2001, February 16). Beta blockers suspected of giving unfair edge. *USA Today,* 10C.

Boje, O. (1939). Doping. *Bulletin of the Health Organization of the League of Nations,* 8, 439-469.

Borell, M. (1976). Brown-Sequard's Organotherapy and its appearance in America at the end of the 19th century. *Bulletin of the History of Medicine,* 50, 309-320.

Bouton, J. (1970). *Ball Four.* New York: World.

Brosnan, J. (1962). *Pennant Race.* New York: Harper & Row.

Brown, J., & Tait, G. (1973). Anabolic steroids—the views of users. *Track Techniques,* 54, 1713-1716.

Brown-Sequard, C.E. (1889). The effects produced in man by subcutaneous injections of a liquid obtained from the testicles of animals. *Lancet,* 2, 105-107.

Buckley, W., Yesalis, C., Friedl, K., Anderson, W., Streit, A., & Wright, J. (1988). Estimated prevalence of anabolic steroid use among male high school seniors. *Journal of the American Medical Association,* 260, 3441-3445.

Burrelle's Information Service. (1992, January 22). Now it can be told.

Butenandt, A., & Hanisch, G. (1935). Über Testosteron Umwandlung des Dehydroandrosterons in Androstenediol und Testosteron; ein Weg zur Darstellung des Testosteron aus Cholesterin. *Zeitschrift Physiologische Chemie,* 237, 89-97.

Catton, B. (1951). *The Army of the Potomac.* Garden City, NY: Doubleday.

Cazeneuve, B., & Layden, T. (2000, August 14). Inside Olympic sport. *Sports Illustrated,* 67.

Champaign News Gazette. (1995, April 9). USOC officials cite test failures.

Chicago Sun-Times. (1994a, January 27). ITF disputes Becker charges.

Chicago Sun-Times. (1994b, July 15). Hulkster admits to steroid use, 109.

Chicago Tribune. (1992, July 22). Drugs still mystery Olympic ingredient, 1, 7.

Connolly, H. (1973). Hearings before the Subcommittee to Investigate Juvenile Delinquency (testimony before the Committee on the Judiciary, United States Senate). Ninety-third Congress, first session, June 18 and July 12 and 13.

Connolly, P. (1989). Hearings on steroids in amateur and professional sports—the medical and social costs of steroid abuse (testimony before Committee on the Judiciary, United States Senate). 101st Congress, first session, April 3 and May 9.

Cotolo, F. (1992). Better racing through chemistry. *Times: In harness* (eight-part series). February 8, 22; March 7, 21; April 4, 18; May 2, 16.

Courson, S. (1988, November 14). Steroids: A different perspective (in Point After). *Sports Illustrated,* 106.

Courson, S. (1991). *False Glory.* Stamford, CT: Longmeadow Press.

Cramer, R.B. (1985, February 14). Olympic cheating: The inside story of illicit doping and the U.S. cycling team. *Rolling Stone,* 25-30.

Csaky, T. (1972). Doping. *Journal of Sports Medicine and Physical Fitness,* 12(2), 117-123.

David, K., Dingemanse, E., Freud, J., & Laqueur, E. (1935). Über Krystallinisches Mannliches Hormon aus Hoden (Testosteron) Wirksamer als aus Harn oder aus Cholesterin Bereitetes Androsteron [Crystalline male hormone from testes (testosterone) more active than androsterone preparations from urine or cholesterol]. *Zeitschrift Physiologische Chemie,* 233, 281-293.

de Kruif, P. (1945). *The Male Hormone.* Garden City, NY: Harcourt, Brace, and Co.

Denver Post. (2000, June 26). Quote of the Day.

Des Moines Sunday Register. (1997, October 5). Athletes live with steroids' toll, 12A.

Donohoe, T., & Johnson, N. (1986). *Foul Play? Drug Use in Sport.* Oxford: Blackwell.

Dubin, C. (1990). Commission of inquiry into the use of drugs and banned practices intended to increase athletic performance (catalogue no. CP32-56/1990E, ISBN 0-660-

13610-4). Ottawa, ON: Canadian Government Publishing Center.

Duchaine, D. (1982). *Underground Steroid Handbook.* Santa Monica, CA: OEM.

Duchaine, D. (1989). *Underground Steroid Handbook II.* Venice, CA: HLR Technical Books.

Dyerson, M. (1998). *Making the American Team: Sport Culture and the Olympic Experience.* Urbana and Chicago: University of Illinois Press.

Edelman, R. (1993). *Serious Fun: A History of Spectator Sports in the USSR.* New York: Oxford University Press.

Fahey, T. (2001). Growth hormone: Muscle-building miracle drug or dark side of the force? *Muscular Development,* 38 (4), 174-177.

Fair, J. (1988). Olympic weightlifting and the introduction of steroids: A statistical analysis of world championship results, 1948-72. *International Journal of the History of Sport,* 5, 96-114.

Fair, J. (1993). Isometrics or steroids? Exploring new frontiers of strength in the early 1960s. *Journal of Sport History,* 20, 1-24.

Ferstle, J. (2000). Evolution and politics of drug testing. In C. Yesalis (Ed.), *Anabolic Steroids in Sport and Exercise,* 2nd ed. Champaign, IL: Human Kinetics.

Finley, M., & Plecket, H. (1976). *The Olympic Games: The First Thousand Years.* London: Chatto and Windus.

Fish, M. (1993, September 29). Experts suspect "a whole country" may be cheating. *Atlanta Journal-Constitution,* E3.

Fish, M. (1994, April 17). China's Olympic obsession. *Atlanta Journal/Atlanta Constitution,* A1, A8-A9.

Fish, M. (2000, September 9). 2000 Olympics: Tests nearly useless as new drugs pop up. *Atlanta Journal-Constitution,* 12F.

Fishbein, M. (1925). *Medical Follies.* New York: Boni & Liverlight.

Fisher, L.M. (1991, May 19). Stamina-building drug linked to athletes' deaths. *New York Times,* 22.

Ford, P. (2000, November 6). Tolerance of sports doping on trial in France. *Christian Science Monitor.*

Fralic, W. (1989). Hearings on steroids in amateur and professional sports—the medical and social costs of steroid abuse (testimony before the Committee on the Judiciary, United States Senate). 101st Congress, first session, April 3 and May 9.

Francis, C. (1990). *Speed Trap.* New York: St. Martin's Press.

Franke, W., & Berendonk, B. (1997). Hormonal doping and androgenization of athletes: A secret program of the German Democratic Republic government. *Clinical Chemistry,* 43(7), 1262-1279.

Fussell, W. (1990). *Muscle.* New York: Poseidon Press.

Gilbert, B. (1969a, June 23). Drugs in sport: Part 1. Problems in a turned-on world. *Sports Illustrated,* 64-72.

Gilbert, B. (1969b, June 30). Drugs in sport: Part 2. Something extra on the ball. *Sports Illustrated,* 30-42.

Gilbert, B. (1969c, July 7). Drugs in sport: Part 3. High time to make some rules. *Sports Illustrated,* 30-35.

Gilmour, J. (1998). Response to: "A comparative analysis of doping scandals: Canada, Russia, China," by Kidd, Brownell, and Edelman. Doping in Elite Sport Conference, Amateur Athletic Foundation of Los Angeles, April 24-25.

Green, G., Uryasz, F., Petr, T., & Bray, C. (2001). NCAA study of substance use and abuse habits of college student-athletes. *Clinical Journal of Sports Medicine,* 11, 51-56.

Hamilton, D. (1986). *The Monkey Gland Affair.* London: Chatto & Windus.

Hart, J., & Wallace, J. (1975). The adverse effects of amphetamines. *Clinical Toxicology,* 8(2), 179-190.

Harvey, R. (2000, October 15). Ignoring steroid issue is a national pastime. *Los Angeles Times.*

Hatfield, F. (1982). *Anabolic Steroids: What Kind and How Many.* Fitness Systems.

Hendershott, J. (1969). Steroids: Breakfast of champions. *Track and Field News,* 22(3).

Henderson, J. (2000, August 7). The ball's not juiced—the players are. *Denver Post,* 1E.

Herman, J. (1982). Rejuvenation: Brown-Sequard to Brinkley. *New York State Journal of Medicine,* 82, 1731-1739.

Hersh, P. (1993a, August 26). Too far, too fast. *Chicago Tribune.*

Hersh, P. (1993b, November 16). China's swimming success raises specter of East Germany. *Chicago Tribune,* Sec. 4, 4.

Hewitt, B. (1993, September 20). NFL players reveal they took cocaine, drank before games. *Chicago Sun-Times,* 100-101.

Hoberman, J. (1992a). The early development of sports medicine in Germany. In J.W. Berryman & R.J. Park (Eds.), *Sport and Exercise Science: Essays in the History of Sports Medicine.* Champaign, IL: University of Illinois Press.

Hoberman, J. (1992b). *Mortal Engines.* New York: Free Press.

Hoberman, J., & Todd, T. (1992, June 7). Chinese regime is hiding atrocities behind a facade of athletic utopia. *Austin American-Statesman,* E16.

Hoberman, J., & Yesalis, C. (1995, February). The history of synthetic testosterone. *Scientific American,* 61-65.

Huffman, S. (1990, August 27). I deserve my turn. *Sports Illustrated,* 26-31.

Humphries, T. (2000, September 13). Late operation on blind eye. *Irish Times,* 63.

Ivy, J. (1983). Amphetamines. In M. Williams (Ed.), *Ergogenic Aids in Sport.* Champaign, IL: Human Kinetics.

Janofsky, M. (1988, November 17). System accused of failing test posed by drugs. *New York Times.*

Johnson, W. (1985, May 13). Steroids: A problem of huge dimensions. *Sports Illustrated,* 38-61.

Johnston, R. (1974, October 14). The men and the myth. *Sports Illustrated,* 106-120.

Jokl, E. (1968). Notes on doping. In E. Jokl & P. Jokl (Eds.), *Exercise and Altitude.* Basel: Karger.

Karpovich, P.V. (1941). Ergogenic aids in work and sports. *Research Quarterly, 12*(Suppl.), 432-450.

Kearns, B., Harkness, R., Hobson, V., & Smith, A. (1942). Testosterone pellet implantation in the gelding. *Journal of the American Veterinary Medicine Association, C/780,* 197-201.

Kelley, S. (1991, July 10). This chapter of Alzado's story is sad. *Seattle Times.*

Kenyon, A., Knowlton, K., Sandiford, I., Koch, F., & Lotwin, G. (1940). A comparative study of the metabolic effects of testosterone propionate in normal men and women and in eunuchoidism. *Endocrinology, 26,* 26-45.

Kenyon, A., Sandiford, I., Bryan, A., Knowlton, K., & Koch, F. (1938). The effect of testosterone propionate on nitrogen, electrolyte, water and energy metabolism in eunuchoidism. *Endocrinology, 23,* 135-153.

Keteyian, A. (1987, January 5). A former Husker fesses up. *Sports Illustrated.*

Keteyian, A. (1998, August). Mass deception: Today's athlete is getting bigger, stronger, faster . . . unnaturally. *Sport.*

Kidd, B., Edelman, R., & Brownell, S. (1998). A comparative analysis of doping scandals: Russia, Canada, China. Doping in Elite Sport Conference, Amateur Athletic Foundation of Los Angeles, April 24-25.

King5.com. (2000, July 1). Armstrong second on first day of Tour de France.

Klecko, J., & Fields, J. (1989). *Nose to Nose: Survival in the Trenches in the NFL.* New York: Morrow.

Klein, A. (1986). Pumping irony: Crisis and contradiction in bodybuilding. *Sociology of Sport Journal, 3,* 112-133.

Klein, A. (1993). Of muscles and men. *The Sciences, 33,* 32-37.

Kochakian, C. (Ed.). (1976). *Anabolic-Androgenic Steroids.* New York: Springer-Verlag.

Kochakian, C., & Murlin, J. (1935). The effect of male hormone on the protein and energy metabolism of castrate dogs. *Journal of Nutrition, 10,* 437-459.

Kruskemper, H. (1968). *Anabolic Steroids.* New York: Academic Press.

Leigh, W. (1990). *Arnold: The Unauthorized Biography.* New York: Congdon-Weed.

Lespinasse, V. (1913). Transplantation of the testicle. *Journal of the American Medical Association, 61*(21), 1869-1870.

Lin, G., & Erinoff, L. (Eds.). (1990). *Anabolic Steroid Abuse* (National Institute on Drug Abuse Research, Monograph 102, DHHS publication no. ADM 90-1720). Rockville, MD: U.S. Department of Health and Human Services, Public Health Service.

Longman, J. (2000a, November 26). Struggles threaten U.S. Olympic movement. *New York Times.*

Longman, J. (2000b, September 10). Samaranch: Olympic savior or spoiler. *New York Times.*

Lucas, J. (1968). Pedestrianism and the struggle for the Sir John Astley belt, 1878-1879. *Research Quarterly, 39*(3), 587-594.

Mandell, A. (1976). *The Nightmare Season.* New York: Random House.

Mandell, A. (1978). The Sunday syndrome. *Psychedelic Drugs, 10,* 379-383.

Mandell, A. (1981). The Sunday syndrome: From kinetics to altered consciousness. *Federation Proceedings, 40,* 2693-2698.

McKinley, J. (2000, October 11). Performance enhancers and baseball. *New York Times.*

Miller, A. (1996, May, 3). Reports of steroid use down, but abuse not over, some say. *Atlanta Journal/Atlanta Constitution,* G4.

Milwaukee Sentinel. (1993, July 12). NFL drug users find invisible assistance.

Mix, R. (1987, October 19). So little gain for the pain. *Sports Illustrated.*

Montville, L. (1994, September 19). Flora and furor. *Sports Illustrated.*

Moore, K. (1993, September 27). Great wall of doubt. *Sports Illustrated.*

Nack, W. (1998, May 18). The muscle murders. *Sports Illustrated.*

National Center on Addiction and Substance Abuse. (2000). *Winning at Any Cost: Doping in Olympic Sport.* A Report by the CASA National Commission on Sports and Substance Abuse. New York: National Center on Addiction and Substance Abuse.

National Steroid Consensus Meeting. (1989, July 30-31). Sponsored by the United States Olympic Committee, the National Collegiate Athletic Association, the National Federation of State High School Associations and the Amateur Athletic Foundation, Los Angeles.

NCAA News. (1997, September 15). Survey shows steroid use on the decline, 1.

NCAA Research Staff. (1997, September). *NCAA Study of Use and Abuse Habits of College Student Athletes.* Kansas City: NCAA.

Newerla, G. (1943). The history of the discovery and isolation of the male hormone. *New England Journal of Medicine, 228*(2), 39-47.

New York Times. (1995, June 25). Ban for steroid user, 14, 10S.

Nightengale, B. (1995, July 15). Many fear performance-enhancing drug is becoming prevalent and believe something must be done. *Los Angeles Times,* 1C.

Noden, M. (1993, March 15). Shot down. *Sports Illustrated.*

Noonan, D. (1997, December 14). Really big football players. *New York Times Magazine,* 64-69.

O'Brien, R. (1993, December 13). Grappling with decline. *Sports Illustrated.*

Osler, T., & Dodd, E. (1979). *Ultra-Marathoning: The Next Challenge.* Mountain View, CA: World.

Padwe, S. (1973, April 30). Get high on sports, not drugs— concern growing over drugs in college sports. *Newsday.*

Parkes, A. (1985). *Off-beat Biologist: The Autobiography of A. S. Parkes* (Vol. 1). Cambridge, England: Galton Foundation.

Parkes, A. (1988). *Biologist at Large: The Autobiography of A. S. Parkes* (Vol. 2). Cambridge, England: Galton Foundation.

Patrick, D. (1993, September 16). Sudden burst encourages drug rumors. *USA Today,* 1-2C.

Patrick, D. (1997, October 24). Breaking the standards. *USA Today,* 3C.

Pausanias. (1959). *Descriptions of Greece,* a second century A.D. work translated by W.H.S. Jones. Cambridge, MA, and London: Loeb Classical Library.

Payne, A.H. (1975). Anabolic steroids in athletics. *British Journal of Sports Medicine,* 9, 83-88.

Phillips, W. (1990). *Anabolic Reference Guide,* 5th ed. Golden, CO: Mile High.

Prokop, L. (1970). The struggle against doping and its history. *Journal of Sports Medicine and Physical Fitness,* 10(1), 45-48.

Ramotar, J. (1990). Cyclists deaths linked to erythropoietin? *Physician and Sportsmedicine,* 18(8), 48-50.

Ray, O., & Ksir, C. (1996). *Drugs, Society, and Human Behavior,* 7th ed. St. Louis: Mosby.

Reid, S. (2000, August 6). The obvious answer. *Orange County Register,* 1D.

Reilly, R. (2000a, August 21). The 'roid to ruin. *Sports Illustrated.*

Reilly, R. (2000b, December 11). Paralympic paradox. *Sports Illustrated,* 98.

Reuter Information Service. (1995, October 12). Rugby: Three players fail World Cup drug test. London.

Robson, P. (1999). *Forbidden Drugs,* 2nd ed. Oxford: Oxford University Press.

Rolleston, H. (1936). *The Endocrine Organs in Health and Disease: With an Historical Review.* London: Oxford University Press.

Rosellini, L. (1992, February 17). The sports factories. *U.S. News & World Report,* 48-59.

Rosenthal, K. (1998). Steroids: Baseball's darkest secret. MSNBC on the Internet.

Santos, L. (1973). Hearings before the Subcommittee to Investigate Juvenile Delinquency (testimony before the Committee on the Judiciary, United States Senate). Ninety-third Congress, first session, June 18 and July 12 and 13.

Scott, J. (1971, October 17). It's not how you play the game, but what pill you take. *New York Times Magazine.*

Shipley, A. (2000, June 15). Drug chief resigns, blasts USOC. *Washington Post,* D10.

Simonson, E., Kearns, W., & Enzer, N. (1941). Effect of oral administration of methyltestosterone on fatigue in eunuchoids and castrates. *Endocrinology,* 28, 506-512.

Simonson, E., Kearns, W., & Enzer, N. (1944). Effect of methyltestosterone treatment on muscular performance and the central nervous system of older men. *Journal of Clinical Endocrinology and Metabolism,* 4, 528-534.

Sports Illustrated. (1991, July 22). The dangers of steroids are becoming more apparent, 10.

Sports Medicine Digest. (1996, September). Drug testing results in Atlanta confound expectations, 103.

Stanley, L. (1922). An analysis of one thousand testicular substance implantations. *Endocrinology,* 6, 787-794.

Starr, B. (1981). *Defying Gravity: How to Win at Weightlifting.* Wichita Falls, TX: Five Starr Productions.

Strauss, R.H., & Curry, T.J. (1987). Magic, science and drugs. In R.H. Strauss (Ed.), *Drugs and Performance in Sports* (3-9). Philadelphia: Saunders.

Struman, M. (1992, December 17). Bulky pigeons face drug-testing. *USA Today,* 2C.

Sullivan, R., & Song, S. (2000, September 11). Are drugs winning the Games? *Time,* 90-92.

Swift, E. (1999, July 5). Drug pedaling. *Sports Illustrated,* 60-65.

Tampa Bay Tribune. (1984, July 2). Steroid information given to athletes.

Tampa Bay Tribune. (1985, January 13 and 23). Player claims druggist used Vandy weight room.

Todd, J., & Todd, T. (2001). Significant events in the history of drug testing and the Olympic movement: 1960-1999. In W. Wilson & E. Derse (Eds.), *Doping in Elite Sport.* Champaign, IL: Human Kinetics.

Todd, T. (1983, August 1). The steroid predicament. *Sports Illustrated,* 62-77.

Todd, T. (1987). Anabolic steroids: The gremlins of sport. *Journal of Sport History,* 14, 87-107.

U.S. Drug Enforcement Administration. (1994). *Conference Report: International Conference on the Abuse and Trafficking of Anabolic Steroids.* Washington, DC: U.S. Department of Justice.

USA Today. (1992, September 9). Briefly, 2C.

USA Today. (1994, October 5). Chinese swimmers, lifters dominate, 9C.

USA Today. (1995, March 21). Drugs detected, 2C.

USA Today. (1997a, April 29). Out of action, 1C.

USA Today. (1997b, October 1). We'll take it, 3C.

USA Today. (1998a, February 20). IOC mum on latest positive drug test, 13E.

USA Today. (1998b, April 8). Lifetime drug ban, 3C.

USA Today. (1998c, July 7). East German says he gave out steroids, 3C.

USA Today. (1998d, July 22). Drug scandal widens, threatens second team, 3C.

Voy, R. (1991). *Drugs, Sport, and Politics.* Champaign, IL: Leisure Press.

Wade, N. (1972). Anabolic steroids: Doctors denounce them, but athletes aren't listening. *Science,* 176, 1399-1403.

Wadler, G., & Hainline, B. (1989). *Drugs and the Athlete.* Philadelphia: Davis.

Whitten, P. (1994). China's short march to swimming dominance: Hard work or drugs? *Swimming World and Junior Swimmer,* 34-39.

Williams, D. (1989). Hearings on steroids in amateur and professional sports—the medical and social costs of steroid abuse (testimony before Committee on the Judiciary, United States Senate). 101st Congress, first session, April 3 and May 9.

Williams, M. (1974). *Drugs and Athletic Performance.* Springfield, IL: Charles C Thomas.

Williams, M. (1980). Blood doping in sports. *Journal of Drug Issues,* 10(3), 331-339.

Wright, J. (1978). *Anabolic Steroids and Sports.* Natick, MA: Sports Science Consultants.

Yaeger, D., & Looney, D. (1993). *Under the Tarnished Dome: How Notre Dame Betrayed its Ideals for Football Glory.* New York: Simon & Schuster.

Yesalis, C. (1993, December 7-10). Epidemiology of anabolic steroid abuse in the U.S. International Conference on the Abuse and Trafficking in Anabolic Steroids, sponsored by the U.S. Drug Enforcement Administration, Prague, Czech Republic.

Yesalis, C. (1995, November 6-8). Misuse of anabolic/androgenic steroids: Epidemiology and public health. Berzelius Symposium on Doping Agents—A Threat Against Sports and Public Health, Stockholm.

Yesalis, C. (1996, August 1). No medals for drug testing. *New York Times,* A27.

Yesalis, C. (2000, September 9). 100% guarantee: No drug-free Olympics now, tomorrow. *USA Today.*

Yesalis, C., Anderson, W., Buckley, W., & Wright, J. (1990). Incidence of the nonmedical use of anabolic-androgenic steroids. In G. Lin & L. Erinoff (Eds.), *Anabolic Steroid Abuse* (National Institute on Drug Abuse Research, Monograph 102, DHHS publication no. ADM 90-1720). Rockville, MD: U.S. Department of Health and Human Services, Public Health Service.

Yesalis, C., & Cowart, V. (1998). *The Steroids Game.* Champaign, IL: Human Kinetics.

Yesalis, C., Kopstein, A., & Bahrke, M. (2001). Difficulties in estimating the prevalence of drug use among athletes. In W. Wilson & E. Derse (Eds.), *Doping in Elite Sport.* Champaign, IL: Human Kinetics.

Zimmerman, P. (1986, November 10). The agony must end. *Sports Illustrated,* 17-21.

Zorpette, G. (2000, September). The chemical games: Blood doping breakthrough. *Scientific American.*

CHAPTER 2

Determining the Efficacy of Performance-Enhancing Substances

Stan Reents, PharmD

The use and abuse of performance-enhancing substances (PES) in international-level competition was first brought to the attention of most spectators by the dramatic victory of Ben Johnson in the 100-m (109 yd) dash at the 1988 Seoul Olympics. Shortly after that race came the report that Johnson had tested positive for the anabolic steroid, stanozolol, a banned substance.

Unfortunately, despite the high-profile nature of the Ben Johnson incident, competitive athletes continue to experiment with substances they believe will enhance performance: even legitimate drug use (i.e., medication) among athletes appears to be suspect: at the 1996 Atlanta Olympics, 383 medical waivers (declarations of use of a medication for a definite health reason) were submitted. This number jumped to 618 for the Sydney Olympics four years later (Wilson S 2000). And there is suspicion that many triathletes are claiming to be asthmatic when in fact they are not, in order to justify the "need" for β-agonist inhalers such as albuterol (Farrey T 1999; Reents S 2000, p. 134; Wilber RL et al. 2000).

Athletes also use dietary supplements. One of the more high-profile examples appeared in 1998 when professional baseball player Mark McGwire admitted to using both androstenedione and creatine. That same year, annual sales of creatine alone were approximately $200 million (Ritter SK 1999). United States Olympic swimmers have been reported to take 15 to 20 supplements per day (NewsEdge, 2000). Abuse of gamma-hydroxybutyric acid (GHB) by bodybuilders has skyrocketed recently (*Washington Post,* March 21, 2000). For some athletes, the will to win overpowers any fear or concern about the risks of using PES.

Athletes also receive much misinformation on this topic. Sport supplements, for example, are promoted to athletes through magazine advertisements, via the Internet, and directly at expositions associated with local-area races. Representatives from these companies are quick to offer advice on why this or that particular ingredient is required, always with the underlying message (either direct or implied) that it enhances performance. And endorsements of these supplements by muscular personal trainers or other athletes fuel the demand.

Unfortunately, for the vast majority of supplements, little or no data exist to either confirm or refute the claims being made concerning their effects on performance (Reents S 2000; Williams MH 1995; Williams MH 1998). But even when published data regarding the ergogenic potential of a particular PES are extensive (for example, quite a lot of good data have been published for creatine [Williams MH et al. 1999]), uncertainty can still exist because of methodological problems in study design, as has been described for anabolic steroids (Elashoff JD et al. 1991; Yesalis CE et al. 1989) and ginseng (Bahrke MS and Morgan WP 2000), or concern over quality control during the production process as is the case with nearly all dietary supplements (see discussion later in this chapter) (Miller MJS 2000).

To provide context, we begin with a brief discussion of supplement regulation and information channels, but the purpose of this chapter is to identify issues that one must consider when reviewing efficacy data for PES. These issues can be categorized into three general groups: study design, factors associated with the substance in question, and type of subjects. The widespread availability of sport supplements, and their use by athletes, demand that we also assess the data (or lack thereof) regarding their effects on performance.

The Dietary Supplement Health and Education Act of 1994

In 1994, Congress passed the Dietary Supplement Health and Education Act (DSHEA), which opened the door to widespread marketing of dietary supplements in the United States. The DSHEA defines a dietary supplement as a food product that contains at least one of the following ingredients: vitamin, mineral, herb or botanical, amino acid, metabolite, constituent, or extract.

Although passage of the DSHEA made life simpler for supplement manufacturers, unfortunately it created problems for consumers. First, DSHEA permits a product to be marketed without any scientific research to support even the most general claims it makes; second, it permits labeling information to be intentionally vague. For manufacturers of dietary supplements, the trade-off is that they (manufacturers) may not claim that their products "cure, mitigate, treat, or prevent" a specific disease; instead, they may make only general statements regarding what the product does. For example, manufacturers of ginkgo cannot make claims that their product is effective in the treatment of Alzheimer's disease, but they can state that it "provides mental energy." As another example, the label on one brand of creatine bears a statement including the phrase "capable of promoting and sustaining muscle mass and repair while helping to prevent the breakdown of muscle tissue." On the opposite side of the label is the footnote: "This statement has not been evaluated by the FDA." (One wonders if placing the footnote in a different area of the label from the statement was intentional!)

The distinction between a supplement and a nonprescription pharmaceutical drug arises not so much from what the compound *is*, but from *how it is marketed*. On the store shelf, a bottle of capsules containing a dietary supplement appears to the average person as indistinguishable from traditional over-the-counter (OTC) drugs. But dietary supplements and OTC drugs are far from similar. The DSHEA allowed manufacturers of dietary supplements to distribute their products without a prescription and, more importantly, outside the domain of good manufacturing practice standards (GMP) as they are applied to drugs. Since these products are considered dietary supplements and not drugs, they are not required to undergo safety and efficacy review, as all OTC and prescription drugs must.

For example, ephedra-containing herbal supplements are abused by athletes (Gruber AJ and Pope HG 1998), and these supplements can lead to serious side effects (Bruno A et al. 1993; Haller CA and Benowitz NL 2000). In June 1997, the FDA proposed capping the amount of ephedra in various dietary supplements, claiming that the agency had received more than 800 reports of adverse events in people taking this supplement. The proposal would have limited use to no more than 8 mg in a 6-hr period or 24 mg in a 24-hr period and would require that the label instruct users not to use the supplement for longer than seven days. The proposal also required that the label state "Taking more than the recommended serving may result in heart attack, stroke, seizure, or death." After an outcry from lawmakers and industry groups, claiming that the FDA did not have enough scientific evidence to support the restrictions, the FDA withdrew the proposals on March 31, 2000. Subsequently, the December 21, 2000 issue of the *New England Journal of Medicine* included a summary of adverse reactions due to ephedra. Note that one of the active alkaloids derived from ephedra is ephedrine, which is marketed as a pharmaceutical drug and, as such, does fall under the more stringent GMP applied to drugs.

Ergogenicity has not been firmly established for many substances that athletes abuse. More disturbing, however, is the realization that athletes will believe the "hype" surrounding a substance's benefit while ignoring reports of its potential to cause serious toxicity as in the example just cited. Table 2.1 lists several substances that athletes mistakenly believe are ergogenic but that have serious potential toxicities.

Thus, athletes are risking serious side effects, if not disqualification (see later), by ingesting substances they believe will enhance performance. Where can an athlete or trainer find reliable information on PES? This text will be a good source. Other texts include *Drugs and the Athlete,* published in 1989 by Wadler and Hainline, and *Sport and Exercise Pharmacology,* published in 2000 by Reents. Regarding sport supplements (i.e., dietary supplements), there are far fewer reliable sources. Occasionally, useful data are published in *Consumer Reports* (see the June 2001 issue). Consumer Union (publishers of *Consumer Reports*) has also created a unique, interactive Web site on androstenedione, creatine, and ephedra at **www.zillions.org** (accessed June 10, 2001).

Table 2.1 Adverse Effects From Substances Used by Athletes

Substance	Ergogenic?	Adverse effects	References
Androstenedione	No	Priapism, elevated estrogen levels	Kachhi & Henderson 2000; King et al. 1999; Leder et al. 2000
Ephedrine	No	Angina, insomnia, stroke, subarachnoid hemorrhage, myocardial infarction, cardiac arrhythmias, death	Bruno et al. 1993; Haller & Benowitz 2000
Gamma-hydroxybutyrate (GHB) *(Date Rape Drug)*	No	Coma, seizures, death	Galloway et al. 1997; Ryan et al. 1997
Growth hormone	No	Left ventricular hypertrophy, diminished exercise capacity	Giustina et al. 1995
Insulin	No	Hypoglycemia, seizures, neuroglycopenia, severe brain damage	Rich et al. 1998
Pseudoephedrine	No	Minimal at recommended doses	Swain et al. 1997

The relatively new *Journal of the American Nutraceutical Association (JANA)* and the Web site **ConsumerLab.com** both publish data on supplements, though these sources do not focus only on sport supplements.

However, athletes themselves are not likely to be reading these texts and articles, particularly not the more scholarly and scientific ones. Yet athletes need to rely on information sources other than ads, Web sites of questionable validity, or trade magazines. Their coaches and physicians, therefore, should keep abreast of current information about PES and pass this information on to the athletes they work with. Reading the following chapters in this book should make it apparent which PES are supported by good data and which are not. In the next section of this chapter we discuss criteria to consider when evaluating studies on PES.

Methodological Issues of Study Design

Regarding study design, a variety of factors can influence the interpretation of results (e.g., placebo controlled? appropriate blinding? adequate sample size? use of multiple substances concurrently? doses and pharmacokinetic issues?). This section addresses these factors.

The "gold standard" in scientific research design is the prospective, double-blind, randomized, placebo-controlled clinical study. Its importance to research is on a par with other scientific dogma such as the four-phase approach to establishing causality for drug side effects (i.e., positive challenge, positive dechallenge, positive rechallenge, and positive dechallenge) and Koch's postulates for verifying the cause of a given infectious disease. Strict adherence to these principles helps to solidify the causality of an observed event. Otherwise, if the process of gathering facts is in question, the results and conclusions are also in question. Williams has summarized the various types of presentation of data on PES in his book *The Ergogenics Edge* (Williams MH 1998).

Prospective Versus Retrospective Design

Several types of study design can be employed effectively if one knows their strengths and limitations. Prospective studies, along with proper randomization and blinding, allow investigators maximum control over potentially confounding variables. Subjects are randomized to either a treatment or a control group and followed from that point forward. On the other hand, retrospective analysis is useful in assessment of trends in disease over a long period of time, which would be difficult to perform in a prospective fashion. Retrospective studies limit the investigators' analysis to data that have been previously recorded. Retrospective analysis is also helpful when one is studying a rare event, a situation in which a prospective design would require the involvement of very large numbers of study subjects. While retrospective analysis may be adequate for analyzing objective data that are well documented historically (e.g., advancements in world records, changes in blood pressure or serum cholesterol), other types of research (for example, the psychological effects of anabolic steroids) would be impossible to perform on a retrospective basis. Finally, retrospective design may be preferable when a prospective design might be unethical (e.g., administration of extremely large doses of anabolic steroids to human subjects).

Crossover Versus Parallel Design

In some studies, subjects are used as their own controls. This type of study is called a "crossover" study. Crossover study design increases the statistical power of the study in comparison to parallel-group design. In crossover studies, however, it is important that enough time elapse between the end of the treatment phase and the beginning of observations after entry into the control group. For example, blood concentrations of exogenously administered epoetin alfa (erythropoietin) decline back to normal range within hours, but the physiologic effects of this hormone last for many weeks (Birkeland KI et al. 2000; Erslev AJ 1991). If the period of time between the end of epoetin alfa administration and the beginning of the control phase is too short, subjects who are crossed over may still demonstrate some of the physiologic effects of the treatment, thus confounding observations obtained from the control phase.

Case-Control Design

Another type of design is the case-control study. This is also a retrospective analysis; however, it utilizes subjects who already possess a given trait (e.g., a specific disease state) and compares them against subjects who are similar but do not have the trait. The case-control study is limited in that it allows for only an approximation of relative and attributable risk, derived from the odds ratio. Calculation of actual incidence of an outcome requires the randomized, prospective design already described.

Case Reports

Sometimes data on PES are provided in the form of a case report. Typically, this involves unique observations and does not represent data generated in a controlled fashion (i.e., utilization of randomization and blinding). While case reports can provide worthwhile data, they cannot answer scientific questions in the same way as the study designs previously described.

Meta-Analysis

More recently, a statistical analysis of a collection of similar studies, known as a "meta-analysis," has evolved. The aim in meta-analysis reviews is to clarify research conclusions when data on a similar issue have been collected by multiple groups of investigators. Validating the conclusions from a meta-analysis requires that the study methods of each group of investigators be highly similar. Since this is often not the case, conclusions from meta-analyses are sometimes questionable. The pitfalls of meta-analyses have been reviewed by Etminan and Levin (Etminan M and Levin M 1999).

Testimonials

Finally, the least reliable "data" (to use the term loosely here) come from unsubstantiated testimonials or anecdotes. Testimonials regarding PES abound on the Internet, which is another phenomenon discussed later. Testimonials should never be regarded as factual; a comparative clinical study is required for that.

Importance of Placebo Controls

Comparing results obtained from an active treatment group with those of a placebo-controlled group helps to evaluate results obtained from a research study. The utilization of a placebo control is crucial when the dependent variable is subjective in nature.

However, a placebo control is also important even when objective data are measured. Athletes can be susceptible to marketing "hype" and testimonials from other athletes. For example, some athletes use β2-agonist inhalers just prior to competition (Farrey T 1999), even though these bronchodilator drugs are generally considered not ergogenic when administered by inhalation (Reents S 2000); others use androstenedione even though there is still no proof that this prohormone enhances performance (King DS et al. 1999; Leder BZ et al. 2000). Thus, despite the selection of an objective parameter (e.g., $\dot{V}O_2$max) as the dependent variable, as well as rigorous documentation of the observations (e.g., assessing cycle ergometer readings every 5 min), a placebo control remains crucial in studies of the effects of PES. An athlete's belief regarding what the ingested supplement might do could influence his performance.

Appropriate Dependent Variable

Selecting the correct dependent variable is a critical factor if one is to draw accurate conclusions about PES. For example, is muscular strength or muscular endurance the better variable to measure in a particular study? What about fine-motor control versus gross-motor control to determine hand-eye coordination? A well-controlled study of effects of dextroamphetamine on athletic performance revealed how conclusions can be affected by selection of the dependent variable. Significant increases were seen in knee extension strength but not elbow flexion strength. Acceleration improved but not peak speed, and time to exhaustion improved but not aerobic power (Chandler JV and Blair SN 1980). Intimately tied to the issue of appropriate dependent variable are the issues of lab- versus field-based research and the type of exercise chosen.

Lab Data Versus Field Data

Investigators must use care when extrapolating lab results to actual competition. For example, is it valid to extrapolate observations of the effect of a drug on $\dot{V}O_2$max to its effects on aerobic performance? Do the effects of caffeine on free fatty acid concentrations explain why an athlete's performance in a triathlon improves? While it may seem logical that documentation of enhanced performance on a bicycle ergometer would readily translate to a competitive cycling event, in fact it may not. Uncontrollable factors such as weather and road conditions, wind resistance, drag, leaning, and turning may each affect cycling performance in the field. Likewise, assessing the effects of creatine supplements on one-repetition maximum (1-RM) bench press exercise may not predict performance in the shot put. Thus, a substance may be ergogenic as a result of its psychological effects but this may not be detectable in the lab, particularly if only changes in muscle strength are measured. Finally, instruments and measurements used in a lab test may not be sensitive enough to detect the small changes that could be responsible for a first-place finish against world-class competition. So, in some cases, lab testing allows for better control of confounding variables; but in other cases, field tests are more readily extrapolated to real-life situations (Williams MH 1998).

Exercise Mode, Intensity, and Duration

When one is designing a study or evaluating the usefulness of a study, the type of exercise selected is significant; it may influence what drug effects occur as the response. For example, anabolic-androgenic steroids may improve muscular strength (Bhasin et al. 1996), but they do not improve aerobic exercise performance. Sodium bicarbonate (Linderman J and Fahey TD 1991) and creatine (Williams MH et al. 1999) appear to be ergogenic in situations requiring short bursts of energy, while caffeine is ergogenic in sustained aerobic exercise (Graham TE and Spriet LL 1991, 1995).

Another significant factor in the design of a study on the efficacy of PES is the duration and intensity of exercise. If endurance exercise is chosen as the mode of exercise, should it be maximal exercise or submaximal exercise? It is important to realize that employing maximal exercise may reveal an ergolytic or ergogenic drug effect not seen during submaximal exercise. The duration of exercise is an important consideration when one is evaluating the effects of creatine on performance. In one study of creatine, military personnel were subjected to high-intensity cycling for various periods of time. Performance improved by roughly 60% when the duration of the test was 20 or 60 sec, but improved by over 100% when the test was conducted for only 10 sec (Prevost MC et al. 1997). Another investigation used a 45-sec continuous jumping test. Creatine improved jumping performance in the first two 15-sec periods, but not in the third (Bosco C et al. 1997).

Study Duration and Timing of Observations

Consider the substances caffeine, creatine, epoetin alfa (erythropoietin), and sodium bicarbonate. An ergogenic effect from caffeine can be measured within an hour or two of a single dose (Flinn S et al. 1990; Graham TE and Spriet LL 1991), but the physiologic response to epoetin alfa is delayed for several weeks (Birkeland KI et al. 2000; Casoni I et al. 1993; Ekblom B 1996). The effects of creatine on performance are intermediate between those of these other two compounds, occurring after a minimum of three to five days of continuous administration. The ergogenic potential of sodium bicarbonate is extremely short-lived. In studies in which the dose was administered 2 hr before testing (Kozak-Collins et al. 1994), no ergogenic effect was seen; however, when an even smaller dose was used but was administered in divided doses just before testing, an ergogenic effect was detected (Iwaoka K et al. 1989). Regarding caffeine, blood concentrations and caffeine-induced increases in epinephrine concentrations rise within 45 min of ingestion of a dose; however, the ergogenic metabolic effects do not peak for several hours.

In summary, it is necessary to consider many elements of study design in order to obtain a reliable assessment of the effects of PES. Other authors have reviewed these issues in greater detail (Bahrke MS and Morgan WP 2000; Williams MH 1998; Yesalis CE et al. 1989; Yesalis CE 2000).

Methodological Issues Regarding the Drug or Substance Being Evaluated

Consider the following:

- Orally administered clenbuterol, a β2-agonist not approved for human use in the United States, has been shown to possess anabolic properties (Dodd SL et al. 1996).

- Albuterol, a related but less potent β2-agonist, has also been shown to be ergogenic after oral administration (van Baak MA et al. 2000), but generally not when administered via inhalation (Reents S 2000).

- Caffeine has been shown to be ergogenic, but the same results were not duplicated when caffeine was ingested as coffee (Graham TE et al. 1998).

- Androstenedione was shown to increase testosterone levels in one study (Leder et al. 2000), but not another (King et al. 1999).

In this section, we examine how and why issues related to the substance being studied can impact the results of a study.

Influence of Dose on Study Results

The dose of a PES administered to the treatment group can also influence the findings, conclusions, and recommendations of a particular study. This has been a factor in studies of anabolic steroids, androstenedione, caffeine, creatine, and sodium bicarbonate, for example.

- **Anabolic steroids.** There does not appear to be a relationship between the use of anabolic steroids and increases in muscle strength (Elashoff JD et al. 1991); however, a major confounding factor is that controlled scientific studies rarely evaluate doses similar to those actually ingested by unethical athletes (Bhasin S et al. 1996). When effects of anabolic steroids on lean body mass are assessed, limited data suggest that the steep portion of the dose-response curve is several orders of magnitude greater than for doses typically used in clinical medicine or in most clinical studies (figure 2.1).

- **Androstenedione.** Serum testosterone concentrations increased when subjects were given 300 mg/day as a single dose (Leder et al. 2000); however, when subjects were administered androstenedione 300 mg/day as three separate 100-mg doses, no increase was observed (King et al. 1999). This illustrates how critical the dose is in relation to the observations and conclusions of a study.

- **Caffeine.** Caffeine, at doses of 6 mg/kg, produced a significant increase in monosynaptic reflex response time in humans, but doses of 3 mg/kg were not different from placebo in their effect (Jacobson BH and Edwards SW 1990). In another caffeine study, doses of 3 and 6 mg/kg improved running performance, but even higher doses of 9 mg/kg did not (Graham TE and Spriet LL 1995). If the investigators studied only a single dose, contradicting results and conclusions would be seen

- **Creatine.** Creatine doses of 2.25 g/day were found to be ergogenic if a loading dose (18.75 g/day × 5 days)

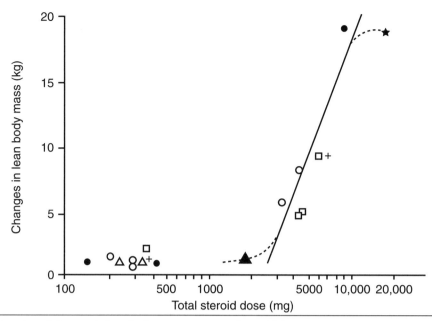

Figure 2.1   Semi-log plot of changes in lean body mass versus total steroid dose.

○ = testosterone; ● = oxandrolone; □ = dianabol; ▲ = androstenelone; △ = nandrolone; + = testosterone; ★ = estimate of the effect of endogenous testosterone production by males during the teen years.

Adapted, by permission, from G.B. Forbes, 1985, The effect of anabolic steroids on lean body mass. In *Metabolism* 34: 571-573.

was given (Prevost MC et al. 1997), but doses of 2 g/day without a loading dose in another study were not ergogenic (Thompson CH et al. 1996). When low doses (2 g/day) were studied, tissue concentrations of creatine did not rise (Harris RC et al. 1992; Thompson CH et al. 1996) and performance was not enhanced (Thompson CH et al. 1996). However, when larger doses (20 g/day) are administered, tissue concentrations do increase (Casey A et al. 1996; Kreis R et al. 1999), and an ergogenic effect is seen (Casey A et al. 1996; Kamber M et al. 1999).

• **Sodium bicarbonate.** Most studies showing an ergogenic effect from sodium bicarbonate have used doses of 300 mg/kg. However, when the dose was 200 mg/kg or less, ergogenic effects were observed less frequently (Linderman J and Fahey TD 1991).

Thus, for some PES, the dose chosen can dramatically affect the results of a study and conclusions about its effect on performance.

Formulation Issues

Albuterol, a β2-agonist commonly used in the management of asthma and exercise-induced bronchoconstriction, has not generally been shown to be ergogenic when administered via inhalation (Reents S 2000); however, some data show that systemic administration has the potential for an ergogenic effect (Caruso JF et al. 1995; van Baak MA et al. 2000). The United States Olympic Committee and the National Collegiate Athletic Association both recognize the impact of route of administration with regard to albuterol:

systemically administered dosage forms are banned, while in some cases inhaled dosage forms are permitted (Fuentes RJ et al. 1999). Another formulation issue to consider is whether the substance in question is produced as a combination product (i.e., a single product with multiple ingredients). This further complicates the evaluation of the effect of a given substance on athletic performance.

Is the Substance in Question Bioavailable?

Bioavailability is the percentage of an administered dose that actually reaches the intended site of action. An issue of concern with regard to dietary supplements is that two formulations of the same active ingredient administered via the same route may exhibit entirely different degrees of bioavailability. Bioavailability is a critical question and is determined by both the nature of the substance (mineral, peptide hormone, etc.) and the formulation of the actual dosage form.

Some endogenous substances such as erythropoietin, growth hormone, and testosterone are not bioavailable after oral administration. Generally, most peptide hormones are destroyed by stomach acid or undergo extensive hepatic extraction (i.e., "first-pass effect") before they can reach the systemic circulation, so it is foolish to consider that oral ingestion of these substances will be ergogenic. To make testosterone bioavailable after oral administration, molecular derivatives, known as 17-α-methyl forms (e.g., fluoxymesterone, oxandrolone, and others), have been developed. Thus, products marketed as oral forms of growth hormone automatically should be considered worthless. Regarding creatine, muscle stores of phosphocreatine do increase after oral administration, and an ergogenic effect has been demonstrated in selected types of physical activity during creatine supplementation (Williams MH et al. 1999). The fact that muscle stores increase after oral administration of creatine supplementation means that it is bioavailable. Thus, even before clinical and/or performance data are generated, we can question whether a given substance marketed as a PES would or would not be ergogenic based on its oral bioavailability profile.

Even if a compound does reach the systemic circulation, however, it still may not be bioavailable at the site of action. Consider L-carnitine: even after two weeks, although plasma concentrations of L-carnitine increased after supplementation, muscle concentrations did not (Williams MH 1998). Issues such as bioavailability, quality control during production (see next section), and clinical documentation are currently being intensely scrutinized with regard to dietary supplements.

Federal "Good Manufacturing Practices"

An issue that is becoming readily apparent as supplements are being more closely examined is the tremendous variation in amount of active ingredient contained in the actual dosage form compared with the amount reported on the label. Obviously, if the amount of active ingredient varies from batch to batch, or brand to brand, there can never be any certainty as to the effects the substance will (or will not) provide. The U.S. FDA has published regulations setting forth minimum current "Good Manufacturing Practice" (GMP) for the production of drugs. The key word in the preceding sentence is "drugs." Most pharmaceutical drugs (i.e., both prescription and OTC drugs) are produced according to these rigid industry standards so that, regardless of the manufacturer, each dosage form contains a predictable and consistent amount of active ingredient(s). For example, consider the standards that exist for production of the oral anabolic steroid oxandrolone:

> "Oxandrolone, USP [bulk powder] . . . contains not less than 97.0% and not more than 100.5% of oxandrolone . . ." and "oxandrolone tablets USP . . . contain the labeled amount, within ±8%." (USP-DI 2000).

This degree of reliability is assured for any oxandrolone products that bear the "USP" designation.

It is important to note that the GMP standard for drugs is currently not mandated for manufacturers of dietary supplements, though some may voluntarily choose to follow it. However, since supplements fall under the food manufacturing standards, production of dietary supplements remains less tightly controlled than for the production of pharmaceutical-grade drugs. As a result, quality control during production is questionable for many supplements, and reports of problems arising from this issue are beginning to emerge in the scientific and clinical literature. Recent examples include the contamination of tryptophan bulk powder with a substance that was linked to the development of over 1500 cases of eosinophilia-myalgia syndrome, 27 of which were fatal (Centers for Disease Control 1989; Swygert LA et al. 1990; Milburn DS and Myers CW 1991); herbal supplements that were contaminated with digitalis glycosides, which led to at least two cases of digitalis toxicity (Slifman NR et al. 1998); and supplements claiming to contain only natural Chinese herbs that actually contained the potent diabetes drugs glyburide and phenformin, which led to symptoms of hypoglycemia (press release obtained from **http://www.dhs.ca.gov**).

Consider the following examples of variation in potency:

- **Carnitine.** Analysis of 12 OTC carnitine products revealed that the actual mean carnitine content was only 52% of the stated label amount and that 5 of 12 products had unsatisfactory pharmaceutical dissolution characteristics (Brass EP 2000; Millington DS and Dubag G 1993).

- **Chondroitin.** Only 5 of 32 brands of chondroitin fell within the target range of ±10% variation in label claim. The authors concluded that "variation greater than 10% suggests poor quality of raw material or poor manufacturing processes and lack of quality control" (figure 2.2, *a* and *b*) (Adebowale AO et al. 2000).

- **Dehydroepiandrosterone (DHEA).** When sample doses from 16 different brands of DHEA were analyzed for DHEA content, 8 of the 16 brands fell outside of the 90% to 110% range of labeled amount, which is commonly applied to pharmaceutical-grade drugs. One of these products contained 150% of the stated label amount, and three of the defective products contained only trace amounts of DHEA or none at all (figure 2.3) (Parasrampuria J et al. 1998).

- **Ephedra.** Two separate lots of 10 commercially available ephedra products were analyzed for amount of active ingredient by high-performance liquid chromatography. Nineteen of 20 tested products contained ephedrine; however, the amount ranged from 1.09 to 15.33 mg per capsule. Pseudoephedrine was detected in 16 samples, and quantities ranged from 0.16 to 9.45 mg per capsule. In several lot-to-lot comparisons, differences in alkaloid content ranged from 44% to 1000% (Gurley BJ et al. 2000).

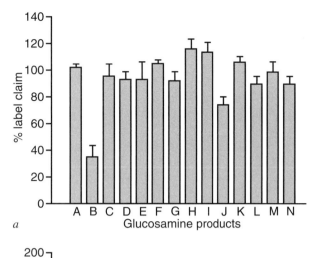

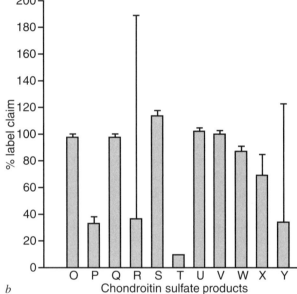

Figure 2.2 Percent actual *(a)* glucosamine and *(b)* chondroitin amounts compared to stated label amount.

Reprinted, by permission, from A.O. Adebowle et al., Spring 2000, *Journal of the American Nutraceutical Association (JANA)* 3 (1):40.

• **Ginseng.** *Consumer Reports* tested 10 different brands of ginseng. The investigators found that when the amount of active ginsenoside was assayed and compared to total amount of ginseng per capsule (as stated on the label), the amount ranged from 0.2% to 7.6%. For three brands each stating that there was 100 mg ginseng per capsule, the amount of ginsenosides was 3.0%, 6.5%, and 7.6% ("Herbal Roulette" November 1995).

Thus, an athlete who uses supplements cannot be certain the product she is ingesting will produce blood levels consistent with those documented in a given research study (assuming a scientific study exists in the first place!) or consistent with the potency of the same product from another manufacturer. This issue completely

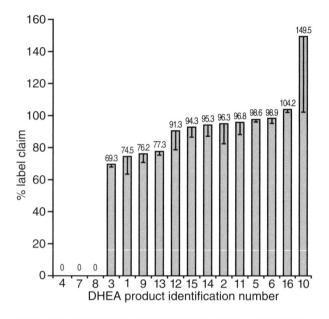

Figure 2.3 Analysis results as a percentage of the label claim for content of dehydroepiandrosterone (DHEA) dietary supplement products. Error bars indicate standard deviations.

Reprinted, by J. Parasrampuria, K. Schwartz, and R. Petesch, 1998, "Quality control of dehydroepiandrosterone dietary supplement products," *Journal of American Medical Association* 280:1565. *Copyrighted 1998, American Medical Association.*

undermines the utility of the few clinical studies published on dietary supplements.

In summary, improved quality control regarding supplements is necessary before any type of reliable clinical study evaluating their effects on athletic performance can ever be conducted. Even if athletes do not sustain adverse effects from supplements, they still risk disqualification. For researchers, any published data involving dietary supplements are suspect until product quality and consistency are documented. Finally, conclusions based on data generated from a study of one dosage form (e.g., oral tablets) should not always be extrapolated to another dosage form (e.g., inhaled) of that drug.

Methodological Issues Involving Study Subjects

In addition to study design and aspects relevant to the PES in question, one needs to take into account the type of subjects included in a study of PES. Factors to consider include level of conditioning/skill level required to complete the test, dietary factors (e.g., protein/caffeine/alcohol intake, state of hydration), concomitant drug use, psychological and social factors (e.g., amount of rest, home field advantage), genetic factors, and gender and age.

Type of Subjects

In any study of PES, study subjects need to be matched for age, sex, training status, and a variety of other factors. For example, growth hormone (GH) has been shown to enhance strength gains in hospitalized patients who are GH deficient (Cuneo RC et al. 1991); however, this same effect has not been seen in athletes who are not GH deficient (Reents S 2000). The issue of trained versus untrained subjects can also be important, as Elashoff and colleagues found in their meta-analysis of studies on anabolic steroids (Elashoff JD et al. 1991). In other cases, the ability to detect any benefit from a PES may be reduced in highly trained subjects because there is a smaller margin for improvement (Clarkson PM and Thompson HS 1997). Research involving androstenedione should account for the fact that the conversion of this substance to testosterone occurs more readily in women than in males (Horton R and Tate JF 1966). The effect of exercise on the metabolic clearance of caffeine is greater in females as compared to males (Duthel et al. 1991). Some investigations have shown that testing exercise capacity in women during the luteal phase of the menstrual cycle produces different responses than during the follicular phase (Pivarnik JM et al. 1992; Schoene RB et al. 1981). These are examples of how the type of subject can influence conclusions of a study of PES.

Dietary Factors

Dietary factors can also influence the evaluation of the efficacy of PES. For example, the epinephrine response to caffeine varies depending on whether the subject being studied is caffeine-naive or caffeine-tolerant (Van Soeren MH et al. 1993). Regular caffeine ingestion can also diminish the ergogenic response to creatine (Vandenberghe K et al. 1996). Protein intake may also affect the response to creatine; some studies suggest that vegetarians demonstrate a more dramatic ergogenic response to creatine supplementation (Harris RC et al. 1992). Similarly, the use of ethanol by study participants is an important variable to control for because of its ergolytic properties (McNaughton LR and Preece D 1986).

Concomitant Drug Use

Many athletes use legitimate drugs for appropriate reasons; but this, too, needs to be controlled for. For example, some volunteers for a study of the effects of marathon running on gastrointestinal blood loss had to be excluded because they routinely used nonsteroidal anti-inflammatory drugs (Stewart JG et al. 1984), which are well known to cause this side effect. Another situation in which concomitant drug use must be considered is in the evaluation of anabolic steroids on performance. It is commonly known that some bodybuilders use these drugs in a variety of combinations (stacking). Finally, many supplements that are promoted for energy or to enhance performance combine ephedrine with caffeine. One should not draw conclusions about these combination products on the basis of research on only one of the components.

Psychological and Social Factors

The great distance runner Steve Prefontaine never lost a race at home. Why? What explanation exists for the phenomenal performance at the 1968 Olympics in Mexico City of black American track athletes like Bob Beamon, Lee Evans, and Tommie Smith, whose records stood for decades? Can it be explained simply by track conditions such as air temperature, humidity, or elevation? More than likely, success was directly related to these athletes' psychological determination to win in this setting. This is a factor that could be better controlled for in a lab-based study than in a field-based study.

The Ideal Study

Many methodologic issues that affect the interpretation of studies of PES have been reviewed here. What, then, are the parameters of an acceptable study? Williams has summarized these in *The Ergogenics Edge* (Williams MH 1998):

- **Logical rationale.** There should be a reasonable, physiologic principle supporting the possibility that the substance in question may possess ergogenic properties. Obviously, if the substance is not bioavailable, then statements that the substance is ergogenic are illogical.

- **Appropriate subjects.** It is important to select the correct type of subjects for study. For example, in some cases highly trained subjects are preferable to untrained subjects in order to avoid the confounding effects of training itself on the observations; in other situations, a substance may not offer ergogenic improvements in an athlete already at the pinnacle of performance.

- **Appropriate testing.** Lab tests or field tests? Submaximal exercise or maximal exercise? One must consider these questions in order to enhance the validity of the study conclusions.

- **"Learning" phase.** The study subjects must be familiar with the testing procedure before the study begins. If not, changes in performance over time might be erroneously attributed to the substance being studied when in fact they are due to a learning-curve effect.

- **Randomization and use of a placebo control.** These factors are critical to ensuring a valid study. The best design is a crossover study whereby subjects serve as their own controls.

- **Blinding.** A double-blind study is the optimum design since it eliminates bias from both the study subjects and the observers.

- **Control of confounding variables.** The number of factors that can introduce doubt into a clinical study are extensive. Investigators must try to anticipate them, and either eliminate them or control for them.

- **Appropriate statistical analysis.** Obviously, all the factors just discussed are meaningless without statistical justification of the data.

Conclusion

It seems that some athletes will try anything if they believe it will enhance their performance. Detection and regulation are necessary to curb this activity, but knowledge and information about what these substances can and cannot do are also important. Well-designed clinical studies are crucial in the effort to evaluate the efficacy of PES. The reader of any health or medical information should be asking "Where is the evidence?" although even for many decisions in clinical medicine, hard-core evidence is still lacking (Levin A 1998). However, when the substance in question is a dietary supplement, the study results (if any exist at all!) are made questionable by the quality control issues discussed in this chapter. In the clinical medicine arena, objective evaluation of supplements and publication of those results have so far been disappointing (Angell M and Kassirer JP 1998). In the sports medicine arena, creatine and caffeine are two PES that have been studied extensively; however, almost no data exist for erythropoietin (epoetin alfa), and most of the research on anabolic steroids does not represent doses used by athletes.

In lieu of solid research data, athletes who use PES need to be educated about the power of the placebo effect and the fact that most supplements either do not enhance performance or have not been studied in this regard (Reents S 2000; Williams MH 1995, 1998). And finally, a healthy dose of skepticism is necessary when one is reading ads or claims regarding the effects of supplements. We hope this book will shed some light on these issues.

References

Adebowale AO, Cox DS, Liang Z, Eddington ND. Analysis of glucosamine and chondroitin sulfate content in marketed products and the caco-2 permeability of chondroitin sulfate raw materials. *JANA* 2000;3:37-44.

Angell M, Kassirer JP. Alternative medicine—the risks of untested and unregulated remedies. *N Engl J Med* 1998;339:839-841.

Bahrke MS, Morgan WP. Evaluation of the ergogenic properties of ginseng. *Sports Med* 2000;29:113-133.

Bhasin S, Storer TW, Berman N, Callegari C, Clevenger B, Phillips J, Bunnell TJ, Tricker R, Shirazi A, Casaburi R.

The effects of supraphysiological doses of testosterone on muscle size and strength in normal men. *N Engl J Med* 1996;335:1-7.

Birkeland KI, Stray-Gundersen J, Hemmersback P, Hallen J, Haug E, Bahr R. Effect of rhEPO administration on serum levels of sTfR and cycling performance. *Med Sci Sports Exerc* 2000;32:1238-1243.

Bosco C, Tihanyi J, Pucspk J, Kovacs I, Gabossy A, Colli R, Pulvirenti G, Tranquilli C, Foti C, Viru M, Viru A. Effect of oral creatine supplementation on jumping and running performance. *Int J Sports Med* 1997;18:369-372.

Brass EP. Supplemental carnitine and exercise. *Am J Clin Nutr* 2000;72(suppl):618S-623S.

Bruno A, Nolte KB, Chapin J. Stroke associated with ephedrine use. *Neurology* 1993;43:1313-1316.

Caruso JF, Kaplan TA, Applegate B, Perry AC. Effects of acute inhalation of the bronchodilator, albuterol, on power output. *Med Sci Sports Exerc* 1995;24:638-642.

Casey A, Constantin-Teodosiu D, Howell S, Hultman E, Greenhaff PL. Creatine ingestion favorably affects performance and muscle metabolism during maximal exercise in humans. *Am J Physiol* 271 (*Endocrinol Metab* 34) 1996;E31-E37.

Casoni I, Ricci G, Ballarin E, Borsetto C, Grazzi G, Guglielmini C et al. Hematological indices of erythropoietin administration in athletes. *Int J Sports Med* 1993;14:307-311.

Centers for Disease Control. Eosinophilia-myalgia syndrome—New Mexico. *MMWR* 1989;38:765-767.

Chandler JV, Blair SN. The effect of amphetamines on selected physiological components related to athletic success. *Med Sci Sports Exerc* 1980;12:65-69.

Clarkson PM, Thompson HS. Drugs and sport: research findings and limitations. *Sports Med* 1997;24:366-384.

Clemons JM, Crosby SL. Cardiopulmonary and subjective effects of a 60 mg dose of pseudoephedrine on graded treadmill exercise. *J Sports Med Phys Fitness* 1993;33:405-412.

Cuneo RC, Salomon F, Wiles CM, Hesp R, Sonksen PH. Growth hormone treatment in growth hormone-deficient adults. I. Effects on muscle mass and strength. *J Appl Physiol* 1991;70:688-694.

Dodd SL, Powers SK, Vrabas IS, Criswell D, Stetson S, Hussain R. Effects of clenbuterol on contractile and biochemical properties of skeletal muscle. *Med Sci Sports Exerc* 1996;28:669-676.

Duthel JM, Vallon JJ, Martin G, Feret JM, Mathieu R, Videman R. Caffeine and sport: role of physical exercise upon elimination. *Med Sci Sports Exerc* 1991;23:980-985.

Ekblom B. Blood doping and erythropoietin. *Am J Sports Med* 1996;24:S40-S42.

Elashoff JD, Jacknow AD, Shain SG, Braunstein GD. Effects of anabolic-androgenic steroids on muscular strength. *Ann Intern Med* 1991;115:387-393.

Erslev AJ. Erythropoietin. *N Engl J Med* 1991;324:1339-1344.

Etminan M, Levin M. Interpreting meta-analyses of pharmacologic interventions: the pitfalls and how to identify them. *Pharmacotherapy* 1999;19:741-745.

Farrey T. Triathletes suck. ESPN.com. Monday, June 14, 1999. 1:35 P.M. EST.

Flinn S, Gregory J, McNaughton LR, Tristram S, Davies P. Caffeine ingestion prior to incremental cycling to exhaustion in recreational cyclists. *Int J Sports Med* 1990;11:188-193.

Forbes GB. The effect of anabolic steroids on lean body mass: the dose response curve. *Metabolism* 1985;34:571-573.

Fuentes RJ, Rosenberg JM. *Athletic drug reference '99*. Clean Data, Inc., Durham, NC, 1999.

Galloway GP, Frederick SL, Staggers FE Jr., Gonzales M, Stalcup SA, Smith DE. Gamma-hydroxybutyrate: an emerging drug of abuse that causes physical dependence. *Addiction* 1997;92:89-96.

Giustina A, Boni E, Romanelli G, Grassi V, Giustina G. Cardiopulmonary performance during exercise in acromegaly, and the effects of acute suppression of growth hormone hypersecretion with octreotide. *Am J Cardiol* 1995;75:1042-1047.

Graham TE, Hibbert E, Sathasivam P. Metabolic and exercise endurance effects of coffee and caffeine ingestion. *J Appl Physiol* 1998;85:883-889.

Graham TE, Spriet LL. Performance and metabolic responses to a high caffeine dose during prolonged exercise. *J Appl Physiol* 1991;71:2292-2298.

Graham TE, Spriet LL. Metabolic, catecholamine, and exercise performance responses to various doses of caffeine. *J Appl Physiol* 1995;78:867-874.

Gruber AJ, Pope HG Jr. Ephedrine abuse among 36 female weightlifters. *Am J Addict* 1998;7:256-261.

Gurley BJ, Gardner SF, Hubbard MA. Content versus label claims in ephedra-containing supplements. *Am J Health Syst Pharm* 2000;57:963-969.

Haller CA, Benowitz NL. Adverse cardiovascular and central nervous system events associated with dietary supplements containing ephedra alkaloids. *N Engl J Med* 2000; 343: 1833-1838.

Harris RC, Soderlund K, Hultman E. Elevation of creatine in resting and exercised muscle of normal subjects by creatine supplementation. *Clin Sci* 1992;83:367-374.

Herbal roulette. *Consumer Reports*, November 1995, pp. 698-705.

Horton R, Tate JF. Androstenedione production and interconversion rates measured in peripheral blood and studies on the possible site of its conversion to testosterone. *J Clin Invest* 1966;45:301-313.

Iwaoka K, Okagawa S, Mutoh Y, Miyashita M. Effects of bicarbonate ingestion on the respiratory compensation threshold and maximal exercise performance. *Jap J Physiol* 1989;39:255-265.

Jacobson BH, Edwards SW. Effects of ingested doses of caffeine on neuromuscular reflex response time in man. *Int J Sports Med* 1990;11:194-197.

Kachhi PN, Henderson SO. Priapism after androstenedione intake for athletic performance enhancement. *Ann Emerg Med* 2000;35:391-393.

Kamber M, Koster M, Kreis R et al. Creatine supplementation—part I: performance, clinical chemistry, and muscle volume. *Med Sci Sports Exerc* 1999;31:1763-1769.

King DS, Sharp RL, Vukovich MD, Brown GA, Reifenrath TA, Uhl NL, Parsons KA. Effect of oral androstenedione on serum testosterone and adaptations to resistance training in young men. *JAMA* 1999;281:2020-2028.

Kozak-Collins K, Burke ER, Schoene RB. Sodium bicarbonate ingestion does not improve performance in women cyclists. *Med Sci Sports Exerc* 1994;26:1510-1515.

Kreis R, Kamber M, Koster M et al. Creatine supplementation—part II: in vivo magnetic resonance spectroscopy. *Med Sci Sports Exerc* 1999;31:1770-1777.

Leder BZ, Longcope C, Catlin DH et al. Oral androstenedione administration and serum testosterone concentrations in young men. *JAMA* 2000;283:779-782.

Levin A. Evidence-based medicine gaining supporters. *Ann Intern Med* 1998;128:334-336.

Linderman J, Fahey TD. Sodium bicarbonate ingestion and exercise performance. *Sports Med* 1991;11:71-77.

McNaughton LR, Preece D. Alcohol and its effects on sprint and middle distance running. *Br J Sports Med* 1986;20:56-59.

Milburn DS, Myers CW. Tryptophan toxicity: a pharmacoepidemiologic review of eosinophilia-myalgia syndrome. *DICP Ann Pharmacother* 1991;25:1259-1262.

Miller MJS. Standardization of herbal medicines: the Pandora's box of quality control. *JANA* 2000;2:44-46.

Millington DS, Dubag G. Dietary supplement L-carnitine: analysis of different brands to determine bioavailability and content. *Clin Res Reg Affairs* 1993;10:71-80.

NewsEdge. XINHUA press release. September 13, 2000.

Parasrampuria J, Schwartz K, Petesch R. Quality control of dehydroepiandrosterone dietary supplement products. *JAMA* 1998;280:1565.

Pivarnik JM, Marichal CJ, Spillman T, Morrow JR Jr. Menstrual cycle phase affects temperature regulation during endurance exercise. *J Appl Physiol* 1992;72:543-548.

Prevost MC, Nelson AG, Morris GS. Creatine supplementation enhances intermittent work performance. *Res Q Exerc Sport* 1997;68:233-240.

Reents S. *Sport and exercise pharmacology*. Human Kinetics, Champaign, IL, 2000.

Rich JD, Dickinson BP, Merriman NA, Thule PM. Insulin use by bodybuilders. *JAMA* 1998;279:1613.

Ritter SK. Faster, higher, stronger. *Chemical & Engineering News,* September 6, 1999, 42-52.

Ryan JM, Stell I. Gamma hydroxybutyrate—a coma inducing recreational drug. *J Accid Emerg Med* 1997;14:259-261.

Schoene RB, Roberson HT, Pierson DJ, Peterson AP. Respiratory drives and exercise in menstrual cycles of athletic and nonathletic women. *J Appl Physiol* 1981;50:1300-1305.

Slifman NR, Obermeyer WR, Aloi BK, Musser SM, Correll WA Jr., Cichowicz SM, Betz JM, Love LA. Contamination of botanical dietary supplements by *Digitalis lanata. N Engl J Med* 1998;339:806-811.

Stewart JG, Ahlquist DA, McGill DB, Ilstrup DM, Schwartz S, Owen RA. Gastrointestinal blood loss and anemia in runners. *Ann Intern Med* 1984;100:843-845.

Swain RA, Harsha DM, Baenziger J, Saywell RM Jr. Do pseudoephedrine or phenylpropanolamine improve maximum oxygen uptake and time to exhaustion? *Clin J Sport Med* 1997;7:168-173.

Swygert LA, Maes EF, Sewell LE, Miller L, Falk H, Kilbourne EM. Eosinophilia-myalgia syndrome: results of national surveillance. *JAMA* 1990;264:1698-1703.

Thompson CH, Kemp GJ, Sanderson AL, Dixon RM, Styles P, Taylor DJ, Radda GK. Effect of creatine on aerobic and anaerobic metabolism in skeletal muscle in swimmers. *Br J Sports Med* 1996;30:222-225.

United States Pharmacopoeia Drug Information [USP-DI], Vol. III, 2000, Micromedex, Englewood, CO, p. IV/367.

van Baak MA, Mayer LHJ, Kempinski RES, Hartgens F. Effect of salbutamol on muscle strength and endurance performance in nonasthmatic men. *Med Sci Sports Exerc* 2000;32:1300-1306.

Vandenberghe K, Gillis N, Van Leemputte M, Van Hecke P, Vanstapel F, Hespel P. Caffeine counteracts the ergogenic action of muscle creatine loading. *J Appl Physiol* 1996;80:452-457.

Van Soeren MH, Sathasivam P, Spriet LL, Graham TE. Caffeine metabolism and epinephrine responses during exercise in users and nonusers. *J Appl Physiol* 1993;75:805-812.

Wadler, G., & Hainline, B. (1989). *Drugs and the athlete.* Philadelphia: F.A. Davis Company.

Wilber RL, Rundell KW, Szmedra L, Jenkinson DM, Joohee IM, Drake SD. Incidence of exercise-induced bronchospasm in Olympic winter sport athletes. *Med Sci Sports Exerc* 2000;32:732-737.

Williams MH. Nutritional ergogenics in athletics. *J Sports Sci* 1995;13(spec no):S63-S74.

Williams MH. *The ergogenics edge.* Human Kinetics, Champaign, IL, 1998.

Williams MH, Kreider RB, Branch JD. *Creatine. The power supplement.* Human Kinetics, Champaign, IL, 1999.

Wilson S. Are Olympic athletes using medication for treating or cheating? Associated Press, November 15, 2000.

Yesalis CE, Kopstein AN, Bahrke MS. Difficulties in estimating the prevalence of drug use among athletes. Chapter 3 in *Doping in elite sport,* Wilson W, Derse E eds. Human Kinetics, Champaign, IL, 2000, pp. 43-62.

Yesalis CE, Wright JE, Bahrke MS. Epidemiological and policy issues in the measurement of the long term health effects of anabolic-androgenic steroids. *Sports Med* 1989;8:129-138.

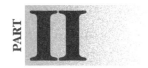
Anabolics

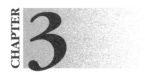
Anabolic-Androgenic Steroids

Michael S. Bahrke, PhD

Charles E. Yesalis, MPH, ScD

Testosterone is the primary natural male hormone (produced primarily by the testes) and is responsible for the androgenic (masculinizing) and anabolic (tissue building) effects observed during male adolescence and adulthood. By 1935, testosterone had been isolated and chemically characterized, and the nature of its anabolic effects elucidated (Kochakian & Yesalis, 2000). Anabolic-androgenic steroids are synthetic derivatives of testosterone.

Since virtually every cell in the body has receptor proteins for anabolic-androgenic steroids, the anabolic or androgenic response is determined by the location (which differs in number of receptors and steroid-metabolizing enzymes) and type of cell, and not by the nature of the steroid (Kruskemper, 1968). Consequently, a pure anabolic steroid has yet to be discovered, and thus the formal, proper name for this group of drugs is anabolic-androgenic steroids. The more common terms "anabolic" and "steroid" are used here for convenience.

Testosterone itself is not effective when taken orally or by injection, because it is susceptible to relatively rapid breakdown by the liver. The chemical structure of testosterone has been modified by pharmaceutical companies and pharmacologists to surmount this problem. Most commonly, testosterone is alkylated at the 17-α position to form oral anabolic steroids, or esterified at the 17-β position to form injectable anabolic steroids; the latter are suspended in oil to help them remain in the body for several weeks, or even months. More recently, transdermal patches, buccal tablets, nasal sprays, gels, and creams are being used by elite athletes as the delivery mechanisms. However, for non-elite athletes, oral tablets and injections remain the typical methods of delivery.

During the past 50 years, anabolic steroids have been used in the treatment of various reproductive dysfunctions, anemia, hereditary angioedema, metastatic breast cancer, and protein deficiency, as well as in patients convalescing from severe infections, surgery, burns, and trauma as well as adjunct therapy for human immunodeficiency virus/acquired immunodeficiency syndrome (HIV/AIDS) patients (Kochakian & Yesalis, 2000). From the late 1930s to the mid-1980s, anabolic steroids were used successfully to treat depression, melancholia, and involutional psychoses (Bahrke, 2000). Why the use of anabolic steroids to treat certain psychiatric disorders has diminished over time is unclear, but the development of other, more efficacious drugs may be the reason.

Effectiveness, Goals, and Methods of Use

Anabolic steroids, as a class, produce weight gain in normal healthy, adult men (Friedl, 2000). Typical weight gains are 6.6 to 11 lb (3-5 kg) after several weeks of high-dose steroid use. This appears to be a permissive action with a threshold effect, where an amount of steroid above the effective dose does not clearly produce more rapid weight gain. The nature of this weight gain is still uncertain, although an increase in muscle size and total body protein accretion is at least one component of the gain. The effects of steroids on strength performance are mostly seen with experienced weight lifters and when strength training is performed concurrently with the steroid administration. Most studies demonstrating strength gains also demonstrate weight gains. The mechanism of action for an effect on skeletal muscle is still not clear.

Although the evidence is incomplete, anabolic steroids may also inhibit or block the catabolic effects of glucocorticoids that are released during intense training. Theoretically, this anticatabolic effect would allow athletes to train more frequently and more intensely, and this may be the most important factor concerning the performance-enhancing effects of anabolic steroids. While there is little evidence to support a beneficial role of anabolic steroids in other types of exercise performance such as muscular endurance or aerobic endurance, anabolic steroids increase the number of red blood cells (RBCs). With the anticatabolic effect and an increase in RBCs, endurance athletes may be able to train more frequently, for longer periods of time, and with greater intensity. In turn, this could produce improved aerobic capacity resulting in quicker running times or in more repetitions of a particular activity.

The goals of individuals who use anabolic steroids in sport and exercise are dependent on the activity in which they participate. Bodybuilders desire more lean body mass and less body fat. Weight lifters desire to lift the maximum amount of weight possible. Field athletes want to put the shot, or throw the hammer, discus, or javelin, farther than their competitors or holders of previous records. Swimmers and runners hope to be able to perform their frequent, high-intensity, long-duration workouts without physical breakdown. Football players want to increase their lean body mass and strength so that they can be successful at the high school, college, or professional level. Other anabolic steroid users simply want to "look good"—which to many people means being big and muscular.

Many athletes use the intramuscular forms of steroids, and needle sharing has been reported. In one study, 25% of adolescent steroid users reported needle sharing (DuRant, Rickert, Ashworth, Newman, & Slavens, 1993). Acquired immunodeficiency syndrome and HIV infection have been reported in bodybuilders sharing needles (Henrion, Mandelbrot, & Delfieu, 1992; Scott & Scott, 1989; Sklarek et al., 1984).

Anabolic steroids have traditionally been taken in "cycles," which are episodes of use lasting 6 to 12 weeks or more (Llewellyn, 2000; Phillips, 1991). Athletes often take more than one steroid at a time; this is referred to as "stacking." In an attempt to avoid developing a tolerance to a particular anabolic steroid ("plateauing"), some users stagger their drugs, taking the anabolic steroids in an overlapping pattern, or stop one drug and start another (Duchaine, 1989; Gallaway, 1997; Phillips, 1991). Often steroid users will "pyramid" their administration patterns, moving from a low daily dose at the beginning of the cycle to a higher dose and then tapering down the dose toward the end of their cycle (Grundig & Bachmann,

1995; Wright, 1982). In addition, individuals may use other drugs concurrently with anabolic steroids to counteract the common adverse effects of steroids. These drugs include diuretics, antiestrogens, human chorionic gonadotrophin, and anti-acne medications (Di Pasquale, 1990). This polypharmacy is termed an "array" (Duchaine, 1989). The frequency of concurrent drug use or the frequency or efficacy of each of these administration patterns is poorly documented.

The dosage of anabolic steroids depends on the sport as well as on the particular needs of the athlete. Endurance athletes use steroids primarily for their alleged catabolism-blocking effects (Friedl, 2000) and use dosages at or slightly below physiological replacement levels, that is, about 7 mg/day of testosterone (Yen & Jaffe, 1978).[1]

Participants in the traditional strength sports, seeking to "bulk up," have generally used dosages that exceed physiological replacement levels by 10 to 100 times or more (Kerr, 1982; Wright, 1982). Administration patterns also vary among athletes within a particular sport, based on each athlete's training goals and response to the drugs, as well as on the biological activity of different anabolic steroids (Di Pasquale, 1990; Kerr, 1982; Kochakian & Yesalis, 2000; Wright, 1982). Women, regardless of sport, are generally thought to use lower dosages of anabolic steroids than men (Elliot & Goldberg, 2000).

Sources of Anabolic-Androgenic Steroids

Most individuals who use anabolic steroids to enhance athletic performance and physical appearance obtain the drugs from the illicit ("black") market (Tolliver, 1998). The U.S. federal government and almost all U.S. state governments currently have laws regarding the distribution, possession, or prescription of anabolic steroids (U.S. Department of Health and Human Services, 1991). The Federal Food, Drug, and Cosmetic Act (FFDCA) of the United States was amended as part of the Anti-Drug Abuse Act of 1988 such that distribution of steroids or possession of steroids with intent to distribute without a valid prescription became a felony. This legislation not only increased the penalties for the illicit distribution of steroids, but also facilitated prosecution under the FFDCA.

In 1990, the Anabolic Steroids Control Act was signed into law by President Bush, adding anabolic steroids to Schedule III of the Controlled Substances Act. This law institutes a regulatory and criminal enforcement system whereby the Drug Enforcement Administration (DEA) controls the manufacture, importation, exportation, distribution, and dispensing of anabolic steroids.

---

[1] Because the bioequivalence of various forms and types of anabolic steroids has not been established, the estimates of dosages used by athletes relative to physiological replacement levels are approximate.

According to the DEA (James Tolliver, personal communication, 2000), the primary source for steroids in the United States remains Mexico. Traffickers come from the United States, purchase prescriptions at the pharmacies and fill them in unlimited quantities, and then smuggle the steroids across the border. Other sources of supply for the U.S. black market are Russia, Poland, Hungary, Spain, Italy, Greece, Canada, and the Netherlands. More recently, however, sources for steroids coming into the United States have expanded: it has been observed that these drugs are now "coming from everywhere!" (James Tolliver, personal communication, 2000).

A significant percentage of black market steroids are counterfeit. Consequently, the actual doses taken by illicit users are often difficult to determine (U.S. Department of Health and Human Services, 1991). Moreover, because some of the drugs are intended for veterinary use (Duchaine, 1989), the equivalent human doses are unknown. A minority of black market steroids are manufactured in the United States by licensed pharmaceutical companies and then diverted by the producers, distributors, pharmacists, veterinarians, or physicians. It is estimated that 10% to 15% of illicit steroid users obtain these drugs by prescription (Kenney,

1994). It is also estimated that approximately 5% to 15% of adolescent steroid users receive these drugs from medical professionals such as physicians, pharmacists, veterinarians, and dentists.

Ergogenic Effects

Although the vast majority of the athletic community accepts that anabolic steroids enhance exercise capacity and performance (Yesalis, Anderson, Buckley, & Wright, 1990), and although there is far more research on the performance-enhancing effects of anabolic steroids than on any other performance-enhancing substance except perhaps amphetamines, the extent to which enhancement occurs and the factors influencing such effects remain incompletely understood and documented (Celotti & Negri-Cesi, 1992). Explanation for the lack of consensus on the effect of anabolic steroids on humans are numerous and complex (table 3.1). Animal studies (using a variety of species) have failed to consistently demonstrate positive effects (i.e., effects exceeding those resulting from exercise alone) on lean body mass or performance variables in healthy young male animals (Lamb, 1984). Animals with lower natural anabolic hormone levels than young males

Table 3.1 Reasons for Lack of Consensus on the Effects of Anabolic Steroids on Performance Variables in Humans

Parameter	Reason
Dosage	Studies used varied dosages. Only a few studies used higher dosages approximating those currently used by competing strength athletes.
Testing methods	Strength was often not measured in the training mode. Body composition was often assessed from skinfold estimates.
Training methods	Volumes and intensities varied between studies.
Drugs	Studies used a variety of drugs. Few studies have reported on athletes self-administering multiple drugs.
Study participants	The number of participants, their experience in weight training, and their physical condition at the start of the studies varied.
Diet	Mostly diet was not controlled or recorded.
Study design	Some studies were crossover, some single blind, some double blind, some not blind; some had no controls.
Mechanisms of action	There are unknown and varying degrees of anabolic and anticatabolic action and of interaction with motivational effects.
Length of study	Studies varied in length and were generally short; reports on prolonged training and self-administration of steroids are lacking.
Placebo effect	It is difficult to assess placebo effect due to easy detection by athletes of steroid administration; consequently blind studies are lacking.
Data interpretation	Interpreters had differing backgrounds (scientific, clinical, athletic, administrative), perspectives, and goals.
Legal and ethical factors	These considerations preclude design and execution of well-controlled studies using doses and patterns of administration of drugs with unknown long-term effects in healthy volunteers in a manner comparable to that of many current steroid users.

Adapted, by permission, from C.E. Yesalis et al., 1989, "Anabolic-androgenic steroids: asynthesis of existing data and recommendations for future research," *Clinical Sports Medicine* 1:120.

(such as castrated males, females, and old animals) do, however, often show substantial increases in muscle mass with steroid administration (Kruskemper, 1968).

From 1977 to 1984, the American College of Sports Medicine (1977, 1984) regarded anabolic steroids as ineffective, sending mixed messages to the athletic community concerning the potential of anabolic steroids to enhance performance. As recently as 1992, other scientists (Celotti & Negri-Cesi, 1992) remained skeptical, also reporting that anabolic steroids were ineffective. However, a study by Bhasin and his colleagues in 1996 quelled much of the residual doubt concerning the effectiveness of anabolic steroids in humans. Using a relatively high dose anabolic steroid (600 mg/wk of testosterone enanthate for 10 weeks), Bhasin et al. (1996) found a 13-lb (6 kg) weight gain and 48.5-lb (22 kg) improvement in the one-repetition maximum (1-RM) bench press in experienced lifters. The results of the Bhasin study (1996) also suggested additive effects of exercise and steroids, with a bench press improvement of approximately 22 lb (10 kg) produced by exercise *or* steroid, and 44 lb (20 kg) produced by exercise *and* steroid.

Despite findings with animals and the methodological and interpretive issues and inconsistencies of human studies (Haupt & Rovere, 1984; Ryan, 1976; Wilson, 1988; Wright, 1980), it appears (as the athletic community has insisted) that steroids used in conjunction with the more anabolic forms of exercise (such as conventional strength training and bodybuilding) do facilitate increases in body mass more than training alone (American College of Sports Medicine, 1984; Bhasin et al., 1996). However, the precise levels of training frequency, duration, and intensity needed to achieve these putative increases have not been documented. At least one study has demonstrated a threshold response of body composition to anabolic steroids, as well as variations in response according to type of steroid (Friedl, Dettori, Hannan, Patience, & Plymate, 1991).

Individuals who are experienced in weight training and who continue training during anabolic steroid administration consistently experience increases in strength beyond those observed in control individuals from training alone (Bhasin et al., 1996; Haupt & Rovere, 1984; Lombardo, 1993; Wright, 1980). However, in the large majority of studies, most participants who were given anabolic steroids but who were not experienced or pretrained with weights gained no more strength than control individuals. The reasons for this result are unknown, as is the basis for differences between research observations (reported in the scientific literature) and self-reports of many athletes and coaches. Additionally, the effects of high doses or prolonged administration of anabolic steroids on physique or physiological capacities

have not been documented. Likewise, the residual effects of anabolic steroids on physiological capacities after the termination of use have not been established. Furthermore, results of any dose on physical/physiological capacities or performance in females are unknown.

Incidence of Use

High levels of use of anabolic steroids have been attributed to professional football players, weight lifters, power lifters, bodybuilders, and throwers in track and field events since the 1960s (Yesalis, Courson, & Wright, 2000). However, until the mid-1970s, all that was known regarding the incidence of nonmedical use of steroids was based on anecdotes, testimonials, and rumors (Yesalis & Bahrke, 1995). Use by high school athletes was rumored to be occurring as early as 1959 (Frazier, 1973; Gilbert, 1969a,b,c). Although rumors still abound, estimates of the incidence of steroid use are now based on the results of systematic surveys. Surveys of steroid use are categorized here as those of (1) adolescent school-age students, (2) college students, and (3) athletes not falling into categories 1 or 2.

We have elected to devote a significant portion of this chapter to discussion of the prevalence and incidence of anabolic steroid use because, except for perhaps amphetamines, anabolic steroids are the one category of performance-enhancing drugs for which we have extensive prevalence and incidence data. Generally, until data become available for other performance-enhancing substances such as human growth hormone, androstenedione, and creatine, we can only speculate as to their prevalence and incidence of use in sport and exercise.

Use Among Adolescent School-Age Students

In 1987, the first U.S. national study of anabolic steroid use at the high school level was conducted by Buckley and associates (Buckley et al., 1988). The investigators found that 6.6% of male high school seniors reported having used these drugs. There was no difference in the level of reported steroid use between urban and rural areas, but there was a small, yet significant, difference by size of enrollment: students at larger high schools had a higher rate of reported steroid use. In addition, among the self-reported steroid users, 38% had initiated use before 16 years of age; and more than one-third of the steroid users did not intend to participate in interscholastic sports.

Multiple U.S. local-, state-, and national-level studies have now confirmed the findings of Buckley et al. (1988), and show that 4% to 6% (with a range of 3% to 12%) of high school males admit to using anabolic steroids at some time in their life (Yesalis, Barsukiewicz, Kopstein, & Bahrke, 1997). Some of these studies also examined the use of anabolic steroids among high school females, generally showing that 1% to 2% reported having used anabolic steroids (Yesalis, Bahrke, Kopstein, & Barsukiewicz, 2000). Likewise, several of the studies confirmed that substantial percentages of steroid users do not participate in traditional school-sponsored sports.

A review of U.S. state- and national-level studies shows mixed trends for anabolic steroid use rates between 1988 and 1997 (Yesalis, Barsukiewicz, Kopstein, & Bahrke, 1997). The findings of multiyear, state-level studies show a decrease in lifetime steroid use rates between 1988 and 1994 for male and female adolescents, although no tests of statistical significance were available. However, since 1991, steroid use by males as measured by two of three U.S. national surveys has generally increased (table 3.2) (Hewitt, Smith-Akin, Higgins, Jenkins, 1998; Johnston, O'Malley, & Bachman, 1996; Kann, Warren, Harris, Collins, Douglas, et al., 1995). Furthermore, since 1991, data from these same three U.S. national surveys point to an increase in anabolic steroid use among adolescent females. In addition, the

1997 Youth Risk and Behavior Surveillance System data (Hewitt et al., 1998) showed that among 9th- to 12th-grade students (ages 13-19) in public and private high schools in the United States, 4.1% of males and 2.0% of females had used anabolic steroids at least once in their lives. Based on 1997 estimates of high school students, these period prevalence rates translate to approximately 375,000 adolescent male and 175,000 adolescent female steroid users in the United States. According to results from the 1999 Monitoring the Future Study, lifetime anabolic steroid use by male high school seniors is at an all-time high, and prevalence of use for 8th-grade students approximates that for 12th-grade students.

We should also note that the use of anabolic steroids by adolescents is not limited to the United States (table 3.3) (Newman, 1994; Yesalis, Ortner, & Bahrke, 1996). Three Canadian studies (Adalf & Smart, 1992; Canadian Centre for Drug-Free Sport, 1993; Killip & Stennett, 1990), two Swedish surveys (Kindlundh, Isacson, Berglund, & Nyberg, 1999; Nilsson, 1995), two South African investigations (Lambert, Titlestad, & Schwellnus,

Table 3.2 U.S. National Studies of Lifetime Anabolic Steroid Use by Adolescents

Report	Year	Sample size	Grade level or age	Total use (%)	Male (%)	Female (%)
YRBSS	1991	12,267	9-12	2.7	4.1	1.2
	1993	16,267	9-12	2.2	3.1	1.2
	1995	10,904	9-12	3.7	4.9	2.4
	1997	16,262	9-12	3.1	4.1	2.0
MTF	1989	2283	12	3.0	4.7	1.3
	1990	2533	12	2.9	5.0	0.5
	1991	2500	12	2.1	3.6	0.4
	1992	2633	12	2.1	3.5	0.7
	1993	2716	12	2.0	3.5	0.6
	1994	2567	12	2.4	3.8	0.9
	1995	2567	12	2.3	3.8	0.8
	1996	2275	12	1.9	3.2	0.6
	1997	2566	12	2.4	4.1	0.9
	1998		12	2.7	4.5	0.8
	1999		12	2.9	5.2	0.8
	2000		12	2.5		
NHSDA	1991	8005	12-17 years	0.6	1.0	0.2
	1992	7254	12-17 years	0.3	0.4	0.1
	1993	6978	12-17 years	0.2	0.3	0.1
	1994	4678	12-17 years	0.7	0.7	0.6

Youth Risk and Behavior Surveillance System (YRBSS); Monitoring the Future Study (MTF); National Household Survey on Drug Abuse (NHSDA).

Adapted, by permission, from C.E. Yesalis, 2000, *Anabolic steroids in sport and exercise* (Champaign, IL: Human Kinetics), 86.

Table 3.3   Self-Reported Anabolic Steroid Use Among International High School-Age Students

Report/Year	Sample size	Age	Male (%)	Female (%)	Total (%)	Time span
Secondary schools, London, Ontario, Canada, 1990	2972	Overall	5.3	0.6	3.0	Past 12 months
		Grade 9	5.5	1.3	3.7	
		Grade 10	5.7	0.0	3.1	
		Grade 11	4.5	0.4	2.4	
		Grade 12	4.6	1.4	2.9	
		Grade 13	5.9	0.0	2.6	
Canadian Centre for Drug-Free Sports, 1992-1993	16,169	Overall	4.1	1.5	2.8	Past 12 months
		11-13 years	2.8	1.1	2.0	
		14-15 years	3.9	2.1	3.1	
		16+ years	5.5	1.5	3.5	
Ontario, Canada, 1992	3915	7, 9, 11, 13 years	2.1	0.2	1.1	Past 12 months
Cape Peninsula, South Africa, 1992	1361	High school	1.2	0.0	0.6	Not specified
U.K. College of Technology, 1992	633	61% <19 years	4.4	1.0	2.8 / 1.4	Lifetime Current
Falkenburg, Sweden, 1993	1383	14-19 years	5.8	1.0	—	Lifetime
New South Wales and Victoria, Australia, 1997	13,355	12-19 years	3.2	1.2	—	Lifetime
			1.7	0.4	—	Past month
Cape Education Authority and Gauteng Province, South Africa, 1998	1136	16-18 years	1.2	0.0	0.6	Not specified
	1411	16-18 years	4.4	0.1	2.3	
Uppsala, Sweden, 1999	2742	16-17 years	2.1	0.2	—	Lifetime
		18-19 years	2.7	0.4	—	Lifetime

Adapted, by permission, from C.E. Yesalis, 2000, *Anabolic steroids in sport and exercise* (Champaign, IL: Human Kinetics), 91.

1998; Schwellnus, Lambert, & Todd, 1992), one British study (Williamson, 1993), and one Australian investigation (Handelsman & Gupta, 1997) have reported overall prevalence rates for high school-aged students to range between 1% and 3% (males and females). Although these rates are slightly lower, they approximate those reported for the United States, reflecting the cross-cultural impact of anabolic steroids on performance and physical appearance.

Risk factors associated with anabolic steroid use among adolescents indicate that adolescent steroid users are significantly more likely to be males and to use other illicit drugs, alcohol, and tobacco (Bahrke, Yesalis, Kopstein, & Stephens, 2000). Student athletes are also more likely than nonathletes to use steroids; and football players, wrestlers, weight lifters, and bodybuilders have significantly higher prevalence rates than students not engaged in these activities. Currently, only a partial profile can be created to characterize the adolescent steroid user. More research is needed to further explore

the possible associations between adolescent steroid use and athletic participation, ethnicity, socioeconomic status, and educational level.

Use Among College Athletes

In 1985, Anderson and McKeag surveyed 2039 National Collegiate Athletic Association (NCAA) male and female athletes at 11 NCAA member colleges and universities regarding alcohol and drug use (table 3.4). The heaviest anabolic steroid use (defined as use in the past 12 months) was among football players (9%), while 4% of the male participants in track and field reported prior use. Overall, 5% of Division I[2] athletes (male and female),

---

[2] Membership in Divisions I, II, or III is determined by NCAA criteria, which include the number of sports the school participates in, the size of the athletic budget, and attendance at sporting events. Division I schools are generally larger, offer more sports, and have the largest athletic budgets, whereas Divisions II and III are smaller, have fewer sports, and so on.

Table 3.4   Self-Reported Anabolic Steroid Use Among U.S. College Athletes

Report/Year	Site and sample	Sample size	Response rate (%)	Group	Incidence of use (%)
Anderson & McKeag 1985	11 universities, intercollegiate athletes	2039	72	Football	9
				Division I	5
				Division II	4
				Division III	2
				Men's track and field	4
				Men's basketball	4
				Men's baseball	3
				Women's swimming	1
Anderson et al. 1991	11 universities, intercollegiate athletes	2282	70	Football	10
				Division I	5
				Division II	5
				Division III	4
				Men's track and field	4
				Women's swimming	1
				Women's track and field	1
				Women's basketball	1
				Men overall	6
				Women overall	1
Anderson et al. 1993	11 universities, intercollegiate athletes	2505	78	Football	5
				Division I	2
				Division II	4
				Division III	2
				Men's track and field	1
				Women's swimming	1
				Women's track and field	3
				Women's basketball	2
				Men overall	3
				Women overall	2

Adapted, by permission, from C.E. Yesalis, 2000, *Anabolic steroids in sport and exercise* (Champaign, IL: Human Kinetics), 92.

4% of Division II athletes, and 2% of Division III athletes reported steroid use in the year prior to the survey.

Anderson and colleagues (1991) repeated their study of athletes during the 1988-1989 academic year (table 3.4). Overall, steroid use had increased only slightly over the proceeding four years. For Division I athletes, reported steroid use remained at 5%. However, for Division II and Division III athletes, anabolic steroid use rose to 5% and 4%, respectively.

Across Divisions I to III, the highest incidence of reported steroid use was again among football players (10%). Anabolic steroid use remained the same for men's track and field events (4%), but declined in baseball (2%), basketball (2%), and tennis (2%).

In 1993, Anderson and his colleagues again repeated their study, observing a significant decline in anabolic steroid use among male athletes, although football players continued to have the highest level of self-reported use (table 3.4). However, female athletes surveyed showed considerable increases in anabolic steroid use relative to the 1985 and 1989 surveys. Yet another survey was conducted in 1997 (National Collegiate Athletic Association Research Staff), using a substantially different sampling method, and showed a further decline in steroid use in most sports. Football players, again, reported the highest levels of use, at 2.2%, although this was a substantial decline from the previous surveys. However, the purported decrease in steroid use among college football players is not consistent with the significant increases in the size of players and a drug-testing program full of loopholes.

Yesalis, Buckley, Anderson, Wang, Norwig, Ott, Puffer, & Strauss (1990) employed projected response survey techniques with collegiate athletes, using indirect questions. Thus, respondents were asked to estimate the level of their competitors' anabolic steroid use. Over 1600 male and female athletes at five NCAA Division I institutions participated in this study during the 1989-1990 academic year. The mean overall projected rate of any prior use of anabolic steroid across all sports surveyed was 14.7% for male and 5.9% for female athletes. Among men's sports, football showed the highest projected lifetime steroid use rates with 29.3%, followed by track and field events with 20.6%. The greatest projected use rate for women's sports was 16.3% for track and field events. The reported overall projected rate of anabolic steroid use during the past 12 months was approximately three times greater than the rate obtained from self-reports by Anderson and colleagues (1991) (table 3.5). The true level of steroid use among athletes probably lies between the lower-bound estimates from self-reports and the upper-bound estimates obtained from the projective response techniques (Yesalis, Buckley, Anderson, Wang, Norwig, Ott, Puffer, & Strauss, 1990).

Other User Groups

Track and field event athletes who participated in the 1972 Olympics were surveyed (Silvester, 1973): 68% of the participants reported prior steroid use, with 61% having used steroids within six months of the Games (table 3.6). In 1975, Ljungqvist surveyed elite Swedish male track and field event athletes and found that 31% admitted prior anabolic steroid use. None of the middle- or long-distance runners admitted to anabolic steroid use, but 75% of the throwers did.

In a survey of 155 U.S. Olympians who participated in the 1992 Winter Games, 80% of the athletes classified steroid use among Olympic competitors as a very serious or somewhat serious problem; just 5% thought that it was not a problem (Pearson & Hansen, 1992). When asked to estimate the level of steroid use in their own sport, 43% of the respondents estimated use by 10% or more of competitors, while 34% estimated use at 1% to 9%. Only 23% of the athletes surveyed believed that there was no steroid use in their sport. In another survey of former Olympians (Pearson, 1994), 75% of the medalists and 63% of the nonmedalists stated that more athletes were using performance-enhancing drugs than when they themselves had competed. In 1988, Yesalis et al. surveyed

Table 3.5   Estimates (%) of Anabolic Steroid Use During the Past 12 Months Among Division I NCAA Athletes (Self-Reported vs. Projected Use)

Sport	Males		Females		Male/Female combined	
	Anderson et al., 1991	Yesalis et al., 1990	Anderson et al., 1991	Yesalis et al., 1990	Anderson et al., 1991	Yesalis et al., 1990
Baseball	2.6	6.67	—	—		
Basketball	1.5	6.86	0	6.25		
Football	9.6	22.43	—	—		
Softball	—	—	0	2.92		
Swimming	—	—	0	5.35		
Tennis	0	2.75	0	5.60		
Track and field	2.3	16.3	1.5	9.53		
Weighted mean	6.2	16.4	0.6	6.37		
All sports					4.8	14.06

Adapted, by permission, from C.E. Yesalis et al., 2000, "Athletes' projections of anabolic steroid use," *Clinical Sports Medicine* 2:168.

Table 3.6   Self-Reported Anabolic Steroid Use Among U.S. Noncollege Athletes

Report/Year	Site and sample size	Response rate (%)	Group	Incidence of use (%)
Silvester 1973	1972 Olympians in track and field from 7 countries	—	Total Past 6 months	68 61
Yesalis et al. 1988	45 elite power lifters	74	Questionnaire (n = 45) Telephone (n = 20)	33 55
Frankle et al. 1984	250 weight lifters in 3 gymnasiums	—	Total	44
Tricker et al. 1989	176 amateur competitive bodybuilders in Missouri and Kansas	46	Males (n = 108) Females (n = 68)	55 10
Kersey 1993	178 weight trainers at 5 health clubs/gymnasiums	—	Males (n = 139) Females (n = 39)	18 2.6

Adapted, by permission, from C.E. Yesalis, 2000, *Anabolic steroids in sport and exercise* (Champaign, IL: Human Kinetics), 96.

elite power lifters using both questionnaires and follow-up telephone interviews (table 3.6). One-third of the questionnaire respondents admitted prior anabolic steroid use; however, 55% of those interviewed later by telephone conceded steroid use.

Weight trainers in three gymnasiums in the Chicago area were questioned (Frankle, Cicero, & Payne, 1984); 44% reported prior steroid use (table 3.6). In a study of amateur competitive bodybuilders (Tricker, O'Neil, & Cook, 1989), over half of the men and 10% of the women reported that they had used anabolic steroids at some time in their life. More recently, of the 185 members of gymnasiums and health clubs, 18% of men and 3% of women acknowledged having used or currently using anabolic steroids (Kersey, 1993).

The level of steroid use appears to have increased significantly over the past three decades (Yesalis, Anderson, Buckley, & Wright, 1990; Yesalis, Kennedy, Kopstein, & Bahrke, 1993), and is no longer limited to elite athletes or to men. Although higher rates of steroid use are reported by competitive athletes, a significant number of recreational athletes and nonathletes appear to be using these drugs, probably to "improve" their appearance. The use of anabolic steroids has cascaded down from the Olympic, professional, and college levels to the high schools and junior high schools, and there are significantly more adolescents using anabolic steroids than elite athletes.

Estimates based on data from the National Household Survey on Drug Abuse indicated that there are more than 1 million current or former steroid users in the United States, with more than half of the lifetime user population being 26 years of age or older (Yesalis, Kennedy, Kopstein, & Bahrke, 1993). More than 300,000 individuals had used steroids in the past year. Males had higher levels of steroid use during their lifetime than females (0.9% and 0.1%, respectively). The median age of first use of steroids for the study population was 18 years; for 12- to 17-year-olds, the median age of initiation was 15 years. Among 12- to 34-year-olds, steroid use was significantly and positively associated with the use of other illicit drugs, cigarettes (12- to 17-year-olds only), and alcohol.

A frequent concern about survey research, especially surveys dealing with illegal or controversial behavior, is the veracity of the responses given by the respondents. Research on the use of self-report methods has shown these methods to be valid for documenting recreational drug use, especially for adolescents (Yesalis, Bahrke, Kopstein, & Barsukiewicz, 2000). However, respondents may have underreported their anabolic steroid use to meet more socially acceptable standards of behavior. The use of anabolic steroids is in violation of U.S. federal and state laws, as well as the rules of virtually all sport federations and the traditional ethics of fair play in sport.

Because of the virilization qualities of steroids, women might be more secretive about their use than men or adolescents. There is no information on individuals who chose not to volunteer information, but it could be hypothesized that a disproportionate number of those who did not participate were steroid users, resulting in an underreporting bias. While it has not been possible to establish what, if any, response bias exists in the measurement of steroid use, it would seem prudent to assume that there is some tangible level of underreporting. Consequently, further research is indicated to better profile adolescent and adult steroid users regarding characteristics such as socioeconomic status, race, educational level, and competitive status. More importantly, we need better understanding of the process involved in initiating anabolic steroid use, including vulnerability factors, age of initiation, and the use of other illicit drugs.

Physical Effects

The short-term health effects of anabolic-androgenic steroids have been increasingly studied, and several authors have reviewed the physiological and health effects of these drugs (Friedl, 2000; Haupt & Rovere, 1984; Lamb, 1984; Wilson, 1988; Wright, 1980). Although anabolic steroid use has been associated (mainly through case reports) with a number of adverse and even fatal effects, the incidence of serious effects thus far reported has been extremely low (Friedl, 2000). However, for several decades experts have consistently stated that the long-term health effects of anabolic steroid use are unknown (Yesalis, Wright, & Bahrke, 1989). Specifically, the long-term health effects as related to type of steroid, dose, frequency of use, age at initiation, and concurrent drug use have not been elucidated. Confounding the assessment of health consequences is the fact that some individuals use large doses of anabolic steroids for prolonged periods of time, while others use therapeutic doses intermittently (Buckley et al., 1988; Duchaine, 1989; Grundig & Bachmann, 1995; Llewellyn, 2000).

Although the role of anabolic steroids in the etiology of various diseases in both animals and humans is still uncertain, steroid use in clinical trials and in laboratory studies has been associated with numerous deleterious changes in risk factors and in the physiology of various organs and body systems, suggesting potential for subsequent health problems (American College of Sports Medicine, 1984; Kruskemper, 1968; Wright, 1980). The best-documented effects are those on the liver, serum lipids, and the reproductive system. Other suspected areas of concern include the psyche and behavior, coronary artery disease, cerebrovascular accidents, prostatic changes, and the immune function (Friedl, 2000).

Steroid use has been related to cardiovascular risk factors. The most important are changes in lipoprotein fraction, increased triglyceride levels and concentrations of several clotting factors, changes in the myocardium itself, and hyperinsulinism and diminished glucose tolerance (Friedl, 2000; Glazer, 1991; Haupt & Rovere, 1984; Sullivan, Martinez, Gennis, & Gallagher, 1998; Wright, 1980). It should be noted, however, that although these effects vary significantly between types and doses of anabolic steroids, and between individuals and situations (Kruskemper, 1968), all of the effects (except postulated changes in the myocardium, which have not been followed) have been demonstrated to be fully reversible within several months after cessation of steroid use (Friedl, 2000; Haupt & Rovere, 1984; Wright, 1980).

Acute thrombotic risk has been linked to steroid use in case reports of nonfatal myocardial infarction and stroke in several athletes who were using anabolic steroids (Rockhold, 1993). Although there is no direct evidence that anabolic steroids are thrombogenic in humans (Ansell, Tiarks, & Fairchild, 1993), the clinical circumstances of these reports suggest a possible causal relationship. These reports further suggest that, if a causal relationship exists, anabolic steroids could have serious short-term effects.

Liver structure and function have also been altered by administration of anabolic steroids; associated conditions include cholestatic jaundice, peliosis hepatis, hepatocellular hyperplasia, and hepatocellular adenomas (Dickerman, Pertusi, Zachariah, Dufour, & McConathy, 1999; Soe, Soe, & Gluud, 1992). Peliosis hepatis is clearly associated with the use of 17-α-alkylated (oral) anabolic steroids, but with unknown frequency. Hepatic tumors are rare in men (1% to 3%), but nearly half of the discovered tumors rupture, and a larger proportion may remain undetected. In two cases, rupture proved fatal (Friedl, 2000). It has not been convincingly demonstrated that anabolic steroids can cause, at least with therapeutic doses, the development of hepatocellular carcinomas. Virtually all histological changes in the liver have been associated with the use of 17-α-alkylated (oral) steroids (Friedl, 2000; Kruskemper, 1968; Wilson, 1988; Wright, 1980); and the cause-and-effect relationship between oral anabolic steroids and these conditions is strengthened by the return of normal blood values and excretory function, the regression of tumors, a general recovery, and a return toward normal liver function after cessation of steroid use (Friedl, 2000).

The effects of anabolic-androgenic steroids on the male reproductive system include reductions in levels of endogenous testosterone, gonadotrophic hormones, and sex hormone-binding globulin (SHBG); reductions in testicle size, sperm count, and sperm motility; and alterations in sperm morphology (Friedl, 2000; Wright, 1980). When steroid use is stopped, the testes resume sperm production. Moreover, there are no reported cases of men with initially normal sperm counts who experienced irreversible sterility as a result of steroid use (Friedl, 2000). Nonetheless, two cases of hypogonadotrophic hypogonadism have been reported that may be associated with anabolic steroid use (Jarrow & Lipshultz, 1990). In neither case, however, was testicular function impaired in the long term: one patient had a normal sperm count at diagnosis, and the other responded favorably to human chorionic gonadotrophic therapy.

In women, anabolic steroids have been associated with a number of adverse effects, some of which are not reversible upon discontinuation of steroid use (Elliot & Goldberg, 2000). These include menstrual abnormalities; deepening of the voice; shrinkage of the breasts; male-pattern baldness; and an increase in sex drive, acne, body hair, and clitoris size. In addition, women using steroids experience dramatically elevated testosterone levels and lowered levels of SHBG, follicle-stimulating hormone, and thyroid-binding proteins (Elliot & Goldberg, 2000; Malarkey, Strauss, & Leizman, 1991). Premature halting of growth in younger users has not been systematically studied, although such effects have been described in case reports for several decades (Rogol & Yesalis, 1992).

Psychological Effects

Previous and current research studies have documented significant positive relationships between testosterone levels, dominance, and aggressive behavior in various species of animals, including nonhuman primates (Bahrke, Yesalis, & Wright, 1990). Relative to the animal literature, fewer studies have assessed the relationship of endogenous or exogenous androgens to aggression or violent behavior in humans. However, a positive pattern of association between endogenous testosterone levels and aggressive behavior in males has been increasingly established (Bahrke, 2000). Also, while random clinical trials using moderate doses of exogenous testosterone for contraceptive and other purposes reveal few adverse effects on male sexual and aggressive behavior, other investigations and case reports of athletes using higher doses suggest the possibility of affective and psychotic syndromes (some of violent proportions), psychological dependence, and withdrawal symptoms.

While several recently published reports support a pattern of association between the use of anabolic steroids by athletes and increased levels of irritability, aggression, personality disturbance, and psychiatric diagnoses, others do not (Bhasin et al., 1996; Millar, 1996; Yates, Perry, MacIndoe, Holman, & Ellingrod, 1999). Only four prospective, blinded studies documenting aggression and adverse overt behavior resulting from steroid use have been reported (Hannan, Friedl, Zold, Kettler, & Plymate, 1991; Pope, Kouri, & Hudson, 2000; Kouri, Lukas, Pope, & Oliva, 1995; Su et al., 1993). As Bjorkqvist and colleagues (1994) point out, much of the psychological and behavioral effect of steroid intake may be placebo. Anticipation of the aggressiveness related to steroid use may lead to actual violent acts and become, in effect, an excuse for aggression.

Although anabolic steroid dependency may be a problem, its prevalence and symptomatology are difficult to reliably establish based on the existing literature. With present estimates of 300,000 yearly anabolic steroid users in the United States (Yesalis, Kennedy, Kopstein, & Bahrke, 1993), an extremely small percentage of users appear to experience psychological dependence requiring clinical treatment. Additional research with larger and more heterogeneous samples will be needed.

In addition to small sample sizes, the variety of anabolic steroids used, and the diversity of techniques employed to assess the psychological and behavioral changes associated with anabolic steroid use, other factors such as the purity and content of steroids and the concomitant use of other drugs further complicate an already complex area. It is also possible that weight training may be a confounding factor in research examining the psychological and behavioral effects of anabolic steroids (Bahrke & Yesalis, 1994). Unfortunately, despite attempts to reduce and eliminate the number of methodological limitations associated with investigating the psychological and behavioral effects of anabolic steroids, these problems persist.

It is interesting to note that with a million or more steroid users in the United States (Yesalis, Kennedy, Kopstein, & Bahrke, 1993), only an extremely small percentage of users appear to experience mental disturbances that result in clinical treatment. Also, of the few individuals who do experience significant changes, most apparently recover without additional problems when the use of steroids is terminated.

Conclusion

Anabolic steroids are synthetic derivatives of testosterone. They are usually administered orally and by injection. Anabolic steroids are used by athletes to enhance performance and appearance. Research findings indicate that anabolic steroid use results in increased body weight and muscular strength. While the long-term effects of anabolic steroids are unknown, the best-documented physiological effects are those on the liver, serum lipids, and the reproductive system. A pattern of association between the use of anabolic steroids and increased levels of irritability, aggression, personality disturbance, and psychiatric diagnoses has been revealed in several reports. The increased arousal and aggression may enable some athletes to train and perform more intensely. Although anabolic steroids are illegal, and their use is banned by virtually every sport governing body, survey and drug-testing data indicate continued use by athletes at all levels and increasing usage by adolescent athletes and nonathletes.

References

Adalf, E.M., & Smart, R.G. (1992). Characteristics of steroid users in an adolescent school population. *Journal of Alcohol and Drug Education, 38(1)*, 43-49.

American College of Sports Medicine. (1977). Position statement on the use and abuse of anabolic-androgenic steroids in sports. *Medicine and Science in Sports, 9*, 11-13.

American College of Sports Medicine. (1984). Position stand on the use of anabolic-androgenic steroids in sports. *Sports Medicine Bulletin, 19*, 13-18.

Anderson, W., Albrecht, M., & McKeag, D. (1993). Second replication of a national study of substance use and abuse habits of college student-athletes. Final report. Overland Park, KS: National Collegiate Athletic Association.

Anderson, W., Albrecht, M., McKeag, D., Hough, D.O., & McGrew, C.A. (1991). A national survey of alcohol and drug use by college athletes. *Physician and Sportsmedicine, 19*, 91-104.

Anderson, W., & McKeag, D. (1985). The substance use and abuse habits of college student-athletes: research paper 2. Mission, KS: National Collegiate Athletic Association.

Ansell, J., Tiarks, C., & Fairchild, V. (1993). Coagulation abnormalities associated with the use of anabolic steroids. *American Heart Journal, 125(2),* 367-371.

Bahrke, M.S. (2000). Psychological effects of endogenous testosterone and anabolic-androgenic steroids. In C.E. Yesalis (Ed.), *Anabolic steroids in sport and exercise.* 2nd ed. (pp. 247-278). Champaign, IL: Human Kinetics.

Bahrke, M.S., & Yesalis, C.E. (1994). Weight training: a potential confounding factor in examining the psychological and behavioral effects of anabolic-androgenic steroids. *Sports Medicine, 18(5),* 309-318.

Bahrke, M.S., Yesalis, C.E., Kopstein, A.N., & Stephens, J.A. (2000). Risk factors associated with anabolic-androgenic steroids use among adolescents. *Sports Medicine, 29(6),* 397-405.

Bahrke, M., Yesalis, C., & Wright, J. (1990). Psychological and behavioral effects of endogenous testosterone levels and anabolic-androgenic steroids among males: a review. *Sports Medicine, 10(5),* 303-337.

Bhasin, S., Storer, T., Berman, N., Callegari, C., Clevenger, B., Phillips, J., Bunnell, T.J., Tricker, R., Shirazi, A., & Casaburi, R. (1996). The effects of supraphysiologic doses of testosterone on muscle size and strength in normal men. *New England Journal of Medicine, 335(1),* 1-7.

Bjorkqvist, K., Nygren, T., Bjorklund, A-C, & Bjorkqvist, S-E. (1994). Testosterone intake and aggressiveness: real effect or anticipation. *Aggressive Behavior, 20,* 17-26.

Buckley, W.E., Yesalis, C.E., Friedl, K.E., Anderson, W.A., Streit, A.L., & Wright, J.E. (1988). Estimated prevalence of anabolic-androgenic steroid use among male high school seniors. *Journal of the American Medical Association, 260(23),* 3441-3445.

Canadian Centre for Drug-Free Sport. (1993). National School Survey on Drugs and Sport. Final report, August. Gloucester, ON, Canada.

Celotti, F., & Negri-Cesi, P.N. (1992). Anabolic steroids: a review of their effects on the muscles, of their possible mechanisms of action and their use in athletics. *Journal of Steroid Biochemistry Molecular Biology, 43(5),* 469-477.

Dickerman, R.D., Pertusi, R.M., Zachariah, N.Y., Dufour, D.R., & McConathy, W.J. (1999). Anabolic steroid-induced hepatotoxicity: is it overstated? *Clinical Journal of Sport Medicine, 9,* 34-39.

Di Pasquale, M.G. (1990). *Anabolic steroid side effects: facts, fiction, and treatment.* Warkworth, ON, Canada: M.G.D. Press.

Duchaine, D. (1989). *Underground steroid handbook II.* Venice, CA: HLR Technical Books.

DuRant, R.H., Rickert, V.I., Ashworth, C.S., Newman, C., & Slavens, G. (1993). Use of multiple drugs among adolescents who use anabolic steroids. *New England Journal of Medicine, 328(13),* 922-926.

Elliot, D.L., & Goldberg, L. (2000). Women and anabolic steroids. In C.E. Yesalis (Ed.), *Anabolic steroids in sport and exercise.* 2nd ed. (pp. 225-246). Champaign, IL: Human Kinetics.

Frankle, M., Cicero, G., & Payne, J. (1984). Use of androgenic anabolic steroids by athletes. Letter. *Journal of the American Medical Association, 252,* 482.

Frazier, S. (1973). Androgens and athletes. *American Journal of Disease of Children, 125,* 479-480.

Friedl, K.E. (2000). Effect of anabolic steroid use on body composition and physical performance. In C.E. Yesalis (Ed.), *Anabolic steroids in sport and exercise.* 2nd ed. (pp. 139-174). Champaign, IL: Human Kinetics.

Friedl, K.E., Dettori, J.R., Hannan, C.J., Patience, T.H., & Plymate, S.R. (1991). Comparison of the effects of high dose testosterone and 19-nortestosterone to a replacement dose of testosterone on strength and body composition in normal men. *Journal of Steroid Biochemistry and Molecular Biology, 40,* 607-612.

Gallaway, S. (1997). *The steroid bible.* 3rd ed. Sacramento, CA: BI Press.

Gilbert, B. (1969a). Drugs in sport, part 1: problems in a turned-on world. *Sports Illustrated,* June 23, 64-72.

Gilbert, B. (1969b). Drugs in sport, part 2: something extra on the ball. *Sports Illustrated,* June 30, 30-42.

Gilbert, B. (1969c). Drugs in sport, part 3: high time to make some rules. *Sports Illustrated,* July 7, 30-35.

Glazer, G. (1991). Atherogenic effects of anabolic steroids on serum lipid levels. *Archives of Internal Medicine, 151,* 1925-1933.

Grundig, P., & Bachmann, M. (1995). *World anabolic review 1996.* Houston: MB Muscle Books.

Handelsman, D.J., & Gupta, L. (1997). Prevalence and risk factors for anabolic-androgenic steroid abuse in Australian high school students. *International Journal of Andrology, 20,* 159-164.

Hannan, C.J., Friedl, K.E., Zold, A., Kettler, T.M., & Plymate, S.R. (1991). Psychological and serum homovanillic acid changes in men administered androgenic steroids. *Psychoneuroendocrinology, 16,* 335-342.

Haupt, H., & Rovere, G. (1984). Anabolic steroids: a review of the literature. *American Journal of Sports Medicine, 12(6),* 469-484.

Henrion, R., Mandelbrot, L., & Delfieu, D. (1992). Contamination par le VIH a la suite d'injections d'anabolisants. *La Presse Medicale, 5,* 21.

Hewitt, S.M., Smith-Akin, C.K., Higgins, M.M., Jenkins, P.M. (1998). Youth Risk Behavior Surveillance: United States, 1997. *MMWR CDC Surveillance Summary, 47,* 61.

Jarrow, J., & Lipshultz, L. (1990). Anabolic steroid-induced hypogonadotropic hypogonadism. *American Journal of Sports Medicine, 18,* 429-431.

Johnston, L., O'Malley, P., & Bachman, J. (1996). National survey results on drug use from the Monitoring the Future Study, volume I (secondary students) 1989-1995. Washington, DC: National Institute on Drug Abuse. U.S. Department of Health and Human Services. National Institutes of Health publication 96-4139.

Kann, L., Warren, C.W., Harris, W.A., Collins, J.L., Douglas, K.A., Collins, M.E., Williams, B.I., Ross, J.G., Kolbe, L.J. (1995). Youth Risk Behavior Surveillance: United States, 1993. *MMWR CDC Surveillance Summary, 44,* 1-55.

Kenney, J. (1994). Extent and nature of illicit trafficking in anabolic steroids. In *Report of the International Conference on the Abuse and Trafficking of Anabolic Steroids* (pp. 34-35). Conference report. Washington, DC: United States Drug Enforcement Administration.

Kerr, R. (1982). *The practical use of anabolic steroids with athletes.* San Gabriel, CA: Kerr.

Kersey, R. (1993). Anabolic-androgenic steroid use by private health club/gym athletes. *Journal of Strength and Conditioning, 7,* 118-126.

Killip, S.M., & Stennett, R.G. (1990). Use of performance enhancing substances by London secondary school students. London, ON, Canada: Board of Education for the City of London.

Kindlundh, A.M.S., Isacson, D.G.L., Berglund, L., & Nyberg, F. (1999). Factors associated with adolescent use of doping agents: anabolic-androgenic steroids. *Addiction, 94(4),* 543-553.

Kochakian, C.D., & Yesalis, C.E. (2000). Anabolic-androgenic steroids: a historical perspective and definition. In C.E. Yesalis (Ed.), *Anabolic steroids in sport and exercise.* 2nd ed. (pp. 17-49). Champaign, IL: Human Kinetics.

Kouri, E.M., Lukas, S.E., Pope, H.G., & Oliva, P.S. (1995). Increased aggressiveness responding in male volunteers following the administration of gradually increasing doses of testosterone cypionate. *Drug and Alcohol Dependence, 40(1),* 73-79.

Kruskemper, H.L. (1968). *Anabolic steroids.* New York: Academic Press.

Lamb, D. (1984). Anabolic steroids in athletics: how well do they work and how dangerous are they? *American Journal of Sports Medicine, 12(1),* 31-38.

Lambert, M.I., Titlestad, S.D., & Schwellnus, M.P. (1998). Prevalence of androgenic-anabolic steroid use in adolescents in two regions of South Africa. *South African Medical Journal, 88(7),* 876-880.

Ljungqvist, A. (1975). The use of anabolic steroids in top Swedish athletes. *British Journal of Sports Medicine, 9,* 82.

Llewellyn, W. (2000). *Anabolics 2000.* Aurora, CO: William Llewellyn.

Lombardo, J. (1993). The efficacy and mechanisms of action of anabolic steroids. In C.E. Yesalis (Ed.), *Anabolic steroids in sport and exercise* (pp. 89-106). Champaign, IL: Human Kinetics.

Malarkey, W., Strauss, R., & Leizman, D. (1991). Endocrine effects in female weight lifters who self-administer testosterone and anabolic steroids. *American Journal of Obstetrics and Gynecology, 165(5),* 1385-1390.

Millar, A.P. (1996). Anabolic steroids—a personal pilgrimage. *Journal of Performance Enhancing Drugs, 1(1),* 4-9.

National Collegiate Athletic Association Research Staff. (1997). Indianapolis.

Newman, S. (1994). Despite warnings, lure of steroids too strong for some young Canadians. *Canadian Medical Association Journal, 151,* 844-846.

Nilsson, S. (1995). Androgenic anabolic steroid use among male adolescents in Falkenberg. *European Journal of Clinical Pharmacology, 48(1),* 9-11.

Pearson, B. (1994). Olympic survey: Olympians of winters past. *USA Today,* February 7, C5.

Pearson, B., & Hansen, B. (1992). Survey of U.S. Olympians. *USA Today,* February 5, 10C.

Phillips, W. (1991). *Anabolic reference guide.* 6th ed. Golden, CO: Mile High.

Pope, H.G., Kouri, E.M., & Hudson, J.I. (2000). Effects of supraphysiologic doses of testosterone on mood and aggression in normal men. *Archives of General Psychiatry, 57,* 133-140.

Rockhold, R. (1993). Cardiovascular toxicity of anabolic steroids. *Annual Review of Pharmacology and Toxicology, 33,* 497-520.

Rogol, A., & Yesalis, C. (1992). Anabolic-androgenic steroids and the adolescent. *Pediatrics Annual, 21(3),* 175-188.

Ryan, A. (1976). Athletics. In C. Kochakian (Ed.). *Anabolic-androgenic steroids* (pp. 515-534). New York: Springer-Verlag.

Schwellnus, M., Lambert, M., & Todd, M. (1992). Androgenic anabolic steroid use in matric pupils. *South African Medical Journal, 82,* 154-158.

Scott, M.J., & Scott, M.J. Jr. (1989). HIV infection associated with injections of anabolic steroids. *Journal of the American Medical Association, 262,* 207-298.

Silvester, L. (1973). Anabolic steroids at the 1972 Olympics. *Scholastic Coach, 43,* 90-92.

Sklarek, H.M., Manovani, R.P., Erens, E., Heisler, D., Niederman, M.S., & Fein, A.M. (1984). AIDS in a bodybuilder using anabolic steroids. *New England Journal of Medicine, 311,* 1701.

Soe, K., Soe, M., & Gluud, C. (1992). Liver pathology associated with the use of anabolic steroids. *Liver, 12,* 73-79.

Su, T-P, Pagliaro, M., Schmidt, P.J., Pickar, D., Wolkowitz, O., & Rubinow, D.R. (1993). Neuropsychiatric effects of anabolic steroids in male normal volunteers. *Journal of the American Medical Association, 269,* 2760-2764.

Sullivan, M.L., Martinez, C.M., Gennis, P., & Gallagher, E.J. (1998). The cardiac toxicity of anabolic steroids. *Progress in Cardiovascular Diseases, 41(1),* 1-15.

Tolliver, J. (1998, February 9-14). Anabolic steroid black-market in the United States. Paper presented at Drugs and Athletes: A Multidisciplinary Symposium. Meeting of the American Academy of Forensic Sciences, San Francisco.

Tricker, R., O'Neil, M., & Cook, D. (1989). The incidence of anabolic steroid use among competitive bodybuilders. *Journal of Drug Education, 19,* 313-325.

U.S. Department of Health and Human Services, Public Health Service. (1991, January). *Interagency Task Force on Anabolic Steroids.* Washington, DC: Author.

Williamson, D.J. (1993). Anabolic steroid use among students at a British college of technology. *British Journal of Sports Medicine, 27(3),* 200-201.

Wilson, J. (1988). Androgen abuse by athletes. *Endocrine Reviews, 9(2),* 181-199.

Wright, J.E. (1980). Steroids and athletics. *Exercise and Sports Sciences Reviews, 8,* 149-202.

Wright, J. (1982). *Anabolic steroids and sport II.* Natick, MA: Sports Science Consultants.

Yates, W.R., Perry, P.J., MacIndoe, J., Holman, T., & Ellingrod, V.L. (1999). Psychosexual effects of three doses of testosterone cycling in normal men. *Biological Psychiatry, 45,* 254-260.

Yen, S., & Jaffe, R. (1978). *Reproductive endocrinology.* Philadelphia: Saunders.

Yesalis, C., Anderson, W., Buckley, W., & Wright, J. (1990). Incidence of the non-medical use of anabolic-androgenic steroids. In G. Lin & L. Erinoff (Eds.), *Anabolic steroid abuse* (National Institute on Drug Abuse Research Monograph Series No. 102) (pp. 97-112). Rockville, MD: U.S. Department of Health and Human Services, Public Health Service, and Alcohol, Drug Abuse, and Mental Health Administration.

Yesalis, C.E., & Bahrke, M.S. (1995). Anabolic-androgenic steroids: current issues. *Sports Medicine, 19,* 326-340.

Yesalis, C.E., Bahrke, M.S., Kopstein, A.N., & Barsukiewicz, C.K. (2000). Incidence of anabolic steroid use: a discussion of methodological issues. In C.E. Yesalis (Ed.), *Anabolic steroids in sport and exercise.* 2nd ed. (pp. 73-115). Champaign, IL: Human Kinetics.

Yesalis, C.E., Barsukiewicz, C.K., Kopstein, A.N., & Bahrke, M.S. (1997). Trends in anabolic-androgenic steroid use among adolescents. *Archives of Pediatric and Adolescent Medicine, 151,* 1197-1206.

Yesalis, C., Buckley, W., Anderson, W., Wang, M.O., Norwig, J.H., Ott, G., Puffer, J.C., & Strauss, R.H. (1990). Athletes' projections of anabolic steroid use. *Clinical Sports Medicine, 2,* 155-171.

Yesalis, C.E., Courson, S.P., & Wright, J.E. (2000). History of anabolic steroid use in sport and exercise. In C.E. Yesalis (Ed.), *Anabolic steroids in sport and exercise.* 2nd ed. (pp. 51-71). Champaign, IL: Human Kinetics.

Yesalis, C., Herrick, R., Buckley, W., Friedl, K., Brannon, D., & Wright, J. (1988). Self-reported use of anabolic-androgenic steroids by elite power lifters. *Physician and Sportsmedicine, 16,* 91-100.

Yesalis, C.E., Kennedy, N., Kopstein, A., & Bahrke, M.S. (1993). Anabolic-androgenic steroid use in the United States. *Journal of the American Medical Association, 270,* 1217-1221.

Yesalis, C.E., Ortner, C.K., & Bahrke, M.S. (1996). Steroidi anabolizzanti mascolinizzanti: dal si dice al quanto: uno sguardo alla situazione internationale. *Sport e Medicina, 5,* 27-35.

Yesalis, C., Wright, J., & Bahrke, M. (1989). Epidemiological and policy issues in the measurement of the long term health effects of anabolic-androgenic steroids. *Sports Medicine, 8(3),* 129-138.

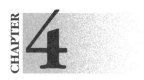

Beta-2 Agonists

Gordon S. Lynch, BSc, PhD

Since the early 1990s, the use of beta-2 adrenoceptor agonists (β2-agonists) for the purpose of enhancing sporting performance has become increasingly prevalent (Delbeke et al. 1995). Although they were traditionally used for the treatment of bronchial ailments, especially asthma (Maltin et al. 1993a), it became apparent that some β2-agonists, including the most well known, clenbuterol, have the ability to increase skeletal muscle mass and decrease body fat (Ricks et al. 1984; Bergen & Merkel 1991). This combination of effects proved desirable for those working in the livestock industry trying to improve meat quality (Sillence et al. 1991b); and not surprisingly, β2-agonists were soon used or abused by those engaged in competitive bodybuilding and soon after by other athletes competing in strength- and power-related sports (Prather et al. 1995; Friedl 2000). Many athletes who use β2-agonists for improving athletic performance claim that they are asthmatics to justify their use (Prather et al. 1995). Despite the so-called desirable effects of increasing muscle bulk and decreasing body fat, many athletes are not aware of the deleterious effects of chronic high-dose β2-agonist administration. This chapter reviews the effects of β2-agonists on skeletal muscle and the reasons for their use by athletes for enhancing physical performance and body appearance. The supposed beneficial effects of β2-agonists on skeletal muscle are weighed against some of the less well reported deleterious effects of these drugs on exercise performance.

Adrenergic Receptors and the Definition of a Beta-2 Agonist

The adrenergic receptors are part of the sympathetic nervous system and are characterized by their interaction with adrenaline (epinephrine) and noradrenaline (norepinephrine). They can be divided into two categories, the α-receptors and the β-receptors. Stimulation of α-receptors is associated with intestinal relaxation; vasoconstriction; and the stimulation of the uterus, nictitating membrane, ureter, and pupil dilation. Stimulation of the β-receptor is associated with myocardial stimulation, vasodilation, and inhibition of the uterine and bronchial smooth muscle (Burgess et al. 1997).

Beta-adrenergic receptors are associated with all tissues involved in growth, including skeletal muscle and adipose tissue, and can be generally differentiated into two subtypes, β1 and β2, based on the receptor affinity for certain compounds (table 4.1). The β1-receptor is traditionally associated with cardiac stimulation and the β2-receptor with bronchial smooth muscle relaxation (Levitzki 1986; Yang & McElligot 1989). However, both β1- and β2-receptors are present and functional in the atrial and ventricular myocardium in all species including humans, although the numbers of the two types of receptors are different across the species (Burgess 1993). The β-receptor on brown adipose tissue is not a mixed population of the two subtypes but a unique receptor, the β3 (Yang & McElligot 1989). The β3-receptor stimulates lipolysis and increases blood flow and thermogenesis in the brown adipose tissue (Yoshida et al. 1998).

A β-agonist is defined simply as a compound that stimulates the β-receptors. Selectivity of β-agonists is defined in terms of the relative effects of isoprenaline, a nonselective agonist at β-receptors that has stimulatory activity at both receptor types for any dose. Agonists selective at the β2-receptor would stimulate that receptor with little or no effect at the β1-receptor. Selectivity can also be dose related such that at high doses a β2-receptor agonist could lose its selective profile (S.R. O'Donnell 1993). Common β-agonists include salbutamol (albuterol), bambuterol, terbutaline, fenoterol, mapenterol, formoterol, tulobuterol, carbuterol, bromobuterol, cimbuterol, zinterol, cimaterol, mabuterol, salmeterol, and the best described of all, clenbuterol

Table 4.1 Distribution of β1- and β2-Receptors and Acute Response to Stimulation in Humans

Tissue	β1-receptor	β2-receptor
Smooth muscle[1]	—	Relaxation
Heart		
Heart rate	Increase	Increase
Contractility	Increase	Increase
Skeletal muscle	—	Tremor

[1]Refers to bronchial smooth muscle and/or vascular smooth muscle.

Adapted from Burgess et al. (1997).

(Burgess et al. 1997). Given the wealth of data on the effects of clenbuterol on skeletal and cardiac muscle, as well as its known effects on exercise performance, the description of the use of β-agonists for performance enhancement will concentrate on clenbuterol.

Clenbuterol: A Powerful Beta-2 Agonist

Clenbuterol (4-amino-α-[t-butylaminomethyl]-3,5-dichlorobenzyl alcohol) is defined as a sympathomimetic amine; that is, its actions mimic that of adrenaline (epinephrine). Clenbuterol, like most β2-agonists, is used primarily for the treatment of asthma and related bronchospasm (Maltin et al. 1993a). It is a powerful bronchodilator and not only has proved useful for hu-mans but also has widespread veterinary applications in the equine and livestock industries (Prather et al. 1995). Brand names for the generic name, clenbuterol, include Clenasma, Monores, Novegam, Prontovent, Spiropent, Broncoterol, Bronchodil, Cesbron, Clenbuter, Pharmachim, Contrasmina, Contraspasmina, Oxyflux, Ventolase, Ventapulmin, and Clenbumar (Duncan 1996; Embleton & Thorne 1998). Clenbuterol is available in tablet form in 10- and 20-μg doses and can be obtained as a powder for use in making solutions of varying clenbuterol concentration. The dose of clenbuterol for use in puffers (inhalers) for the treatment of asthma in humans ranges between 0.02 and 0.03 mg twice daily (Prather et al. 1995). With infrequent use and at such low dosages, asthmatics experience few side effects of β2-agonist administration (Anstead et al. 2001). Surprisingly, clenbuterol is not approved for use by humans as a bronchodilator in the United States, nor does it have Federal Drug Administration approval. Albuterol (salbutamol) is listed as the alternative drug to clenbuterol for use by asthmatics (Prather et al. 1995). Only recently has an orally administered syrup containing clenbuterol (Ventapulmin) been made available in the United States for use in horses affected with airway obstruction, such as that associated with chronic obstructive pulmonary disease (COPD) (Torneke et al. 1998; Kearns et al. 2001). In Europe, Australia, Canada, and South America, Ventapulmin has been available for at least 10 years. The duration of clenbuterol treatment recommended for horses is 30 days (at a dose of 0.8 μg/kg).

The Rise of Beta-2 Agonist Usage by Athletes

The use of clenbuterol and related β2-agonists in the livestock industry revealed a number of interesting and beneficial side effects, namely that in high doses, β2-agonist administration produced an increase in skeletal muscle mass and a concomitant decrease in body fat (Ricks et al. 1984; Hamby et al. 1986; Reeds et al. 1986; Beerman et al. 1987; Miller et al. 1988; Schiavetta et al. 1990; Koohmarie et al. 1991; Chwalibog et al. 1996; Hulot et al. 1996; Hansen et al. 1997a,b; Bell et al. 1998; Li et al. 2000; Pan et al. 2001). As such, β2-agonists such as clenbuterol (and cimaterol) became known as a "repartitioning agents" (Kim et al. 1992; Mersmann 1989). Clenbuterol is one of the few anabolic compounds that increases growth primarily through reducing muscle protein degradation (Sillence et al. 2000). Many involved in the livestock industry quickly took advantage of the repartitioning effects of clenbuterol and used it in the feeding of cattle, sheep, pigs, and poultry for the purpose of improving meat production (Moore et al. 1994). It is therefore not surprising that there have been several reports in humans of clenbuterol poisoning after the ingestion of meat from animals fed excessive doses of clenbuterol (Salleras et al. 1995; Garay et al. 1997; Mitchell & Dunnavan 1998; Sporano et al. 1998; Brambilla et al. 2000; Smith 2000). These ill effects of excess clenbuterol intake are discussed later (see "Side Effects of the Chronic Use of Beta-2 Agonists" on p. 54).

The so-called repartitioning effects of clenbuterol are what make it so desirable for athletes, such as those involved in strength- and power-related sports and especially those involved in competitive bodybuilding (Delbeke et al. 1995). Although clenbuterol has powerful muscle anabolic effects, it also has potent lipolytic effects. This has also made clenbuterol a drug of choice for many athletes in sports involving weight restrictions for competing in specific weight classes, for example, rowing (Duncan 1996). Traditionally, the use of anabolic steroids and growth hormone (GH) dominated the world of performance-enhancing drugs (Prather et al. 1995). However, in the last decade, the use of β2-agonists, particularly clenbuterol, for athletic and cosmetic purposes has been increasing steadily (Delbeke et al. 1995; Duncan 1996).

Clenbuterol became notorious during the 1992 Summer Olympic Games in Barcelona, Spain, when two athletes tested positive for its use. Clenbuterol has a long half-life of approximately 35 hr (Tschan et al. 1979), and subsequently the drug will accumulate with repeated doses (Murugaiah & O'Donnell 1994). It can be detected via urine analysis, but 97% of the drug is removed from the body within approximately eight days (Duncan 1996). Clenbuterol was banned by the International Olympic Committee (IOC) on April 21, 1992. Nevertheless, many athletes still abuse this substance, with most not aware of its potentially lethal side effects when taken in excessive dosages.

The fact that clenbuterol is not approved by the Food and Drug Administration for use on humans means that little information is available in the scientific literature concerning the use and abuse of β-agonists by athletes (Maltin et al. 1993a; Clarkson & Thompson 1997; Embleton & Thorne 1998). The dramatic effects of clenbuterol administration observed in livestock served as the basis for its application by male and female bodybuilders in gymnasiums throughout the world. Advances in the development of muscle anabolic agents are quickly incorporated into drug regimens employed by bodybuilders, often with dire consequences. In many cases, scientific research into the effects of such muscle anabolic compounds lags far behind the ad hoc knowledge acquired by dubious trial-and-error experiments conducted by the bodybuilders on themselves. The "catch-up" knowledge obtained from rigorous scientific experimentation is often too late to prevent the often irreversible effects of these drugs.

Clenbuterol is an extremely attractive drug for athletes because of its ability to modify body structure and function in addition to the fact that it is administered orally, is freely available (in many countries), and is relatively cheap (Duncan 1996). However, even though clenbuterol is promoted as the "safe" alternative to anabolic steroids, it does have deleterious side effects, although these do not appear to act as a deterrent to the large number of athletes abusing this drug (Duncan 1996). Anecdotal reports regarding the use of clenbuterol by bodybuilders indicate that they use it primarily as a precontest "cutting-up" drug, taking advantage of its lipolytic actions. Unfortunately, many of these athletes take multiple drugs in varying combinations in order to maximize muscle mass and reduce their body fat (Prather et al. 1995). Sadly, the combination of clenbuterol use with diuretics (for example) has been thought responsible for the deaths of several prominent professional bodybuilders (Prather et al. 1995; Embleton & Thorne 1998). Before we return to the application of β-agonists for performance enhancement, it is important to understand the basis for the use of β-agonists, such as clenbuterol, among athletes.

Beta-2 Agonists and Muscle Growth

Studies have demonstrated that when β2-agonists are given in high (mg/kg) doses, extended use produces significant increases in muscle mass in mice (Hayes & Williams 1994; Lynch et al. 1999, 2000b), rats (Deshaies et al. 1980; Emery et al. 1984; Rothwell & Stock 1985; Reeds et al. 1986; Maltin et al. 1987; McElligott et al. 1987, 1989; Zeman et al. 1988, 1991; MacLennan & Edwards 1989; Yang & McElligott 1989; Agbenyega & Wareham 1990; Palmer et al. 1990; Carter et al. 1991;

Sillence et al. 1991a; Choo et al. 1992; Kim & Sainz 1992; Torgan et al. 1993; Waterfield et al. 1995; Guggenbuhl 1996; Cepero et al. 2000; Duncan et al. 2000), sheep (Baker et al. 1984; Beerman et al. 1987; MacRae et al. 1988), and cattle (Ricks et al. 1984; Bardsley et al. 1992), on the order of 10% to 25% following 10 to 20 days of administration. These doses of clenbuterol are much higher than what could be tolerated by humans. At these mg/kg doses, clenbuterol would cause muscle tremors, heart palpitations, and severe sweating in humans (Embleton & Thorne 1998). The clenbuterol-induced increase in muscle protein is considered "true" muscle hypertrophy (Yang & McElligott 1989) since hyperplasia (increased cell number) and satellite cell division are not associated with the protein increases (Maltin et al. 1986). Other β2-agonists that have proved effective in producing a muscle hypertrophic response include cimaterol, salbutamol, isoproterenol, and ractopamine, although clenbuterol ranks as one of the most potent of these compounds (Moore et al. 1994).

That β2-adrenoceptors mediate the anabolic effects of clenbuterol was confirmed by the actions of the nonselective β1/β2-adrenoceptor antagonist, sotalol, which attenuated both the muscle growth response and the reduction in β2-adrenoceptor density. Further confirmation was obtained from the use of the antagonist ICI118551, which has a ~100-fold greater affinity for β2-adrenoceptors than for β1-adrenoceptors (Sillence et al. 1991a). ICI118551 reduced the anabolic effects of clenbuterol, and when administered alone caused muscle atrophy. These studies confirmed that β2-adrenoceptors mediate the pharmacological effects of clenbuterol and indicate that they are involved in the control of muscle growth (Sillence et al. 1991a).

The effectiveness of clenbuterol as an anabolic agent has been attributed to its ability to promote muscle protein synthesis (Ricks et al. 1984; Emery et al. 1984; Reeds et al. 1986; Maltin et al. 1987; Claeys et al. 1989; Inkster et al. 1989; Choo et al. 1992) as well as reduce muscle protein degradation (Reeds et al. 1986; Bohorov et al. 1987; Maltin et al. 1987; Wang & Beerman 1988; MacRae et al. 1988; Forsberg et al. 1989; Benson et al. 1991). Although there has been much debate whether the increase in muscle mass is more a result of one mechanism or the other (Bell et al. 1998), the most recent studies attribute the anabolic properties primarily to the ability of clenbuterol to inhibit protein degradation (Sillence et al. 2000). The exact mechanism for the protein accretion following β2-agonist administration appears to differ between species.

Anecdotal reports indicate that the muscle anabolic effects of clenbuterol in humans are much less pronounced than those observed in livestock. In fact, studies on cattle, sheep, and pigs have shown that the mechanism controlling tissue responsiveness to β2-agonists varies from species to species, and even among different tissues within a species, primarily because of differences in the densities of the receptor subtypes (Hill et al. 1998; Sillence et al. 2000). Although the muscle anabolic effects of clenbuterol appear to be much less powerful in humans compared with livestock, it is the lipolytic effects of clenbuterol that have the greatest appeal for bodybuilders.

Thermogenesis

Studies in both humans and animals have shown that clenbuterol has powerful lipolytic effects due to its thermogenic (heat producing) properties (Blum & Fluekiger 1988; Arch et al. 1984; Rothwell & Stock 1985; Reeds et al. 1986; Bohorov et al. 1987; MacRae et al. 1988; Choo et al. 1989; Bergen & Merkel 1991; Belahsen & Deshaies 1992). Adipose tissue is a major site for thermogenesis. White adipose tissue is a major site for fat storage, and β-agonists act on the adrenoceptors in this tissue to increase lipolysis (Mills 2000). Beta-2 agonists such as clenbuterol stimulate the breakdown of fat and increase energy expenditure. Brown adipose tissue is almost nonexistent in humans soon after birth. Other mammals have greater brown adipose stores. The β3-adrenoceptors are primarily involved with this tissue. Disruption of β3-adrenoceptors is thought to contribute to a predisposition to the development of obesity (Revelli et al. 1997; Weyer et al. 1999).

Desensitization of Beta-Adrenoceptors

In animals the density of β2-adrenoceptors is higher in slow muscles than in fast muscles (Martin et al. 1989; Williams et al. 1984), and this distribution is similar in humans (Elfellah et al. 1989; Martin et al. 1989). However, studies have indicated that the density of β2-adrenoceptors appears not to be related to skeletal muscle growth (Choo et al. 1989; Sillence et al. 2000). Adrenergic receptor desensitization occurs within two weeks of continuous clenbuterol stimulation (Reeds et al. 1986; Yang & McElligott 1989; Bruckmaier & Blum 1992), and the rapid increases in muscle mass and decreases in body fat are attenuated (Rothwell et al. 1987; McElligott et al. 1989; Greife et al. 1989; Sillenee et al. 1991a,b; Torgan et al. 1993; Kim & Kim 1997). This reduced efficacy following continued β2-agonist administration has been attributed to the reduction in skeletal muscle β-adrenoceptor density (Rothwell et al. 1987; Sillence et al. 1991a). It should be noted that even though the response to a drug or hormone is dependent partly on the density of the tissue receptors, researchers who studied β-adrenoceptor densities in the skeletal muscles of livestock found that β-adrenoceptor density was not a useful predictor of growth, carcass quality, or meat quality in cattle (Hoey et al. 1995).

There are reports that an atypical β-adrenergic receptor site is located in particularly high concentrations in the soleus muscle, with some of the characteristics of β3-receptors (Molenaar et al. 1991; Arch & Kaumann 1993). The β3-receptor differs from β2-receptor in that it lacks the phosphorylation sites involved in down-regulation or desensitization (Liggett et al. 1988, 1993; Liggett & Green 1997), and therefore it is possible that the desensitization evident in fast-twitch muscles results from the down-regulation of β2-receptors.

Can the Desensitization of Adrenoceptors During Chronic Administration of Beta-Agonists Be Offset?

Much debate exists regarding the issue of β-adrenoceptor down-regulation or desensitization (Huang et al. 2000). In studies on animals (Yang & McElligott 1989), it has been reported that the down-regulation of the β-receptors may be overcome if the β-agonist is administered intermittently rather than continuously. Early studies using clenbuterol suggested that the effects of the β-agonist could be prolonged if it was administered using a "two days on followed by two days off" approach (Yang & McElligott 1989). Although anecdotal reports indicate that such a strategy is recommended for athletes taking clenbuterol and other β2-agonists, evidence for the efficacy of such an approach is scant. Numerous combinations of treatment "days on" and "days off" have been employed successfully in animals (Yang & McElligott 1989), but virtually no scientific evidence exists for the efficacy of such an approach by human athletes. Anecdotal reports indicate that the "two days on, two days off" approach is rarely followed, simply because the long half-life of β-agonists such as clenbuterol would mean that there is insufficient time to clear the drug from the system. As such, a "two days on, two days off" approach would do little to reduce the problem of β-adrenoceptor down-regulation. Longer periods of nonuse have also been advocated, for example "one week on, one week off" or "two weeks on, two weeks off"; and variations on this theme have appeared to be successful in increasing muscle mass in animals even when clenbuterol was given for one year (Lynch et al. 1999).

Some researchers have tried to increase the number of β-adrenoceptors in skeletal muscle using corticosteroids that increase the number of β2-adrenoceptors and enhance the effects of β-adrenergic agonists in lung tissue (Huang et al. 1998). Studies indicate that in clenbuterol-treated rats, dexamethasone had the opposite effect on β2-adrenoceptors in skeletal muscle, and it did not enhance the anabolic effects of β-adrenergic agonist treatment (Huang et al. 2000).

Use of Clenbuterol Among Athletes

Clenbuterol usage is highest among bodybuilders, both for its muscle anabolic properties and for its lipolytic effects (Duncan 1996; Embleton & Thorne 1998). The exact dosage of clenbuterol that results in the greatest improvements in muscle mass and reductions in body fat has not yet been identified. These criteria are especially important for bodybuilders before competitions, when the maintenance of muscle mass during periods of strict dieting is critical. The dosages used by bodybuilders exceed that recommended for asthmatics for therapeutic purposes. Typically, the dose of clenbuterol used by athletes ranges from 50 to 100 μg/day or 80 to 140 μg/day taken over the course of the day, but the maximum dose is usually dependent on the individual's tolerance (Embleton & Thorne 1998). To prevent receptor down-regulation, clenbuterol is often used in two- or three-week "on and off" cycles. Comparing the doses that are effective in rats and then translating these for use in humans is obviously difficult because of the differences in size, growth, and metabolism between the species. However, some authors have made interspecies comparisons based on metabolic measurements. For example, Maltin et al. (1993a) suggested that a dose of 10 μg/kg for the rat was equivalent to 1.0 μg/kg for humans, a dose considered to be safe (Duncan 1996). Even if a theoretical safe dosage of clenbuterol was prescribed for promoting muscle mass in humans, it is unlikely that bodybuilders would adhere to this level given that some of these athletes are notorious for taking anabolic steroids in excess of 26 times the therapeutic dose (Brower et al. 1991; Duncan 1996). Another confounding issue is the fact that many bodybuilders take more than one drug at any one time (Delbeke et al. 1995; Prather et al. 1995); and the supposed increases in muscle mass following clenbuterol administration are hard to gauge when, for example, it is taken in conjunction with one or more anabolic steroids.

Effects of Beta-2 Agonists on Skeletal Muscle Structure and Muscle Fiber Type Composition

The exact mechanisms by which β-agonists such as clenbuterol exert their effects at the cellular level are not understood completely. When β-agonists bind to β-adrenoceptors they increase the intracellular concentration of the second messenger cyclic adenosine monophosphate (cAMP), leading to the activation of adenylate cyclase (Roberts & Summers 1998). Activation of the β-adrenoceptors influences several metabolic and physiological processes in skeletal muscle (table 4.2), including glucose uptake and metabolism, growth, heat production, and contractility (Yang & McElligot 1989). Proteins phosphorylated following elevation of cAMP and protein kinase A in skeletal muscle include glycolytic enzymes, sarcolemmal Na^+/K^+ pumps, phospholamban, and voltage-sensitive and sarcolemmal Ca^{2+} channels (Roberts & Summers 1998; Navegantes et al. 2000). An in-depth analysis of the underlying mechanisms of β-agonist action on β-adrenergic receptors is beyond the scope of this review. There are many good reviews on various topics within this broad field that the reader should consult where necessary, including the molecular biology of β-adrenoceptors (Liggett & Green 1997), the coupling of β-adrenergic receptors to adenylate cyclase (Levitzki 1986), the pharmacokinetics of β2-adrenoceptor-stimulating drugs (Nyberg 1997), and the regulation of action by G-proteins (Bowman & Nott

Table 4.2 Some Effects and Potential Adverse Side Effects of Chronic β-Adrenergic Agonist Administration

System	Effect/Side effect
Cardiovascular	Tachycardia (increased heart rate)
	Vasodilation
	Electrocardiogram changes[1]
	Cardiac arrhythmia
	Myocardial ischemia
	Myocardial necrosis[2]
	Potential inotropy[3]
Skeletal muscle	Tremor
	Spasms/cramps
Other metabolic parameters	Glycogenolysis
	Gluconeogenesis[4]
	Insulin production[5]
	Hypokalemia (decreased potassium)[6]
	Decreased magnesium[7]
	Lipolysis
	Increased lactate production
Central nervous system	Nervousness
	Insomnia
	Migraine
	Paresthesia
	Psychosis[8]

[1]Prolongation of QT interval; [2]infiltration of noncontractile material following chronic, high-dose administration; [3]some reports of increased contractile force following acute high-dose treatment; [4]overall effect of stimulating glycogenolysis and gluconeogenesis is to increase glucose production; [5]possibly due to stimulation of pancreatic islet cells; [6]linked to cardiac arrhythmia; [7]also linked to cardiac arrhythmia; [8]in extreme cases.

Adapted from Kendall & Haffner (1993).

1969; Gilman 1995; Strader et al. 1995; Rens-Domiano & Hamm 1995). In high doses, clenbuterol alters thyroid status, blocking the conversion of T4 to the active T3 (Zeman et al. 1988), which helps explain the alterations in body temperature and increased lipolysis. Alterations in intracellular Na^+ and K^+ are also thought to be implicated in the process of clenbuterol-induced muscle growth (Cartana & Stock 1995). Clenbuterol has also been reported to be a potent inhibitor of the inflammatory cytokines TNF-α and IL-6 (Izeboud et al 1999).

Clenbuterol treatment has been shown to produce hypertrophy of both fast- and slow-twitch muscle fibers (Apseloff et al. 1993), although the literature is divided on whether the effects are greater in type II (fast-twitch) muscle fibers (Maltin et al. 1986; Kim et al. 1992; Beerman et al. 1987; Miller et al. 1988; Zeman et al. 1988; Palmer et al. 1990; Smith et al. 1995) or in type I (slow-twitch) muscle fibers (Maltin et al. 1986; Beerman et al. 1987; Palmer et al. 1990).

Clenbuterol treatment in rats and mice produces slow-to-fast muscle fiber transitions within the predominantly slow soleus muscle (Maltin et al. 1986; Zeman et al. 1987; Beerman et al. 1987; Agbenyega & Wareham 1990; Palmer et al. 1990; Hayes & Williams 1994; Criswell et al. 1996; Stevens et al. 2000b; Rajab et al. 2000; Gregorevic 2000; Gregorevic et al. 2002). Fiber transitions can also occur within the subtypes of the fast fiber populations—for example, the conversion of fast-oxidative glycolytic (type IIa) fibers toward those having more glycolytic metabolism (i.e., fast glycolytic or type IIb muscle fibers; Maltin et al. 1986). This means that in animals, chronic clenbuterol treatment will cause typically slow muscles to become more fastlike in terms of their fiber type composition—not just their biochemical makeup (oxidative to glycolytic), but also their myosin heavy chain isoform composition and hence their contractile properties (Lynch et al. 1996). Similar fiber type transitions within the skeletal muscles of animals are usually possible only after chronic high-frequency electrical stimulation, and to a very limited extent after exercise (Lynch et al. 1995). Significant slow-to-fast transitions in the expression of myosin heavy chain isoforms and significant increases in the myofibrillar adenosine triphosphatase (ATPase) activity were found in the diaphragm and soleus muscles of young rats administered clenbuterol (1.5 mg/kg/day for 4 weeks) during the 21- to 49-day period of postnatal development (Polla et al. 2001).

Effects of Beta-2 Agonists on Muscle Strength

There have been numerous studies on animals regarding the use of β2-agonists and their effects on skeletal muscle. These studies have primarily focused on therapeutic applications of the anabolic properties of β2-agonists, such as clenbuterol, for reversing the muscle atrophy observed with aging (Carter et al. 1991; Chen & Alway 2000, 2001); denervation (Agbenyega & Wareham 1990; Maltin et al. 1987; Zeman et al. 1987; Babij & Booth 1988; Sneddon et al. 2000); muscle unloading (Delday & Maltin 1997; Ricart-Firinga et al. 2000; Stevens et al. 2000a; Canu et al. 2001) and muscle-wasting diseases such as muscular dystrophy (Maltin et al. 1987; Choo et al. 1989; Maltin et al. 1993b; Zeman et al. 1994; Agbenyega et al. 1995; Dupont-Versteegden 1996; Tawil 1999; Lynch 2001a, b); emphysema and COPD (Van der Heijden et al. 1998a,b); and amyotrophic lateral sclerosis (Puls et al. 1999). Although clenbuterol and other β2-agonists increase skeletal muscle mass in a variety of species (Kim & Sainz 1992), major inconsistencies exist regarding their effects on the functional properties of normal and diseased skeletal muscle (Zeman et al. 1988; Cairns & Dulhunty 1993; Hayes and Williams 1994; Zeman et al. 1994; Dupont-Versteegden et al. 1995; Dodd et al. 1996; Lynch et al. 1999, 2000b; Zhang et al. 1996). All of these studies on rats and mice have employed high doses of clenbuterol (~2 mg/kg) administered to the animals daily over a period of several weeks or months. The majority of studies show only minor (or no) improvement in the force-producing capacity and maximal power output of isolated muscles after chronic clenbuterol administration (Lynch et al. 2000a,b). In many cases, the force output per muscle cross-sectional area is actually reduced after clenbuterol administration, indicating that the intrinsic force-producing capacity of the muscles after treatment does not keep pace with the obvious increases in muscle mass (Gregorevic et al. 2002). Beta-2 agonists including clenbuterol and salbutamol have been used to increase the muscle tissue mass for cardiac assist surgery in which, in conjunction with electrical stimulation, a portion of the latissimus dorsi muscle is wrapped around the heart and stimulated to aid contraction of the ventricle (Petrou et al. 1999; Wright et al. 1999; Guldner et al. 2000).

There have been only a few studies on the effects of therapeutic doses of β2-agonists on exercise performance and skeletal muscle function in humans (Martineau et al. 1992; Maltin et al. 1993a; Kissel et al. 1998). Morton and colleagues (1996) tested 10-sec and 30-sec sprint cycling performance and leg flexion and leg extension muscular strength in nonasthmatic athletes and found that an acute dose of 50% μg of inhaled salmeterol had no performance-enhancing effects. Caruso and colleagues (1995) reported that nonasthmatic subjects receiving therapeutic doses of albuterol (given as 16 mg/day) for six weeks had improved strength in some exercises compared with untreated subjects, whereas Lemmer and colleagues

(1994) found no improvement with albuterol in nonasthmatic well-trained cyclists subjected to a 30-sec Wingate anaerobic power test. Healthy male subjects receiving a therapeutic dose of the β-agonist salbutamol (given as 8 mg twice a day) for three weeks showed only minor improvements in the strength of their quadriceps muscles compared with subjects given a placebo (Martineau et al. 1992). Whether these minor alterations in strength would be beneficial to athletes remains untested.

Beta-2 agonists have also been evaluated in human patients as a means of improving the size and strength of muscles affected by neuromuscular diseases or following orthopedic surgery. Orthopedic patients administered clenbuterol 20 μg twice daily for four weeks did not exhibit any improvement in the absolute strength of their knee extensor muscles compared with patients given placebo (Maltin et al. 1993a). A three-month pilot trial of albuterol (16 mg/day) given to 15 patients with facioscapulohumeral muscular dystrophy led to improved maximum voluntary isometric contractile performance (Kissel et al. 1998). Patients with muscle atrophy after spinal cord injury who were given a β-agonist, metaproterenol (80 mg/day), for four weeks showed increased forearm muscle size and strength, whereas three patients with spinal cord injury given salbutamol (2 mg/day) for two weeks showed improvements in the cross-sectional area of their vastus lateralis muscles but no improvement in contractile function (Murphy et al. 1999). In another study, treatment with the β2-agonist metaproterenol (80 mg/day) for four weeks increased muscle size and strength in patients with muscular atrophy following spinal cord injury (Signorile et al. 1995). Patients with low skeletal muscle strength and exercise capacity due to chronic heart failure showed no improvement in quadriceps muscle mass, maximal isometric strength, or muscle fatigue following treatment with salbutamol (8 mg twice daily) for three weeks (Harrington et al. 2000).

Effects of Beta-2 Agonists on Other Parameters of Exercise Performance

Studies on the effects of chronic use of β2-agonists in high doses on exercise performance have been conducted on animals. Ingalls and colleagues (1996) subjected mice to a combination of eight weeks of treadmill running (three sets of 3 min, 36-40 m/min, 10-17% grade, 30-sec recovery, 4 days/week) and clenbuterol treatment (1.6 mg/kg, 4 days/week) and found that clenbuterol treatment decreased total work performance. Although clenbuterol increased muscle mass, it had antagonistic effects on running performance (Ingalls et al. 1996). Clenbuterol

administration in rats altered the normal adaptations of skeletal muscle to endurance exercise training (Yaspelkis et al. 1999). Clenbuterol treatment (0.8 mg/kg for 8 weeks) decreased glucose transporter (GLUT-4) content and decreased citrate synthase activity in the skeletal muscles of obese Zucker rats (Kuo et al. 1996). For athletes involved in sports with a major endurance component, it would be predicted that clenbuterol treatment would impair muscle oxidative capacity. Other researchers have investigated the effects of clenbuterol and exercise training on skeletal muscle but have not reported changes in exercise performance directly (Torgan et al. 1995; Murphy et al. 1996).

Further evidence for the negative impact of clenbuterol on exercise performance comes from a recent study showing that long-term clenbuterol administration significantly decreased the sprint running, endurance swimming, and voluntary running training performance of rats (Duncan et al. 2000). These detrimental effects of clenbuterol on exercise performance have important implications for athletes involved in similar modes of training who are taking β2-agonists to increase muscle mass and/or decrease body fat. In addition to the clenbuterol-induced decreases in exercise performance, the findings of significant cardiac hypertrophy and localized collagen infiltration in the left ventricular wall in the hearts of some clenbuterol-treated rats highlight some of the undesirable adaptations following chronic (high dose) clenbuterol treatment (see "Side Effects of the Chronic Use of Beta-2 Agonists" on p. 54). Other studies have shown that clenbuterol treatment can reduce citrate synthase activity in skeletal muscles (Torgan et al. 1993) as well as decrease capillary density in the left ventricle and skeletal muscles of rats, increasing the diffusion distance for oxygen in the heart and skeletal muscles (Suzuki et al. 1997).

The IOC permits administration of the β2-agonist salbutamol only by inhalation for the management of asthma and exercise-induced asthma in athletes. It is interesting to note that about one of every five athletes who participated in the 1996 Summer Olympic Games in Atlanta had a past history of asthma, had symptoms that suggested asthma, or took asthma medications (Weiler et al. 1998; Weiler & Ryan 2000). Media reports after the 2000 Summer Olympic Games in Sydney revealed that 618 athletes had medical waivers to use drugs; of those waivers, 561 were for salbutamol (albuterol). This number of waivers was almost double that recorded at the Olympic Games in Atlanta four years earlier. Much attention has been devoted to distinguishing between the IOC-authorized use (inhaled) and the IOC-prohibited use (oral) of salbutamol by athletes (Berges et al. 2000; Ventura et al. 2000). Asthmatic patients given either salmeterol (50 μg) or salbutamol (200 μg) had improved cardiorespiratory responses (such as forced expiratory volume) compared with placebo-treated asthmatic subjects. However, cardiorespiratory, hemodynamic, or subjective responses to progressive maximum exercise tests were not different with salmeterol, salbutamol, or placebo, nor did endurance capacity change following any treatment (Robertson et al. 1994). Similarly, in studies on nonasthmatic cross-country skiers, acute salmeterol treatment did not have any beneficial effect on heart rate, blood lactate concentration, respiratory exchange ratio, running time to exhaustion, oxygen uptake, or minute ventilation during exercise. This lack of enhancement of exercise performance in healthy endurance athletes further supports the recent approval of salmeterol for prophylactic use by asthmatic athletes during training and competition (Sue-Chu et al. 1999; Sansund et al. 2000). Interestingly, most studies indicate that asthma is more common among athletes than in the general population (Nystad et al. 2000).

Beta-2 agonists are frequently used by elite cross-country skiers, a group of athletes with a high prevalence of asthma (Larsson et al. 1997; Wilber et al. 2000). Healthy, nonasthmatic athletes (cyclists, cross-country skiers, middle- and long-distance runners) with normal bronchial responsiveness tested the effect of an inhaled β-agonist, terbutaline, while exercising on a treadmill to exhaustion in a climate chamber maintained at 10 °C. Inhalation of terbutaline at a dose that produced significant bronchodilation did not influence physical performance at low temperature in healthy elite athletes (Larsson et al. 1997). Other researchers investigated the possible improvement in endurance performance in healthy well-trained athletes (17-30 years of age) after administration of inhaled salmeterol (long-acting β2-agonist) or salbutamol (short-acting β2-agonist) compared with placebo treatment (Carlsen et al. 1997). The authors reported no significant differences for ventilation, oxygen uptake, or heart rate at anaerobic threshold or at maximum performance between placebo and the β2-agonist-treated groups (Carlsen et al. 1997). Although lung function was increased significantly after exercise, there were no differences between the β2-agonist-treated and placebo groups. Of significance was the fact that running time to exhaustion was reduced significantly in both the long- and the short-acting β2-agonist treatment groups compared with the placebo group (Carlsen et al. 1997).

Apart from clenbuterol, terbutaline, and salmeterol, salbutamol also has been reputedly used by athletes for the purpose of athletic enhancement, especially by cyclists. Prominent cyclists have tested positive for salbutamol in Europe, where it is a banned substance (Delbeke et al. 1995). Most evidence would indicate that the ergogenic properties of salbutamol are far less than that of clenbuterol and that acute administration of a therapeutic dose of salbutamol is not ergogenic at all (Norris et al. 1996). Apart from potentially improving ventilatory capacity (Fleck et al. 1993), salbutamol is presumably being taken by endurance cyclists to enhance blood flow. An acute therapeutic effect of β2-receptor stimulation is to inhibit the contraction of smooth muscle, including that surrounding blood vessels. This would cause vasodilation, which in turn would reduce peripheral resistance and enhance blood flow. The increased venous return and greater preload on the heart would cause cardiac output to be increased. Such effects are not likely to result after therapeutic use (for asthmatics), but instead only when the β2-agonists are taken in large doses and for extended periods. Such a strategy is likely to lead to adverse side effects that will, in turn, decrease exercise performance.

Side Effects of the Chronic Use of Beta-2 Agonists

The side effects associated with long-term therapeutic use of β2-agonists have been detailed previously (Kendall & Haffner 1993; Burgess et al. 1997). Excluding athletes, there are two groups of individuals exposed to β2-agonists: patients being treated with the drugs, and individuals who eat the meat of animals that have been treated with the drugs (Baldi et al. 1994; Embleton & Thorne 1998; Sporano et al. 1998). The most frequently reported side effects associated with the use of β2-agonists include nausea, headaches, and insomnia (see table 4.2). Excessive clenbuterol intake (in high μg-mg/kg doses) leads to symptoms such as muscle tremor, palpitations, muscle cramps, headache, and peripheral vasodilatation (Prather et al. 1995). The most serious side effects of excessive β2-agonist intake are those associated with the heart (Au et al. 2000).

There are four β-adrenoceptors in the heart (Kaumann 1997), so it is not surprising that adrenergic stimulation from β2-agonists has major effects on cardiac as well as skeletal muscle (Deshaies et al. 1980; Rothwell & Stock 1985; Reeds et al. 1986; MacLennan & Edwards 1989; Palmer et al. 1990). Although the exact mechanisms responsible for cardiac growth following β2-agonist administration have not been determined, it appears that they are different from those responsible for skeletal muscle hypertrophy (Duncan 1996). Cardiac adaptations are mediated by the cyclooxygenase metabolite of arachidonic acid (Emery et al. 1984; Reeds et al. 1986; Maltin et al. 1987), meaning that the cardiac hypertrophy should be preventable by administration of fenbufen, a nonsteroidal anti-inflammatory drug that inhibits the cyclooxygenase pathway. This would inhibit the release of prostaglandins and protein synthesis without inhibiting the skeletal muscle response (Palmer et al. 1990; Duncan

1996). Studies by Sillence and colleagues (1991a) showed that the effects of clenbuterol on the heart are also mediated by β2-adrenoceptor stimulation, a finding that supported earlier reports of the presence of functional β2-adrenoceptors in the myocardium (Kaumann 1997).

Tachycardia (rapid heartbeat) is one of the first indications that β2-agonists such as clenbuterol are having an effect. Sudden death due to cardiac failure has been reported among bodybuilders suspected of using clenbuterol in conjunction with diuretics (Embleton & Thorne 1998) and also in clenbuterol-treated rats during high-intensity swimming exercise (Duncan et al. 2000). Chronic use of high doses of clenbuterol or salbutamol in rats almost invariably produces significant cardiac hypertrophy (Cepero et al. 1998; Duncan et al. 2000). Clenbuterol treatment in rats has also been shown to increase cortisol and corticosterone secretions, and to increase the size of the adrenal glands due to hyperplasia of adrenocortical cells (Illera et al. 1998).

Athletes apparently stop using clenbuterol because of headaches, nervousness, insomnia, rapid heartbeat/ palpitations, increased blood pressure, nausea, significantly elevated body temperatures, sweating, alternating fevers and chills, nosebleeds, hives, uncontrolled muscle tremor, serious muscle cramps, or a combination of these (Prather et al. 1995; Duncan 1996). There appears to be great variety in the tolerance levels for this drug among humans, with some athletes reporting no side effects and others finding the same doses unbearable (Duncan 1996). Clenbuterol administration has been linked to alterations in animal behavior including increased aggression in mice (Matsumoto et al. 1994) and suppression of feeding following acute treatment in rats (Yamashita et al. 1994). Interestingly, data from Benelli and colleagues (1990) indicated that clenbuterol negatively affected the copulatory behavior of sexually vigorous male rats but improved that of sexually sluggish ones, providing evidence that central β-receptor activation produces behavioral effects. Clenbuterol has been shown to produce effects on behavior similar to those seen after administration of clinically active antidepressant drugs, indicating that clenbuterol and related β2-agonists may possess antidepressant activity (J.M. O'Donnell 1990; Murugaiah & O'Donnell 1994).

Bodybuilders using clenbuterol are especially susceptible to muscle cramps in the time leading up to a contest. At these times many bodybuilders also use diuretics to aid the removal of excess body water. During this process they also inevitably remove important ions (such as K+) and electrolytes critical for normal organ function (Embleton & Thorne 1998). Anecdotal reports have advised bodybuilders to take potassium supplements when using clenbuterol in order to control their electrolyte status and reduce muscle cramping. The advice given to

bodybuilders to monitor their blood pressure regularly when using clenbuterol is also important but trivializes the hidden dangers of excessive clenbuterol use—namely, its "silent" and deleterious effects on cardiac structure and function.

Previous studies have shown that chronic use of β2-agonists in high doses can have toxic effects on the heart (Kendall & Haffner 1993). Histological examination of the myocardium of dogs after chronic treatment with isoprenaline in mg/kg doses revealed severe necrosis (Kendall & Haffner 1993). Congestion, interstitial edema, hypertrophy of muscle fibers, and myocardial necrosis were evident in rats given very large doses (between 17 and 150 mg/kg daily) of another β2-agonist, salbutamol, for one month (Libretto 1994). Increases in cardiac mass of up to 27% have been reported (Duncan 1996). Severe myocardial lesions were found in the hearts of sheep given intravenous doses of either salbutamol, fenoterol, or isoprenaline (128 μg/kg at 15-min intervals) for four days (Pack et al. 1994). Isoproterenol treatment produced necrosis and an increase in collagen content in the hearts of rats (Beznak 1962) even when applied in low doses (Benjamin et al. 1989).

Shorter periods of clenbuterol administration did not appear to affect cardiac function despite a 26% increase in left ventricular hypertrophy (Wong et al. 1998). Similar findings of little or no change in cardiac function have been reported in rats treated with low doses (0.2-0.4 mg/ kg body mass) of isoproterenol (Baldwin et al. 1982; Taylor & Tang 1984), although a recent study suggests that in rats, the changes to the heart during isoproterenol-induced cardiac hypertrophy are not homogenous and that myocardial mass, myocardial relaxation, left ventricular stiffness, and systolic function differ between subgroups of animals (Murad & Tucci 2000).

On the contrary, rats given high doses of clenbuterol (2 mg/kg) daily for several months showed significant cardiac hypertrophy, infiltration of collagen in the left ventricular walls (Duncan et al. 2000), and impaired cardiac mechanics, including reductions in left ventricular pressure (Duncan et al. 1996). Clearly, the dosages of clenbuterol administered in these studies are higher than those used by athletes. However, the doses of clenbuterol employed by bodybuilders exceed typical therapeutic recommendations. The adverse effects of high-dose β2-agonists on the heart highlight the often forgotten side effects and dangers associated with these drugs. In addition, bodybuilders often use clenbuterol in conjunction with anabolic steroids, a combination that has proved lethal (Goldstein et al. 1998). The adverse side effects associated with chronic adrenergic stimulation are summarized in table 4.2.

Because of these adverse side effects, the suitability of clenbuterol as an animal growth promoter has been questioned (Sillence et al. 1991a), with cimaterol and ractopamine suggested as alternatives for use in animal production. It is clear that athletes taking clenbuterol in excessive doses and for extended periods are placing themselves at risk. Although many of the side effects (i.e., sweating, tachycardia, and tremor) cease when the athlete goes off clenbuterol, the question whether the deleterious effects on the heart are reversible is difficult to answer. Evidence from clenbuterol-treated animals indicates that the deposition of noncontractile fibrotic material in the ventricular walls is likely to affect cardiac mechanics and impair exercise performance (Duncan et al. 1996). On the basis of its deleterious and potentially lethal side effects, athletes would be wise to stay clear of clenbuterol altogether. A summary of the proposed effects of clenbuterol administration on striated muscle and potential implications for sports performance is presented in table 4.3.

Latest Research on Beta-2 Agonists for Promoting Muscle Growth

The latest research involving the muscle anabolic potential of β2-agonists is based on the development of antibodies that can activate β2-adrenoceptors and hence mimic the effects of β2-agonists such as clenbuterol (Hill et al. 1998). Immunological approaches are potentially alternative methods to the direct administration of growth-promoting compounds to manipulate growth and body composition (Kim & Kim 1997). This research is being led by those involved in the livestock industry, where the immunoneutralization of somatostatin has already improved growth rate in lambs (Spencer & Oliver 1996; Laarveld et al. 1986). It is clear that muscle growth, carcass composition, and feed efficiency can be improved

through the use of β2-agonists (Sillence et al. 1993). These researchers have faced two major setbacks: the difficulty in administering these compounds to large herds that graze on extensive pastures and, as discussed already, the very serious side effects of clenbuterol poisoning that have occurred when humans have eaten the flesh of animals treated (illegally) with clenbuterol (Hill et al. 1998).

Researchers are developing vaccines for use in livestock that cause the production of antibodies that activate tissue β2-adrenoceptors. They claim that only one or two doses of the vaccine would be needed; that the antibodies would not accumulate in muscle or fat stores; and that gentle cooking would destroy any of the antibodies or, failing this, would be easily degraded in the gut (Hill et al. 1998). A vaccine was developed that caused rabbits to produce antibodies with "β-agonist-like" activity, recognizing β-adrenoceptors in isolated bovine muscle as well as enhancing the relaxant effects of a β-agonist in smooth muscle (Hill et al. 1998).

Although such vaccine research has legitimate application for improving growth rate, feed efficiency, and body composition in the livestock industry, it is not too difficult to predict that if this research has any possible application for enhancing muscle growth for human athletes, it will be exploited.

Reducing some of the side effects of clenbuterol, particularly its effects on the heart, is another major area of β-agonist research. Clenbuterol is available commercially as a racemic mixture (1:1 ratio) of two enantiomers, (−)-R and (+)-S, but whether one or both of the enantiomers produce the undesirable side effects has received little attention. Recent work by Von Deutsch and colleagues (2000) showed that both clenbuterol enantiomers produced significant increases in skeletal

---

Table 4.3 Summary of Proposed Effects of Extended Clenbuterol Administration on Striated Muscle Properties and Potential Implications for Sport Performance

Parameter	Effect of clenbuterol	Implications for performance
Muscle fiber size	Significant hypertrophy	Increased muscle mass desirable for body-building as well as strength and power sports
Muscle regeneration	Enhanced muscle regenerative capacity	Increased recovery from injury, improved recovery from training
Muscle force and power	May be increased under some (but not all) circumstances	Desirable for strength- and power-related sports/activities
Muscle endurance	Decreased aerobic enzyme activities and decreased GLUT-4 protein levels	May prevent endurance training adaptations and therefore not desirable for such athletes
Heart size	May cause hypertrophy and some fibrosis	Increased risk for cardiovascular disease
Heart function	Possible decrease in left ventricular pressure	Impairment of normal cardiac function is clearly very dangerous

The predictions relating to the effect of clenbuterol on striated muscle and sporting performance derive primarily from animal-based studies.

muscle mass, but that both were less active in producing cardiac muscle hypertrophy than the racemic mixture. If clenbuterol is to be used clinically as a therapeutic anabolic agent, addressing the issue of these deleterious side effects must be a priority area of research.

Conclusion and Legal Implications

Of all the β2-agonists that have been shown to have anabolic properties on skeletal muscle, clenbuterol is the most notorious. In laboratory animals, clenbuterol has been shown to produce significant increases in skeletal muscle mass; and clenbuterol is used illegally by athletes to maintain the anabolic effects after steroid use is discontinued (Schwenk 1997). In addition to its muscle anabolic effects, clenbuterol is a potent lipolytic agent capable of decreasing fat deposition and increasing lean body mass. As such, clenbuterol is often referred to as a repartitioning agent. Clenbuterol use by athletes is banned by the IOC, the United States Olympic Committee (USOC), and the National Collegiate Athletic Association.

Except for approved use in the medical treatment of asthma, all β-agonists are generally banned by the USOC. Some inhaled β-agonists such as albuterol, terbutaline, and salmeterol are now permitted by the IOC for medical purposes, since their anabolic effects are negligible compared with those of the more powerful clenbuterol. Despite the lack of evidence that inhaled β-agonists have any significant ergogenic effect, an ever increasing number of athletes are claiming to be asthmatic and using β-agonists for their purported ergogenic properties (Eichner 1997). The extensive animal-based research makes it clear that the administration of β-agonists (especially in high doses) can produce significant undesirable physiological side effects that are likely to deleteriously affect athletic performance in the long term. Despite this warning, it is clear that athletes will continue to use β-agonists if they perceive that these drugs will improve performance.

Acknowledgments

The author is grateful to the Australian Research Council, the National Health and Medical Research Council (Australia), the Rebecca L. Cooper Medical Research Foundation, and the Muscular Dystrophy Association (USA) for grant support.

References

Agbenyega, E.T., Morton, R.H., Hatton, P.A. & Wareham, A.C. (1995). Effect of the β2-adrenergic agonist clenbuterol on the growth of fast- and slow-twitch skeletal muscle of the dystrophic (C57BL6J dy2J/dy2J) mouse. Comparative Biochemistry and Physiology 111C:97-103.

Agbenyega, E.T. & Wareham, A.C. (1990). Effect of clenbuterol on normal and denervated muscle growth and contractility. Muscle & Nerve 13:199-203.

Anstead, M.J., Hunt, T.A., McConnell, J.W., & Burki, N.K. (2001). Effects of therapeutic doses of albuterol on β2 adrenergic receptor density and metabolic change. Journal of Asthma 38:59-64.

Apseloff, G., Girten, B., Walker, M., Shepard, D.R., Krecic, M.E., Stern, L.S. & Gerber, N. (1993). Aminohydroxybutane bisphosphonate and clenbuterol prevent bone changes and retard muscle atrophy respectively in tail-suspended rats. Journal of Pharmacology and Experimental Therapeutics 264:1071-1078.

Arch, J.R., Ainsworth, A.T., Cawthorne, M.A., Piercy, V., Sennitt, M.V., Thody, V.E., Wilson, C. & Wilson, S. (1984). Atypical beta-adrenoceptor on brown adipocytes as target for anti-obesity drugs. Nature 309:163-165.

Arch, J.R. & Kaumann, A.J. (1993). β3 and atypical β-adrenoceptors. Medical Research Reviews 13:663-729.

Au, D.H., Lemaitre, R.N., Curtis, J.R., Smith, N.L. & Psaty, B.M. (2000). The risk of myocardial infarction associated with inhaled beta-adrenoceptor agonists. American Journal of Respiratory & Critical Care Medicine 161:827-830.

Babij, P. & Booth, F.W. (1988). Clenbuterol prevents or inhibits loss of specific mRNAs in atrophying rat skeletal muscle. American Journal of Physiology 254:C657-C660.

Baker, P.K., Dalrymple, R.H., Ingle, D.L. & Ricks, C.A. (1984). Use of a β-adrenergic agonist to alter muscle and fat deposition in lambs. Journal of Animal Science 59:1256-1261.

Baldi, A., Bontempo, V., Cheli, F., Corino, C. & Polidori, F. (1994). Hormonal and metabolic responses to the stress of transport and slaughterhouse procedures in clenbuterol-fed pigs. Journal of Veterinary Medicine 41:189-196.

Baldwin, K.M., Ernst, S.B., Mullin, W.J., Schrader, L.F. & Herrick, R.E. (1982). Exercise capacity and cardiac function of rats with drug-induced cardiac enlargement. Journal of Applied Physiology 52:591-595.

Bardsley, R.G., Allcock, S.M., Dawson, J.M., Dumelow, N.W., Higgins, J.A., Lasslet, Y.V., Lockley, A.K., Parr, T. & Buttery, P.J. (1992). Effect of beta-agonists on expression of calpain and calpastatin in skeletal muscle. Biochimie 74:267-273.

Beerman, D.H., Butler, W.R., Hogue, D.E., Fishell, V.K., Dalrymple, R.H., Ricks, C.A. & Scanes, C.G. (1987). Cimaterol-induced muscle hypertrophy and altered endocrine status in lambs. Journal of Animal Science 65:1514-1524.

Belahsen, R. & Deshaies, Y. (1992). Modulation of lipoprotein lipase activity in the rat by the beta 2-adrenergic agonist clenbuterol. Canadian Journal of Physiology and Pharmacology 70:1555-1562.

Bell, A.W., Bauman, D.E., Beerman, D.H. & Harrell, R.J. (1998). Nutrition, development and efficacy of growth modifiers in livestock species. Journal of Nutrition 128:360S-363S.

Benelli, A., Zanoli, P. & Bertolini, A. (1990). Effect of clenbuterol on sexual behavior in male rats. Physiology & Behavior 47:373-376.

Benjamin, I.J., Jalil, J.E., Tan, L.B., Cho, K., Weber, K.T. & Clark, W.A. (1989). Isoproterenol-induced myocardial fibrosis in relation to myocyte necrosis. Circulation Research 65:657-670.

Benson, D.W., Foley-Nelson, T., Chance, W.T., Zhang, F.S., James, J.H. & Fischer, J.E. (1991). Decreased myofibrillar protein breakdown following treatment with clenbuterol. Journal of Surgical Research 50:1-5.

Bergen, W.G. & Merkel, R.A. (1991). Body composition of animals treated with partitioning agents—implications for human health. FASEB Journal 5:2951-2957.

Berges, R., Segura, J., Ventura, R., Fitch, K.D., Morton, A.R., Farre, M., Mas, M. & de la Torre, X. (2000). Discrimination of prohibited oral use of salbutamol from authorized inhaled asthma treatment. Clinical Chemistry 46:1365-1375.

Beznak, M. (1962). Hemodynamics during the acute phase of myocardial damage caused by isoproterenol. Canadian Journal of Biochemistry and Physiology 40:25-30.

Blum, J.W. & Fluekiger, N. (1988). Early metabolic and endocrine effects of perorally administered β-adrenoceptor agonists in calves. European Journal of Pharmacology 151:177-194.

Bohorov, O., Buttery, P.J., Correia, J.H. & Soar, J.B. (1987). The effect of the β2-adrenergic agonist clenbuterol or implantation with oestradiol plus trenbolone acetate on protein in wether lambs. British Journal of Nutrition 57:99-107.

Bowman, W.C. & Nott, M.W. (1969). Actions of sympathomimetic amines and their antagonists on skeletal muscle. Pharmacological Reviews 21:27-72.

Brambilla, G., Cenci, T., Franconi, F., Galarini, R., Macri, A., Rondoni, F., Strozzi, M. & Loizzo, A. (2000). Clinical and pharmacological profile in a clenbuterol epidemic poisoning of contaminated beef meat in Italy. Toxicology Letters 114:47-53.

Brower, K.J., Blow, F.C., Young, J.P. & Hill, E.M. (1991). Symptoms and correlates of anabolic-androgenic steroid dependence. British Journal of Addiction 86:759-768.

Bruckmaier, R.M. & Blum, J.W. (1992). Responses of calves to treadmill exercise during beta-adrenergic agonist administration. Journal of Animal Science 70:2809-2821.

Burgess, C.D. (1993). An overview of experimental methods. In (eds) Beasley, R. & Pearce, N.E., The Role of Beta Receptor Agonist Therapy in Asthma Mortality, CRC Press, Boca Raton, Florida, pp127-148.

Burgess, C.D., Beasley, R., Crane, J. & Pearce, N. (1997). Adverse effects of beta2-agonists. In (eds) Pauwels, R. & O'Byrne, P.M., Beta2-Agonists in Asthma Treatment, Marcel Dekker, New York, pp257-282.

Cairns, S.P. & Dulhunty, A.F. (1993). β-adrenergic potentiation of E-C coupling increases force in rat skeletal muscle. Muscle & Nerve 16:1317-1325.

Canu, M.H., Stevens, L., Ricart-Firinga, C., Picquet, F. & Falempin, M. (2001). Effect of the β2-agonist clenbuterol on the locomotor activity of rat submitted to a 14-day period of hypodynamia-hypokinesia. Behavioural Brain Research 122:103-112.

Carlsen, K.H., Ingjer, F., Kirkegaard, H. & Thyness, B. (1997). The effect of inhaled salbutamol and salmeterol on lung function and endurance performance in healthy well-trained athletes. Scandinavian Journal of Medicine and Science in Sports 7:160-165.

Cartana, J. & Stock, M.J. (1995). Effects of clenbuterol and salbutamol on tissue rubidium uptake in vivo. Metabolism 44:119-125.

Carter, W.J., Dang, A.Q., Faas, F.H. & Lynch, M.E. (1991). Effects of clenbuterol on skeletal muscle mass, body composition, and recovery from surgical stress in senescent rats. Metabolism 40:855-860.

Caruso, J.F., Signorile, J.F., Perry, A.C., Leblanc, B., Williams, R., Clark, M. & Bamman, M.M. (1995). The effects of albuterol and isokinetic exercise on the quadriceps muscle group. Medicine and Science in Sports and Exercise 27:1471-1476.

Cepero, M., Cubría, J.C., Reguera, R., Balaña-Fouce, R., Ordóñez, C. & Ordóñez, D. (1998). Plasma and muscle polyamine levels in aerobically exercised rats treated with salbutamol. Journal of Pharmacy and Pharmacology 50:1059-1064.

Cepero, M., Pérez-Pertejo, Y., Cubría, J.C., Reguera, R., Balaña-Fouce, R., Ordóñez, C. & Ordóñez Escudero, D. (2000). Muscle and serum changes with salbutamol administration in aerobically exercised rats. Comparative Biochemistry and Physiology 126C:45-51.

Chen, K.D. & Alway, S.E. (2000). A physiological level of clenbuterol does not prevent atrophy or loss of force in skeletal muscle of old rats. Journal of Applied Physiology 89:606-612.

Chen, K.D. & Alway, S.E. (2001). Clenbuterol reduces soleus muscle fatigue during disuse in aged rats. Muscle & Nerve 24:211-222.

Choo, J.J., Horan, M.A., Little, R.A. & Rothwell, N.J. (1989). Muscle wasting associated with endotoxemia in the rat: modification by the β2-adrenoceptor agonist clenbuterol. Bioscience Reports 9:615-621.

Choo, J.J., Horan, M.A., Little, R.A. & Rothwell, N.J. (1992). Anabolic effects of clenbuterol on skeletal muscle are mediated by β2-adrenoceptor activation. American Journal of Physiology 263:E50-E56.

Chwalibog, A., Jensen, K. & Thorbek, G. (1996). Quantitative protein and fat metabolism in bull calves treated with β-adrenergic agonist. Archives of Animal Nutrition 49:159-167.

Claeys, M.C., Mulvaney, D.R., McCarthy, F.D., Gore, M.T., Marple, D.N. & Sartin, J.L. (1989). Skeletal muscle protein synthesis and growth hormone secretion in young lambs treated with clenbuterol. Journal of Animal Science 67:2245-2254.

Clarkson, P.M. & Thompson, H.S. (1997). Drugs and sport—research findings and limitations. Sports Medicine 24:366-384.

Criswell, D.S., Powers, S.K. & Herb, R.A. (1996). Clenbuterol-induced fiber type transition in the soleus of adult rats. European Journal of Applied Physiology and Occupational Physiology 74:391-396.

Delbeke, F.T., Desmet, N. & Debackere, M. (1995). The abuse of doping agents in competing bodybuilders in Flanders (1988-1993). International Journal of Sports Medicine 16:66-70.

Delday, M.I. & Maltin, C.A. (1997). Clenbuterol increases the expression of myogenin but not myoD in immobilized rat muscles. American Journal of Physiology 35:E941-E944.

Deshaies, Y., Willemot, J. & LeBlanc, J. (1980). Protein synthesis, amino acids uptake, and pools during isoproterenol-induced hypertrophy of the rat heart and tibialis muscle. Canadian Journal of Physiology and Pharmacology 59:113-121.

Dodd, S.L., Powers, S.K., Vrabas, I., Criswell, D., Stetson, S. & Hussain, R. (1996). Effects of clenbuterol on contractile and biochemical properties of skeletal muscle. Medicine and Science in Sports and Exercise 28:669-676.

Duncan, N.D. (1996). Striated muscle adaptations resulting from exercise and clenbuterol administration. Ph.D. thesis, Department of Physiology, The University of Melbourne, Victoria, Australia.

Duncan, N.D., Lynch, G.S., Jones, D.L. & Williams, D.A. (1996). Cardiac muscle contractility following chronic clenbuterol administration and exercise. Medicine and Science in Sports and Exercise (Supplement) 28:S167.

Duncan, N.D., Williams, D.A. & Lynch, G.S. (2000). Deleterious effects of clenbuterol treatment on endurance and sprint exercise performance in rats. Clinical Science 98:339-347.

Dupont-Versteegden, E.E. (1996). Exercise and clenbuterol as strategies to decrease the progression of muscular dystrophy in mdx mice. Journal of Applied Physiology 80:734-741.

Dupont-Versteegden, E.E., Katz, M.S. & McCarter, R.J. (1995). Beneficial versus adverse effects of long-term use of clenbuterol in mdx mice. Muscle & Nerve 18:1447-1459.

Eichner, E.R. (1997). Ergogenic aids: what athletes are using—and why. The Physician and Sportsmedicine 25:70.

Elfellah, M.S., Dalling, R., Kantola, I.M., & Reid, J.L. (1989). Beta-andrenoceptors and human skeletal muscle characterization of receptor subtype and effect of age. British Journal of Clinical Pharmacology 27:31-38.

Embleton, P. & Thorne, G. (1998). Anabolic primer. MuscleMag International, Ontario, Canada.

Emery, P.W., Rothwell, N.J., Stock, M.J. & Winter, P.D. (1984). Chronic effects of β2-adrenergic agonists on body composition and protein synthesis in the rat. Bioscience Reports 4:83-91.

Fleck, S.J., Lucia, A., Storm, W.W., Vint, P.F. & Zimmerman, S.D. (1993). Effects of acute inhalation of albuterol on submaximal and maximal VO_2 and blood lactate. International Journal of Sports Medicine 14:235-243.

Forsberg, N.E., Ilian, M.A., Ali-Bar, A., Cheeke, P.R. & Wehr, H.A. (1989). Effects of cimaterol on rabbit growth and myofibrillar protein degradation and on calcium-dependent proteinase and calpastatin activities in skeletal muscle. Journal of Animal Science 67:3313-3321.

Friedl, K.E. (2000). Performance-enhancing substances: effects, risks, and appropriate alternatives. In (eds) Baechle, T.R. & Earle, R.W., Essentials of Strength Training and Conditioning, Human Kinetics, Champaign, Illinois, pp209-228.

Garay, J.B., Jimenez, J.E.H., Jimenez, M.L., Sebastian, M.V., Matesanz, J.P., Moreno, P.M. & Galiana, J.R. (1997). Clenbuterol poisoning—clinical manifestations and analytical findings in an epidemic outbreak in Mosteles, Madrid. Revista Clinica Espanola 197:92-95.

Gilman, A.G. (1995). G proteins and regulation of adenyl cyclase. Bioscience Reports 15:65-97.

Goldstein, D.R., Dobbs, T., Krull, B. & Plumb, V.J. (1998). Clenbuterol and anabolic steroids: a previously unreported cause of myocardial infarction with normal coronary arteriograms. Southern Medical Journal 91:780-784.

Gregorevic, P. (2000). Aspects of skeletal muscle regeneration and adaptation. Ph.D. thesis, Department of Physiology, The University of Melbourne, Victoria, Australia.

Gregorevic, P., Williams, D.A. & Lynch, G.S. (2002). Effects of LIF on fast and slow muscle fibers of the rat are modulated with clenbuterol treatment. Muscle & Nerve 25:194-201.

Greife, H.A., Klotz, G. & Berschauer, F. (1989). Effects of the phenethanolamine clenbuterol on protein and lipid metabolism in growing rats. Journal of Animal Physiology and Animal Nutrition 61:19-27.

Guggenbuhl, P. (1996). Evaluation of β2-adrenergic agonists repartitioning effects in the rat by a non-destructive method. Journal of Animal Physiology and Animal Nutrition 75:31-39.

Guldner, N.W., Klapproth, P., Grossherr, M., Stephan, M., Rumpel, E., Noel, R. & Sievers, H.H. (2000). Clenbuterol-supported dynamic training of skeletal muscle ventricles against systemic load—a key for powerful circulatory assist? Circulation 101:2213-2219.

Hamby, P.L., Stouffer, J.R. & Smith, S.B. (1986). Muscle metabolism and real-time ultrasound measurement of muscle and subcutaneous adipose growth in lambs fed diets containing a beta-agonist. Journal of Animal Science 63:1410-1417.

Hansen, J.A., Yen, J.T., Nelssen, J.L., Nienaber, J.A., Goodband, R.D. & Wheeler, T.L. (1997a). Effects of somatotropin and salbutamol in three genotypes of finishing barrows: growth, carcass, and calorimeter criteria. Journal of Animal Science 75:1798-1809.

Hansen, J.A., Yen, J.T., Nelssen, J.L., Nienaber, J.A., Goodband, R.D. & Wheeler, T.L. (1997b). Effects of somatotropin and salbutamol in three genotypes of finishing barrows: blood hormones and metabolites and muscle characteristics. Journal of Animal Science 75:1810-1821.

Harrington, D., Chua, T.P. & Coats, A.J.S. (2000). The effect of salbutamol on skeletal muscle in chronic heart failure. International Journal of Cardiology 73:257-265.

Hayes, A. & Williams, D.A. (1994). Long-term clenbuterol administration alters the isometric contractile properties of skeletal muscle from normal and dystrophin-deficient mdx mice. Clinical and Experimental Pharmacology and Physiology 21:757-765.

Hill, R.A., Hoey, A.J. & Sillence, M.N. (1998). Functional activity of antibodies at the bovine β2-adrenoceptor. Journal of Animal Science 76:1651-1661.

Hoey, A.J., Reich, M.M., Davis, G., Shorthose, R. & Sillence, M.N. (1995). Beta (2)-adrenoceptor-densities do not correlate with growth, carcass quality, or meat quality in cattle. Journal of Animal Science 73:3281-3286.

Huang, H., Gazzola, C., Pegg, G.G. & Sillence, M.N. (1998). Effect of corticosterone on beta-adrenoceptor density in rat skeletal muscle. Journal of Animal Science 76:999-1003.

Huang, H., Gazzola, C., Pegg, G.G. & Sillence, M.N. (2000). Differential effects of dexamethasone and clenbuterol on rat growth and on β2-adrenoceptors in lung and skeletal muscle. Journal of Animal Science 78:604-608.

Hulot, F., Ouhayoun, J. & Manoucheri, M. (1996). Effect of clenbuterol on productive performance, body composition and muscle biochemistry in the rabbit. Meat Science 42:457-464.

Illera, J.C., Silvan, G., Blass, A., Martinez, M.M. & Illera, M. (1998). The effect of clenbuterol on adrenal function in rats. Analyst 123:2521-2524.

Ingalls, C.P., Barnes, W.S. & Smith, S.B. (1996). Interaction between clenbuterol and run training: effects on exercise performance and MLC isoform content. Journal of Applied Physiology 80:795-801.

Inkster, J.E., Deb Hovell, F.D., Kyle, D.J., Brown, D.S. & Lobley, G.E. (1989). The effects of clenbuterol on basal protein turnover and endogenous nitrogen loss in sheep. British Journal of Nutrition 62:285-296.

Izeboud, C.A., Monshouwer, M., van Miert, A.S. & Witkamp, R.F. (1999). The beta-adrenoceptor agonist clenbuterol is a potent inhibitor of the LPS-induced production of TNF-alpha and IL-6 in vitro and in vivo. Inflammation Research 48:497-502.

Kaumann, A.J. (1997). Four β-adrenoceptor subtypes in the mammalian heart. Trends in the Pharmacological Sciences 18:70-76.

Kearns, C.F., McKeever, K.H., Malinowski, K., Struck, M.B. & Abe, T. (2001). Chronic administration of therapeutic levels of clenbuterol acts as a repartitioning agent. Journal of Applied Physiology 91:2064-2070.

Kendall, M.J. & Haffner, C.A. (1993). The acute unwanted effects of β2 receptor agonist therapy. In (eds) Beasley, R.

& Pearce, N.E., The Role of Beta Receptor Agonist Therapy in Asthma Mortality, CRC Press, Boca Raton, Florida, pp163-199.

Kim, Y.H. & Kim, Y.S. (1997). Effects of active immunization against clenbuterol on the growth promoting effect of clenbuterol in rats. Journal of Animal Science 75:446-453.

Kim, Y.S. & Sainz, R.D. (1992). β-adrenergic agonists and hypertrophy of skeletal muscles. Life Sciences 50:397-407.

Kim, Y.S., Sainz, R.D., Summers, R.J. & Molenaar, P. (1992). Cimaterol reduces beta-adrenergic receptor density in rat skeletal muscles. Journal of Animal Science 70:115-122.

Kissel, J.T., McDermott, M.P., Natarajan, R., Mendell, J.R., Pandya, S., King, W.M., Griggs, R.C. & Tawil, R. (1998). Pilot trial of albuterol in facioscapulohumeral muscular dystrophy. Neurology 50:1402-1406.

Koohmarie, M., Shackleford, S.D., Muggli-Cockett, N.E. & Stone, R.T. (1991). Effect of the β-adrenergic agonist L644,969 on muscle growth, endogenous proteinase activities, and postmortem proteolysis in wether lambs. Journal of Animal Science 69:4823-4835.

Kuo, C.H., Ding, Z.P. & Ivy, J.L. (1996). Interaction of exercise training and clenbuterol on GLUT-4 protein in muscle of obese Zucker rats. American Journal of Physiology 34:E847-E854.

Laarveld, B., Haplin, R.K. & Kerr, D.E. (1986). Somatostatin immunization and growth of lambs. Canadian Journal of Animal Science 66:77-84.

Larsson, K., Gavhed, D., Larsson, L., Holmer, I., Jorfelt, L. & Ohlsen, P. (1997). Influence of a beta(2)-agonist on physical performance at low temperature in elite athletes. Medicine and Science in Sports and Exercise 29:1631-1636.

Lemmer, J.T., Fleck, S.J., Wallach, J.M., Fox, S., Burke, E.R., Kearney, J.T. & Storms, W.W. (1994). The effects of albuterol on power output in non-asthmatic athletes. International Journal of Sports Medicine 16:243-249.

Levitzki, A. (1986). β-adrenergic receptors and their mode of coupling to adenylate cyclase. Physiological Reviews 66:819-854.

Li, Y.Z., Christopherson, R.J., Li, B.T. & Moibi, J.A. (2000). Effects of a beta-adrenergic agonist (L-644,969) on performance and carcass traits of growing lambs in a cold environment. Canadian Journal of Animal Science 80:459-465.

Libretto, S.E. (1994). A review of the toxicology of salbutamol (albuterol). Archives of Toxicology 68:213-216.

Liggett, S.B., Freedman, N.J., Schwinn, D.A. & Lefkowitz, R.J. (1993). Structural basis for receptor subtype-specific regulation revealed by a chimeric β3/β2-adrenergic receptor. Proceedings of the National Academy of Sciences (USA) 90:2665-3669.

Liggett, S.B. & Green, S.A. (1997). Molecular biology of the beta2-adrenergic receptor. In (eds) Pauwels, R. & O'Byrne, P.M., Beta2-Agonists in Asthma Treatment, Marcel Dekker, New York, pp19-34.

Liggett, S.B., Shah, S.D. & Cryer, P.E. (1988). Characterisation of β-adrenergic receptors of human skeletal muscle obtained by needle biopsy. American Journal of Physiology 254:E795-E798.

Lynch, G.S. (2001a). Novel therapies for muscular dystrophy. Expert Opinion on Therapeutic Patents 11:587-601.

Lynch, G.S. (2001b). Therapies for improving muscle function in neuromuscular disorders. Exercise and Sport Sciences Reviews 29:141-148.

Lynch, G.S., Hayes, A., Campbell, S.P. & Williams, D.A. (1996). Effects of β2-agonist administration and exercise on contractile activation of skeletal muscle fibers. Journal of Applied Physiology 81:1610-1618.

Lynch, G.S., Hinkle, R.T & Faulkner, J.A. (1999). Yearlong treatment with clenbuterol increases muscle mass but not force or power output of skeletal muscles of mice. Clinical and Experimental Pharmacology and Physiology 26:117-120.

Lynch, G.S., Hinkle, R.T. & Faulkner, J.A. (2000a). Force and power output of diaphragm muscle strips from mdx and control mice after clenbuterol treatment. Neuromuscular Disorders 11:192-196.

Lynch, G.S., Hinkle, R.T. & Faulkner, J.A. (2000b). Power output of skeletal muscles of control and mdx (dystrophic) mice after clenbuterol treatment. Experimental Physiology 85:294-298.

Lynch, G.S., Stephenson, D.G. & Williams, D.A. (1995). Analysis of Ca^{2+}- and Sr^{2+}-activation characteristics in skinned muscle fibre preparations with different proportions of myofibrillar isoforms. Journal of Muscle Research and Cell Motility 16:65-78.

MacLennan, P.A. & Edwards, R.H.T. (1989). Effects of clenbuterol and propranolol on muscle mass. Evidence that clenbuterol stimulates muscle β-adrenoceptors to induce hypertrophy. Biochemical Journal 264:573-579.

MacRae, J.C., Skene, P.A., Connell, A., Buchan, V. & Lobley, G.E. (1988). The action of the β-agonist clenbuterol on protein and energy metabolism in fattening wether lambs. British Journal of Nutrition 59:457-465.

Maltin, C.A., Delday, M.I. & Reeds, P.J. (1986). The effect of a growth promoting drug, clenbuterol, on fiber frequency and area in hind limb muscles from young male rats. Bioscience Reports 6:293-299.

Maltin, C.A., Delday, M.I., Watson, J.S., Heys, D., Nevison, I.M., Ritchie, I.K. & Gibson, P.H. (1993a). Clenbuterol, a β-adrenoceptor agonist, increases relative muscle strength in orthopaedic patients. Clinical Science 84:651-654.

Maltin, C.A., Hay, S.M., Delday, M.I., Smith, F.G., Lobley, G.E. & Reeds, P.J. (1987). Clenbuterol, a beta-agonist induces growth in innervated and denervated rat soleus muscle via apparently different mechanisms. Bioscience Reports 7:525-532.

Maltin, C.A., Jones, P. & Mantle, D. (1993b). Effect of protease inhibitors and clenbuterol on the in vitro degradation of dystrophin by endogenous proteases in human skeletal muscle. Bioscience Reports 13:159-167.

Martin, W.H. III, Murphree, S.S. & Saffitz, J.E. (1989). β-adrenergic receptor distribution among muscle fiber types and resistance arterioles of white, red, and intermediate skeletal muscle. Circulation Research 64:1096-1105.

Martineau, L., Horan, M.A., Rothwell, N.J. & Little, R.A. (1992). Salbutamol, a β2-adrenoceptor agonist, increases skeletal muscle strength in young men. Clinical Science 83:615-621.

Matsumoto, K., Ojima, K., Ohta, H. & Watanabe, H. (1994). Beta 2- but not beta 1-adrenoceptors are involved in desipramine enhancement of aggressive behavior in long-term isolated mice. Pharmacology, Biochemistry and Behavior 49:13-18.

McElligott, M.A., Barreto, A. Jr. & Chaung, L.Y. (1989). Effect of continuous and intermittent clenbuterol feeding on rat growth rate and muscle. Comparative Biochemistry and Physiology 92C:135-138.

McElligott, M.A., Mulder, J.E., Chaung, L.Y. & Barreto, A. Jr. (1987). Clenbuterol-induced muscle growth: investigation of possible mediation by insulin. American Journal of Physiology 253:E370-E375.

Mersmann, H.J. (1989). Potential mechanisms for repartitioning of growth by β-adrenergic agonists. In (eds) Campion, D.R., Hausman, G.J. & Martin, R.J., Animal Growth Regulation, Plenum Press, New York, pp337-357.

Miller, M.F., Garcia, D.K., Coleman, M.E., Ekeren, P.A., Lunt, D.K., Wagner, K.A., Procknor, M., Welsh Jr., T.H. & Smith, S.B. (1988). Adipose tissue, longissimus muscle and anterior pituitary growth and function in clenbuterol-fed heifers. Journal of Animal Research 66:12-20.

Mills, S. (2000). Beta-adrenergic receptor subtypes mediating lipolysis in porcine adipocytes. Studies with BRL-37344, a putative β3-adrenergic agonist. Comparative Biochemistry and Physiology (Part C) 126:11-20.

Mitchell, G.A. & Dunnavan, G. (1998). Illegal use of beta-adrenergic agonists in the United States. Journal of Animal Science 76:208-211.

Molenaar, P., Roberts, S.J., Kim, Y.S., Pak, H.S., Sainz, R.D. & Summers, R.J. (1991). Localisation and characterisation of two propranolol resistant (-) [125I] cyanopindolol binding sites in rat skeletal muscle. European Journal of Pharmacology 209:257-262.

Moore, N.G., Pegg, G.G. & Sillence, M.N. (1994). Anabolic effects of the β2-adrenoceptor agonist salmeterol are dependent on route of administration. American Journal of Physiology 267:E475-E484.

Morton, A.R., Joyce, K., Papalia, S.M., Carroll, N.G. & Fitch, K.D. (1996). Is salmeterol ergogenic. Clinical Journal of Sport Medicine 6:220-225.

Murad, N. & Tucci, P.J.F. (2000). Isoproterenol-induced hypertrophy may result in distinct left ventricular changes. Clinical and Experimental Pharmacology and Physiology 27:352-357.

Murphy, R.J.L., Béliveau, L., Seburn, K.L. & Gardiner, P.F. (1996). Clenbuterol has a greater influence on untrained than previously trained skeletal muscle in rats. European Journal of Applied Physiology and Occupational Physiology 73:304-310.

Murphy, R.J.L., Hartkopp, A., Gardiner, P.F., Kjaer, M. & Beliveau, L. (1999). Salbutamol effect in spinal cord injured individuals undergoing functional electrical stimulation training. Archives of Physical Medicine & Rehabilitation 80:1264-1267.

Murugaiah, K.D. & O'Donnell, J.M. (1994). Clenbuterol increases norepinephrine release from rat brain slices by a calcium- and receptor-independent mechanism. Research Communications in Molecular Pathology and Pharmacology 86:311-324.

Navegantes, L.C.C., Resano, N.M.Z., Migliorini, R.H. & Kettelhut, I.C. (2000). Role of adrenoceptors and cAMP on the catecholamine-induced inhibition of proteolysis in rat skeletal muscle. American Journal of Physiology 279:E663-E668.

Norris, S.R., Petersen, S.R. & Jones, R.L. (1996). The effect of salbutamol on performance in endurance cyclists. European Journal of Applied Physiology and Occupational Physiology 73:364-368.

Nyberg, L. (1997). Pharmacokinetics of beta2-adrenoceptor-stimulating drugs. In (eds) Pauwels, R. & O'Byrne, P.M., Beta2-Agonists in Asthma Treatment, Marcel Dekker, New York, pp87-130.

Nystad, W., Harris, J. & Borgen, J.S. (2000). Asthma and wheezing among Norwegian elite athletes. Medicine and Science in Sports and Exercise 32:266-270.

O'Donnell, J.M. (1990). Behavioral effects of beta adrenergic agonists and antidepressant drugs after down-regulation of beta-2 adrenergic receptors by clenbuterol. Journal of Pharmacology and Experimental Therapeutics 254:147-157.

O'Donnell, S.R. (1993). The development of beta receptor agonist drugs. In (eds) Beasley, R. & Pearce, N.E., The Role of Beta Receptor Agonist Therapy in Asthma Mortality, CRC Press, Boca Raton, Florida, pp3-26.

Pack, R.J., Alley, M.R., Dallimore, J.A., Lapwood, K.R., Burgess, C. & Crane, J. (1994). The myocardial effects of fenoterol, isoprenaline and salbutamol in normoxic and hypoxic sheep. International Journal of Experimental Pathology 75:357-362.

Palmer, R.M., Delday, M.I., McMillan, D.N., Noble, B.S., Bain, P. & Maltin, C.A. (1990). Effects of the cyclo-oxygenase inhibitor, fenbufen, on clenbuterol-induced hypertrophy of cardiac and skeletal muscle of rats. British Journal of Pharmacology 101:835-838.

Pan, S.J., Hancock, J., Ding, Z.P., Fogt, D., Lee, M.C. & Ivy, J.L. (2001). Effects of clenbuterol on insulin resistance in conscious obese Zucker rats. American Journal of Physiology 280:E554-E561.

Petrou, M., Clarke, S., Morrison, K., Bowles, C., Dunn, M. & Yacoub, M. (1999). Clenbuterol increases stroke power and contractile speed of skeletal muscle for cardiac assist. Circulation 99:713-720.

Polla, B., Cappelli, V., Morello, F., Pellegrino, M.A., Boschi, F., Pastoris, O. & Reggiani, C. (2001). Effects of the β2-agonist clenbuterol on respiratory and limb muscles of weaning rats. American Journal of Physiology 280:R862-R869.

Prather, I.D., Brown, D.E., North, P. & Wilson, J.R. (1995). Clenbuterol: a substitute for anabolic steroids. Medicine and Science in Sports and Exercise 27:1118-1121.

Puls, I., Beck, M., Giess, R., Magnus, T., Ochs, G. & Toyka, K.V. (1999). Clenbuterol in amyotrophic lateral sclerosis. No evidence for therapeutic efficacy. Nervenarzt 70:1112-1115.

Rajab, P., Fox, J., Riaz, S., Tomlinson, D., Ball, D. & Greenhaff, P.L. (2000). Skeletal muscle myosin heavy chain isoforms and energy metabolism after clenbuterol treatment in the rat. American Journal of Physiology 279:R1076-R1081.

Reeds, P.J., Hay, S.M., Dorward, P.M. & Palmer, R.M. (1986). Stimulation of muscle growth by clenbuterol: lack of effect on muscle protein biosynthesis. British Journal of Nutrition 56:249-258.

Rens-Domiano, S. & Hamm, H.E. (1995). Structural and functional relationships of heterotrimeric G-proteins. FASEB Journal 9:1059-1066.

Revelli, J.P., Preitner, F., Samec, S., Muniesa, P., Kuehne, F., Boss, O., Vassalli, J.D., Dulloo, A., Seydoux, J., Giacobino, J.P., Huarte, J. & Ody, C. (1997). Targeted gene disruption reveals a leptin independent role for the mouse beta(3)-adrenoceptor in the regulation of body composition. Journal of Clinical Investigation 100:1098-1106.

Ricart-Firinga, C., Stevens, L., Canu, M.H., Nemirovskaya, T.L. & Mounier, Y. (2000). Effects of beta(2)-agonist clenbuterol on biochemical and contractile properties of unloaded soleus fibers of rat. American Journal of Physiology 278:C582-C588.

Ricks, C.A., Dalrymple, R.H., Baker, P.K. & Ingle, D.L. (1984). Use of a β-agonist to alter fat and muscle deposition in steers. Journal of Animal Science 59:1247-1255.

Roberts, S.J. & Summers, R.J. (1998). Cyclic AMP accumulation in rat soleus muscle: stimulation by β2- but not β3-adrenoceptors. European Journal of Pharmacology 348:53-60.

Robertson, W., Simkins, J., Ohickey, S.P., Freeman, S. & Cayton, R.M. (1994). Does single dose salmeterol affect exercise capacity in asthmatic men. European Respiratory Journal 7:1978-1984.

Rothwell, N.J. & Stock, M.J. (1985). Modification of body composition by clenbuterol in normal and dystrophic (mdx) mice. Bioscience Reports 5:755-760.

Rothwell, N.J., Stock, M.J. & Sudera, D.K. (1987). Changes in tissue blood flow and β-receptor density of skeletal muscle in rats treated with β2-adrenoceptor agonist clenbuterol. British Journal of Pharmacology 90:601-607.

Salleras, L., Dominguez, A., Mata, E., Taberner, J.L., Moro, I. & Salva, P. (1995). Epidemiologic study of an outbreak of clenbuterol poisoning in Catalonia. Public Health Reports 110:338-342.

Sandsund, M., Sue-Chu, M., Reinertsen, R.E., Helgerud, J., Holand, B. & Bjermer, L. (2000). Treatment with inhaled beta(2)-agonists or oral leukotriene antagonist do not enhance physical performance in nonasthmatic highly trained athletes exposed to –15 degrees C. Journal of Thermal Biology 25:181-185.

Schiavetta, A.M., Miller, M.F., Lunt, D.K., Davis, S.K. & Smith, S.B. (1990). Adipose tissue cellularity and muscle growth in young steers fed the β-adrenergic agonist clenbuterol for 50 days and after 78 days of withdrawal. Journal of Animal Science 68:3614-3623.

Schwenk, T.L. (1997). Psychoactive drugs and athletic performance. The Physician and Sportsmedicine 25:32.

Signorile, J.F., Banovac, K., Gomez, M., Flipse, D., Caruso, J.F. & Lowensteyn, I. (1995). Increased muscle strength in paralyzed patients after spinal cord injury—effect of a beta-2 adrenergic agonist. Archives of Physical Medicine & Rehabilitation 76:55-58.

Sillence, M.N., Hunter, R.A., Pegg, G.G., Brown, M.L., Matthews, M.L., Magner, T., Sleeman, M. & Lindsay, D.B. (1993). Growth, nitrogen metabolism, and cardiac responses to clenbuterol and ketoclenbuterol in rats and underfed cattle. Journal of Animal Science 71:2942-2951.

Sillence, M.N., Matthews, M.L., Badran, T.W. & Pegg, G.G. (2000). Effects of clenbuterol on growth in underfed cattle. Australian Journal of Agricultural Research 51:401-406.

Sillence, M.N., Matthews, M.L., Spiers, W.G., Pegg, G.G. & Lindsay, D.B. (1991a). Effects of clenbuterol, ICI118551 and sotalol on the growth of cardiac and skeletal muscle and on β2-adrenoceptor density in female rats. Archives of Pharmacology 344:449-453.

Sillence, M.N., Pegg, G.G. & Lindsay, D.B. (1991b). Affinity of clenbuterol analogues for β2-adrenoceptors in bovine skeletal muscle and the effect of these compounds on urinary nitrogen excretion in female rats. Archives of Pharmacology 344:442-448.

Smith, D.J. (2000). Total radioactive residues and clenbuterol residues in swine after dietary administration of [C-14]clenbuterol for seven days and preslaughter withdrawal periods of zero, three, or seven days. Journal of Animal Science 78:2903-2912.

Smith, S.B., Davis, S.K., Wilson, J.J., Stone, R.T., Wu, F.Y., Garcia, D.K., Lunt, D.K. & Schiavetta, A.M. (1995). Bovine fast-twitch myosin light chain 1: cloning and mRNA amount in muscle of cattle treated with clenbuterol. American Journal of Physiology 268:E858-E865.

Sneddon, A.A., Delday, M.I. & Maltin, C.A. (2000). Amelioration of denervation-induced atrophy by clenbuterol is associated with increased PKC-α activity. American Journal of Physiology 279:E188-E195.

Spencer, G.S.G. & Oliver, M.H. (1996). Suppression of immune response in lambs during treatment with the beta-adrenergic agonist clenbuterol. Journal of Animal Science 74:151-153.

Sporano, V., Grasso, L., Chem, M.E., Chem, G.O., Brambilla, G. & Loizzo, A. (1998). Clenbuterol residues in non-liver containing meat as a cause of collective food poisoning. Veterinary & Human Toxicology 40:141-143.

Stevens, L., Firinga, C., Gohlsch, R., Bastide, B., Mounier, Y. & Pette, D. (2000a). Effects of unweighting and clenbuterol on myosin light and heavy chains in fast and slow muscles of rat. American Journal of Physiology 279:C1558-C1563.

Stevens, L., Gohlsch, B., Mounier, Y. & Pette, D. (2000b). Upregulation of myosin heavy chain MHCl alpha in rat muscles after unweighting and clenbuterol treatment. Biochemical & Biophysical Research Communications 275:418-421.

Strader, C.E., Fong, T.M., Graziano, M.P. & Tota, M.R. (1995). The family of G-protein-coupled receptors. FASEB Journal 9:745-754.

Sue-Chu, M., Sandsund, M., Helgerud, J., Reinertsen, R.E. & Bjermer, L. (1999). Salmeterol and physical performance at –15 degrees C in highly trained nonasthmatic cross-country skiers. Scandinavian Journal of Medicine and Science in Sports 9:48-52.

Suzuki, J., Gao, M., Xie, Z. & Koyama, T. (1997). Effects of the β2-adrenergic agonist clenbuterol on capillary geometry in cardiac and skeletal muscles in young and middle-aged rats. Acta Physiologica Scandinavica 161:317-326.

Tawil, R. (1999). Outlook for therapy in the muscular dystrophies. Seminars in Neurology 19:81-86.

Taylor, P.B. & Tang, Q. (1984). Development of isoproterenol-induced cardiac hypertrophy. Canadian Journal of Physiology and Pharmacology 62:384-389.

Torgan, C.E., Etgen Jr., G.J., Brozinick Jr., J.T., Wilcox, R.E. & Ivy, J.L. (1993). Interaction of aerobic exercise training and clenbuterol: effects on insulin-resistant muscle. Journal of Applied Physiology 75:1471-1476.

Torgan, C.E., Etgen Jr., G.J., Kang, H.Y. & Ivy, J.L. (1995). Fiber type-specific effects of clenbuterol and exercise training on insulin-resistant muscle. Journal of Applied Physiology 79:163-167.

Torneke, K., Larsson, C.I., & Appelgren, L.E. (1998). A comparison between clenbuterol, salbutanol and terbutaline in relation to receptor binding and in vitro relaxation of equine tracheal muscle. Journal of Veterinary Pharmacology and Therapeutics 21:388-392.

Tschan, M., Perrochoud, A. & Herzog, H. (1979). Dose response relationship of clenbuterol (NAB 365) as a solution for inhalation. European Journal of Clinical Pharmacology 15:159-162.

Van der Heijden, H.F.M., Dekhuijzen, P.N.R., Folgering, H., Ginsel, L.A. & Van Herwaarden, C.L.A. (1998a). Long-term effects of clenbuterol on diaphragm morphology and contractile properties in emphysematous hamsters. Journal of Applied Physiology 85:215-222.

Van der Heijden, H.F.M., Dekhuijzen, P.N.R., Folgering, H., Ginsel, L.A. & Van Herwaarden, C.L.A. (1998b). Salbutamol enhances the isotonic contractile properties of rat diaphragm muscle. Journal of Applied Physiology 85:525-529.

Ventura, R., Segura, J., Berges, R., Fitch, K.D., Morton, A.R., Berruezo, S. & Jimenez, C. (2000). Distinction of inhaled and oral salbutamol by urine analysis using conventional screening procedures for doping control. Therapeutic Drug Monitoring 22:277-282.

Von Deutsch, D.A., Abukhalaf, I.K., Wineski, L.E., Aboul-Enein, H.Y., Pitts, S.A., Parks, B.A., Oster, R.A., Paulsen, D.F. & Potter, D.E. (2000). β-agonist-induced alterations in organ weights and protein content: composition of racemic clenbuterol and its enantiomers. Chirality 12:637-648.

Wang, S.Y. & Beerman, D.H. (1988). Reduced calcium-dependent proteinase activity in cimaterol-induced muscle hypertrophy in lambs. Journal of Animal Science 66:2545-2550.

Waterfield, C.J., Jairath, M., Asker, D.S. & Timbrell, J.A. (1995). The biochemical effects of clenbuterol: with particular reference to taurine and muscle damage. European Journal of Pharmacology 293:141-149.

Weiler, J.M., Layton, M. & Hunt, M. (1998). Asthma in United States Olympic athletes who participated in the 1996 Summer Games. Journal of Allergy & Clinical Immunology 102:722-726.

Weiler, J.M. & Ryan, E.J. (2000). Asthma in United States Olympic athletes who participated in the 1998 Olympic Winter Games. Journal of Allergy & Clinical Immunology 106:267-271.

Weyer, C., Gautier, J.F. & Danforth Jr., E. (1999). Development of beta3-adrenoceptor agonists for the treatment of obesity and diabetes—an update. Diabetes & Metabolism 25:11-21.

Wilber, R.L., Rundell, K.W., Szmedra, L., Jenkinson, D.M., Im, J. & Drake, S.D. (2000). Incidence of exercise-induced bronchospasm in Olympic winter sport athletes. Medicine and Science in Sports and Exercise 32:732-737.

Williams, R.S., Caron, M.G. & Daniel, K. (1984). Skeletal muscle β-adrenergic receptors: variations due to fiber type and training. American Journal of Physiology 246:E160-E167.

Wong, K., Boheler, K.R., Bishop, J., Petrou, M. & Yacoub, M.H. (1998). Clenbuterol induces cardiac hypertrophy with normal functional, morphological and molecular features. Cardiovascular Research 37:115-122.

Wright, L.D., Zhang, K.M., McClain, L.C., Hsia, P.W.E., Briggs, F.N. & Spratt, J.A. (1999). Salbutamol and the conditioning of latissimus dorsi for cardiomyoplasty. Journal of Surgical Research 81:209-215.

Yamashita, J., Onai, T., York, D.A. & Bray, G.A. (1994). Relationship between food intake and metabolic rate in rats treated with beta-adrenoceptor agonists. International Journal of Obesity & Related Metabolic Disorders 18:429-433.

Yang, Y.T. & McElligott, M.A. (1989). Multiple actions of β-adrenergic agonists on skeletal muscle and adipose tissue. Biochemical Journal 261:1-10.

Yaspelkis, B.B., Castle, A.L., Ding, Z. & Ivy, J.L. (1999). Attenuating the decline in ATP arrests the exercise training-induced increases in muscle GLUT4 protein and citrate synthase activity. Acta Physiologica Scandinavica 165:71-79.

Yoshida, T., Umekawa, T., Kumamoto, K., Sakane, N., Kogure, A., Kondo, M., Wakabayashi, Y., Kawada, T., Nagase, I. & Saito, M. (1998). β3-adrenergic agonist induces a functionally active uncoupling protein in fast and slow-twitch muscle fibers. American Journal of Physiology 274:E469-E475.

Zeman, R.J., Hirschman, A., Hirschman, M.L., Guo, G. & Etlinger, J.D. (1991). Clenbuterol, a β2-receptor agonist, reduces net bone loss in denervated hindlimbs. American Journal of Physiology 261:E285-E289.

Zeman, R.J., Ludemann, R., Easton, T.G. & Etlinger, J.D. (1988). Slow to fast alterations in skeletal muscle fibres caused by clenbuterol, a β2-receptor agonist. American Journal of Physiology 254:E726-E732.

Zeman, R.J., Ludemann, R. & Etlinger, J.D. (1987). Clenbuterol, a β2-agonist, retards atrophy in denervated muscles. American Journal of Physiology 252:E152-E155.

Zeman, R.J., Zhang, Y. & Etlinger, J.D. (1994). Clenbuterol, a β-agonist, retards wasting and loss of contractility in irradiated dystrophic mdx muscle. American Journal of Physiology 267:C865-C868.

Zhang, K.M., Hu, P., Wang, S.W., Feher, J.J., Wright, L.D., Wechsler, A.S., Spratt, J.A. & Briggs, F.N. (1996). Salbutamol changes the molecular and mechanical properties of canine skeletal muscle. Journal of Physiology 496:211-220.

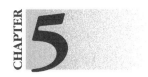

CHAPTER 5

Growth Hormone: Physiological Effects of Exogenous Administration

William J. Kraemer, PhD

Bradley C. Nindl, PhD

Martyn R. Rubin, MS

As athletes strive for excellence in sport, they explore many avenues for a competitive advantage (Davies et al. 1997; Deysigg and Frisch 1993; Knopp et al. 1997; Macintyre 1987; Neely and Rosenfeld 1994; Spalding 1991; Wadler 1994). Growth hormone (GH) is a common pharmacological tool that athletes use. In addition, GH has become one of the most popular anti-aging drugs. Pharmacological interventions have always been of interest to the athlete, and now such strategies are moving into the general public (Janssen et al. 1999). In general, GH and growth factors promote protein accretion, increase muscle fiber hypertrophy, and improve physical performance. Specifically, the GH/insulin-like growth factor-I (IGF-I) axis is thought to play a pivotal role by serving as a systemic mediator orchestrating nutrient partitioning away from fat deposition and toward protein synthesis. Anecdotally, many bodybuilders use GH each week during a cycle (e.g., 1-2 IU every other day). In the competitive environment (e.g., bodybuilding), GH is often not used alone; and when it is used with various combinations of synthetic testosterone administrations, a synergistic effect appears to occur. Thus, while one can examine the effects of GH, the "real world" presents a complex picture of different combinations of anabolic drugs that anecdotally appear to be more effective than single-drug use. However, the desired result of increased muscularity is not without unwanted adverse side effects (Clarkson 1997).

Anecdotally, when GH has been added to the mix of anabolic drug use in athletes, an improved muscularity is often achieved. This result is supported by one of the few studies examining highly conditioned athletes using a progressive resistance training program accompanied by met-hGH (human growth hormone) administration in a double-blind fashion (2.67 mg/0.5 ml diluent, 3 days per week for 6 weeks). In this study, met-hGH use augmented performance increases during the resistance training program and high protein diet used by the athletes and resulted in an increased fat-free weight, decreased percent body fat, and improvement in the ratio of fat-free weight to fat weight. In addition, the endogenous circulating concentrations of IGF-I were elevated (Crist et al. 1988). Thus GH, despite a lack of understanding of exactly how this hormone mediates effects at the molecular and cellular levels, is thought to be a potent drug for enhancing body composition contributing to athletic performance.

The combination of drug therapies now available for the athlete is dramatic, and at this point a method to effectively test for many of these polypeptide drugs remains unclear both scientifically and at the level of legal challenges. The complex interactions of these anabolic agents in the body can make scientific understanding of the compounds difficult to achieve through experimentation. It is our hope that by understanding the fundamental cybernetics of the GH/IGF axis and the factual basis of hormonal supplementation, the coach, clinician, and athlete can make clinical speculations regarding possible rationales and reasons for use of the drugs by athletes. It is crucial to understand that while natural training methods are valid and noble, they will never produce the same level of results as physical conditioning supplemented by pharmacological agents. There are also difficulties in attempting to test and to legislate competitions simply due to the costs of test development, issues regarding implementation, and inability to deter users given the dramatic financial rewards related to athletic performance.

This chapter summarizes the endocrine physiology of the GH/IGF-I axis and overviews the relevant human studies that have experimentally examined the somatotrophic influences of exogenous GH/IGF-I administration, including orally active GH secretagogues.

Growth Hormone/Insulin-Like Growth Factor-I Axis

Not surprisingly, the complexity of the GH polypeptide makes the supplementation of the hormone an even more complex phenomenon. Many of the unknown and potentially interesting effects of exogenous GH may relate to complexities of the GH family of polypeptides and interactions that are only beginning to be understood scientifically, much less clinically. Thus, it is important to understand the various aspects of GH endocrinology in order to put the exogenous use into a new context.

Growth Hormone Release

Human growth hormone (i.e., somatotropin) is a pleiotropic polypeptide hormone that mediates myriad metabolic and growth processes, with potent effects on lipid, carbohydrate, and protein metabolism in nearly all body tissues. Growth hormone is secreted from the anterior pituitary gland in an episodic and pulsatile manner throughout the day, with a dramatic surge of release during slow-wave sleep. This pulsatile release is under the regulatory control of the two hypothalamic hormones that serve to stimulate (GH-releasing hormone [GHRH]) or inhibit (somatostatin) hGH release. The balance between these two hormones determines the relative magnitude of initial release from the anterior pituitary (Muller et al. 1999). Many other factors are also known to affect hGH secretion. For example, age, gender, diet and nutrients, stress, other hormones (e.g., gonadal steroids, thyroid hormones, catecholamines, and IGF-I), adiposity, fitness level, and exercise have all been implicated as factors that influence hGH concentrations in the blood (figure 5.1) (Harvey et al. 1995).

Growth Hormone Heterogeneity

Endogenous GH exhibits a great deal of molecular heterogeneity, thereby making exogenous GH administration much more complex than once thought. The main pituitary molecular weight variant of the GH family is the 22-kD form. This protein is 191 amino acids in length and represents ~21% of all circulating plasma GH. However, hGH can undergo various post-translational and/or postsecretory modifications to form aggregates (i.e., dimers, trimers, pentamers) or fragments that exist in significant quantity in the circulation (Baumann 1991; Lewis et al. 2000; Hymer et al. 2001). The existence of high- and low-affinity GH-binding proteins adds further complexity to the nature and spatial arrangement of circulating hGH moieties. This molecular heterogeneity appears to have physiological significance, as the different forms have been shown to possess different biological activities and immunodetectabilities. For example, recent research has shown that specific fragments of the 191-amino acid parent hormone (i.e., 22

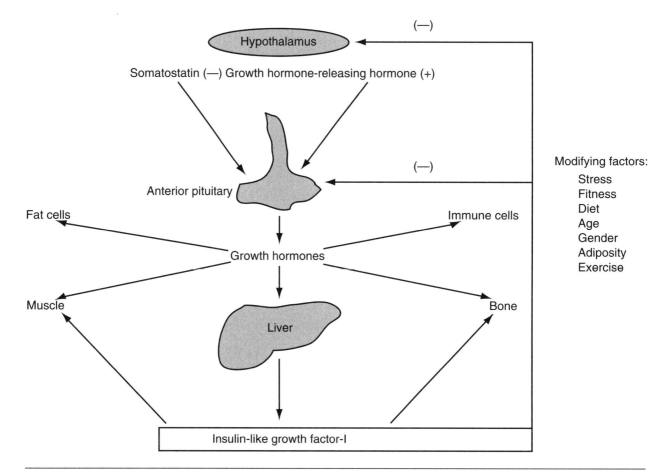

Figure 5.1   Cybernetic interactions of growth hormone with other target sites in the body.

kD) may have independent and very specific roles in the metabolism of carbohydrates and lipids (Lewis et al. 2000). Furthermore, the formation of GH aggregates in the pituitary prior to secretion may have tremendous implications for the biological activity of hGH in terms of tissue growth (Hymer et al. 2000). Indeed, what this means for the future of exogenous GH administration will be determined only as biotechnology advances in concert with a greater understanding of the different molecular hGH forms and their respective functions. Nevertheless, current understanding of the molecular heterogeneity of hGH already suggests that it is a gross oversimplification merely to administer the 22-kD parent hormone.

The Insulin-Like Growth Factor-I System

Many GH effects are thought to occur indirectly through the actions of hepatically produced IGF-I (i.e., the somatomedin hypothesis). The IGF-I system is composed of IGF-I itself (a 7.6-kD polypeptide), a family of six binding proteins (BPs; i.e., BP-1 through -6, ranging in size from 22.8 to 31.4 kD), an acid labile subunit (ALS; 80-86 kD), and an IGF-I protease. Insulin-like growth factor-I can circulate either unbound (i.e., free) or bound to one of the binding proteins. The majority of IGF-I (~75%) circulates primarily in a ternary complex (~150 kD) consisting of IGF-I, IGFBP-3, and ALS. In addition to its well-known mitogenic, anabolic, and cell cycle progression properties, the IGF-I system has been implicated in the mediation of the growth-promoting actions of physical activity.

Recombinant Human Growth Hormone

A number of pharmaceutical companies have developed and marketed a multitude of recombinant human growth hormone (rhGH) products with the generic name somatropin. Companies and their products include Genentech (Protropin, Nutropin, and Nutropin AQ), Novo Nordisk (Norditropin), Pharmacia/Upjohn (Genotropin), Eli Lilly (Humatrope), and Serono (Serostim and Saizen). These rhGH products are typically administered intramuscularly or subcutaneously. The prescribed dose is typically 0.30 mg/kg/week with an associated cost upward of $200/5.0 mg (average wholesale cost of $42/mg) (Windisch et al. 1998). Thus, for a 176-lb (80 kg) person, the cost of rhGH administration for three months is approximately $12,096. Administration of GH by encapsulated biodegradable microspheres is an alternative means of delivery. The advantage to this method appears to be more prolonged and sustained effect (Johnson et al. 1996, 1997). However, we should

note that all recombinantly produced GH products are synthetic versions of the 22-kD GH form. Again, even though this form seems to be the predominant form in the human circulation, it is quite possible that there are a number of physiological actions mediated by GH variants that are not accomplished by exogenous administration of the parent 22-kD form of the hormone.

Adverse Side Effects of Growth Hormone Excess

The clinical condition in which the pituitary oversecretes GH is known as *acromegaly*. This condition is associated with increases in total body water, calcium, sodium, potassium, and phosphorous retention. According to Harvey et al. (1995), retention of these elements can result in physical discomfort to include facial and aural soft-tissue swelling; profuse sweating; deepening of the voice; skeletal and articular changes such as gigantism; costal growth; mandibular growth; frontal bossing; frontal sinus overgrowth; vertebral bony overgrowth; phalangeal bony overgrowth; articular cartilage growth; widening joint space; accelerated osteoarthritis; visceral growth of cardiac, heptic, renal, pulmonary, and thyroidal tissue growth; insulin resistance; hyperinsulinemia; impaired glucose tolerance; diabetes mellitus; increase in 1,25-dihydroxycholecalciferol; hypercalciuria; hyperprolactinemia; menstrual irregularity; amenorrhea; impotence; thyroid-stimulating hormone, adrenocorticotropic hormone, and vasopressin hyper- or hyposecretion; headache; vision loss; sleep apnea; entrapments, hypertrophic neuropathy; and myopathy. At least one study has shown that the incidence of leukemia is greater during rhGH therapy (Watanabe et al. 1989). Most of the known side effects of GH excess have been obtained by clinical evaluation of acromegaly. Few data are available in populations abusing GH. Pierard-Franchimont et al. (1996) reported that in eight bodybuilders who were rhGH abusers, dermal viscosity was increased. Rudman et al. (1990) have also reported an increase in skin thickness after 24 weeks of rhGH administration in older men.

Physiological Effects of Growth Hormone Administration

Growth hormone can exert both a transitory insulin-like effect and an anti-insulin diabetogenic effect (i.e., raises circulating glucose). The mechanism for the diabetogenic effect appears to be a reduced peripheral uptake and utilization of glucose. Growth hormone decreases the sensitivity to insulin downstream from the insulin receptor, possibly via reduced synthesis of GLUT 1 (the major glucose transporter in the cell membrane of adipocytes). Conversely, the insulin-like or glucose transport-stimulating effects of GH are identical to those of insulin involving translocation of GLUT 4.

Growth hormone exerts potent lipolytic effects. The possible mechanisms accounting for these include (1) direct effect, (2) increase in other lipolytic hormones such as catecholamines and glucagon, and (3) influence on adipocyte (i.e., fat cell) responsiveness to other hormones. Growth hormone can directly blunt lipogenesis by decreasing the transcription and synthesis of key lipogenic enzymes: acetyl-CoA carboxylase, glucose-6-phosphate dehydrogenase, fatty acid synthase, 6-phosphogluconate dehydrogenase, and isocitrate dehydrogenase. Indirectly, GH may increase adrenergic receptor number or reduce inhibitory factors. In addition, as was observed in a study by Crist et al. (1988), dramatic decreases in percent body fat accompany GH drug use. Indeed, this effect may be even more dramatic in premenopausal women, who have much greater fat stores than other populations. This reduction in body fat in women may have implications for performance concomitant with the increased lean tissue mass. The effects of GH drug use on women's menstrual status, fat deposition, and body development remain speculative, but are of concern with respect to normal physiological function and interplay with other hormones (e.g., estrogen, IGF-I).

Perhaps the most glamorized effects of GH are on muscle protein synthesis. Growth hormone enhances amino acid uptake and transport, thereby increasing the capacity for protein synthesis. Growth hormone optimizes the efficiency and utilization of nitrogen by increasing protein synthesis and decreasing protein degradation. Mechanistically, many of the GH effects on protein are thought to occur indirectly via IGF-I; however, direct effects are also possible.

Effects On Body Composition and Physical Performance

Much of the recent work on GH administration in normal subjects has come from Yarasheski and colleagues. This group has performed a number of investigations on GH administration combined with exercise training in normal populations. In Yarasheski's first experiment (Yarasheski et al. 1992), 16 men were randomly assigned to a resistance-trained group supplemented with GH (40 g rhGH/kg/day) or a resistance-trained group supplemented with placebo. Both groups performed a total body resistance training program for 12 weeks. Fat-free mass and total body water increased in both groups, but to a larger extent in the group that received GH. Whole-body protein synthesis and protein balance were higher in the GH group. However, quadriceps muscle protein synthesis rate, torso and limb circumferences, and muscle strength

did not increase to a greater extent in the GH-treated group. Consequently the authors concluded that the large increase in fat-free mass (FFM) with GH treatment was probably attributable to an increase in lean tissue other than skeletal muscle (e.g., connective tissue). Furthermore, resistance training supplemented with GH did not increase muscle hypertrophy or strength better than resistance training alone.

The next study by Yarasheski et al. (1993) involved experienced weight lifters. Fractional rate of skeletal muscle protein synthesis and the whole-body rate of protein breakdown were determined in seven male weight lifters before and after 14 days of GH administration (40 g rhGH/kg/day). Administration of GH increased serum IGF-I, but did not increase the fractional rate of muscle protein synthesis or reduce the rate of whole-body protein breakdown. This study showed that short-term GH treatment did not lead to metabolic adaptations that would augment further increases in muscle mass. However, it is likely that the duration of GH supplementation (14 days) was too short to elicit a significant effect.

Yarasheski et al. (1995) next evaluated the effect of GH administration in conjunction with resistance training in older men. Twenty-three healthy sedentary older men (mean age 67 years) underwent a 16-week progressive resistance training program with GH administration (n = 8) or placebo (n = 15). The GH-treated group received 12.5-24 micrograms/kg/day. As with the younger men, the GH-treated group experienced greater increases in FFM and total body water than the placebo group. Whole-body protein synthesis and breakdown rates increased in the GH group. However, vastus lateralis muscle protein synthesis rate, urinary creatinine excretion, and training-specific muscle strength were similar in the two groups. As in the study with younger men, Yarasheski et al. concluded that daily GH treatment does not further augment strength and anabolism associated with a resistance training program. In addition, the increase in FFM was attributed to an increase in noncontractile protein and fluid retention.

It is important to note that these are short-term studies, and as with most short-term resistance training studies, a large window for adaptation is available, making it difficult to separate out intervention effects. Most researchers to date have been able to examine GH supplementation only within the confines of limited short-term training programs as well as within a limited dose duration and range, the latter relating to approval for use of human subjects.

Taaffe et al. (1994) also researched the effects of rhGH supplementation in conjunction with resistance exercise in older men. Eighteen healthy older men (65-82 years) were trained for 14 weeks to establish a conditioned state. Subjects were then randomized to receive either 0.02 mg/kg body weight/day rhGH or placebo. Subjects then underwent an additional 10 weeks of resistance training. Absolute body mass was not altered in either group; however, changes in body composition were observed, with an increase in FFM and a decrease in fat mass in the GH-supplemented group. No systemic difference in muscle strength was observed between the two conditions.

Deyssig et al. (1993) administered rhGH in power athletes for a period of six weeks. Twenty-two men (mean age 23 years) were assigned in a double-blind manner to either GH treatment (0.09 IU/kg body weight per day) or placebo. Growth hormone, IGF-I, and IGF-binding protein (IGFBP) increased significantly in the treated group. Fasting insulin increased and thyroxine decreased in the GH-treated group. There was no effect of GH treatment on maximal strength, body weight, or body fat. The authors concluded that in highly trained power athletes with low fat mass there were no effects of GH treatment on strength or body composition. However,

the increase in fasting insulin does indicate a reduced glucose tolerance consistent with the diabetogenic properties of GH, while the reduced thyroxine concentrations may be indicative of alterations in basal metabolic rate.

In summary, rhGH supplementation combined with resistance training in healthy younger and older men does not appear to augment muscle strength (Zachwieja and Yarasheski 1999). The increases in FFM do not appear to be attributable to contractile protein but rather to noncontractile protein, possibly due to fluid retention or connective tissue (Frisch 1999). Furthermore, GH administration may potentially have profound adverse effects on other hormonal systems and metabolic processes. Again it is crucial to note that with the current understanding of the molecular weight variants of GH, it is possible that simple administration of the synthetic 22-kD form of GH does not fully tap the potential of GH as a growth-promoting hormone. Table 5.1 summarizes the various studies and the effects of GH administration.

Table 5.1 Summary of Studies on Somatotrophic Effects of Exogenous Human Growth Hormone (GH) Administration

Authors	Subjects	Growth hormone administration dose/duration	Dependent variables	Salient findings
Mauras et al. 2000	10 adult subjects with profound insulin-like growth factor (IGF)-I deficiency due to a mutation in the GH receptor gene	Twice-daily subcutaneous injections of 60 μ/kg of rhIGF-I	Body compositions via DEXA and measurements of growth factor concentrations	Plasma IGF-I concentrations increased and there was a significant positive effect on body composition.
Murphy et al. 1999	187 elderly adults (65 years)	Oral doses of 10 or 25 mg of MK-677	Bone resorption, serum osteocalcin and bone-specific alkaline phosphatase (BSAP), and serum IGF-I	Serum IGF-I, serum osteocalcin, BSAP, and bone resorption increased.
Svensson et al. 1999	24 obese males (18-50 years) with BMI >30 kg/m^2 and waist/hip ratio >.95	25 mg of MK-677 orally with 150 ml of water	Lipoprotein (a), apolipoprotein A and E, total cholesterol, LDL, HDL, serum triglycerides, and lipoprotein lipase activity	Serum lipoprotein did not change. Apolipoprotein A and E changed at 2 weeks but were unchanged at 8 weeks, as were HDL and serum triglycerides. LDL and lipoprotein lipase activity were unchanged.
Wallace et al. 1999	17 healthy males (18-40 years)	Subcutaneous abdominal injection of .15 IU/kg/day for 7 days	GH/(IGF) axis	Increased serum GH, GH-binding protein, total IGF-I, IGFBP-3, and acid-labile subunit. IGFBP-1 increased after exercise was completed. Free IGF-I did not change.

(continued)

Table 5.1 *(continued)*

Authors	Subjects	Growth hormone administration dose/duration	Dependent variables	Salient findings
Karila et al. 1998	9 healthy, non-obese and noncompeting male power lifters who were aggressive substance abusers	Self-administered hormonal substances	Serum IGF-I and IGFBP-3 concentration	Anabolic steroids decreased both the basal and GH-stimulated IGFBP-3 concentrations, whereas its effects on serum IGF-I concentration were variable and affected by low-calorie diet.
Murphy et al. 1998	8 healthy volunteers (24-39 years)	During last 7 days of each diet period (2), 25 mg of MK-677 orally; 14-21 day washout interval between periods	Diet-induced negative nitrogen balance	Improved nitrogen balance, peak GH response, mean IGF-I concentration, mean IGFBP-3. No differences were found for IGFBP-2 and cortisol.
Svensson et al. 1998b	24 obese males (18-50 years) with BMI >30 kg/m^2 and waist/hip ratio >.95	25 mg of MK-677 orally with 150 ml of water	Serum IGF-I, IGFBP-3, GH, and prolactin	Serum IGF-I, IGFBP-3, GH, and prolactin were all increased after treatment.
Svensson et al. 1998a	24 healthy obese males (19-49 years) with BMI >30 kg/m^2	25 mg of MK-677 for 8 weeks	Bone formation and bone resorption	Increased markers of bone formation and bone resorption. Increase in serum levels of osteocalcin, IGF-I, IGFBP-5, and IGFBP-4.
Copinschi et al. 1997	9 healthy young men (18-39 years), 6 older subjects (65-71 years)	5 and 25 mg of MK-677 orally for three 7-day treatments; older subjects: 2 and 25 mg of MK-677 for two 14-day treatments	Sleep and hormonal data	Increase in stage IV sleep and an increase in REM sleep. In older subjects there was a decrease in REM latency. The frequency of deviations from normal sleep decreased.
Yarasheski et al. 1997	18 healthy elderly men (67 years)	12.5 or 18 μg/kg/day subcutaneous injection	Whole-body and regional BMD via DEXA and serum osteocalcin and IGF-I	Serum IGF-I and osteocalcin increased, and there was no change in BMD.
Chapman et al. 1996	15 women, 17 men (healthy, 64-81 years)	2, 10, or 25 mg of MK-677 orally once daily for 2 separate study periods of 14 and 28 days	GH, prolactin, and cortisol	GH concentrations increased in a dose-dependent manner. GH pulse height increased significantly without significant changes in the number of pulses. Serum IGF-I, fasting glucose, IGFBP-3, and prolactin increased. There was no change in cortisol.

Authors	Subjects	Growth hormone administration dose/duration	Dependent variables	Salient findings
Copinschi et al. 1996	9 healthy young men (18-39 years) weighing 65-80 kg	5 and 25 mg of MK-677 orally	IGF-I, IGFBP-3, GH, and cortisol	GH pulse frequency, plasma IGF-I levels, and IGFBP-3 levels were increased; and there was no effect on cortisol profiles.
Pierard-Franchimont et al. 1996	8 adult bodybuilders who abused GH	Self-administered GH	Mechanical properties of skin	Skin deformability and biological elasticity remained within the normal range; an increase in dermal viscosity was noted.
Yarasheski et al. 1995	23 sedentary, healthy elderly (64-75 years) men with low serum IGF-I levels	Strength training plus subcutaneous injection of placebo (15) or 12.5-24 µg rhGH/kg/day (8) for 7 days/week after each exercise session for 16 weeks	Serum IGF-I and antibodies to rhGH, whole-body protein turnover, body composition and anthropometry, and muscle strength	Despite variation in GH dose, anthropometric, muscle strength, and serum IGF-I response to GH were similar. IGF-I remained unchanged in placebo group while increasing twofold in GH group with increases in fat-free mass (FFM).
Taaffe et al. 1994	18 healthy elderly men (65-82 years)	.02 mg/kg/day	Muscle strength, body composition, circulating levels of IGF-I, IGFBP-3	IGF-I and IGFBP-3 increased. There was no effect on muscle strength. Body weight did not change, but lean mass increased and fat mass decreased.
Deyssig et al. 1993	22 healthy non-obese male power athletes	.09 IU/kg/day subcutaneously	GH, IGF-I, IGF-II, IGFBP-3, insulin, thyroxine, free thyroxine, triiodothyronine, TSH, LH, FSH, testosterone, blood glucose, and skinfolds	GH, IGF-I, and IGF-binding proteins increased significantly. Fasting insulin concentrations increased significantly and thyroxine levels decreased significantly. Body weight and body fat were unchanged.
Yarasheski et al. 1993	7 young, healthy, experienced male weight lifters (23 ± 2 yrs)	40 µg/kg/day subcutaneous injection	Fasting rate of whole-body protein breakdown and the fractional rate of muscle protein synthesis	Increased fasting serum IGF-I but did not increase the fractional rate of muscle protein synthesis or reduce the rate of whole-body protein breakdown.
Hartman et al. 1992	10 normal men	Oral doses of placebo or 30, 100, or 300 µg GHRP/kg and an i.v. injection of 1.0 µg GHRP/kg at weekly intervals.	Serum GH concentraions obtained at 5-min intervals for 1 hr before and 4 hr after each dose	Increases in GH concentrations and secretion rates.

(continued)

Table 5.1 *(continued)*

Authors	Subjects	Growth hormone administration dose/duration	Dependent variables	Salient findings
Yarasheski et al. 1992	16 men (21-34 years)	40 μg/kg/day subcutaneous injection	OGTT, body composition, muscle strength, overnight GH profile and serum IGF-I, whole-body and skeletal muscle protein kinetics	FFM and total body water increased along with whole-body protein synthesis rate and whole-body protein balance. Quadriceps muscle protein synthesis rate, torso and limb circumferences, and muscle strength did not increase.
Yarasheski et al. 1992	16 young healthy untrained men (27 years)	Strength training plus subcutaneous injection of placebo (9) or 40 μg rhGH/kg/day (7) after each exercise session, 5 days/week for 12 weeks	GH, IGF-I, OGTT, insulin levels, body composition and anthropometry, muscle strength, whole-body protein turnover, leucine turnover, and muscle biopsy	Serum GH curve and serum IGF-I remained unchanged in placebo, while GH curve in treated subjects increased. Glucose and insulin were unaffected by training or treatment. Body weight and FFM increased in both groups, but the increment of FFM was greater in the GH-treated group.
Zuliani et al. 1989	15 male bodybuilders	Self-administered hormonal substances	Anthropometric data, total cholesterol, triglycerides, HDL cholesterol and apolipoproteins B and A-1	Significant decrease of HDL cholesterol and apolipoprotein A-1.
Crist et al. 1988	8 well-trained adults	Double-blind, placebo crossover design, high-protein diet, administered hormonal substances, 2.67 mg/0.5 ml diluent 3 days/week, progressive resistance training program, 6 weeks in length	Underwater weighing, IGF-I concentrations, L-dopa/arginine, and submaximal stimulation of natural GH tests	Significant increase of FFM and decrease in body fat; 5 of 7 subjects had depressed GH response to stimulation after treatment.

IGFBP = insulin-like growth factor binding protein; rhIGF-I = recombinant human IGF-I; rhGH = recombinant human GH; GHRP = growth hormone releasing peptide; DEXA = dual energy x-ray absorptiometry; LDL = low density lipoproteins; HDL = high-density lipoproteins; BMD = bone mineral density; TSH = thyroid stimulating hormone; LH = leutinizing hormone; FSH = follicle stimulating hormone; OGTT = oral glucose tolerance test.

Physiological Effects of Insulin-Like Growth Factor Administration

In comparison to the research on GH administration, far fewer studies have addressed the effects of IGF-I supplementation in humans (Botfield et al. 1997; Fryburg 1994; Liao et al. 2000; Van Wyk and Smith 1999). A recent study by Mauras et al. (2000) demonstrated that recombinant human IGF-I (rhIGF-I) administration had significant anabolic effects in adults with a GH receptor

deficiency. Subjects were IGF-I deficient as a result of a mutation in the GH receptor gene. Baseline measures included infusion of stable tracers ($[^{13}C]$leucine, $[^2H_2]$glucose, and d_5-glycerol) and indirect calorimetry, dual energy X-ray absorptiometry-assessed body composition, and evaluation of growth factors. Subjects received rhIGF-I (60 g/kg) twice daily for eight weeks. Plasma IGF-I increased, fat mass decreased, and FFM increased. Protein turnover increases were accompanied by decreased protein oxidation and increased whole-body protein synthesis. All measures of lipolysis and fat oxidation were augmented, including glycerol turnover rate, free fatty acid and β-hydroxybutyrate, and fat oxidation. Administration of rhIGF-I had positive effects on body composition and measures of intermediate metabolism independent of GH, suggesting that this type of therapy may be beneficial for adult patients with Laron's syndrome.

Butterfield et al. (1997) examined the effects of both rhGH and rhIGF-I on protein metabolism in older women. Fourteen women (66-82 years) were randomly assigned to either 0.025 mg rhGH/kg once daily or rhIGF-I at 0.015, 0.03, or 0.06 mg/kg twice daily for one month. Both protein synthesis and breakdown, measured by a primed constant infusion of [^{15}N]glycine, were increased with rhGH and with the low and high dose of rhIGF-I. Net protein synthesis was significantly increased with rhGH and with the mid- and high-dose rhIGF-I. Muscle protein synthesis measured by incorporation of [$^{1-13}$C]leucine increased with the rhGH and the mid and high rhIGF-I doses. This was the first study to demonstrate that, contrary to results in other reports, GH and IGF-I were both able to stimulate muscle protein synthesis in older subjects.

Growth Hormone Secretagogues

According to classical endocrinology, GHRH positively stimulates the pituitary release of GH (Muller et al. 1999). However, since the seminal work of Bowers in the late 1970s, much work has concentrated on GH secretagogues (GHS) that are also known to positively stimulate GH release. Growth hormone secretagogues stimulate GH release through a separate and unique receptor and in a synergistic fashion with GHRH (Pong et al. 1996). Thus, the traditional view of GH release now has to be reconsidered. Growth hormone secretagogues remain an active and promising area of research (Argente et al. 1996; Bowers 1993; Bowers et al. 1984; Copinschi et al. 1996, 1997; Ghigo et al. 1997, 1998; Johansen et al. 1999; Patchett et al. 1995, 1998; Raun et al. 1998; Svensson 1999; Thorner et al. 1997).

The synthetic hexapeptides, GH-releasing peptides (GHRP-1 [a heptapeptide], -2, and -6 and hexarelin), are known to act at the level of the hypothalamus and may be acting directly on GHRH or somatostatin neurons or through a modulation of other hypothalamic factors that influence GH secretion. These peptides have been recognized for some time and may also act at the level of the anterior pituitary through receptors separate from the GHRH. Growth hormone-releasing peptide-6 was the first hexapeptide to be studied in humans. These peptides exhibit a robust dose-response relationship and are effective through a number of administration routes. For example, Hartman et al. (1992) evaluated GH responses in normal men after oral doses of hexarelin. In this study,

10 normal men received oral doses of placebo or 30, 100, or 300 g/kg of hexarelin. Deconvolution analysis assessed the pulsatile release of GH in blood samples obtained at five minute intervals for one hour before and after each condition. This analysis indicated that increasing doses of hexarelin progressively stimulated GH secretion. The increase in GH secretion was mainly due to an increase in the amplitude of GH secretory pulses with no change in GH pulse frequency.

Merck Laboratories developed an orally active GH-releasing peptide known as mimetic (MK-677). Administration of MK-677 was examined in normal, healthy younger and older adults; GH-deficient men; persons who were obese; and a population undergoing diet-induced catabolism. Chapman et al. (1996) studied the effects of MK-677 in healthy elderly adults. Thirty-two subjects (15 women and 17 men, aged 64-81 years) received a placebo or 2, 10, or 25 mg of MK-677 for two separate study periods of 14 and 28 days in a randomized, double-blind, placebo-controlled trial. Growth hormone pulse amplitude, interpulse nadir, and 24-hr mean concentrations were increased in a dose-response manner. This increase in GH also translated to an 87% increase in IGF-I concentrations, thereby making the mean IGF-I concentration comparable to those of young adults. Chapman et al. (1997) next evaluated MK-677 in GH-deficient adults. Subjects were nine men aged 17 to 34 with lifelong GH deficiency. Treatment was one daily oral dose of MK-677 at either 10 or 50 mg or placebo for four days over two treatment periods. Following treatment with 10 mg MK-677, 24-hr mean GH concentrations increased by 78% and IGF-I concentrations rose by 52%. Following treatment with 50 mg MK-677, 24-hr GH concentrations rose by 82% and IGF-I concentrations rose by 79%, indicating a dose-response relationship for MK-677 on circulating GH and IGF-I. Svensson et al. (1998b) studied 24 obese men taking either 25 mg of MK-677 or placebo daily for eight weeks. Treatment with MK-677 increased serum GH, IGF-I, IGFBP-3, and FFM and produced a transient increase in basal metabolic rate. In another study, Svensson et al. (1999) reported that 25-mg MK-677 administration in obese men positively influenced circulating lipoprotein concentrations via decrease in the low-density lipoprotein/high-density lipoprotein cholesterol ratio. Murphy et al. (1998) explored the efficacy of MK-677 for reversing diet-induced protein catabolism. Eight healthy subjects aged 24 to 39 years were calorically restricted (18 kcal/kg/day) for two 14-day periods. During the last seven days of each period, the subjects received either 25 mg of MK-677 or placebo. MK-677 improved nitrogen balance, indicating that short-term anabolic effects are maintained in patients who are in a catabolic state. Murphy et al. (1999) have also demonstrated that oral administration of MK-677 increases markers of bone turnover in healthy and functionally impaired older adults.

Another orally active GH secretagogue derived from ipamorelin, NN703, has also been recently studied. Hansen et al. (1999) initially characterized NN703 and reported that it had a different receptor than GHRP-6 and MK-677. Zdravkovic et al. (2000) subsequently investigated the pharmacodynamic and pharmacokinetic safety as well as tolerability of a single dose in healthy men. The study was double blind, randomized, and placebo controlled, with eight escalating doses (0.05 to 12 mg/kg body weight). Growth hormone area under the curve was significantly higher than control for the three highest doses, and GH maximal concentrations were higher at the four highest doses than with placebo. Furthermore, IGF-I concentrations were higher than with placebo for the 6.0 and 12.0 mg/kg body weight doses. No difference between treatment and placebo were observed for adrenocorticotropic hormone, luteinizing hormone, follicle-stimulating hormone, thyroid-stimulating hormone, prolactin, or cortisol. NN703 was well tolerated by the subjects, illustrating that NN703 may have promise for treating GH-deficient populations.

Insulin-Like Growth Factor Displacers

Recently, attention has been given to the indirect IGF-I-promoting activity of IGF displacers (Clark 1998). Lowman et al. (1998) have shown that it is possible to produce small molecules that act as "releasing factors" for IGFs. IGF-I binds to a family of at least six different binding proteins (including the ternary complex composed of IGF-I, IGFBP-3, and ALS). The bioavailability of IGF-I is limited in its bound form since the complexed molecules are too large to escape the circulation. Novel synthetic peptides have been produced that bind to the IGFBPs, which displace or prevent IGF binding, thus serving as IGF agonists. The complexity of this cascade is shown in figure 5.2. Most studies thus far have used animal models, with these molecules exhibiting some potential as therapeutic agents.

Measurement and Testing of Systemic Growth Hormone

Use of rhGH by athletes is banned by the International Olympic Committee and other sport governing bodies. However, there is no current valid or accepted method to test for rhGH use (Bradley and Sodeman 1990; Birkeland and Hemmersbach 1999; Clarkson and Thompson 1997; Healy and Russel-Jones 1997; Kicman and Cowan 1992). Despite recent assay developments, the ability to discern endogenous forms from exogenous molecules of GH remains dependent on both scientific methods and longitudinal testing prior to any GH supplementation. As this chapter has suggested, GH may be more important as a stimulator of other endogenous compounds than as a direct anabolic substance itself in its basic form. This concept has moved the debate and therapeutic array to other peptide compounds that may be the primary mediators of many of the 22-kD effects observed with injection studies. Measurement of GH can be problematic because of the pulsatile release and molecular heterogeneity of the hormone. Normal GH concentrations

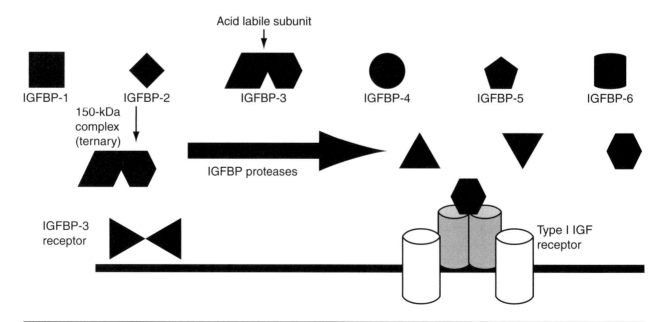

Figure 5.2 Insulin-like growth factor-I receptor sequence and interactions. IGFBP = insulin-like growth factor-binding protein.

can change dramatically during the day because of the episodic nature of the release as well as GH's sensitivity to exercise or stress—making the rather insensitive urinary measurement of GH futile. Alternatives for GH testing are biomarkers known to be influenced by GH action, such as the IGF-I system (Kicman et al. 1997).

Wallace et al. (1999) tested the hypothesis that components of the IGF-I system are potential markers of GH abuse. They evaluated serum GH, GH-binding protein (GHBP), total IGF-I, free IGF-I, IGFBP-3, and ALS after endurance exercise during GH administration (0.15 IU/kg/day) and GH withdrawal. One week of rhGH administration exaggerated the response of total IGF-I, IGFBP-3, and ALS. After GH withdrawal, the GH response to exercise was suppressed. The authors concluded that GH pretreatment augmented the exercise-induced changes in ternary complexes and that serum total IGF-I, IGFBP-3, and ALS may be suitable biomarkers of GH abuse. Saugy et al. (1996) have reported that an enzyme-linked immunoabsorbent assay (Norditest) is able to detect, without extraction, urinary hGH in a dynamic range of 2 to 50 ng hGH/L. In this study, after rhGH treatment for one week, urinary hGH excretion showed increases of 50 to 100 times the basal values and returned to near the mean normal level after 24 hr. Thus, the timing of the test (i.e., random testing vs. staged testing) will impact the results.

Tests of peripheral growth factors and other hormones influenced by rhGH will also depend on the determination of normal values of these factors and on determination of extremes in biological levels. However, since there is tremendous interindividual variation of hormonal levels, definitive interpretation of one random test result is difficult. Thus, testing is not a simple or easy solution to peptide hormone doping. Consequently no test for GH/IGF-I anabolic drug use has been put forth that is ready for legal or scientific challenges in a court of law.

Conclusion

The use of GH and IGF-I compounds has become popular over the past 10 years in both the general and athletic populations. Although the major sport governing bodies have made attempts to test for GH use by athletes, we are still far from a reliable test for exogenous GH use. There is still question as to the beneficial performance effects, if any, of exogenous GH administration. The equivocal nature of many of the human studies may be due to the complex nature of polypeptide interactions with the many target tissues in the body, as can be seen in the molecular heterogeneity of endogenous GH. Adverse side effects undoubtedly relate to this phenomenon of multiple targets. Crist et al. (1988) demonstrated that five of seven subjects had a suppressed GH response to stimulation from either L-dopa/arginine or submaximal exercise after their treatment period of six weeks, indicating a down-regulation

of endogenous GH production. In addition, it is clear that the use of many other types of synthetic polypeptide hormones and growth factors is likely to increase over the next decade as we continue to discover the complexities of the hormonal mechanisms related to growth (Hymer et al. 2000). Still, use of the many current forms of GH and IGF-I remains a legitimate health concern, since the effects on the body's general environment in the absence of constant monitoring and individualized dosing remains unknown. Use of GH for the purposes of performance enhancement remains more an art than a true medical science. Undoubtedly as science continues to discover new forms of the primary polypeptides of the pituitary and IGF axis, more interest will focus on these nonsteroidal compounds and their potential for anabolic effects and performance enhancement.

References

Argente, J., L.M. Garcia-Segura, J. Pozo, J.A. Chowen. Growth hormone-releasing peptide: clinical and basic aspects. *Horm Res* 46: 155-159, 1996.

Baumann, G. Growth hormone heterogeneity: genes, isohormones, variants, and binding proteins. *Endocrinol Rev* 12(4): 424-449, 1991.

Birkeland, K.I., P. Hemmersbach. The future of doping control in athletes. Issues related to blood sampling. *Sports Med* 28(1): 25-33, 1999.

Botfield, C., R.J. Ross, C.J. Hinds. The role of IGFs in catabolism. *Bailliere's Clin Endocrinol Metab* 11: 679-697, 1997.

Bowers, C.Y. GH Releasing Peptides – Structure and Kinetics. *J Ped Endocrinol.* 6: 21-31, 1993.

Bowers, C.Y., F.A. Momany, G.A. Reynolds, A. Hong. On the in vitro and in vivo activity of a new synthetic hexapeptide that acts on the pituitary to specifically release growth hormone. *Endocrinology* 114: 1537-1545, 1984.

Bradley, C.A., T.M. Sodeman. Human growth hormone. Its use and abuse. *Clin Lab Med* 10(3): 473-477, 1990.

Butterfield, G.E., J. Thompson, M.J. Renie, R. Marcus, R.L. Hintz, A.R. Hoffman. Effect of rhGH and rhIGF-I treatment on protein utilization in elderly women. *Am J Physiol* 272: E94-99, 1997.

Chapman, I.M., M.A. Bach, E. Van Cauter, M. Farmer, D. Krupa, A.M. Taylor, L.M. Schilling, K.Y. Cole, E.H. Skiles, S.S. Pezzoli, M.L. Hartman, J.D. Veldhuis, G.J. Gormley, M.O. Thorner. Stimulation of the growth hormone (GH)-insulin-like growth factor I axis by daily oral administration of a GH secretagogue (MK-677) in healthy elderly subjects. *J Clin Endocrinol Metab* 81: 4249-4257, 1996.

Chapman, I.M., O.H. Pescovitz, G. Murphy, T. Treep, K.A. Cerchio, D. Krupa, B. Gertz, W.J. Polvino, E.H. Skiles, S.S. Pezzoli, M.O. Thorner. Oral administration of growth hormone (GH) releasing peptide-mimetic MK-677 stimulates the GH/insulin-like growth factor-I axis in selected GH-deficient adults. *J Clin Endocrinol Metab* 82: 3455-3463, 1997.

Clark, R. Molecules that bind to insulin-like growth factor binding proteins. *Proc Fourth Int Sci Meeting* 217-229, 1998.

Clarkson, P.M., H.S. Thompson. Drugs and sport. Research findings and limitations. *Sports Med* 24: 366-384, 1997.

Copinschi, G., R. Leproult, A. Van Onderbergen, A. Caufriez, K.Y. Cole, L.M. Schilling, C.M. Mendel, I. De Lepeleire, J.A. Bolognese, E. Van Cauter. Prolonged oral treatment with MK-677, a novel growth hormone secretagogue, improves sleep quality in man. *Neuroendocrinology* 66: 278-286, 1997.

Copinschi, G., A. Van Onderbergen, M. L'Hermite-Baleriaux, C.M. Mendel, A. Caufriez, R. Leproult, J.A. Bolognese, M. De Smet, M.O. Thorner, E. Van Cauter. Effects of a 7-day treatment with a novel, orally active, growth hormone (GH) secretagogue, MK-677, on 24-hour GH profiles, insulin-like growth factor I, and adrenocortical function in normal young men. *J Clin Endocrinol Metab* 81: 2776-2782, 1996.

Crist, D.M., G.T. Peake, P.A. Egan, D.L. Waters. Body composition response to exogenous GH during training in highly conditioned adults. *J Appl Physiol* 65(2): 579-584, 1988.

Davies, J.S., C.L. Morgan, C.J. Currie, J.T. Green. Growth hormone use by body builders. *Br J Sports Med* 31(4): 352-353, 1997.

Deysigg, R., H. Frisch. Self-administration of cadaveric growth hormone in power athletes. *Lancet* 341(8847): 768-769, 1993.

Deyssig, R., H. Frisch, W.F. Blum, T. Waldhr. Effect of growth hormone treatment on hormonal parameters, body composition and strength in athletes. *Acta Endocrinologica* 128: 313-318, 1993.

Frisch, H. Growth hormone and body composition in athletes. *J Endocrinol Invest* 22(5 Suppl): 106-109, 1999.

Fryburg, D.A. Insulin-like growth factor I exerts growth hormone- and insulin-like actions on human muscle protein metabolism. *Am J Physiol* 267(2 Pt 1): E331-E336, 1994.

Ghigo, E., E. Arvat, F. Camanni. Orally active growth hormone secretagogues: state of the art and clinical perspectives. *Ann Med* 30: 159-168, 1998.

Ghigo, E., E. Arvat, G. Muccioli, F. Camanni. Growth hormone-releasing peptides. *Eur J Endocrinol* 136: 445-460, 1997.

Hansen, B.S., K. Raun, K.K. Nielsen, P.B. Johanseb, T.K. Hansen, B. Peschke, J. Lau, P.H. Anderson, M. Ankersen. Pharmacological characterization of a new oral GH secretagogue NN703. *Eur J Endocrinol* 141: 180-189, 1999.

Hartman, M.L., G. Farello, S.S. Pezzoli, M.O. Thorner. Oral administration of growth hormone (GH)-releasing peptide stimulates GH secretion in normal men. *J Clin Endocrinol Metab* 74: 1378-1384, 1992.

Harvey, S., C.G. Scanes, W.H. Daughaday. *Growth hormone.* Boca Raton, FL: CRC Press. 1995.

Healy, M.L., D. Russel-Jones. Growth hormone and sport: abuse, potential benefits, and difficulties in detection. *Br J Sports Med* 31(4): 267-268, 1997.

Hymer, W., K. Kirshnan, W.J. Kraemer, J. Welsch, W. Lanham. Mammalian pituitary growth hormone: applications of free flow electrophoresis. *Electrophoresis* 21: 311-317, 2000.

Hymer, W.C., W.J. Kraemer, B.C. Nindl, J.O Marx, D.E. Benson, J.R. Welsch, S.A. Mazzetti, J.S. Volek, D.R. Deaver. Characteristics of circulating growth hormone in women following acute heavy resistance exercise. *Amer J Physiol: Endocrinol Metab.* 281(4): E878-E887, 2001.

Janssen, Y., J.H. Doornbos, F. Roeltsema. Changes in muscle volume, strength, and bioenergetics during recombinant human Growth Hormone (GH) therapy in adults with GH deficiency. *J Clin Endocrinol Metab* 84(1): 279-284, 1999.

Johansen, P.B., J. Nowak, C. Skjaerbaek, A. Flyvbjerg, T.T. Andreassen, M. Wilken, H. Orskov. Ipamorelin, a new growth-hormone-releasing peptide, induces longitudinal bone growth in rats. *Growth Horm IGF Res* 9(2): 106-113, 1999.

Johnson, O.L., J.L. Cleland, H.J. Lee, M. Charnis, E. Duenas, W. Jaworowicz, D. Shepard, A. Shahzamani, A.J. Jones, S.D. Putney. A month-long effect from a single injection of microencapsulated human growth hormone. *Nat Med* 2: 795-799, 1996.

Johnson, O.L., W. Jaworowicz, J.L. Cleland, L. Bailey, M. Charnis, E. Duenas, C. Wu, D. Shepard, S. Magil, T. Last, A.J. Jones, S.D. Putney. The stabilization and encapsulation of human growth hormone into biodegradable microspheres. *Pharm Res* 14: 730-735, 1997.

Karila, T., H. Koistinen, M. Seppala, R. Koistinen, T. Seppala. Growth hormone induced increase in serum IGFBP-3 level is reversed by anabolic steroids in substance abusing power athletes. *Clin Endocrinol* 49(4): 459-463, 1998.

Kicman, A.T., D.A. Cowan. Peptide hormones and sport: misuse and detection. *Br Med Bull* 48(3): 496-517, 1992.

Kicman, A.T., J.P. Miell, J.D. Teale, J. Powrie, P.J. Wood, P. Laidler, P.J. Milligan, D.A. Cowan. Serum IGF-I and IGF binding proteins 2 and 3 as potential markers of doping with human GH. *Clin Endocrinol* 47(1): 43-50, 1997.

Knopp, W.D., T.W. Wang, B.R. Bach Jr. Ergogenic drugs in sports. *Clin Sports Med* 16(3): 375-392, 1997.

Lewis, U.J., Y.N. Sinha, G.P. Lewis. Structure and properties of members of the hGH family: a review. *Endocrinology J* 47: S1-S8, 2000.

Liao, W., M. Rudling, B. Angelin. Insulin-like growth factor I for growth hormone therapy. *Lancet* 355: 148, 2000.

Lowman, H.B., Y.M. Chen, N.J. Skelton, D.L. Mortenson, E.E. Tomlinson, M.D. Sadick, I.C. Robinson, R.G. Clark. Molecular mimics of insulin-like growth factor-I (IGF-I) for inhibiting IGF-I:IGF-binding protein interactions. *Biochemistry* 37: 8870-8878, 1998.

Macintyre, J.G. Growth hormone and athletes. *Sports Med* 4: 129-142, 1987.

Mauras, N., V. Martinez, A. Rini, J. Guevara-Aquirre. Recombinant human insulin-like growth factor I has significant anabolic effects in adults with growth hormone receptor deficiency: studies on protein, glucose, and lipid metabolism. *J Clin Endocrinol Metab* 85: 3036-3042, 2000.

Muller, E.E., V. Locatelli, D. Cocchi. Neuroendocrine control of growth hormone secretion. *Physiol Rev* 79: 511-607, 1999.

Murphy, M.G., M.A. Bach, MK-677 Study Group, D. Plotkin, J. Bolognese, J. Ng, D. Krupa, K. Cerchio, B.J. Gertz. Oral administration of the growth hormone secretagogue MK-677 increases markers of bone turnover in healthy and functionally impaired elderly adults. *J Bone Miner Res* 14: 1182-1188, 1999.

Murphy, M.G., L.M. Plunkett, B.J. Gertz, W. He, J. Wittreich, W.M. Polvino, D.R. Clemmons. MK-677, an orally active growth hormone secretagogue, reverses diet-induced catabolism. *J Clin Endocrinol Metab* 83: 320-325, 1998.

Neely, E.K., R.G. Rosenfield. Use and abuse of human growth hormone. *Ann Rev Med* 45: 407-420, 1994.

Patchett, A.A., R.P. Nargund, J.R. Tata, M.H. Chen, K.J. Barakat, D.B. Johnston, K. Cheng, W.W. Chan, B. Butler, G. Hickey. Design and biological activities of L-163,191 (MK-0677): a potent, orally active growth hormone secretagogue. *Proc Natl Acad Sci USA* 92: 7001-7005, 1995.

Patchett, A.A., R.G. Smith, M.J. Wyvratt. Orally active growth hormone secretagogues. *Pharm Biotechnol* 11: 525-554, 1998.

Pierard-Franchimont, C., F. Henry, J.M. Crielaard, G.E. Pierard. Mechanical properties of skin in recombinant human growth factor abusers among adult bodybuilders. *Dermatology* 192(4): 389-392, 1996.

Pong, S.S., L.Y. Chaung, D.C. Dean. R.P. Nargund, A.A. Patchett, R.G. Smith. Identification of a new G-protein-linked receptor for growth hormone secretagogues. *Mol Endocrinol* 10(1): 57-61, 1996.

Raun, K., B.S. Hansen, N.L. Johansen, H. Thogersen, K. Madsen, M. Ankersen, P.H. Andersen. Ipamorelin, the first selective growth hormone secretagogue. *Eur J Endocrinol* 139: 552-561, 1998.

Rudman, D., A.G. Fellar, H.S. Nagraj et al. Effects of human growth hormone in men over 60 years old. *New Engl J Med* 323: 1-6, 1990.

Saugy, M., C. Cardis, C. Schweizer, J.L. Veuthey, L. Rivier. Detection of human growth hormone doping in urine: out of competition tests are necessary. *J Chromatogr B Biomed Appl* 687(1): 201-211, 1996.

Spalding, B.J. Black-market biotechnology: athletes abuse EPO and HGH. *Biotechnology* 9(11): 1150, 1152-1153, 1991.

Svensson, J. Growth hormone secretagogues as therapeutic agents. *Growth Horm IGF Res* 9 (Suppl A): 107-109, 1999.

Svensson, J., J.O. Jansson, M. Ottosson, G. Johannsson, M.R. Taskinen, O. Wiklund, B.A. Bengtsson. Treatment of obese subjects with the oral growth hormone secretagogue MK-677 affects serum concentrations of several lipoproteins, but not lipoprotein (a). *J Clin Endocrinol Metab* 84: 2028-2033, 1999.

Svensson, J., L. Lonn, J.O. Jansson, G. Murphy, D. Wyss, D. Krupa, K. Cerchio, W. Polvino, B. Gertz, I. Boseaus, L. Sjostrom, B.A. Bengtsson. Two-month treatment of obese subjects with the oral growth hormone (GH) secretagogue MK-677 increases GH secretion, fat-free mass, and energy expenditure. *J Clin Endocrinol Metab* 83: 362-369, 1998a.

Svensson, J., C. Ohlsson, J.O. Jansson, G. Murphy, D. Wyss, D. Krupa, K. Cerchio, W. Polvino, B. Gertz, D. Baylink, S. Mohan, B.A. Bengtsson. Treatment with the oral growth hormone secretagogue MK-677 increases markers of bone formation and bone resorption in obese young males. *J Bone Miner Res* 13: 1158-1166, 1998b.

Taaffe, D.R., L. Pruitt, J. Reim, R.L. Hintz, G. Butterfield, A.R. Hoffman, R. Marcus. Effect of recombinant human growth hormone on the muscle strength response to resistance exercise in elderly men. *J Clin Endocrinol Metab* 79(5): 1361-1366, 1994.

Thorner, M.O., I.M. Chapman, B.D. Gaylinn, S.S. Pezzoli, M.L. Hartman. Growth hormone-releasing hormone and growth hormone releasing peptide as therapeutic agents to enhance growth hormone secretion in disease and aging. *Recent Prog Horm Res* 52: 215-246, 1997.

Van Wyk, J.J., E.P. Smith. Insulin-like growth factors and skeletal growth: possibilities for therapeutic interventions. *J Clin Endocrinol Metab* 84: 4349-4354, 1999.

Wadler, G.I. Drug use update. *Med Clin North Am* 78(2): 439-455, 1994.

Wallace, J.D., R.C. Cuneo, R. Baxter, H. Orskov, N. Keay, C. Pentecost, R. Dall, T. Rosen, J.O. Jorgensen, A. Cittadini, S. Longobardi, L. Sacca, J.S. Christiansen, B. Bengtsson, P.H. Sonksen. Responses of the growth hormone (GH) and insulin-like growth factor axis to exercise, GH administration, and GH withdrawal in trained adult males: a potential test for GH abuse in sport. *J Clin Endocrinol Metab* 84(10): 3591-3601, 1999.

Watanabe, S., N. Yamaguchi, Y. Tsunematsu, A. Komiyama. Risk factors for leukemia occurrence among growth hormone users. *Jpn J Cancer* 80: 822-825, 1989.

Windisch, P.A., F.J. Papatheofanis, K.A. Matuszewski. Recombinant human growth hormone for AIDS-associated wasting. *Ann Pharmacother* 32: 437-445, 1998.

Yarasheski, K.E. Growth hormone effects on metabolism, body composition, muscle mass, and strength. *Ex Sports Sci Rev* 22: 285-312, 1994.

Yarasheski, K.E., J.A. Campbell, W.M. Kohrt. Effect of resistance exercise and growth hormone on bone density in older men. *Clin Endocrinol.* 47(2):222-229, 1997.

Yarasheski, K.E., J.A. Campbell, K. Smith, M.J. Rennie, J.O. Holloszy, D.M. Bier. Effect of growth hormone and resistance exercise on muscle growth in young men. *Am J Physiol* 262(3 Pt 1): E261-E267, 1992.

Yarasheski, K.E., J.J. Zachwieja, T.J. Angelopoulos, D.M. Bier. Short-term growth hormone treatment does not increase muscle protein synthesis in experienced weight lifters. *J Appl Physiol* 74: 3073-3076, 1993.

Yarasheski, K.E., J.J. Zachwieja, J.A. Campbell, D.M. Bier. Effect of growth hormone and resistance exercise on muscle growth and strength in older men. *Am J Physiol* 268(2 Pt 1): E268-E276, 1995.

Zachwieja, J.J., K.E. Yarasheski. Does growth hormone therapy in conjunction with resistance exercise increase muscle force production and muscle mass in men and women aged 60 years or older? *Phys Ther* 79: 76-82, 1999.

Zdravkovic, M., B. Sogaard, L. Ynddal, T. Christiansen, H. Agerso, M.S. Thomsen, J.E. Falch, M.M. Iiondo. The pharmacokinetics, pharmacodynamics, safety and tolerability of a single dose of NN703, a novel orally active growth hormone secretagogue in healthy male volunteers. *Growth Horm IGF Res* 10(4): 193-198, 2000.

Zuliani, U., B. Bernardini, A. Catapano, M. Campana, G. Cerioli, M. Spattini. Effects of anabolic steroids, testosterone, and hGH on blood lipids and echocardiographic parameters in bodybuilders. *Int. J. Sports Med.* 10(1): 62-66, 1989.

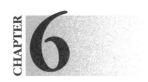

Physiological Effects of Testosterone Precursors

William J. Kraemer, PhD

Martyn R. Rubin, MS

Duncan N. French, MS

Michael R. McGuigan, PhD

The popularity of the use of supplements containing precursors to the male hormone testosterone is attributable in part to exposure gained from Mark McGwire's experimentation with androstenedione during his chase for the all-time home run record. In addition, treatments with such compounds as a part of anti-aging strategies have contributed to the use of these supplements. This popularity relates primarily to the goal of enhancing muscle mass or athletic performance without the need for use of exogenous testosterone or other synthetic forms of the hormone known as anabolic steroids. Supplement use is based on the concept of augmenting the body's own natural anabolic hormonal status. Classically, the anabolic environment has been associated with such hormones as testosterone, growth hormone, insulin, and insulin-like growth factors (IGF) (Kraemer et al., 1990, 2000). Protein and carbohydrate supplements during a resistance training program have been used to increase the concentrations of growth hormone, insulin, and IGF-I in the body following a workout in an attempt to augment recovery and promote muscular development; and recent research points toward the efficacy of this method (Kraemer et al., 1998). However, the precursor hormones are thought to play a more direct role in promoting an increase in the basal concentrations of testosterone itself, and thus can be considered a more potent means of adaptation.

The ingestion of a variety of testosterone precursors (i.e., androstenedione, dehydroepiandrosterone [DHEA]) has become popular within the context of the attempt to enhance endogenous testosterone production. This is especially so for men in resistance training programs who hope to promote and support the anabolic processes that evoke muscular development. At present, the efficacy of precursor hormonal substances as a direct cause of muscle hypertrophy remains unknown, though there is evidence that the efficacy is not as dramatic as that of testosterone itself or of its synthetic derivatives (Kraemer, 2000). The amount of information on use of these compounds can be considered limited at this time.

Biochemical Properties of Testosterone Precursors

Each of the precursor substances (often called prohormones) used in supplementation today is found primarily in the biosynthetic pathway of testosterone. In addition, each substance has its own biological potency as a weak androgen-anabolic compound. Figure 6.1 indicates that each of these prohormones has an integral role to play as precursors to the end product of testosterone.

Among the prohormone supplements, androstenedione has gained the most exposure. Androstenedione is a steroid produced endogenously primarily in the Leydig cells of the testes in men, in the ovaries in women, and in the adrenal cortex (Goodman, 1994; Guyton and Hall, 2000). In the male testes, the primary role of androstenedione is in the biosynthesis pathway of testosterone. Luteinizing hormone from the pituitary, in concert with cholesterol, initiates a cascade of events leading to gonadal steroid hormone synthesis. This pathway involves the enzymatic conversion of cholesterol to pregnenolone, which leads to DHEA, androstenedione, and ultimately testosterone. The normal pathway of gonadal steroidogenesis in the testes ends with the conversion of androstenedione to testosterone via the enzyme 17β-hydroxysteroid dehydrogenase, whereas normal ovarian steroidogenesis continues one step further with the enzymatic conversion of testosterone to estradiol via aromatase (Goodman, 1994; Guyton and Hall, 2000). The conversion of testosterone to estradiol has been one of the more dramatic effects with precursor hormonal supplement use. Figure 6.2 shows the further processing of testosterone. This bioprocessing of extra amounts of testosterone to maintain homeostatic balances in the body remains a prominent problem with the theoretical use of testosterone precursors.

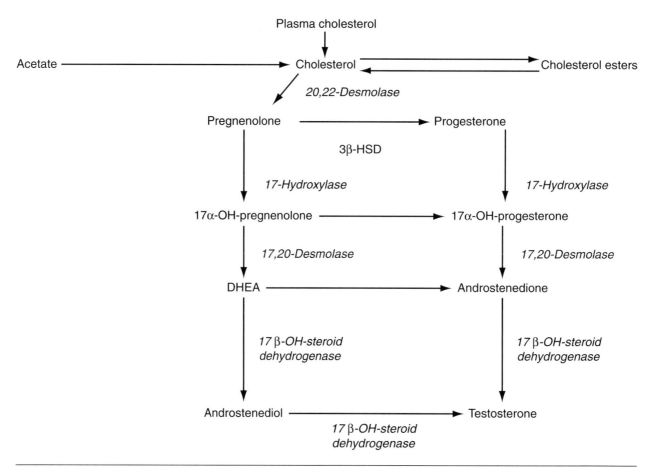

Figure 6.1 Pathways of testosterone biosynthesis in the human testis. 3β-HSD = 3β-hydroxysteroid dehydrogenase; DHEA = dehydroepiandrosterone.

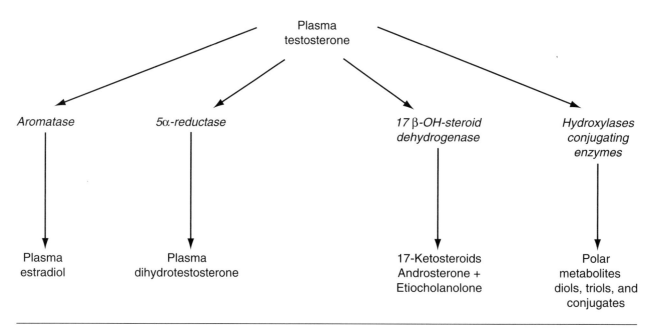

Figure 6.2 Pathways of peripheral metabolism of plasma testosterone. DHEA = dehydroepiandrosterone.

Again, the rationale behind ingestion of testosterone precursors such as androstenedione and DHEA is that increasing the concentrations of the primary precursors of testosterone will increase the total amount of testosterone synthesized at a basal rate, thereby helping to augment muscle protein synthesis. Recently, a number of studies (Mortola and Yen, 1990; Morales et al., 1994; Brown et al., 2000a,b) have examined the role of androstenedione and/or DHEA in the context of endogenous testosterone levels, muscular strength, and aging. Aging models provide a unique opportunity to examine the efficacy of testosterone precursor ingestion, since androgen production has been classically shown to decline with age. This has been termed "andropause" in men due to hypogonadal function. This is synonymous to the hormonal changes seen during menopause in women.

Hormonal Responses to Androstenedione Ingestion

Androstenedione has been marketed as a means of increasing blood testosterone concentrations in order to increase muscle mass and strength. Table 6.1 outlines the studies that have addressed hormonal responses to

androstenedione ingestion. Results of the effects of oral intake on serum testosterone concentrations are mixed. Ballantyne et al. (2000) recently examined the effects of androstenedione supplementation on the hormonal profiles of 10 men and its interaction with resistance exercise. Subjects ingested 200 mg of androstenedione or placebo in a crossover design for two days, also participating in heavy resistance training on the second day. Blood samples were taken before, after, and at 90 min after exercise. The supplement elevated the primary concentrations of androstenedione and luteinizing hormone, but did not change plasma testosterone concentrations significantly. Exercise in the supplemented condition significantly increased only estradiol levels, thus providing comparisons suggesting that androstenedione supplementation is unlikely to provide any anabolic benefits in association with heavy resistance exercise.

The theories behind the use of oral supplementation of androstenedione or DHEA as an effective means of increasing available free androgenic hormonal levels in humans are, however, developed from a sound biochemical rationale. Following an oral dosage in adult men of 300 mg/day of androstenedione for seven days,

Table 6.1   Androstenedione/Dehydroepiandrosterone (DHEA) and Hormonal Response Studies

Author/Year	Subjects	Treatment	Dependent variables	Results
Brown et al., 2000a	Adult men 30-56 years	Double-blind; 100 mg 3 times/day for 28 days	T, free T, andro, estradiol	↑ free T, estradiol, andro; ↔ T
Ballantyne et al., 2000	Adult men	Crossover design; 200 mg/day or placebo for 2 days; on day 2 subjects performed heavy resistance training	Andro, serum T, E_2, exercise	Andro group ↑ andro; ↑ T with no difference between conditions; ↑ plasma E_2 in andro group with exercise
Earnest et al., 2000	Young men	Crossover design; acute ingestion of 200 mg of 4-androstene-3, 17-dione (delta-4), 4-androstene-3β, 17β-diol (delta 4-diol), or placebo	T, free T, delta-4	T and free T AUC higher with delta-4 treatment than placebo but not delta 4-diol treatment
Leder et al., 2000	Adult men	Oral androstenedione ingestion (100 mg/day or 300 mg/day for 7 days) or no andro for 7 days	Serum T, andro, estrone, estradiol	Changes in T AUC significant for 300 mg/day only; E_2 AUC significant for 100 mg/day and 300 mg/day
Bosy et al., 1998	Adult men	50 mg/day for 30 days	T/EPIT	↔ urine T/EPIT
Labrie et al., 1997	Adult men and women	10 ml DHEA solution/day for 2 weeks (skin application)	DHEA, DHEA-S, andro, E_1 and E_2	↑ DHEA, DHEA-S, andro; ↔ serum T, DHT, E_1, E_2

T = testosterone; E_2 = estradiol; Andro = androstenedione; EPIT = epitestosterone; DHT = dihydrotestosterone; E_1= estrone; AUC = area under the curve

Leder et al. (2000) observed a significant increase in serum testosterone levels above baseline values. This rise in available testosterone, however, was not observed following 100 mg/day of androstenedione under the same conditions. Significant increases in hormonal estrogen concentrations were observed for both treatment dosages. These findings indicate that it is possible to increase androgenic hormone concentrations with an oral supplement of androstenedione when the dosage is large enough to initiate a response. Therefore, it appears that there is a dose-response curve with the use of these supplements when ingested orally. Leder et al. (2000) do suggest, however, that there is a marked variability between individual responses to the supplement for all measures of the sex steroids.

In an attempt to further determine the extent to which orally ingested androgenic hormone precursors for testosterone can be readily transformed to testosterone, Earnest et al. (2000) investigated the functional responses of a group of young men during supplementation of 200 mg of androstene-3,17-dione (delta-4) or 4-androstene-3β,17β-diol (delta-4 diol) over seven days. Free testosterone concentrations following the intervention were significantly higher than in a placebo control group for delta-4 supplementation, whereas no differences were observed following the ingestion of delta-4 diol. Again, these results may indicate that delta-4 is capable of producing increases in testosterone concentration within healthy young men following an oral supplementation period.

The trend continues for recent studies to show that the dosages recommended by manufacturers of androgenic supplements are insufficient to bring about significantly increased levels of free testosterone. Bosy et al. (1998) followed a group of adult men who received 50 mg of DHEA per day for 30 days. Results indicated that administration of DHEA at this dose, for this period of time, had minimal effects on the urinary ratio of testosterone to epitestosterone (an inactive synthetic byproduct), which indicates increased testosterone biosynthesis. After these negative results were obtained, a single subject agreed to take a single dosage of 250 mg for comparative purposes. This acute high dosage caused positive responses in the testosterone:epitestosterone ratio, which showed a 40% increase relative to pre-dose values.

In a short-term study by King et al. (1999), 10 subjects were randomly assigned to take a 100-mg dose of either androstenedione or a placebo in order to assess the acute effects of a single supplementation on circulating hormonal concentration. Baseline blood samples were collected prior to ingestion of the supplement and then every 30 min afterward for 6 hr. As has been seen in most cases, oral ingestion significantly increased andro-stenedione levels within the serum. However, this single dose did not change any of the serum concentrations for luteinizing hormone, follicle-stimulating hormone, or free or total testosterone. These findings contradict those of Bosy et al. (1998), who did see an active increase in testosterone activity following supplementation.

In a group of young men, Brown et al. (2000b) studied the effects of androgen precursors combined with herbal extracts designed to enhance testosterone formation and reduce conversion of androgens to estrogens. Subjects performed three days of resistance training per week for eight weeks. They consumed either placebo (n = 10) or a supplement (n = 10) that contained daily doses of 300 mg androstenedione, 150 mg DHEA, 750 mg *Tribulus terrestris,* 625 mg Chrysin, 300 mg indole-3-carbinol, and 540 mg saw palmetto. Serum androstenedione concentrations were significantly higher in the supplement group after two, five, and eight weeks, while serum concentrations of free and total testosterone were unchanged in both groups. Serum estradiol was significantly elevated at weeks 2, 5, and 8 in the supplement group; serum estrone was significantly elevated at weeks 5 and 8. Muscle strength significantly increased from weeks 0 to 4 and again from weeks 4 to 8 in both treatment groups. These data provided evidence that the addition of herbal extracts to androstenedione does not result in increased serum testosterone concentrations or reduce the estrogenic effect of androstenedione. Furthermore, there was no augmentation in the adaptations to resistance training.

A recent study addressed the effects of 100-mg androstenedione intake in healthy 30- to 56-year-old-men (Brown et al., 2000a). In a double-blind, random assignment design, subjects ingested androstenedione (n = 28) or placebo (n = 27) three times daily for 28 days. Ingestion of androstenedione did not alter serum total testosterone concentrations but significantly elevated serum free testosterone, estradiol, and androstenedione concentrations. There was no change in perceived mood, heath, or libido with androstenedione ingestion. Some speculate that consumers of androstenedione take much higher dosages than have been used in research studies. However, the effects of higher doses of androstenedione on muscle mass, strength, and hormone levels are unknown. The potential for greater conversion to other end products with such doses also remains a distinct possibility (see figure 6.1). For example, ingestion of higher doses of androstenedione, which may induce circulating concentrations far above physiological norms, may further enhance aromatase activity and the subsequent conversion of androstenedione to estrogen (King et al., 1999, Leder et al., 2000).

The use of androgenic prohormone substances in young women and children has not been studied for obvious reasons. Because of the androgenic nature of these compounds, the promotion of potentially higher-than-normal testosterone concentrations, and the fact that androstenedione may have a more dramatic impact as a natural anabolic mediator in response to resistance exercise in women, such studies are not considered ethical (Weiss et al., 1983). The use of these compounds in premenopausal women and children is considered potentially harmful due to the resulting abnormal concentration of these substances that would result. Such high amounts of these weak androgens would produce androgenic-anabolic effects that would be detrimental to normal functioning of a host of physical systems (e.g., endocrine, immune, and neuromuscular).

The interaction of weak androgens with the androgen receptor on the regulatory unit of the DNA chromatin proceeds is shown in figure 6.3. Testosterone and dihydrotestosterone bind to the androgen receptor (Goodman, 1994). The impact of the weaker androgens in the biosynthetic pathway of testosterone and dihydrotestosterone is due to a less dramatic impact on the primary binding sites for these other two hormones. Yet, the weaker androgens do have effects where these compounds may not be typically found due to tissue differences in biosynthetic processing and such acute conversions within the body would affect the natural amounts of these hormones. Such impact may be more prominent in premenopausal women and young children, who have only low blood concentration of endogenous androgens naturally (Goodman, 1994; Guyton and Hall, 2000). Thus, the external effects (e.g., bone, hair) of androgenic-anabolic steroids may be more dramatic with exogenous administration of testosterone precursors.

Many questions about androgen actions remain unanswered. The acceptor sites for the androgen-receptor complexes in the nuclei (called the hormone regulatory element) are palindromes in the DNA sequences located 5' to the genes under control of the hormone, and they recognize specific sequences in the DNA-binding domains of the receptors (Goodman, 1994; Guyton and Hall, 2000). Exactly how the weak precursor androgens impact this binding phenomenon remains unclear, but direct effects as they relate to the primary domains of the receptors for testosterone and dihydrotestosterone in

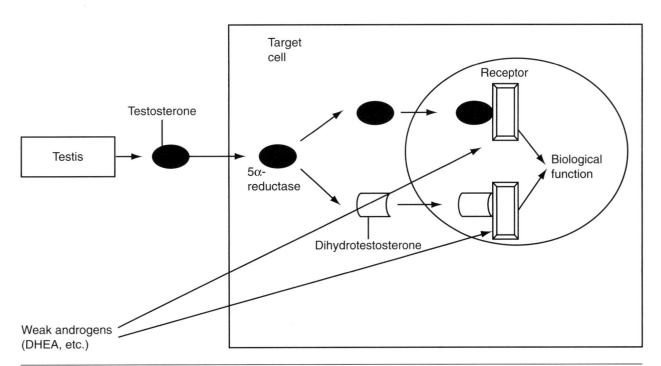

Figure 6.3 Diagram of androgen-binding physiology. Testosterone binds to the androgen receptor in the target cell, either directly or after conversion to dihydrotestosterone. The primary binding for muscle is testosterone, and that for sex-linked tissues (e.g., prostate) is dihydrotestosterone. Weak androgens interact with these receptor sites to a lesser extent through partial binding on the primary receptor sequences and allosteric sites. In addition, they bind to other receptors and stimulate production of other hormones such as insulin-like growth factor-I.

tissues are different (Goodman, 1994; Guyton and Hall, 2000). For example, the primary hormone, which binds to a reactor, varies between sex-linked tissues (PHT) versus skeletal muscle (T). Each tissue will have its own preference for the testosterone molecule it binds with maximally to produce physiological effects. Hormone specificity may be related to the location of the hormone regulatory element with respect to the coding sequence under hormonal control, differences in binding affinities of the complex, or participation of additional transcription regulatory proteins in the active transcription complex. Androgen actions are limited in most tissues if gene-based growth has occurred as in puberty. Thus, our understanding of the interactions of the precursor steroids is complicated by the fact that many aspects of the two primary hormones, testosterone and dihydrotestosterone, remain unresolved. In addition, it has been shown in an exercise rat model that exercise-induced changes do not affect the affinities for testosterone but rather the maximal binding, making certain strategies for precursor interactions less clear at the level of the muscle, which is the primary target for anabolic effects with training (Deschenes et al., 1994).

Muscle Development in Response to Androstenedione Supplementation

Results from recent studies on the use of androstenedione as a dietary supplement to increase protein synthesis and muscle growth have largely conflicted with the messages promoted by the companies that market this product for muscle hypertrophy purposes. Table 6.2 summarizes the studies on muscle changes in response to androstenedione supplementation. These studies have generally involved younger healthy men. The effect of ingestion of oral androstenedione on muscle growth and strength levels has been inconsistent, and no direct evidence suggests that it is an effective anabolic agent.

In a five-day study designed to examine the effects of androstenedione on skeletal muscle anabolism, Rasmussen et al. (2000) concluded that 100-mg oral supplementation per day had no significant effect on the rate of protein metabolism in young men. In six healthy young men, plasma levels of testosterone and luteinizing hormone did not change from basal levels following administration, whereas plasma concentrations of

Table 6.2   Androstenedione/Dehydroepiandrosterone (DHEA) and Muscle Growth Studies

Author/Year	Subjects	Treatment	Dependent variables	Results
Rasmussen et al., 2000	Young men	100 mg/day for 5 days; androstenedione	Protein turnover with infusion of L-[ring-2H5] phenalanine, plasma T, andro, LH, E_2	↑ andro, E_2; ↔ T, LH; no effect on protein synthesis or breakdown
King et al., 1999	Young men	8 weeks resistance training; androstenedione/placebo	Serum T, E_2, muscle fiber CSA	↔ T, ↑ E_2 with andro; ↑ muscle fiber CSA, no difference between groups
Wallace et al., 1999	Trained adult men	12 weeks androstenedione vs. DHEA, 100 mg/day for 12 weeks; nonsupervised resistance training	LBM, strength, plasma T, DHEA, DHEA-S, andro, IGF-I	Small ↑ in LBM (no effect of supplementation); ↑ in DHEA-S from baseline and placebo with DHEA; ↑ IGF-I from baseline with DHEA (no difference between groups)
Brown et al., 1999	Young men	8 weeks resistance training; DHEA/placebo	Serum T, E_2, estrone, estriol, strength, LBM	No change in any hormones; ↑ LBM similar with DHEA and placebo
Welle et al., 1990	Healthy males	4 weeks supplementation, 1600 mg/day DHEA/placebo	Plasma DHEA-sulphate, T, cholesterol, body weight, LBM, energy expenditure, leucine flux, rate of leucine incorporation	↑ in DHEA; ↔ body weight, LBM; ↔ energy and protein metabolism (i.e., nonoxidized portion of leucine flux); ↔ cholesterol, T

T = testosterone; LH = luteinizing hormone; E_2 = estradiol; CSA = cross sectional area; LBM = lean body mass; Andro = androsteredione androstenedione and estradiol did increase significantly. When protein synthesis or breakdown was compared to values in a nontreatment control group, results clearly showed that oral androstenedione had no anabolic effect on protein metabolism.

In a similar effort to establish the role that oral androstenedione supplementation may play in muscle hypertrophy and skeletal muscle fiber development, King et al. (1999) examined the effect of ingestion of androstenedione in conjunction with resistance training exercise. Brown et al. (1999) studied the use of an androgenic supplement during resistance training but with the precursor DHEA. Both studies tracked a group of sedentary young men through eight weeks of whole-body resistance training, with King et al. administering 300-mg doses of androstenedione per day and Brown et al. administering only 150 mg/day of DHEA. Both studies showed little change in free hormone levels following the treatment period, except that King et al. saw a significant rise in estradiol after supplementation, suggesting aromatization of the ingested supplement. Most notably, in the context of muscle hypertrophy, significant increases in muscular strength and muscle fiber cross-sectional area were not different between groups receiving androstenedione, DHEA, or placebo. Also, significant increases in lean body mass and decreased fat mass following the resistance training program were not different between supplement and placebo groups in either study. The findings of both studies support the stand that androstenedione, or its precursor DHEA, has little or no effect in enhancing skeletal muscle adaptations when ingested as an oral supplement.

Current research has continued to question the practical benefits of androstenedione supplementation on muscle growth. The volume of studies that show few or no positive characteristics of hypertrophy following a prolonged period of ingestion continues to increase. Indeed, more effort has been focusing on this area since the rise in the popularity of prohormone supplementation among both professional and recreational athletes. In a study of trained subjects with an active history of strength training exercise, Wallace et al. (1999) sought to discover the extent to which androstenedione or DHEA can be used to augment the characteristic changes in muscular profiles brought about by resistance exercise. There were small increases in lean body mass and mean strength following 12-week supplementation (100 mg androstenedione or DHEA per day), but neither change was shown to be a direct result of the androgenic agent. When the results were compared to placebo results from the same group of subjects, there were no significant differences in either of these measures.

The failure of certain orally ingested supplementary androgenic agents to influence energy or protein metabolism in humans was demonstrated in early research done by Welle et al. (1990). In this study of high dosages (1600 mg/day) of DHEA over a four-week period, the parameters of lean body mass, energy expenditure, and protein metabolism were compared to placebo results. Ingestion of DHEA caused a ninefold increase in DHEA sulfate concentrations but had no significant effect on body weight or on two parameters of lean body mass. Furthermore, DHEA supplementation caused no significant changes in any of the parameters of energy expenditure and protein metabolism, including resting metabolic rate, total energy expenditure, and an index of whole-body protein synthesis (leucine flux). All these findings suggest that oral ingestion of DHEA does not play an important regulatory role in energy or protein metabolism in humans.

In the context of oral administration of androstenedione as a means of augmenting protein synthesis and the development of skeletal muscle, studies have presented conflicting evidence with respect to the underlying theories. In view of the potent anabolic effect that testosterone can have in the growth of skeletal muscle, strength and power athletes view any means of manipulating endogenous testosterone levels as a potential ergogenic aid. Because of the role androstenedione plays in the schema of gonadal steroid hormone synthesis, the hypotheses for its use as a means of enhancing protein synthesis are indeed founded in basic science. The findings from the limited amount of research discussed here suggest that the use of androstenedione for ergogenic purposes remains highly questionable.

Androstenedione Ingestion With Age

Interestingly, aging in women and men is characterized by a progressive decline of circulating DHEA levels. Research has shown improvement in well-being and an absence of adverse effects with replacement doses of DHEA in older men and women (Mortola and Yen, 1990; Morales et al., 1994). Restoring DHEA to young-adult levels in older persons appears to increase the bioavailability of IGF-I as shown by increased IGF-I and a decrease in IGF-binding protein-1 levels (Morales et al., 1994). The improvement in well-being described in post-menopausal women treated with DHEA suggests that the steroid may exert beneficial effects on the central nervous system. The decreases in circulating levels of beta-endorphins are considered to be hormonal markers of the neuroendocrine modifications. More recently, Stomati et al. (1999) investigated the neuroendocrine and behavioral effects of three months of DHEA supplementation in postmenopausal women. After each treatment, the beta-endorphin response was completely restored, suggesting that DHEA and its active metabolites modulate the neuroendocrine control of pituitary beta-endorphin secretion.

The study by Brown et al. (2000) did not show a significant differential response with respect to age after androstenedione supplementation, apart from dihydrotestosterone. There was no relationship between age and changes in serum androstenedione, free testosterone, or estradiol concentrations. The results showed that ingestion of 100 mg of androstenedione three times each day is unlikely to provide a hormonal profile for promoting muscle size in older adults. However, the research with androstenedione and older adults is limited, and no studies have addressed the long-term effects of supplementation in any population.

Bioavailability of Dehydroepiandrosterone Products

One of the greatest concerns surrounding the use of prohormones is the purity of the compounds in a supplement (Parasrampuria et al., 1998). This concern relates directly to the uncontrolled production of these compounds in many corporate laboratories that do not achieve the quality of a pharmaceutical standard. The primary adverse effect associated with use of androstenedione appears to be a reduction in the "good" cholesterol (high-density lipoproteins) (King et al., 1999). In addition, as reviewed earlier, increases in the circulating concentrations of estrogen in men have been observed in androstenedione ingestion studies (King et al., 1999; Leder et al., 2000). This potentiation of estrogen is presumably a result of peripheral conversion of androstenedione to estrogen via the enzyme aromatase. In this light, the anabolic environment may actually be compromised as a result of ingestion of testosterone precursors. Rather than the desired increases in testosterone production with the aim of enhancing performance and optimizing the anabolic environment, there may be an attenuation in muscular strength and exercise performance. Other side effects have not been noted in clinical studies, but given that the content of a supplement is often unknown and that positive drug tests have been obtained in athletes using these supplements, their use as anabolic agents for enhanced performance remains unclear (Myhal and Lamb, 2000).

Conclusion

Androstenedione is an anabolic-androgenic steroid produced primarily in the Leydig cells of the testes in men, the ovaries in women, and the adrenal cortex. Androstenedione is an immediate precursor to testosterone and estrogen; and it has been suggested that increasing the level of the primary precursors of testosterone will increase the total amount of testosterone synthesized at a basal rate, thereby augmenting muscle protein synthesis. However, the findings of the research discussed in this chapter indicate that the use of androstenedione for ergogenic purposes remains highly questionable. Studies in healthy men taking oral androstenedione have had varying outcomes regarding the effects on serum testosterone concentrations, strength, and muscle mass. Little evidence exists concerning the use of androstenedione by older adults or children, and the long-term health effects of androstenedione supplementation are unknown. Androstenedione is on the list of banned substances for the National Collegiate Athletic Association (NCAA), U.S. Olympic Committee (USOC), and International Olympic Committee (IOC) and will produce positive drug tests.

Current discussion of the use of androstenedione seems to have resulted in a controversy concerning how to classify this and other similar testosterone precursors. For instance, if androstenedione is officially classified as an "anabolic steroid," similar to other synthetic pharmacological forms of testosterone, by not only the NCAA, USOC, and IOC but also the Drug Enforcement Agency, this would make it an illegal drug (i.e., a Schedule III controlled substance). Thus, the use of testosterone precursors may have tremendous legal implications. As a result, up to now there has been uncertainty as to how to classify testosterone precursors in light of the question whether testosterone precursors are in fact steroids. The underlying issue is whether the substance produces anabolic growth of tissue. Such direct evidence remains to be demonstrated in the scientific literature within the moral confines of such experimentation (as discussed previously in relation to women and children).

Biologically speaking, there is little question that androstenedione, DHEA, and other testosterone precursors are steroid hormones, based on the molecular biology of these compounds. Again, the legal classification will not be simple. If androstenedione is officially classified as an "anabolic steroid" by law, thereby making possession illegal, the implications for androstenedione use may go beyond the physiological and performance effects of testosterone precursor ingestion; there will be additional legal and ethical questions as well. The fact that testosterone precursors are considered "weak androgens" speaks to the lesser physiological potency of these compounds relative to testosterone itself and its synthetic forms—a fact that clinicians and sports medicine professionals must consider when addressing this issue.

References

Ballantyne C.S., S.M. Philips, J.R. MacDonald, M.A. Tarnopolsky, and J.D. MacDougal. The acute effects of androstenedione supplementation in healthy young males. *Canadian Journal of Applied Physiology* 25(1): 68-78. 2000.

Bosy T.Z., K.A. Moore, and A. Poklis. The effect of oral dehydroepiandrosterone (DHEA) on the urine testosterone/epitestosterone (T/E) ratio in human male volunteers. *Journal of Analytical Toxicology* 22(6): 455-459. 1998.

Brown G.A., M.D. Vukovich, E.R. Martini, M.L. Kohut, W.D. Franke, D.A. Jackson, and D.S. King. Endocrine responses to chronic androstenedione intake in 30-56-year-old men. *Journal of Clinical Endocrinology and Metabolism* 85: 4074-4080. 2000a.

Brown G.A., M.D Vukovich, T.A Reifenrath, N.L Uhl, K.A Parsons, R.L.Sharp, and D.S. King. Effects of anabolic precursors on serum testosterone concentrations and adaptations to resistance training in young men. *International Journal of Sports Nutrition, Exercise and Metabolism* 10(3): 340-359. 2000b.

Brown G.A., M.D. Vukovich, R.L. Sharp, T.A. Reifenrath, K.A. Parsons, and D.S. King. Effect of oral DHEA on serum testosterone and adaptations to resistance training in young men. *Journal of Applied Physiology* 87(6): 2274-2283. 1999.

Deschenes M.R., C.M. Maresh, L.E. Armstrong, J.M. Covault, W.J. Kraemer, and J.F. Crivello. Endurance and resistance exercise induce muscle fiber type specific responses in androgen binding capacity. *Journal of Steroid Biochemistry and Molecular Biology* 50(3/4): 175-179. 1994.

Earnest C.P., M.A. Olson, C.E. Broeder, K.F. Breuel, and S.G. Beckham. In vivo 4-androstene-3, 17-dione and 4-androstene-3 beta, 17 beta-diol supplementation in young men. *European Journal of Applied Physiology* 81(3): 229-232. 2000.

Goodman H.M. *Basic Medical Endocrinology,* 2nd ed. Lippencott-Raven, Philadelphia. 1994.

Guyton A.C., and J.E. Hall. *Textbook of Medical Physiology,* 10th ed. Saunders, Philadelphia. 2000.

King D.S., R.L. Sharp, M.D. Vukovich, G.A. Brown, T.A. Reifenrath, N.L. Uhl, and K.A. Parsons. Effect of oral androstenedione on serum testosterone and adaptations to resistance training in young men: a randomized controlled trial. *Journal of the American Medical Association* 281(21): 2020-2028. 1999.

Kraemer, W.J. Endocrine responses to resistance exercise. In *Essentials of Strength and Conditioning,* 2nd ed., T.R. Baechle (ed.). Human Kinetics, Champaign, IL, 91-114. 2000.

Kraemer W.J., L. Marchitelli, D. McCurry, R. Mello, J.E. Dziados, E. Harman, P. Frykman, S.E. Gordon, and S.J. Fleck. Hormonal and growth factor responses to heavy resistance exercise. *Journal of Applied Physiology* 69(4): 1442-1450. 1990.

Kraemer W.J., J.S. Volek, J.A. Bush, M. Putukian, and W.J. Sebastianelli. Hormonal responses to consecutive days of heavy-resistance exercise with or without nutritional supplementation. *Journal of Applied Physiology* 85(4): 1544-1555. 1998.

Labrie, F., A. Belanger, L. Cusan, and B. Candas. Physiological changes in dehydroepiandrosterone are not reflected by serum levels of active androgens and estrogens but of their metabolites: intraconology. *Journal of Clinical Endocrinological Metabolism* 82(2): 2403-2409. 1997.

Leder B.Z., C. Longcope, D.H. Catlin, B. Ahrens, D.A. Schoenfeld, and J.S. Finkelstein. Oral androstenedione administration and serum testosterone concentrations in young men. *Journal of the American Medical Association* 283(6): 779-782. 2000.

Morales A.J., J.J. Nolan, J.C. Nelson, and S.S. Yen. Effects of replacement dose of dehydroepiandrosterone in men and women of advancing age. *Journal of Endocrinology Metabolism* 78(6): 1360-1367. 1994.

Mortola J.F., and S.S. Yen. The effects of oral dehydroepiandrosterone on endocrine-metabolic parameters in postmenopausal women. *Journal of Clinical Endocrinology and Metabolism* 71(3): 696-704. 1990.

Myhal M., and D.R. Lamb. Hormones as performance enhancing drugs. In *Sports Endocrinology,* M.P. Warren and N.W. Constantini (eds.). Humana Press, Totowa, NJ, 433-476. 2000.

Parasrampuria J., K. Schwartz, and R. Petesch. Quality control of dehydroepiandrosterone dietary supplement products. *Journal of the American Medical Association* 280(18): 1565. 1998.

Rasmussen B.B., E. Volpi, D.C. Gore, and R.R. Wolfe. Androstenedione does not stimulate muscle protein anabolism in young healthy men. *Journal of Clinical Endocrinology and Metabolism* 85(1): 55-59. 2000.

Stomati M., S. Rubino, A. Spinetti, D. Parrinni, S. Luisi, E. Casarosa, F. Petraglia, and A.R. Genazzani. Endocrine, neuroendocrine and behavioral effects of oral dehydroepiandrosterone sulfate supplementation in postmenopausal women. *Gynecological Endocrinology* 13(1): 15-25. 1999.

Wallace M.B., J. Lim, A. Cutler, and L. Bucci. Effects of dehydroepiandrosterone vs androstenedione supplementation in men. *Medicine and Science in Sports and Exercise* 31(12): 1788-1792. 1999.

Welle S., R. Jozefowicz, and M. Statt. Failure of dehydroepiandrosterone to influence energy and protein metabolism in humans. *Journal of Clinical Endocrinology and Metabolism* 71(5): 1259-1264. 1990.

Weiss L.W., K.J. Cureton, and F.N. Thompson. Comparison of serum testosterone and androstenedione responses to weight lifting in men and women. *European Journal of Applied and Occupational Physiology* 50(3): 413-419. 1983.

Human Chorionic Gonadotropin

R. Craig Kammerer, PhD

Human chorionic gonadotropin (hCG) is a naturally occurring hormone produced primarily by the placenta. It is a member of the glycoprotein hormone family, which includes luteinizing hormone (LH), follicle-stimulating hormone (FSH), and thyroid-stimulating hormone (TSH). All these hormones consist of a common α-subunit and a unique β-subunit, the latter of which helps confer specific activity in the body. Each of these molecules has a large molecular weight, making it a formidable task to detect and analyze for any of them in a tissue or fluid sample. The levels of hCG rise dramatically in the female human beginning about 10 days after fertilization of the egg by a sperm cell. Along with estrogen, hCG helps maintain the pregnancy, with the levels of hCG doubling (Pittaway et al., 1986) every two days during the first 60 days of a pregnancy. Because of the rapid rise in hCG levels very soon after fertilization or conception, hCG has served as the basis for the most commonly utilized pregnancy tests in the human, which have been on the market as a variety of home test kits since 1977. Over 100 different pregnancy test kits exist, and 19 million tests were sold for home use in 1999 (Lipsitz, 2000). Human chorionic gonadotropin also has recently been shown to directly stimulate the Leydig cells to produce testosterone, and to block the effects of physical exercise in lowering testosterone production by directly stimulating endocrine testicular function (DeLeo et al., 2000). Therein lie the main reasons why athletes consider abuse of hCG.

Human Chorionic Gonadotropin, the Drug

For many years, hCG was considered a female hormone not found in the male, and present only at low levels in the female until the initiation of pregnancy. As test methods improved, low levels of hCG were found in nonpregnant females and at much lower levels in males (Robertson et al., 1978; Braunstein et al., 1979), with definitive studies appearing that showed the presence of hCG both in nonpregnant females and in males (Alfthan et al., 1992a; Stenman et al., 1987; Odell & Griffin, 1987).

Data also emerged to indicate that there was a relationship between the presence of the hormone hCG and certain malignancies. These cases included nontrophoblastic disease, like pancreatic and biliary

cancer (Alfthan et al., 1992b) and testicular cancer (Mann & Karl, 1983), as well as gestational trophoblastic disease (Stenman et al., 1985; Ozturk et al., 1988). In the latter cases, the levels of hCG were higher than the levels found during a normal pregnancy.

Besides being a large polypeptide molecule made up of two large subunits, hCG, like the other glycoprotein hormones, is glycosylated to varying degrees. Glycosylation is simply the linking of each subunit molecule to varying numbers of sugar molecules. The resulting molecule, with added sugar moieties, then has higher specificity for certain regions in the body; in other words, the process of sugar addition helps direct the hormone to various action sites (receptors) and/or determine its clearance rate (elimination of the hormone from the tissue after its action is finished). Research has shown that the presence of hyperglycosylated hCG indicates an abnormal pregnancy and that the presence of a specific variant of hyperglycosylated hCG indicates Down's syndrome. Prenatal urine testing for this variant of hyperglycosylated hCG is becoming the prevailing screening test for the presence of Down's syndrome in a developing human fetus.

Today, it appears that hCG, once thought to be exclusively a female hormone needed only to maintain pregnancy, now has several functions, depending upon the sex and the disease status of the person.

Use and Abuse in Sport

Since hCG is basically a female hormone and not a stimulant, hallucinogen, or sedative, not until recently had it seemed likely that members of the public would have any reason to abuse the drug, as there were no apparent "beneficial" effects from use of the compound. However, athletes state that hCG increases natural testosterone levels, particularly after the long-term suppression of testosterone synthesis that results from anabolic steroid abuse. In addition, athletes also claim that use of hCG enhances fat burning/loss, stimulates the testes (which would increase the natural synthesis of testosterone), and increases the libido. Data have appeared to indicate that hCG administration may enhance endogenous testosterone production and/or normalize production of testosterone after it has been suppressed (DeLeo et al., 2000).

It is clear that the primary therapeutic use for hCG is to stimulate gonadal steroid production (Dunkel et al., 1985; Martikainen et al., 1986). In the recently disclosed secret East German National Doping program, which was in place for decades, hCG use was a part of many of the protocols used in the doping of athletes (Franke & Berendonk, 1997). Natural levels of hCG increase during circumstances in which rapid growth is needed (e.g., for the obvious purpose of sustaining a pregnancy, with a side effect of helping sustain growth of some tumor tissues that might be present). Thus, a reasonable result of hCG use would be to stimulate testosterone production and/or normalize the testosterone/epitestosterone ratio in man, either after or during administration of anabolic steroids. As a result, hCG usage has grown in athletes who wish to increase their performance while avoiding any conviction for drug abuse.

Any potential side effects of hCG usage are difficult to predict. In men, it is unclear what processes supplementation with hCG would induce, as hCG is a female placental hormone that is present in extremely small amounts in the male and whose presence in the male at all is not yet clear. Human chorionic gonadotropin is obviously often involved in the induction of cell proliferation, as its presence in many malignant tissues and any pregnancy indicates. It also stimulates testosterone production, particularly in cases in which the levels of testosterone are below normal, as discussed later in the chapter. In females, the question of any side effects is less relevant, as hCG use is not banned in women—obviously because it would be ridiculous, as well as legally untenable, to ban pregnancy. Side effects in women are again difficult to predict, aside from the induction of the menstrual cycle.

Testing Methods

The International Olympic Committee (IOC, 2001) has banned hCG usage only in males, because of the extremely small levels found in the male, with larger levels detectable only in the case of malignancy. Acceptable methods listed by the IOC for detection of hCG abuse are immunoassay for screening of samples, with a different immunoassay required for a confirmation test. This use of immunoassay for both screening and confirmation tests, without any use of mass spectrometry in the confirmation test, does raise a major question of scientific and legal validity.

Mass spectrometry involves the ionization (induction of charge into the molecule by removal of electrons from the structure) of the drug molecule by a variety of techniques, which usually yields information about the molecular weight of the molecule and often information about some or many of the pieces that are formed when gentle fragmentation of the molecule is induced by the ionization process. This molecular-structural information, when coupled with chromatographic or separation information, is usually definitive for the identification of a molecule. When this information is compared with the known drug, analyzed under identical conditions, and yields the same results, the identification of the drug is certain.

While it is certainly true that the use of two different immunoassay tests on the same suspicious sample, both of which give the same positive result, indicates a higher degree of certainty in the result than does the use of only a single test (Leinenon et al., 1999), the specificity of a mass spectrometric test has still not been reached. In the past, it was required that *all* confirmation tests for *all* drugs be based upon a mass spectrometric detection method in order to achieve the level of certainty necessary for conviction of an athlete for drug abuse. The use of a mass spectrometric confirmation test, when performed under the correct conditions, with proper control sample comparisons, confers a degree of certainty unequaled by any other testing method. One has to remember that such a positive drug test has the effect of ruining the entire future of the individual and removing most of the financial rewards of being a world-class athlete.

Many immunoassays have been developed for the detection of hCG, yet it has been known for many years that they can produce discordant results (Cole & Kardana, 1992). Although immunoprocedures for hCG detection in both clinical treatment and doping control were reviewed recently (Stenman et al., 1997), and a detailed description of the value of hCG testing for detection of Down's syndrome appeared (Cole et al., 1999a), recent studies have reported a disturbing number of false-positive results with the use of hCG immunoassays. These disturbing results include false diagnosis of malignancy (Rotmensch & Cole, 2000) and false-positive results leading to unnecessary surgery (Cole et al., 1999b; Cole, 2000). Ayed has also described several general analytical interferences with hCG immunoassays (Ayed et al., 2000). Thus, there are still many problems with immunoassay results for hCG levels, despite an increased level of research.

Research on mass spectrometric methods (MS) for hCG detection has yielded variable results to date. As hCG has a very large molecular weight, it is impossible to utilize the standard GC-MS (gas chromatography–mass spectrometry) method of analysis. This is the case because even with derivatization, the hCG molecule cannot be made volatile enough to vaporize into the GC-MS system without decomposition. Thus, liquid chromatographic and/or direct introduction of a more purified sample extract into the MS is required to obtain useful results. Initial liquid chromatography–mass spectrometry (LC-MS) research has shown some promise

(Liu & Bowers, 1995, 1996, 1997a,b) for developing a method of detecting hCG, but issues still remain both about interpretation of results and about what form(s) of hCG to monitor for a valid test. The technique of matrix-assisted laser desorption/ionization time-of-flight mass spectrometry (MALDI-TOF-MS) was first described by Karas and Hillencamp (1988) for determining the mass of a macromolecule such as hCG. Recent studies have applied the technique of MALDI-TOF-MS to the analysis of hCG (Laidler et al., 1995; Jacoby et al., 2000) and detected the molecule in various forms, but the existence of a large variety of variant forms of hCG (Kardana et al., 1991), coupled with a lack of data on what concentrations of hCG under various conditions constitute normal levels, leaves the exact details of how to distinguish a drug positive undefined. Even though there are studies (Laidler et al., 1994) directed toward defining criteria for the detection of hCG abuse, data do not yet exist that permit evaluation of the effects of age, disease state (such as thyroid conditions), and other variables impacting the level of naturally occuring hCG.

Philosophy of Human Chorionic Gonadotropin Testing

Although several early reviews and preliminary studies suggested that hCG abuse in sport would be a problem (Cowan et al., 1991; DeBoer et al., 1991; Kicman et al., 1991; Kicman & Cowan, 1992), neither definitive testing methods, nor the definition of levels of hCG that constitute abuse rather than just normal variation of endogenous levels, has been elucidated. Studies have been directed toward defining criteria by which a positive test result could be reached, but even a recent study of 5663 male athletes (Delbeke et al., 1998) did not take into account the difficult issues of differentiating between malignancy induced and/or "abnormal" hCG levels.

It has always been the philosophy of the IOC and other responsible sport organizations that no competitor should be accused or convicted of drug abuse unless the test results are absolutely certain. This philosophy was based on the premise that it was much better to have some drug abusers go without detection than to have even one innocent athlete convicted of drug use. Today, it appears, sport organizations are clearly stating that it does *not* matter how the agent got into the athlete; the athlete is guilty until proven innocent. This attitude is utterly ridiculous and is becoming commonplace also in various forms of government. Difficult as it is to handle the issue of a drug positive, it has to matter how the level of the agent reached the illegal level. Especially in the case of an agent that is formed naturally, disease, genetics, contamination of legitimate market materials or drugs, and sabotage are all reasons why an agent may have

reached the level found. There is no point in ruining an athlete's life unless procedure or convenience of the officials in charge is the only concern, rather than the athlete's welfare. Today, the personal as well as financial ramifications of an incorrect or false accusation for drug abuse are overwhelming.

References

Alfthan, H., Haglund, C., Dabek, J., & Stenman, U.H. (1992a). Concentrations of HCG, β-HCG and cβ-HCG in serum and urine of nonpregnant women and men. Clinical Chemistry, 38: 1981-1987.

Alfthan, H., Haglund, C., Roberts, P., & Stenman, U.H. (1992b). Elevation of free β subunit of HCG and core β fragment of HCG in serum and urine of patients with malignant pancreatic and biliary disease. Cancer Research, 52: 4628-4633.

Ayed, B., Benkirane, A., Godet, G., Foglietti, M., & Bernard, M.A. (2000). Analytical interference in HCG immunoassays: an in vivo and in vitro study. Clinical Chemistry, 46: #6 Supplement, A36.

Braunstein, G.D., Kamdar, V., Rasor, J., Swaminathan, N., & Wade, M.E. (1979). Widespread distribution of chorionic gonadotropin-like substance in normal human tissues. Journal of Clinical Endocrinology and Metabolism, 49: 917-925.

Cole, L.A. (2000). False positive HCG/HCG-β test results leading to needless surgery and chemotherapy. Clinical Chemistry, 46: #6 Supplement, A125.

Cole, L.A., & Kardana, A. (1992). Discordant results in HCG assays. Clinical Chemistry, 38: 263-270.

Cole, L.A., Rinne, K.M., Shahabi, S., & Omrani, A. (1999b). False positive HCG assay results leading to unnecessary surgery and chemotherapy and needless occurrences of diabetes and coma. Clinical Chemistry, 45: 313-314.

Cole, L.A., Shahabi, S., Oz, U.A., Singh, R.A.B., & Mahoney, M.J. (1999a). Hyperglycosylated human chorionic gonadotropin (Invasive Trophoblast Antigen) immunoassay: a new basis for gestational Down syndrome screening. Clinical Chemistry, 45: 2109-2119.

Cowan, D.A., Kicman, A.T., Walker, C.J., & Wheeler, M.J. (1991). Effect of administration of human chorionic gonadotrophin on criteria used to assess testosterone administration in athletes. Journal of Endocrinology, 131: 147-154.

DeBoer, D., DeJong, E.G., Van Rossum, J.M., & Maes, R.A.A. (1991). Doping control of testosterone and HCG: a case study. International Journal of Sports Medicine, 12: 46-51.

Delbeke, F.T., Eenoo, P.V., & Backer, P.D. (1998). Detection of human chorionic gonadotrophin misuse in sport. International Journal of Sports Medicine, 19: 287-290.

DeLeo, V., La Marca, A., Pasqui, I., Zhu, B., & Morgante, G. (2000). Effects of human chorionic gonadotropin administration on testicular testosterone secretion during prolonged exercise. Fertility & Sterility, 73(4): 864-866.

Dunkel, L., Perheentupa, J., & Apter, D. (1985). Kinetics of the steroidogenic response to single versus repeated doses of human chorionic gonadotropin in boys in prepuberty and early puberty. Pediatric Research, 19(1): 1-4.

Franke, W.W., & Berendonk, B. (1997). Hormonal doping and androgenization of athletes: a secret program of the German Democratic Republic government. Clinical Chemistry, 43: 1262-1279.

International Olympic Committee (IOC). (2001). Prohibited classes of substances and methods, Lausanne, Switzerland, September 1.

Jacoby, E.S., Kicman, A.T., Laidler, P., & Iles, R.K. (2000). Determination of the glycoforms of human chorionic gonadotropin β-core fragment by matrix-assisted laser desorption/ionization time-of-flight mass spectrometry. Clinical Chemistry, 46(11): 1796-1803.

Karas, M., & Hillencamp, F. (1988). Laser desorption ionization of proteins with molecular masses in excess of 10000 daltons. Analytical Chemistry, 60: 2299-2301.

Kardana, A., Elliott, M.M., Gawinowicz, M.A., Birken, S., & Cole, L.A. (1991). The heterogeneity of human chorionic gonadotropin (HCG) I. Characterization of peptide heterogeneity in thirteen individual preparations of HCG. Endocrinology, 129: 1541-1550.

Kicman, A., Brooks, R., & Cowan, D. (1991). HCG & sport. British Journal of Sports Medicine, 25: 73-80.

Kicman, A.T., & Cowan, D.A. (1992). Peptide hormones and sport: misuse and detection. British Medical Bulletin, 48: 496-517.

Laidler, P., Cowan, D.A., Hider, R.C., Keane, A., & Kicman, A.T. (1995). Tryptic mapping of human chorionic gonadotropin by matrix-assisted laser desorption/ionization mass spectrometry. Rapid Communications in Mass Spectrometry, 9: 1021-1026.

Laidler, P., Cowan, D.A., Hider, R.C., & Kicman, A.T. (1994). New decision limits and quality-control material for detecting human chorionic gonadotropin misuse in sports. Clinical Chemistry, 40(7 Pt. 1): 1306-1311.

Leinonen, A., Tahtela, R., & Karjalainen, E. (1999). Detection of HCG in urine by two different immunoassays. In Schaenzer, W., Geyer, H., Gotzmann, A., & Mareck-Engelke, U. (Eds.), Recent Advances in Dope Analysis 6; Proceedings of the 16th Cologne Workshop on Dope Analysis (pp. 313-320). Cologne: Sport & Buch Strauss.

Lipsitz, R. (2000). Pregnancy tests. Scientific American, No. 11, 110-111.

Liu, C., & Bowers, L.D. (1995). Studies towards confirmation of HCG using HPLC/MS. In Donike, M., Geyer, H., Gotzmann, A., & Mareck-Engelke, U. (Eds.), Proceedings of the 12th Cologne Workshop on Dope Analysis (pp. 235-242). Cologne: Sport & Buch Strauss.

Liu, C., & Bowers, L.D. (1996). Immunoaffinity trapping of urinary human chorionic gonadotropin and its high-performance liquid chromatographic-mass spectrometric confirmation. Journal of Chromatography Biomedical Applications, 687(1), 213-220.

Liu, C., & Bowers, L.D. (1997a). Mass spectrometric characterization of the β-subunit of human chorionic gonadotropin. Journal of Mass Spectrometry, 32: 33-42.

Liu, C., & Bowers, L.D. (1997b). Mass spectrometric characterization of nicked fragments of the β-subunit of human chorionic gonadotropin. Clinical Chemistry, 43: 1172-1181.

Mann, K., & Karl, H.J. (1983). Molecular heterogeneity of human chorionic gonadotropin and its subunits in testicular cancer. Cancer, 52: 654-660.

Martikainen, H., Alen, M., Rahkila, P., & Vihko, R. (1986). Testicular responsiveness to human chorionic gonadotrophin during transient hypogonadotrophic hypogonadism induced by androgenic/anabolic steroids in power athletes. Journal of Steroid Biochemistry, 25(1): 109-112.

Odell, W.D., & Griffin, J. (1987). Pulsatile secretion of human chorionic gonadotropin in normal adults. New England Journal of Medicine, 317(27): 1688-1691.

Ozturk, M., Berkowitz, R., Goldstein, D., Bellet, D., & Wands, J.R. (1988). Differential production of human chorionic gonadotropin and free subunits in gestational trophoblastic disease. American Journal of Obstetrics and Gynecology, 158: 193-198.

Pittaway, D.E., Reish, R.L., & Wentz, A.C. (1986). Doubling times of human chorionic gonadotropin increase in early viable intrauterine pregnancies. American Journal of Obstetrics & Gynecology, 152: 299-302.

Robertson, D.M., Suginami, H., Hernandez, M.H., Puri, C.P., Choi, S.K., & Diczfalusy, E. (1978). Studies on a human chorionic gonadotropin-like material present in non-pregnant subjects. Acta Endocrinologia, 89: 492-505.

Rotmensch, S., & Cole, L.A. (2000). False diagnosis and needless therapy of presumed malignant disease in women with false positive human chorionic gonadotropin concentrations. The Lancet, 355: 712-715.

Stenman, U.H., Alfthan, H., & Halila, H. (1985). Determination of chorionic gonadotropin in serum of non-pregnant subjects and patients with trophoblastic cancer by time-resolved immunofluorimetric assay. Tumor Biology, 5: 97.

Stenman, U.H., Alfthan, H., Ranta, T., Vartiainen, E., Jalkanen, J., & Seppala, M. (1987). Serum levels of HCG in nonpregnant women and men are modulated by gonadotropin releasing hormone and sex steroids. Journal of Clinical Endocrinology and Metabolism, 64: 730-736.

Stenman, U.H., Kallio, L.U., Korhonen, J., & Alfthan, H. (1997). Immunoprocedures for detecting human chorionic gonadotropin: clinical aspects and doping control. Clinical Chemistry, 43: 1293-1298.

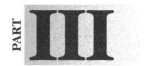
Blood Doping

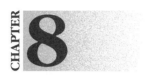
Blood Doping

Björn T. Ekblom, MD

Human physical performance is determined by a combination of several anatomical, physiological, and psychological factors. The relative importance of each of these depends on the nature of the exercise. For instance, in endurance sports such as running, rowing, cycling, or cross-country skiing, which involve the use of large muscle groups, often during fairly long periods of time, maximal aerobic power ($\dot{V}O_2$max) is a prerequisite for elite physical performance, although other factors such as aerobic exercise efficiency ("running economy"), aerobic-anaerobic balance, anaerobic capacity, substrate availability, muscle strength, and psychological factors may influence or modify the performance capacity (2).

In elite athletes from these endurance events, $\dot{V}O_2$max of >7.0 $L \cdot min^{-1}$ or >90 $ml \cdot kg$ body weight$^{-1} \cdot min^{-1}$ have frequently been obtained (17, 39). Studies of the central circulation during maximal exercise in these athletes show that these extremely high values are due to a large maximal cardiac output ($\dot{Q}$max) in combination with a large arteriovenous oxygen difference (a-$\bar{v}O_2$diff). For $\dot{Q}$max, more than 40 $L \cdot min^{-1}$ has been measured (17). Since the peak heart rate (HRmax) in these athletes is not different from that obtained in untrained or moderately trained individuals of the same sex and age, the main cause for the high $\dot{Q}$max is a large stroke volume (SV). Values >200 ml during maximal exercise are frequently obtained in these athletes (17).

The a-$\bar{v}O_2$diff is also of interest in this discussion. Basically it is determined by the hemoglobin concentration ([Hb]) and its saturation (SaO_2) on the one hand and the oxygen content of the mixed venous blood ($C\bar{v}O_2$) on the other. In well-trained athletes, [Hb] at rest and during exercise is not different from that obtained in

untrained individuals of the same sex and age (17, 41, 42). Although regular physical training can reduce $C\bar{v}O_2$ to a minor extent during maximal exercise in previously untrained individuals (15), the [Hb] mainly determines the magnitude of the a-$\bar{v}O_2$diff between different individuals. Therefore it is clear that unless factors other than those related to the central circulation do not limit $\dot{V}O_2$max (see discussion further on), changes in [Hb] during exercise will have a direct influence on $\dot{V}O_2$max and physical performance.

It is worth mentioning that although physical performance in many endurance sports has improved a great deal over the last 40 to 50 years, the highest values of $\dot{V}O_2$max have not changed during the same period of time (2, 17, 39). Therefore, there is no doubt that since $\dot{V}O_2$max is a prerequisite for elite performance, manipulations of factors determining $\dot{V}O_2$max—for instance, increasing [Hb] by infusion of erythrocytes ("blood doping")—will change physical performance, as discussed later on in this chapter.

What Limits $\dot{V}O_2$max?

This important question was first addressed by Hill and Lupton in 1923, when they observed a plateau phenomenon of oxygen consumption above which additional rate of work did not increase $\dot{V}O_2$max (24). The limitation of the pathway of oxygen from ventilation and site of uptake of oxygen in the lungs to the final step in the electron transport system chain in the muscle mitochondria includes a series of steps, each of which is still discussed in relation to the limiting factors for $\dot{V}O_2$max (3, 4, 32, 44). In short, the principal views are that of a single-step limitation (for instance, the heart functional capacity) and that of an integrated limitation over the whole oxygen transport system chain, as indicated by the hypothesis of "symmorphosis" (44). A central part of this discussion is the role of the red blood cell (RBC) and [Hb], both for the level of individual $\dot{V}O_2max$ and for the regulation of regional blood flow at rest and during exercise.

In elite athletes as well as in untrained individuals, the arterial blood is fairly well saturated by the pulmonary system during heavy exercise (13, 17), even if there is some arterial hypoxemia (desaturation) compared to resting values in some (but not all) well-trained athletes (14, 36). The reason for hypoxemia in well-trained athletes is not fully understood, but it does not contradict the well-accepted understanding that the pulmonary system has very little influence on and is not a main limiting factor for $\dot{V}O_2max$ in most healthy individuals (4).

This is an important point in our discussion of how changes in [Hb] affect the performance of heavy exercise. If the diffusion capacity, or pulmonary ventilation, limits arterial oxygen saturation during heavy exercise, and is thus an important regulator of $\dot{V}O_2max$, then increases in [Hb] will have very little or no effect on $\dot{V}O_2max$ and physical performance.

Since the beginning of the 1970s, arguments have been advanced to suggest that factors related to peripheral oxygen transport and utilization, such as capillary density, mitochondria mass, enzyme concentrations, or muscle mass, might limit $\dot{V}O_2max$ (26). This is certainly true for heavy exercise carried out with small muscle groups, such as dynamic arm work. In this situation these "peripheral" factors are of the utmost importance for, and certainly do limit, aerobic energy turnover, performance, and endurance (40). However, during exercise with large muscle groups (e.g., running, combined arm and leg work, and cross-country skiing), there are several reasons for theorizing that the "periphery" does not limit $\dot{V}O_2max$. The following are some of these reasons:

• Increasing muscle mass during maximal exercise—for example, adding maximal arm work to maximal leg work—does not increase $\dot{V}O_2max$ above the level obtained by working maximally with legs only (5, 43).

• There is no relation between muscle enzyme activity and $\dot{V}O_2max$ (25, 26, 40).

• Endurance training may increase, and inactivity reduces, mitochondria enzyme concentrations considerably without any changes or only minor changes in $\dot{V}O_2max$ (22, 33, 34, 40).

• Calculations of the maximal aerobic energy turnover for a well-defined muscle group, such as quadriceps femoralis, show that peak $\dot{V}O_2$/kg muscle mass for this muscle far exceeds that of the whole-body $\dot{V}O_2max$ (1, 37).

It is obvious from these data that the central circulation, including the blood volume (BV) and [Hb], has a crucial role in establishing high values of $\dot{V}O_2max$. If the periphery limited $\dot{V}O_2max$, acute or chronic increase in [Hb] would not increase aerobic power, endurance, and performance during maximal exercise.

Despite these facts, some have questioned whether or not an increased [Hb] during heavy exercise could improve $\dot{V}O_2max$ and physical performance. Furthermore, it has been argued that from a rheological point of view, the individual [Hb] is already "optimal" for each person—especially in athletes. According to these objections, an elevated [Hb] would cause an increased viscosity, which in turn would enhance arterial blood pressure (BP), reduce $\dot{Q}$ during heavy exercise, and ultimately impair $\dot{V}O_2max$ and physical performance.

The Importance of Hemoglobin Concentration

It is well known that acute blood loss and chronic and acute anemia cause increased heart rate (HR), blood lactate concentration, and rate of perceived exertion during submaximal exercise (10, 20). $\dot{V}O_2max$ is reduced and the time to exhaustion is shortened during heavy dynamic physical exercise (16, 20). Furthermore, blocking hemoglobin (Hb) with carbon monoxide causes the same types of effects (18, 45). The reduced arterial oxygen content during maximal exercise cannot be compensated for by some other factor within the central circulation (19, 20). Thus, during both submaximal and maximal exercise, the reduced arterial oxygen content causes an increased stress on various energy systems.

As mentioned earlier, the [Hb] at rest in well-trained endurance athletes is well within the normal range reported for the general population. As a consequence, in healthy individuals there is no positive relation between $\dot{V}O_2max$ and [Hb] at rest or during exercise. It should also be pointed out that regular physical training does not increase [Hb] at rest or during exercise, although total Hb mass may increase considerably (15). In fact, since plasma volume increases slightly more than red cell mass with exercise training, [Hb] is often reduced, causing a dilutional pseudoanemia or "sports anemia" (41, 42, 47). It is important to emphasize that such a reduction in [Hb] cannot be used as an argument for infusion of whole blood or packed RBCs in order to correct a pathological anemia situation in the trained athlete.

Process and Effects of Blood Doping

In blood doping, two to four units (one unit corresponds to 450 ml of whole blood) are collected from the individual. Red blood cells are separated from plasma, frozen, and stored in glycerol. At least two to three months is needed in order for the erythropoiesis to restore normal [Hb] in hard-training endurance athletes. Three to five days before the competition, the RBCs are washed with saline and infused. As a consequence of the modern freezing method, the RBC concentration of 2,3-diphosphoglycerate is unchanged, and thus the oxygen-carrying capacity and effectiveness of the RBCs are preserved (16). Heterologous whole blood can also be used instead of the stored autologous blood, but with some risk of complications such as infections and transfusion complications.

In the future, Hb solutions and other artificial substitutes may very well be used for enhancing oxygen-carrying capacity of the blood. However, the more artificial the methods are, the greater the risks for complications and the easier the detection will be.

Effects of Red Blood Cell Infusion

The first experiment on the physiological effect of infusion of 2 L of whole blood was done in 1947 (35). Although $\dot{V}O_2$max was not measured, performance was enhanced, indicating a clear positive effect of this first "blood-doping" experiment. Subsequent studies (e.g., 9, 10, 16, 20, 21, 27, 28, 50) on the physiological and performance consequences of infusion of 1000 to 1200 ml of whole blood or 400 to 500 ml of packed RBCs have shown concordant effects at rest and during submaximal and maximal exercise. These are the main conclusions:

• There are essentially no differences between infusion of whole blood and of packed RBCs in the physiological response to rest and submaximal or maximal exercise. Thus, the important element of the procedure is the change in oxygen-carrying capacity.

• Blood volume is more or less unchanged or only slightly increased, depending on the volume of blood infused and the time of determination of BV after infusion (16, 20). This indicates that the body tends to keep the total BV more or less unchanged despite an acute accumulated increase of about 1 L of packed erythrocytes within 12 to 14 days, increasing [Hb] considerably (10). It should also be pointed out, as discussed further on, that an increased BV can increase "preload" and cause a rise in SV during submaximal and maximal exercise (27, 29, 31, 38).

• Hemoglobin concentration and hematocrit (Hct) at rest and during exercise increase. However, there are some individual variations in the Hct and [Hb] responses. Part of the individual variation is due to the effect of infusion on the BV response, but other presently unknown factors have an influence. Since there was no evident hemolysis during or after the infusion experiments, this factor cannot explain the interindividual variations in the [Hb]/Hct responses.

• During a standard submaximal rate of work, $\dot{V}O_2$, as a marker of mechanical efficiency, was unchanged after infusion of RBCs compared to before, which was expected. However, $\dot{Q}$ was reduced in accordance with the increased oxygen content of the arterial blood (20). Heart rate was also lower after reinfusion compared to the control value. Thus, SV was unchanged or slightly increased presumably due to increased preload (see discussion further on). Blood lactate concentration was also reduced, indicating a lesser stress on the anaerobic energy systems after reinfusion of RBCs compared to before. Thus, even fairly small changes in oxygen-carrying capacity of the blood lead to alterations in the circulatory and metabolic adaptation to submaximal exercise. Therefore, one must consider changes in [Hb] when evaluating the effects of various external and internal factors, such as training programs and diet manipulations, on physical performance and the physiological adaptation to submaximal exercise.

• During submaximal exercise, systolic blood pressure has been shown not to be increased after infusion of RBCs compared to control values (20). Thus, there seemed to be no evident effect of the increased [Hb], and presumably viscosity, on BP during either submaximal or maximal exercise.

• The most evident effect of reinfusion of RBCs and the increased [Hb] is the enhanced $\dot{V}O_2$max and prolonged time to exhaustion during a standard maximal test (figure 8.1). Calculations based on the results from seven well-trained subjects, in whom $\dot{V}O_2$, $\dot{Q}$, and [Hb] were measured during maximal exercise in our laboratory before and after reinfusion of RBCs, showed that although there were large individual variations, the average increase in [Hb] was 9 g·L^{-1} at a $\dot{Q}$max of about 27 L·min^{-1}. Thus, the oxygen availability was increased by 0.33 L·min^{-1}, which was about the same as the measured increased $\dot{V}O_2$max of 0.31 L·min^{-1}. Another point to emphasize is that there appears to be no difference between an increased $\dot{V}O_2$max from an anemic situation to normal [Hb] (e.g., from 120 to 160 g·L^{-1}) and from normal [Hb] up to a higher value (e.g., from 160 to 200 g·L^{-1}) in the same subject. Thus, there seems to be no deflection or "plateau phenomenon" for the increase in $\dot{V}O_2$max with increasing [Hb] up to at least 200 g·L^{-1} (10).

• The total increase in $\dot{V}O_2$max per gram increase in [Hb] was about 20 ml O$_2$·min^{-1} in these young, trained subjects and was not influenced by the variation in baseline [Hb] between 130 and 170 g·L^{-1} (10). However, as already mentioned, there are some individual variations in the change in $\dot{V}O_2$max with increasing [Hb]. The reason for this is not known.

• Peak values for SV and HR, and thus $\dot{Q}$, during maximal exercise were about the same in the postinfusion studies as in the preinfusion control experiments. Thus, the amount of "offered" oxygen to the peripheral tissues during maximal exercise ($\dot{Q}max \times C_aO_2$) is increased after infusion of RBCs, which is an important explanation and a prerequisite for an increase in $\dot{V}O_2max$ after the infusion.

• Performance-related applied studies have shown that 5- or 10-km (3.1 or 6.2 miles) race times are reduced after infusion of RBCs or whole blood (8, 49). The increased amount of "offered" oxygen to the periphery during intense exercise (increased $\dot{V}O_2max$) was evidently used in the active muscles to improve performance. It must be mentioned that there is at least one study in which no positive effect of infused RBCs could be documented (48). The [Hb] was increased, but $\dot{V}O_2max$ was not measured. Therefore the infusion of erythrocytes may have been too close in time to the withdrawal of blood so that the effect of the increased [Hb] could have been masked by other factors.

Effects of Blood Volume Expansion

Cross-sectional studies show that BV and total amount of hemoglobin (THb), but not [Hb], are positively related to $\dot{V}O_2max$ (28). Although BV is more or less unchanged by infusion of whole blood or packed RBCs, the question arises: What are the effects on $\dot{V}O_2max$ and physical performance of an acute BV increase through plasma volume (PV) expansion?

Acute PV expansion (using Macrodex) increases SV during submaximal and maximal exercise in well-trained individuals (27, 29, 31, 38, 46). The explanation is that the enhanced BV causes an enhanced diastolic filling pressure (preload), which through a direct Frank-Starling mechanism increases SV (12, 29, 38). Since peak HR is unchanged, $\dot{Q}max$ is increased. However, this increase is just about enough to compensate for the reduced [Hb] and C_aO_2 during maximal exercise, so the $\dot{V}O_2max$ is mainly unchanged in well-trained athletes after PV expansion compared to that in control experiments (27, 28).

Conversely, in untrained or moderately trained individuals, a corresponding PV expansion with Macrodex may offset the reduction of [Hb] during maximal exercise and thus increase $\dot{V}O_2max$ (11, 12, 31). It seems, therefore, that an acute expansion of PV and

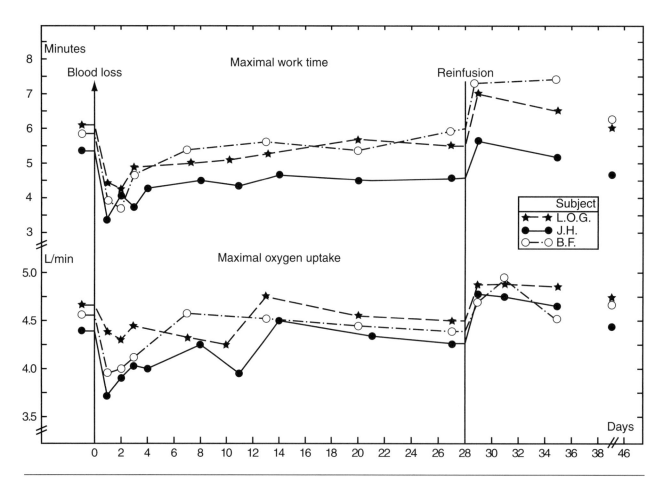

Figure 8.1 Maximal oxygen uptake before and after infusion of 400 ml of packed red blood cells.

Reprinted, by permission, from A. Goldberg and B. Gullbring, 1972, "Response to exercise after blood loss and reinfusion," *Journal of Applied Physiology* 33: (2)175-180.

BV may have a potential ergogenic effect only in untrained or moderately trained individuals, while in well-trained athletes there is no such positive effect on $\dot{V}O_2$max. The latter is supported by the fact that the physical performance, evaluated as time to exhaustion on a standard maximal workload, was slightly reduced after PV expansion in trained athletes (27). The reason is not known.

Risks

There is no increase in arterial BP at rest and during exercise after the infusion of RBCs compared to before infusion (20). On the other hand, heterologous infusion of whole blood or packed RBCs always includes risks of transfusion complications such as allergic reactions and infections of different kinds. To the author's knowledge there is no report on any complication connected to infusion with autologous whole blood or packed RBCs carried out for scientific purposes in healthy subjects. However, it cannot be ruled out that complications during both auto- and heterologous transfusions carried out for "doping" purposes in sport could have occurred, since it is clear and understandable that such an incident would not be reported unless the subject became severely ill.

Detection of Blood Doping

There is no doubt—although scientific experiments have not been published—that infusion of heterologous blood can be detected using sophisticated hematological methods and DNA techniques. Autologous infusion of whole blood or packed RBCs causes an increase in [Hb], increased RBC fragility, increased bilirubin and iron content, and reduced concentration of erythropoietin in plasma. However, detection methods based on these consequences of reinfusion of RBCs cannot be used unless multiple blood samples can be obtained before and after the infusion. If such a procedure could be applied, then the use of blood doping to improve physical performance might be detected in approximately every second person (6, 7). However, there would be many logistical problems related to such a detection method, and therefore no practical method is available today for detection of autologous infusion of whole blood or packed RBCs (blood doping).

Blood Doping in Sport

Blood doping as a method for enhancing performance was banned by the International Olympic Committee Medical Commission in 1984; but the method was evidently used by many athletes, mainly in various endurance sports, before 1984 and has apparently also been used since. No figures are available on the prevalence of blood doping in sport, but there are some case reports. Athletes on a cycling team in the 1984 Olympic Games (30), a track and field runner in the 1990 Olympic Games (23), and others have confessed that they used blood doping to improve performance. Evidently the procedure was effective. The use of plasma expanders was detected in the Finnish cross-country ski team during the world championships in Lathi, Finland, in 2001. Thus, despite information campaigns, lifetime suspensions after repeated disclosures of use of forbidden substances, increased testing programs carried out by international sport federations, and other efforts against doping, there is no doubt that world-class athletes have used forbidden substances and procedures, including blood doping, on various occasions and won gold medals and other titles.

Conclusion

Increasing [Hb] through infusion of erythrocytes or whole blood increases $\dot{V}O_2$max. Since cardiac output and BP at rest and during submaximal and maximal exercise are the same in pre- and postinfusion experiments, physical performance and endurance are increased in accordance with the increased oxygen availability in the blood. Time trials in running and cycling verify the positive effects of blood boosting. Although the prevalence of blood doping in sport is not known, there are several cases of confessed use of this method for enhancing physical performance in sport. However, no practical methods are available today to detect blood doping.

References

1. Andersen P, Saltin B. Maximal perfusion of skeletal muscles in man. J Physiol (London) 366:233-249, 1985.

2. Åstrand P-O, Rodahl K. Textbook of Work Physiology. McGraw-Hill, New York, 1986.

3. Basset DR Jr., Howley ET. Maximal oxygen uptake: Classical versus contemporary viewpoints. J Appl Physiol 29:591-603, 1997.

4. Bergh U, Ekblom B, Åstrand P-O. Maximal oxygen uptake: "Classical" versus "contemporary" viewpoints. Med Sci Sports Exerc 32:85-88, 2000.

5. Bergh U, Kanstrup-Jensen I-L, Ekblom B. Maximal oxygen uptake during exercise with various combinations of arm and leg work. J Appl Physiol 41:191-196, 1976.

6. Berglund B. Development of techniques for the detection of blood doping in sport. Sports Med 5:127-135, 1988.

7. Berglund B, Hemmingsson P, Birgegård G. Detection of autologous blood transfusions in cross-country skiers. Int J Sports Med 8:66-70, 1987.

8. Brian AJ, Simon TL. The effects of red blood cell infusion on 10 km race time. JAMA 257:2761-2765, 1987.

9. Buick FJ, Gledhill N, Froese AB, Spriet L, Meyers EC. Effect of induced erythrocythaemia on aerobic work capacity. J Appl Physiol 48:636-642, 1980.

10. Celsing F, Svedenhag J, Pihlstedt P, Ekblom B. Effect of anaemia and stepwise-induced polycythaemia on maximal aerobic power in individuals with high and low hemoglobin concentration. Acta Physiol Scand 129:47-54, 1987.

11. Coyle EF, Hemmert MK, Coggan AR. Effects of detraining on cardiovascular responses to exercise: Role of blood volume. J Appl Physiol 60: 95-99, 1986.

12. Coyle EF, Hopper MK, Coggan AR. Maximal oxygen uptake relative to plasma volume expansion. Int J Sports Med 11:116-119, 1990.

13. Dempsey JA. Is the lung built for exercise? Med Sci Sports Exerc 18:143-155, 1986.

14. Dempsey JA, Wagner PD. Exercise-induced arterial hypoxemia. J Appl Physiol 87:1997-1999.

15. Ekblom B, Åstrand P-O, Saltin B, Stenberg J, Wallström BM. Effect of training on circulatory response to exercise. J Appl Physiol 24:518-528, 1968.

16. Ekblom B, Goldberg AN, Gullbring B. Response to exercise after blood loss and infusion. J Appl Physiol 33:175-180, 1972.

17. Ekblom B, Hermansson L. Cardiac output in athletes. J Appl Physiol 25: 619-625, 1968.

18. Ekblom B, Huot R. Response to submaximal and maximal exercise at different levels of carboxyhemoglobin. Acta Physiol Scand 86:474-482, 1972.

19. Ekblom B, Huot R, Stein E, Thorstensson A. Effect of changes in arterial oxygen content on circulation and physical performance. J Appl Physiol 39:71-75, 1975.

20. Ekblom B, Wilson G, Åstrand P-O. Central circulation during exercise after venesection and infusion of red blood cells. J Appl Physiol 40:379-383, 1976.

21. Gledhill N. The influence of altered blood volume and oxygen-transport capacity on aerobic performance. Exerc Sports Sci Rev 13:75-93, 1985.

22. Henriksson J, Reitman JS. Time course of changes in human skeletal muscle succinate dehydrogenase and cytochrome oxidase activities and maximal oxygen uptake with physical activity and inactivity. Acta Physiol Scand 99:91-97, 1977.

23. Higdon H. Blood doping among endurance athletes. Am Med News 37:39-41, 1985.

24. Hill AV, Lupton H. Muscular exercise, lactic acid and the supply and utilisation of oxygen. Q J Med 16:135-171, 1923.

25. Hollozy JO. Biochemical adaptations to exercise: Aerobic metabolism. Exerc Sport Sci Rev 1:45-71, 1973.

26. Hoppeler H, Lindstedt SL. Malleability of skeletal muscle tissue in overcoming limitations: Structural elements. J Exp Biol 115:355-364, 1985.

27. Kanstrup I-L, Ekblom B. Acute hypervolemia, cardiac performance and aerobic power during exercise. J Appl Physiol 52:1186-1191, 1982.

28. Kanstrup I-L, Ekblom B. Blood volume and hemoglobin concentration as determinants of maximal aerobic power. Med Sci Sports Exerc 16:256-262, 1984.

29. Kanstrup I-L, Marving J, Hoilund-Carlsen PF. Acute plasma expansion: Left ventricular hemodynamics and endocrine function during exercise. J Appl Physiol 73:1791-1796, 1992.

30. Klein HG. Blood transfusion and athletics. N Engl J Med 312:854-856, 1985.

31. Krip B, Gledhill N, Jamnik V, Warburton D. Effect of alterations in blood volume on cardiac function during maximal exercise. Med Sci Sports Exerc 29:1469-1476, 1997.

32. Noakes, TD. Maximal oxygen uptake: "Classical" versus "contemporary" viewpoints. A rebuttal. Med Sci Sports Exerc 30:1381-1398, 1998.

33. Örlander J, Kiessling KH, Ekblom B. Time course of adaptation to low intensity training in sedentary men: Dissociation of central and local effects. Acta Physiol Scand 108:85-90, 1980.

34. Örlander J, Kiessling KH, Karlsson J, Ekblom B. Low intensity training, inactivity and resumed training in sedentary men. Acta Physiol Scand 101:351-362, 1977.

35. Pace N, Lozner EL, Consolalazio WV. The increase in hypoxia tolerance of normal men accompanying the polycytemia induced by transfusion of erythrocytes. Am J Physiol 148:152-163, 1947.

36. Powers SK, Lawler J, Dempsey JA, Dodd S, Landry G. Effects of incomplete pulmonary gas exchange of VO_2max. J Appl Physiol 66:2491-2495, 1989.

37. Rådegran G, Blomstrand E, Saltin B. Peak muscle perfusion and oxygen uptake in humans: Importance of precise estimates of muscle mass. J Appl Physiol 87:2375-2380, 1999.

38. Robinsson B, Epstein S, Kahler R, Braunwald E. Circulatory effects of acute expansion of blood volume. Circ Res 29:26-32, 1966.

39. Saltin B, Henriksson J, Nygaard E, Andersen P. Fiber types and metabolic potentials of skeletal muscle in sedentary men and endurance runners. Ann New York Acad Sci 301:3-29, 1977.

40. Saltin B, Nazar K, Costill DL, Stein E, Jansson E, Essén B, Gollnick PD. The nature of the training response; peripheral and central adaptations to one-legged exercise. Acta Physiol Scand. 96:289-305, 1976.

41. Saris W, Senden J, Brouns F. What is a normal red-blood cell mass for professional cyclists? Lancet 352:1758, 1998.

42. Smith J. Exercise, training and RBC turnover. Sport Med 19:9-31, 1995.

43. Stenberg, J, Åstrand P-O, Ekblom B, Royce J, Saltin B. Hemodynamic response to work with different muscle groups, sitting and supine. J Appl Physiol 22:61-70, 1967.

44. Taylor CR, Weibel ER. Design of the mammalian respiratory system. I. Problem strategy. Respir Physiol 44:1-10, 1981.

45. Vogel JA, Gleser MA. Effect of carbon monoxide on oxygen transport during exercise. J Appl Physiol 32:234-239, 1972.

46. Warburton DER, Gledhill N, Jamnik VK, Kirp B, Card N. Induced hypervolemia, cardiac function, VO_2max and performance of elite cyclists. Med Sci Sports Exerc 31:800-808, 1999.

47. Weight L. Sports anaemia—does it exist? Sports Med 16:1-4, 1993.

48. Williams MH, Lindhejm M, Schuster R. The effect of blood infusion upon endurance capacity and ratings of perceived exertion. Med Sci Sports 10:113-118, 1978.

49. Williams MH, Wesseldine S, Somma T, Schuster R. The effect of induced erythrocythemia upon 5-mile treadmill run time. Med Sci Sports Exerc 13:169-175, 1981.

50. Young A, Sawka M, Musa S, Boushel R, Luons T, Rock P, Freund B, Waters R, Cymerman A, Pandolf K, Valeri R. Effects on erythrocyte infusion on $\dot{V}O_2$max at high altitude. J Appl Physiol 81:252-259, 1996.

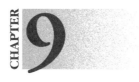

Erythropoietin

Björn T. Ekblom, MD

Chapter 8 dealt with the importance of hemoglobin concentration ([Hb]) for physical performance and circulatory response to submaximal and maximal exercise. The main conclusion was that all changes in the oxygen-carrying capacity of the blood in healthy individuals will ultimately cause corresponding changes in $\dot{V}O_2$max and consequently physical performance in endurance sports. This chapter presents a discussion of the effects of exogenous administration of a hemopoiesis-stimulating substance, erythropoietin (EPO).

Basic Considerations

The red blood cell (RBC), 7 μm in diameter and including about 280 million hemoglobin (Hb) molecules, is the main oxygen carrier from the lungs to the muscles and is also an important part of the transport of carbon dioxide from the muscles back to the lungs. Calculations indicate that the Hb in the RBCs accounts for about 70% of the total acid-base buffering capacity of the body, which is important to emphasize from an exercise point of view. Thus, changes in [Hb] will not only increase oxygen transport but may also improve anaerobic physical performance.

The entrance of the hemopoietic stem cell into the cell cycle is promoted by several factors such as interleukin 1, 3, and 6. In the progression of red bone marrow cells (erythropoiesis) from erythroblasts and reticulocytes to the mature adult erythrocyte, which has lost its nucleus and other organelles, granulocyte-macrophage colony stimulation and EPO are essential components. Presently it is not known whether the entire erythropoiesis process can be manipulated by each of these factors, but it is clear that any stimulation may generate ethical and moral problems in the sporting world. Erythropoiesis is also dependent on the availability of sufficient amounts of iron (as indicated by a serum ferritin concentration >15 $\mu g \cdot L^{-1}$), vitamins (e.g., vitamin B12), and various amino acids.

Normally about 2 to 3 million RBCs are produced per second depending on body size, level of training, blood loss of various kinds, hypoxia stress, and other factors. The average lifetime of an RBC is about 120 days. However, it is shorter in the athlete as a consequence of metabolic, osmotic, and mechanical stress during training and competition. This means that the RBC population in the training athlete includes a relatively higher number of young mature RBCs with good capacity for oxygen transport—for instance, the possibility of good deformation for passing through the muscle capillary, which has a diameter of about 3 to 4 μm.

It should be pointed out that during erythropoiesis, surface transferrin receptors (sTrR) binding the iron carrier ferritin are released to the plasma. A stimulated production of RBCs (e.g., through injections of EPO) can be indicated in part by an increased number of reticulocytes in the blood, the content of reticulocyte Hb, increased reticulocyte volume, increased number of hypochromic RBCs, increased serum concentration of sTrR, and certain other indicators (10, 24). However, [sTrR] is also increased during iron deficiency, among other situations, but is unaffected by inflammation, so this specific marker might be used together with other signs and markers of increased erythropoiesis for evaluation of possible abuse of EPO. In the post-erythropoietic stimulated phase, other changes occur, among them depression of [EPO] and increase in hematocrit (Hct)/[Hb].

Erythropoietin

Erythropoietin is a glycoprotein (40% carbohydrate) with a molecular weight of about 34,000 daltons, produced mainly in the tubular cells of the kidneys but also, importantly, in the liver (7). Oxygen availability in the kidneys and liver is the main regulator of EPO production. Hypoxia due to anemia or low plasma oxygen pressure leads to an increase of EPO secretion. Erythropoietin receptors in the bone marrow enhance the mitosis and differentiation of the RBC precursors, leading to production of RBCs. Normally, serum [EPO], measurable via immunoassays or bioassays, is low in the early morning, peaks during the day, and remains high in the late afternoon.

Concentration of EPO is increased or decreased as a consequence of changes in the oxygen availability at the renal site. Thus, hemodilution, various types of hypoxia, and anemia are known causes for an enhanced production and concentration of EPO. Consequently, [EPO] is reduced in polycythemia, which is an important fact in the search for unethical use of the hormone. Short-term submaximal or maximal exercise has no immediate effects on [EPO], while long-term exhaustive and strenuous physical activity may cause complex changes in serum [EPO] (7). A prolonged or intermittent state of hypoxia, which is very common among endurance athletes, increases [EPO] gradually over the first three or four days. The EPO concentration subsequently declines, reaching sea level values after about two weeks of hypoxia. After return to sea level living and training, [EPO] decreases to lower-than-normal values but is normalized after about 10 days (6).

It is important to emphasize that [EPO] exhibits large individual and interindividual variation during the day and also in different physiological situations (6, 7). These variations in [EPO] are so great that a single quantitative determination of [EPO] for detection of unethical administration of recombinant human EPO (rhEPO) is difficult unless multiple blood samplings and determinations of other hematological structures over time can be obtained.

Today EPO is available through recombinant DNA techniques. Injections of rhEPO to patients with certain diseases have restored their physical performance to near-normal levels, primarily through increased [Hb]. It is important to stress that EPO is one of the best drugs manufactured during the last 20 years. Erythropoietin has changed the quality of life of millions of people with various illnesses and diseases (14, 18). It can now be used in clinical settings instead of blood transfusions (17, 25) and for other indications (11).

Effects of Exogenous Administration of Erythropoietin

In relation to healthy individuals and sport, the pertinent questions are as follows:

- Will increased serum [EPO] increase [Hb] in the normal athlete?
- If so, will increased [Hb] enhance $\dot{V}O_2$max and thereby improve aerobic physical performance?
- What are other physiological and medical consequences of rhEPO injection?
- Can exogenous administration of rhEPO be detected in doping tests?

These questions have been addressed in a series of studies using trained male subjects (3, 5, 8, 12, 24). In the first three studies (3, 5, 12) from our laboratory, baseline values of $\dot{V}O_2$max of 4.56 ± 0.43 L·min^{-1} were established after preliminary submaximal and maximal pre-experimental testing. Thereafter, injections of rhEPO were administered subcutaneously, on average three times per week, over six weeks, at a dose of 20 or 40 IU·kg body weight^{-1}. The physiological effects of

the administration of exogenous EPO were evaluated at rest, during both a low (100 W) and a high (200 W) submaximal rate of work on a cycle ergometer, and during a standard maximal running test on a treadmill. Finally, in one study the effects of injection of EPO were evaluated during intermittent high-intensity exercise (3).

Rest and Submaximal Exercise

In summary, the effects observed in the studies just described were as follows:

- Hemoglobin concentration and Hct increased in all subjects, but with wide variation between individuals. The reason for this individual variation is unknown.
- Blood volume remained basically unchanged or increased only slightly.
- Resting heart rate (HR) remained unchanged.
- There were no changes in $\dot{V}O_2$ or ventilation per liter $\dot{V}O_2$ ($\dot{V}_E / \dot{V}O_2$) during the standard submaximal workloads after the EPO injection period compared to before.
- During the standard submaximal workloads, HR was reduced from an average of 114.7 to 108.4 bpm on the low submaximal workload and from 145.5 to 137.4 bpm on the high submaximal workload (both $p < 0.05$).
- As a consequence of the unchanged $\dot{V}O_2$ and the reduced HR during submaximal exercise, oxygen pulse increased significantly from 15.5 to 16.4 ml·beat^{-1} on the low submaximal workload and from 18.6 to 19.9 ml·beat^{-1} on the high submaximal workload.

One unexpected finding was that neither blood lactate concentration ([Hla]) nor subjective rate of perceived exertion (RPE) as evaluated on the Borg scale showed significant changes as a consequence of the increased Hct and [Hb] after the injection period. The reason for this is not known, but the rate of submaximal work might have been too low for some subjects, causing no decrease in these subjects and thus nonsignificant group changes in these physiological responses. However, subjects with initial high [Hla] and RPE values had lower values during the submaximal tests after the injection period, showing that increased oxygen availability in the blood can lower the stress on anaerobic energy systems and also lead to less perceived exertion.

However, medically the most important finding was that the arterial systolic blood pressure during the higher submaximal workload (200 W) was significantly increased from an average of 177 to 191 mmHg, with large interindividual variations (figure 9.1). This finding is in

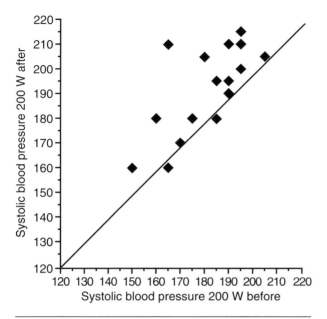

Figure 9.1 Systolic blood pressure at 200 W before and after seven weeks of injection of 20 to 40 IU·kg body weight^{-1} recombinant human erythropoietin (n = 25).

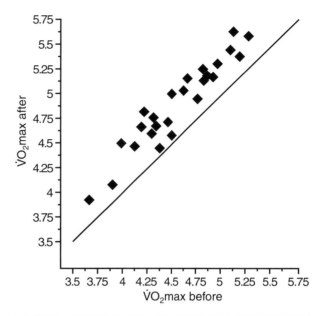

Figure 9.2 Maximal oxygen uptake before and after seven weeks of injection of 20 to 40 IU·kg body weight^{-1} recombinant human erythropoietin (n = 25).

accordance with observations in other studies (20, 23). The reason for this result is not known, but the fact that the hormone EPO is related to the renin-angiotensin hormone system may have relevance. Thus, it is possible that EPO might have a vasoconstrictor effect on peripheral vessels.

Maximal Exercise

Maximal tests performed on a motor-driven treadmill demonstrated that all subjects in our studies (3, 5, 12) increased their $\dot{V}O_2$max, irrespective of their baseline values, on average from 4.56 ± 0.43 to 4.90 ± 0.44 L·min^{-1} (+7.5%, p < 0.05) (figure 9.2). The average increase was 0.34 ± 0.13 (range 0.11-0.62) L·min^{-1}. In the study of Parisotto et al. (24), the average increase in $\dot{V}O_2$max, with the same amount of EPO injected, was 6.5%. In the studies from our laboratory the average increase in $\dot{V}O_2$max per gram [Hb] was 14.8 ml O_2·g^{-1}·min^{-1}, which is statistically not different from the corresponding increase in $\dot{V}O_2$max per gram increase in [Hb] after blood infusion (see chapter 8).

These findings are in line with results from a study by Birkeland and coworkers (8). In a double-blind, placebo-controlled study on 20 healthy, well-trained, mainly endurance athletes, Birkeland et al. showed that 5000 IU of rhEPO three times a week for four weeks increased the group mean Hct from 42.7% to 50.8%, peaking on the day after the last injection. $\dot{V}O_2$max increased from an average of 63.6 to 68.1 ml·min^{-1}·kg body weight^{-1}. Ferritin and sTrR values increased as expected. Thus, even in well-trained athletes, rhEPO

injections speed up erythropoiesis and enhance physical performance.

Since there was no difference in the increase in $\dot{V}O_2$max per gram increase in [Hb] after RBC infusion compared with rhEPO in these studies, the slow (rhEPO treatment) and the acute (blood infusion) increase in [Hb] resulted in a similar pattern in increase in $\dot{V}O_2$max. In parallel with the increased $\dot{V}O_2$max, physical performance, evaluated as time to exhaustion at a standard maximal rate of work on the treadmill, increased after the EPO injection period from 493 ± 74 sec to 567 ± 82 sec, or 15% (p < 0.05). This shows that the increased $\dot{V}O_2$max following the EPO administration period improved physical performance similarly to the way it did after blood reinfusion. Thus, the increased oxygen delivery from the heart during maximal exercise was used in the working muscles for increasing physical performance.

However, as soon as a week after the last rhEPO injection, $\dot{V}O_2$max was lower in some subjects compared to the peak value at the end of the injection period (12). This is probably attributable to a decreased endogenous production of EPO during the injection period as a result of normal inhibition. Endogenous EPO production returned to normal levels when the individual's [Hb] was back to baseline level (27).

High-Intensity Intermittent Exercise

The effects of rhEPO administration on high-intensity intermittent exercise have also been evaluated (3). This is the most common type of exercise in sport. During a single bout of intense exercise for a duration of a few seconds, adenosine triphosphate (ATP) is normally resynthesized by the splitting of creatine phosphate and anaerobic glycolysis. However, if the exercise is too intense or if the rest period is too short, the ATP may also be resynthesized through the formation of one ATP from two adenosine diphosphates. The metabolites of, and markers for, this adenonucleotide energy pathway are hypoxanthine and uric acid (19).

Thus, if maximal running for a few seconds is repeated (e.g., every 30th second), there is evidently a large stress on these anaerobic energy systems. In this situation, however, the aerobic energy metabolism may also become important. In a study on this issue (3), six healthy men performed fifteen 6-sec high-intensity bouts of uphill running on a treadmill, interspersed with 24 sec of passive rest, before and after seven weeks of rhEPO administration, during which $\dot{V}O_2$max increased 8% (from 4.76 to 5.14 L·min^{-1}).

Comparison of peak values after the intermittent running test on the treadmill before and after EPO administration showed that plasma [Hla], hypoxanthine, and uric acid concentrations, markers of anaerobic glycolysis and adenonucleotide energy metabolism, respectively, were significantly reduced (3). This finding indicates that an enhanced oxygen transport capacity and availability may improve the recovery process during rest periods between short-time intense bouts of exercise, and might possibly also increase the aerobic energy yield during the exercise bouts. The study shows that the circulation and arterial oxygen content and transport play important roles, even during short-term, high-intensity exercise such as in most ball sports.

Muscle Biopsy Findings

Biopsies from the vastus lateralis of the quadriceps muscle were taken and analyzed before and after the EPO administration period. There were no significant changes either in fiber type composition and myoglobin concentration or in the concentration of any enzyme from the mitochondrial aerobic or anaerobic energy pathways.

The increase in physical performance during continuous maximal treadmill exercise, as well as during maximal intermittent high-intensity sprinting, can therefore not be explained by changes in the peripheral characteristics of the muscles. The most probable explanation for the increased physical performance is the increased $\dot{V}O_2$max. It is also noteworthy that the change in [Hb] was probably too small to account for any important changes in total buffering capacity.

Erythropoietin Doping in Sport

Undoubtedly rhEPO doping has been used from the first day commercial EPO became available. Riders on a French Tour de France cycling team in 1998 and several other athletes have confessed to the use of EPO for increasing physical performance. These cases may be only the tip of the iceberg.

The prevalence of EPO use in sport is unknown. There are no published studies supporting the general view that unethical use of the drug is fairly common in mainly endurance-type sports. However, as discussed further on, the steady increase over a period of a few years in resting [Hb] among cross-country skiers (which after a decision by the International Ski Federation [FIS] decreased again in many skiers) might be an indirect indication of EPO use in at least cross-country skiers. Furthermore, several runners in track and field have been caught in doping tests for EPO use.

There have been media reports, but no scientific reports, of a number of unexpected deaths in well-trained endurance athletes during the past 10 years (1). In some cases, EPO use was confirmed. Since up to now (see section on detection later in the chapter), no practical doping test method has been available, one can only assume that extensive abuse still occurs despite large anti-doping efforts on the part of many national and international organizations.

Since the end of the 1980s, cross-country skiers have been required to undergo tests for [Hb] determination in connection with competitions. In 1996, FIS was notified that the average [Hb] had increased over the years from 1988 (26). There were also several extremely high individual values. Therefore, FIS decided in 1996 that skiers whose tests showed a [Hb] value above 165 and 185 g·L^{-1} for women and men, respectively, would not be allowed to enter the following competition. The International Cycling Union (ICU) made the same decision. However, the ICU set the highest accepted [Hb] at 170 g·L^{-1} or 50% Hct.

Suspected doping is not the reason for suspending athletes. The official reason is that a high [Hb] value is a threat to the athlete's health. It is interesting that the average [Hb] at rest in both male and female elite cross-country skiers competing in the World Cup increased gradually from 1987 to 1996, but that after the FIS decision in 1996 it decreased again (26). The extremely high individual values found regularly before the 1996 season are not found today. Even skiers, who in the past had high individual values, have had more "normal" values since the 1996 season. Some of these athletes have not been as successful since the 1996 season as before, but there could be various explanations for this change.

It is known that there are athletes who normally have high resting [Hb] values for whom the FIS limit on [Hb] is a problem, since day-to-day variations may increase [Hb] up to and over the limits. Since there are no exemptions, at least in cross-country skiing, these athletes simply are not allowed to start in a race.

It should be pointed out that prolonged training at high altitude (e.g., 2000-2500 m [2187-2734 yd] above sea level) or staying in houses with low oxygen content does not increase [Hb] to the limit values of 165 (women) and 185 g·L^{-1} (men) in most people who usually have normal [Hb] values (4). In addition, after an individual returns to sea level following a time at altitude, [Hb] is normally reduced to sea level values within a couple of days. Thus, high [Hb] values at sea level cannot be explained by a prolonged stay and/or training at altitude.

Risks

It is known that high EPO values can enhance thrombotic activity through endothelial and platelet activation. On the other hand, endurance athletes generally have reduced thrombolytic risk as a consequence of the positive medical effects of endurance training. Still, the increased risk with high doses of EPO should not be overlooked. It is well known that athletes combine injections of EPO with injections of iron. Very high values of serum ferritin are regularly found in elite endurance athletes. The excess iron is taken up in parenchymal cells and can cause an entire series of problems in various organs, not least in the liver.

Studies have shown that compared with the pre-EPO-administration period, arterial systolic and diastolic blood pressure (BP) at rest remained unaltered after an rhEPO administration period. However, during submaximal exercise at 200 W (corresponding to an average of about 50% of $\dot{V}O_2$max in the fairly well trained subjects in these studies), there was a marked increase in arterial systolic BP from an average of 177 to 191 mm Hg (5). In corresponding studies on the effects of increased [Hb] after erythrocyte infusion, there was no increase in systolic blood pressure during exercise compared to that measured in preinfusion experiments (13).

The difference in the BP response to submaximal exercise between experiments using infusion of packed RBCs and injection of rhEPO to increase [Hb] shows that the increased arterial BP cannot simply be explained by an increased Hct and, presumably, increased viscosity. The reason for the increased BP after the rhEPO injection period is presently not known, although some have suggested that EPO may have a direct effect on peripheral vessels, increasing peripheral resistance during exercise (7, 20, 23).

Even if HR is reduced during submaximal exercise, the stress on the heart during heavy strenuous and prolonged exercise is greater after rhEPO administration because of the increase in BP (increased "double product"). During a competition in cycling and running, the average energy turnover is often in the range of 75% to 85% of $\dot{V}O_2$max, or even higher, for long periods of time. Thus, it is obvious that the elevated arterial BP due to rhEPO injections during exercise can be part of the explanation for the unexpected deaths of some young athletes that have been reported in the media during the past decade (1).

Can Recombinant Human Erythropoietin Doping Be Detected?

Since EPO is a hormone that is very similar to the one produced by the body itself, some have doubted that there will ever be any anti-doping method for detecting unethical use of EPO in sport. Despite this, in 1989 the International Olympic Committee placed EPO on its doping list—only a few years after its appearance on the market. Since then, there has been an urgent need for a good EPO detection doping test. In principle, there are two possibilities—direct and indirect doping tests.

Direct Detection of Doping

Regarding direct detection, apart from a possibly high [EPO] in the blood hours after an injection, the interindividual variation, as well as the effects of different stresses on the athlete, might be so great that quantitative determinations of [EPO] cannot be used for doping control. However, Professor Leif Wide in Uppsala, Sweden, has developed a unique electrophoretic detection method that sidesteps the barrier erected by large interindividual differences in plasma EPO. This method discriminates between endogenous EPO and exogenous rhEPO, both in blood and in urine, as the rhEPO—manufactured from hamster ovary and kidney cells and mouse fibroblasts—has a lesser negative electric charge than natural endogenous EPO (27). Thus, this method makes it possible to measure a mean value for electrophoretic mobility of EPO in samples from both plasma and urine. A biphasic curve can also be seen when both endogenous EPO and rhEPO are present in a sample.

With this method it is also possible to detect exogenous rhEPO administration in 100% of subjects within a 24-hr time span and in 75% of subjects after 48 hr. Within two weeks of the cessation of injections, most of the effect of exogenous administration on $\dot{V}O_2$max (and presumably on physical performance) has disappeared (12, 27). Because of the differences in electrophoretic mobility, this qualitative method is very safe. There are no false positives. However, the method takes a long time and is very costly. Furthermore, it has been difficult to reproduce the results of the Wide method, mainly because of difficulties in obtaining sufficient amounts of antibodies. For the moment it is not possible to use this method for doping control purposes in sport, since the results of doping tests must be available in fairly short periods of time.

Therefore, development of direct methods for detection of rhEPO in plasma and urine for use in doping control in sport has been urgently needed. In extending the Wide method, a French research team has recently carried out very promising work (21). This method also discriminates between endogenous and exogenous EPO, with no false-positive cases. This direct method was accepted by the Medical Commission of the International Olympic Committee at a meeting in Lausanne in August 2000 and was used in the Sydney Olympic Games the same year.

Indirect Detection of Doping

Indirect methods must also be used to detect exogenous EPO in the blood or the urine in situations in which the athlete has stopped using EPO well in advance but a positive physiological and performance effect of the EPO use is still possible.

Bressolle and coworkers (2, 9) suggest that an increased Hct, with a concomitant increased sTrR value (>10 mg·L^{-1}) and an increased [sTrR]:ferritin ratio (measured in mg·L^{-1}), more than 403, may allow identification of rhEPO users. Another possibility for increasing sensitivity to identify rhEPO users is to employ messenger RNA for transferrin receptors, since transferrin mRNA seem to be very sensitive (16, 22). However, this latter method must be validated against other possible erythropoietic stress situations.

At a Paris workshop in May 1999 (15), indirect methods for detecting the abuse of rhEPO in sport were discussed. The participants agreed on the parameters shown in table 9.1.

If any of the parameters in table 9.1 are abnormal, then more extensive testing is called for. In the meantime, an observation period should begin and at least three further

Table 9.1 Suggested Parameters and Value Limits for Detection of Manipulated Erythropoiesis

Parameter	Suggested suspect value
sTrR	>normal range of the assay
Hematocrit	
Men	>47%
Women	>44%
Hypochromic red cells	>5%
Reticulocyte number	>150 × 10^9·L^{-1}
Reticulocyte hemoglobin	>4.5 g·L^{-1}

follow-up samples should be collected under the same conditions as before. Additional, unannounced samples will also be harvested. Previously collected data for that athlete could also be used in determining whether the observed variations in parameters reflect an abnormal stimulation.

In order to find indirect markers for EPO abuse in sport, Parisotto and coworkers (24) have extended these data and continue with the work mentioned earlier, conducting very ambitious studies in athletes and others during many different conditions. The program is based on either one, or two to three, blood samples during a follow-up period of up to two weeks. It includes measurement of five separate blood parameters: Hct, percent reticulocyte and macrocyte volume in blood, [EPO], and [sTrR]. Blood samples from more than 1000 athletes have been obtained in order to achieve statistical variation in these parameters (24). Statistical analyses of the results from placebo and rhEPO groups have been used to form two different formulas:

- An "On" model that aims at finding current rhEPO users
- An "Off" model to identify those who recently stopped injecting rhEPO

Each formula has been tested against various situations that may cause false-positive and false-negative results. Results from these tests have not yet been published in international journals but were presented at the International Olympic Committee's Lausanne meeting in August 2000. After extensive discussions with several international hematological experts, the results were judged to be scientifically solid. Therefore the decision was made to use this indirect method in combination with the direct urine test discussed earlier (21) for discrimination between endogenous and exogenous EPO at the Sydney Olympic Games in 2000.

Conclusion

Today, one direct and one indirect method for detecting rhEPO abuse in sport are available. Even so, it is important that athletes be tested frequently. Relevant hematological data can be obtained and reported to independent scientific committees. It is obvious that multiple samplings of [Hb] and Hct, for instance, in the same athlete will sooner or later detect EPO users, since individual data of [Hb] and Hct are very stable over time. However, further research is necessary before the indirect detection method (probably the best method with respect to practicality, time, and cost) can be used more widely for testing. There are hematological and medical abnormalities in healthy individuals that may cause changes in various parameters of interest; there also may be changes due to medication. Finally, the blood values indicated earlier must be obtained in athletes who are using other methods to stimulate erythropoiesis, such as high-altitude training, intermittent or continuous normobaric hypoxia ("hypoxia flats"), or various hypoxia devices. An additional possibility is a system in which all athletes are asked to carry a "blood passport," just as they carry an international travel passport, that includes several measurements of their blood profile factors. In this situation athletes who are cheating may have difficulty undergoing doping tests without being caught.

Conclusion

Injections of rhEPO to healthy subjects increase [Hb], Hct, $\dot{V}O_2$max, and physical performance in continuous as well as intermittent exercise. A negative side effect is the increased systolic blood pressure during exercise, which might have been the cause of unexpected deaths in several young athletes. The prevalence of unethical EPO use in sport is not known. There are both direct and indirect methods that can be used for doping detection of rhEPO use in sport.

References

1. Adamson JW, Vapnek D. Recombinant human erythropoietin to improve athletic performance. N Engl J Med 324:689-699, 1991.

2. Audran M, Garneau R, Matecki S, Durand, Chenard C, Sicart M-T, Marion B, Bressolle F. Effects of erythropoietin in training athletes and possible indirect detection in doping control. Med Sci Sports Exerc 31:639-645, 1999.

3. Balsom PD, Ekblom B, Sjödin B. Enhanced oxygen availability during high intensity intermittent exercise decreases anaerobic metabolite concentrations in blood. Acta Physiol Scand 150:455-456, 1994.

4. Berglund B. High-altitude training. Sports Med 14:289-303, 1992.

5. Berglund B, Ekblom B. Effect of recombinant human erythropoietin treatment on blood pressure and some hematological parameters in healthy males. J Int Med 229:125-130, 1991.

6. Berglund B, Fleck SJ, Kearney JT, Wide L. Serum erythropoietin in athletes at moderate altitude. Scand J Med Sci Sports 2:21-25, 1992.

7. Bergström J. Frontiers in medicine. New aspects of erythropoietin treatment. J Int Med 233:1-18, 1993.

8. Birkeland KI, Stray-Gundersen J, Hemmersbach P, Hallén J, Haug E, Bahr R. Effect of rhEPO administration on serum levels of sTrR and cycling performance. Med Sci Sports Exerc 32:1238-1243, 2000.

9. Bressolle F, Audrian M, Guidicelli C, Garneau R, Baynes RD, Gomeni R. Population pharmacodynamics for monitoring Epoetin Athletes. Clin Drug Invest 14:233-242, 1997.

10. Brugnara C, Zelmanovic D, Sorette M, Ballas SK, Platt O. Reticulocyte hemoglobin. An integrated parameter for evaluation of erythropoietic activity. Am J Clin Pathol 108:133-142, 1997.

11. Cazzola M, Mercuriali F, Brugnara C. Use of recombinant human erythropoietin outside the setting of uremia. Blood 89:4248-4267, 1997.

12. Ekblom B, Berglund B. Effect of erythropoietin administration on maximal aerobic power in man. Scand J Med Sci Sports 1:125-130, 1991.

13. Ekblom B, Wilson G, Åstrand P-O. Central circulation during exercise after venesection and infusion of red blood cells. J Appl Physiol 40:379-383, 1976.

14. Eschbach J, Egrie J, Downing M, Browne J, Adamson L. Correction of the anaemia of end-stage renal disease with recombinant human erythropoietin. N Engl J Med 316:73-78, 1987.

15. French Cycling Federation. Workshop on the detection of abnormal activation of erythropoiesis by pharmacological doses of human recombinant EPO, Rosny-sous-Bois, Paris, France, May 11, 1999.

16. Gareau R, Gagnon MG, Thellend C. Transferrin soluble receptor: a possible probe for detection of erythropoietin abuse in athletes. Horm Metab Res 26:311-312, 1994.

17. Geissler RG, Schulte P, Ganser A. Clinical use of hematopoietic growth factors in patients with myelodysplastic syndromes. Int J Hemat 65:339-354, 1997.

18. Glapsy J. The impact of epoietin alfa on quality of life during cancer chemotherapy: a fresh look at an old problem. Sem Hemat 34:20-26, 1997.

19. Hellsten-Westing Y, Ekblom B, Sjödin B. The metabolic relationship between hypoxanthine and uric acid in man following maximal short distance running. Acta Physiol Scand 137:341-345, 1989.

20. Huang C, Davis G, Johns EJ. The effect of chronic erythropoietin treatment on blood pressure and renal haemodynamics in the rat. J Physiol 473:273, 1993.

21. Lasne F, de Ceaurriz J. Recombinant erythropoietin in urine. Nature 405:635, 2000.

22. Magnani M, Corsi D, Bianchi M, Paiardini M, Galluzzi L, Pigozzi F, Parisi A. A new approach for the detection of rhEPO abuse in athletes. Fourth Ann Cong Eur Coll Sports Science, Rome, 1999.

23. Maschio G. Erythropoietin and systemic hypertension. Nephrol Dial Transpl 10:74-79, 1995.

24. Parisotto R, Gore CJ, Emslie KR, Ashenden MJ, Brugnara C, Howe C, Martin DT, Trout GJ, Hahn AG. A novel method for the detection of recombinant human erythropoietin abuse in athletes utilising markers of altered erythropoiesis. Haematol 85:564-572, 2000.

25. Spence RK. Emerging trends in surgical blood transfusions. Sem in Hemat 34:48-53, 1997.

26. Videman T, Lereim I, Hemmingsson P, Turner MS, Rousseau-Bianchi MP, Jenoure P, Raas E, Schonhuber H,

Rusco H, Stray-Gundersen J. Changes in hemoglobin values in elite cross-country skiers from 1987-1999. Scand J Med Sci Sports 10:98-102, 2000.

27. Wide L, Bengtsson C, Berglund B, Ekblom, B. Detection in blood and urine of recombinant erythropoietin administrated to healthy men. Med Sci Sports Exerc 27:1569-1576, 1995.

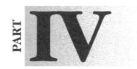
Diuretics

10

Diuretics

Lawrence E. Armstrong, PhD, FACSM

Numerous diuretic agents are available with a prescription, but most of this chapter involves research conducted on furosemide (Lasix). The technical chemical name for this compound is 4-chloro-N-(2-furylmethyl)-5-sulfamoylanthranilic acid. Its chemical formula is $C_{12} H_{11} C_1 N_2 O_5 S$. The usual oral adult dose of furosemide is 20 to 80 mg as a single dose, which may be repeated and increased at 6- to 8-hr intervals, not to exceed a maximum of 600 mg daily (U.S. Pharmacopeial Convention, 1997). Other commonly prescribed diuretics include acetazolamide (Diamox), amiloride (Midamor), ethacrynic acid (Edecrin), hydrochlorothiazide (Oretic), spironolactone (Aldactone), and triamterene (Dyrenium). Although intravenous administration of diuretics is used in hospitals and other clinical settings, most diuretics are taken orally.

The Kidneys: Target Organ for Diuretic Action

Figure 10.1 depicts a nephron, the functional unit of filtration. Each kidney contains approximately 1.2 million of these structures, which are hollow tubes consisting of a single cell layer. To understand the way diuretics affect the body, it is important to understand the segments of a typical nephron. Figure 10.1a shows that each nephron protrudes into the kidney, from the cortex to the medulla. Capillary blood enters Bowman's capsule, and the resulting filtrate passes through the proximal (e.g., near) tubule, descending limb, ascending limb, distal (e.g., distant) tubule, and collecting duct; from this point to the bladder, the filtrate is considered to be urine. Different compounds enter and leave the nephron at various sites along this course, including bicarbonate, glucose, amino acids (proximal tubule), and urea (ascending limb and collecting duct). However, water and sodium chloride

(NaCl; e.g., table salt) move across the nephron at all points (figure 10.1b).

Diuretics alter the water and NaCl reabsorption of the cells that line the nephron's tubular system and are classified by their sites of action or mechanisms, as follows: osmotic diuretics, carbonic anhydrase inhibitors, loop diuretics (acting at the loop of Henle), thiazide diuretics, and potassium-sparing diuretics. Because the use of the first two types is generally limited, their importance in exercise and sport is relatively minor (Caldwell, 1987).

Loop diuretics block the reabsorption of sodium (Na^+) in the thick ascending loop of Henle (figure 10.1) by binding to the Na^+-K^+-$2Cl^-$ transport protein in the membrane of renal nephrons (Hinchcliff & Muir, 1991). Because water follows salt (e.g., sodium) movement, a large volume of fluid accumulates in the distal tubule and passes into the collecting duct. Urinary excretion of Na^+, potassium (K^+), calcium (Ca^{++}), and magnesium (Mg^{++}) also increases. The loop diuretics are extremely powerful and rapid acting, so their potential for abuse is great. Marked increases in urine output can be achieved within minutes (Caldwell, 1987) and reach maximum during the initial 3 hr of use. Furosemide (Lasix), azosemide, bumetandine, ethacrynic acid, and piretanide are examples of loop diuretics.

The thiazide diuretics derive their name from their chemical structure. They act on the early distal tubule of the nephron (see figure 10.1) to block Na^+ absorption, causing Na^+ excretion to increase during the initial 48 hr of use. This loss of Na^+ typically results in a 1.6- to 2.1-quart (1.5-2.0 L) water loss from the extracellular fluid compartment and a 15% contraction of plasma volume (Freis, 1983). Fluid shifts of this magnitude can affect

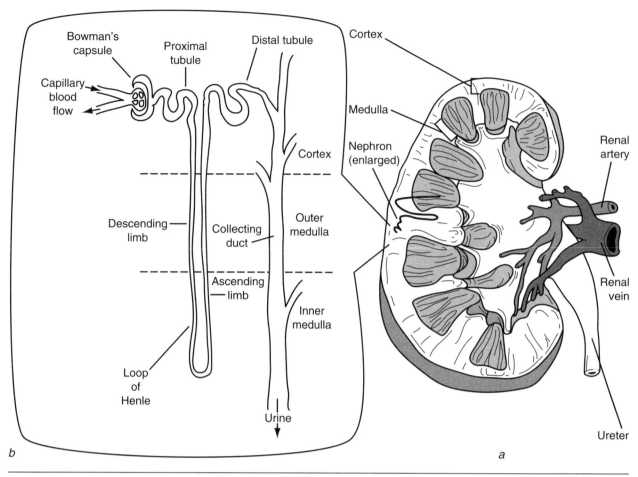

Figure 10.1 *(a)* A cross-section of the human kidney and *(b)* detail of a nephron.

cardiovascular performance markedly (Armstrong, 1992). Continual use of this agent may result in a decreased blood concentration of K^+ (hypokalemia) and serious clinical illness. Benzthiazide, cyclothiazide, hydrochlorothiazide, and polythiazide are examples of drugs in this diuretic class.

The potassium-sparing diuretics act on the late distal tubule and collecting duct (see figure 10.1) to block K^+ and hydrogen ion (H^+) secretion, as well as Na^+ and water uptake. This results in diuresis with an excess of K^+ in the blood and extracellular fluid compartment (hyperkalemia). Because both K^+ and Na^+ are vital to muscle contraction and nerve conduction, prolonged use of such drugs can alter neuromuscular function. In rare, advanced cases (i.e., incidence of 10-19%), the clinical symptoms may include muscle weakness, paralysis, or fatal cardiac arrhythmias (Caldwell, 1987).

Following diuretic use, dramatic and rapid changes occur in renal function, urine volume, and the concentration of excreted substances. Figure 10.2 illustrates this phenomenon in humans. The top panel depicts the rate of urine formation, and the bottom panel shows urine specific gravity, at the same time points.

Specific gravity refers to the density of urine sample (mass per unit volume) in comparison to that of pure water. Any fluid that is denser than water has a specific gravity greater than 1.000. Normal adult values for the rate of urine production and specific gravity are 45 to 60 ml·hr^{-1} and .013 to 1.029, respectively.

Diuretic Use by Athletes

Although it is not likely that an elite athlete would have a valid medical need for a diuretic (e.g., for hypertension), the International Olympic Committee (IOC) reported that diuretics are among the most commonly abused compounds. After anabolic steroids, stimulants, and narcotics, diuretics were the fourth most commonly abused drug group (Benzi, 1994).

A recent study of diuretic use among National Collegiate Athletic Association (NCAA) Division I athletes surveyed 371 females with a mean age of 19.5 years. The authors (Martin et al., 1998) reported that 7.9% of all athletes in three sports utilized diuretics to lose weight and that 7.2% utilized laxatives. Diuretic use was greatest among volleyball competitors (23.6%, 30 of 127 players), followed by players of softball (3.6%) and

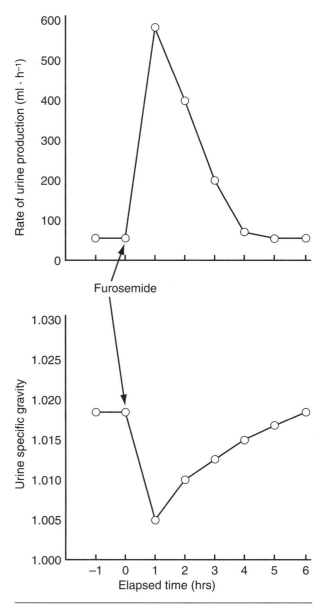

Figure 10.2 Typical changes in rate of urine production (top graph) and urine specific gravity (bottom graph) following oral consumption of 40 mg furosemide. A low specific gravity (<1.010) indicates dilute urine.

basketball (1.0%). It is likely that the incidence of diuretic use is much greater in sports such as wrestling, because among the 400,000 athletes who compete annually in the United States, about 60% lose weight through dehydration using various methods (Anonymous, 1998).

Therefore, to safeguard health and to give all athletes similar competitive advantages, the NCAA and the U.S. Olympic Committee (USOC) ban the use of all diuretics. For example, all of the diuretics named in the first paragraph of this chapter are illegal under the rules of the NCAA, USOC, and IOC (Reents, 2000). This means that the vast majority of collegiate and Olympic athletes who use diuretics do so illicitly.

Sports such as wrestling, boxing, power lifting, and judo contain levels of competition determined by weight (Patterson, 1981). This often encourages athletes to attempt to reduce body weight, to qualify for (or excel in) an established weight class, just prior to competition. Besides using starvation diets, athletes attempt to lower body weight quickly by losing water. This typically is accomplished via diuretics and other drugs or methods that induce diarrhea, vomiting, and/or dehydration (i.e., exercise in impermeable suits or hot rooms).

In sports that emphasize appearance and slender body types, such as gymnastics and ballet, weight loss is encouraged. Bodybuilders also utilize diuretics to achieve greater muscle definition and to appear "cut" (Hickson et al., 1990). But diuretic use can be fatal when taken to an extreme. In 1992, bodybuilder Mohammed Benaziza died suddenly of cardiac arrest, just days after placing fourth in the Mr. Olympia contest in Finland. The medical report cited "heart failure due to use of diuretics" as the cause of death. Benaziza had been using furosemide to prepare for competition (Vest, 1993). Indeed, diuretics have been described as the most dangerous drugs in the sport of bodybuilding today because of their widespread abuse.

Jockeys also strive to lose weight to reduce the load that racing horses carry because the potential of a winning effort holds the promise of financial reward. Although jockeys in previous generations utilized dieting, fluid deprivation, and sweating, the abuse of diuretics now is commonplace. Considering that muscle weakness and loss of mental acuity are possible side effects of severe food and fluid deprivation, it is sobering to contemplate someone in these conditions controlling a 1000-lb (454 kg) animal running at full speed in a field of 15 to 20 horses (Robinson, 1974).

A Russian ski jumper became the first person in the history of his sport to fail a drug test, in January 2001. He tested positive for the prescription diuretic furosemide at a World Cup event in Innsbruck, Austria, an event in which he was among the top three skiers (Associated Press, 2001). The International Ski Federation banned him from competition for two years. Light ski jumpers usually can stay aflot longer and cover greater distances than their nondoping competitors.

Diuretics also have been used improperly to dilute the urine so that the presence of performance-enhancing drugs, or their metabolic counterparts, cannot be detected. This most commonly occurs when a competitor is likely to undergo a drug detection test. A Bulgarian power lifter was the first athlete to be disqualified from the 2000 Summer Olympic Games in Sydney, Australia. He lost the silver medal in the 56-kg (123 lb) weightlifting class because he tested positive for furosemide (Associated Press, 2000). News reports suggested that this athlete used furosemide in an attempt to mask anabolic steroids or other performance-enhancing compounds.

Detecting Diuretic Use

The procedure to determine whether an athlete has used diuretics follows a protocol similar to that for drug tests performed in government and industry. The athlete provides a urine sample, in the presence of a witness, that is sealed and marked to verify authenticity. A witness is used because athletes have previously sent impersonators to drug-testing stations, introduced "clean" urine into the bladder through a catheter, consumed chemicals to mask or reduce elimination of banned substances, and introduced chemicals into the sample at the time of voiding (Di Pasquale, 1984).

The urine sample is delivered to a laboratory, where a sophisticated, accurate analysis is conducted via either radioimmunoassay or liquid chromatography. Radio-immunoassay is a technique that measures the levels of specific radioactive antibodies to identify illegal ergogenic aids. Liquid chromatography separates the individual components of urine during a period of several minutes and signals their presence as a pen deflection on a chart recorder.

Analysis of a urine sample involves three phases: extraction, screening, and confirmation (Di Pasquale, 1984). The initial step, the extraction, involves isolation of the chemicals in urine that are relevant to the testing process. Typically, multiple extractions are required because many other drugs are excreted in urine, in their original form and as metabolic by-products. The second stage, the screening, involves a search for traces of banned substances within the extracted solutions. The IOC and NCAA laboratory technicians do not screen for one suspected compound; they attempt to identify all chemicals that are banned by the governing body. The third phase, confirmation, is accomplished with use of the gas chromatography–mass spectroscopy technique. Although the results of this technique are scientifically valid, if the concentration of the compound is low, mass spectroscopy will not be able to confirm its presence.

In the event of a positive test, the athlete is notified and asked to provide a second urine sample. The athlete, or his representative, may observe the second laboratory test as it is conducted. If a diuretic is found in the athlete's urine, the individual will be disqualified from competition for the period determined by the governing sport federation.

Diuretic Use and Physical Performance in Humans

As already noted, many types of athletes utilize diuretics to enhance their athletic performance (Reents, 2000). Even skiers and mountain climbers sometimes take the diuretic acetazolamide to ward off symptoms of acute mountain sickness (Caldwell, 1987). Thus, acute dehydration has been the focus of most investigations involving diuretics. Table 10.1 provides a summary of several studies that have evaluated diuretic effects in humans. At least one deleterious effect of performance or physiologic function was observed in all studies shown. This included maximal isometric leg strength and the rate of force development.

Figure 10.3 illustrates the effects of furosemide (Lasix) on running performance. In this study (Armstrong et al., 1985), eight male distance runners ran six randomized competitive trials (e.g., two trials at each of three distances—1500 m, 5000 m, and 10,000 m (1640, 5468,

Table 10.1 Effects of Diuretic Use on Physical Performance and Physiological Function in Humans

Level of dehydration (% body weight), dose, and diuretic type	Effects of diuretic administration	Author and year
–2% 40 mg furosemide	Performance in 1500-m, 5000-m, and 10,000-m footraces declined; no change in $\dot{V}O_2$max occurred.	Armstrong et al., 1985
–3% 40-80 mg furosemide	Cycling performance (35% $\dot{V}O_2$max) decreased, heart rate increased, rectal and muscle temperatures increased.	Claremont et al., 1976
–3% 50 mg triamterene + 25 mg hydrochloric-thiazide for 4 days	During cycling, the cardiac output and stroke volume decreased but rectal temperature increased; a 50% reduction of forearm skin blood flow was observed.	Nadel et al., 1980
–4% 126 mg furosemide	$\dot{V}O_2$max and cycling work output declined.	Caldwell et al., 1984
–4% 40 mg furosemide	No change in $\dot{V}O_2$max; heart rate during cycling fell at low exercise intensities but increased at a high exercise intensity.	Baum et al., 1986
–4% 80 mg furosemide	Maximal isometric leg strength and the rate of force development decreased[1].	Viitasalo et al., 1987

$\dot{V}O_2$max—maximal oxygen consumption or maximal aerobic power.

[1]Maximal vertical jump height improved after diuretic use due to the decrease in body weight.

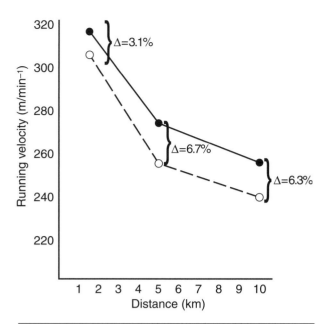

Figure 10.3 Group mean velocities of hydrated (closed circles) and furosemide-dehydrated (open circles) running trials conducted on a synthetic outdoor track.

Reprinted, by permission, from L.E. Armstrong, D.L. Costill, and W.J. Fink, 1985, "Influence of diuretic-induced dehydration on competitive running performance," *Medicine and Science in Sports and Exercise* 17 (4):456-461.

and 10,936 yd)—on an outdoor synthetic track. Prior to three of the trials, runners consumed 40 mg of furosemide that induced an average dehydration (see open circles in figure 10.3) of 1.3 to 1.7 quarts (1.2-1.6 L) of urine in 5 hrs. Prior to three other trials (i.e., on control days), they were normally hydrated (see closed circles in figure 10.3). Because the usual daily adult dose of furosemide is 20 to 80 mg, the experimental dose was likely equal to or less than the dose that athletes utilize to enhance performance. The influence of diuretic-induced dehydration on performance was greater in the longer events, despite the absence of a measurable change in maximal oxygen consumption ($\dot{V}O_2$max). The authors attributed this result primarily to the reduced plasma volume (as discussed further on) and consequent negative effects on cardiovascular function. Their experimental method allowed the authors to evaluate the effects of diuretic use alone, without interference from elevated body temperature or water loss via sweating. This was made possible by the fact that furosemide and some other diuretics produce urine that has essentially the same electrolyte concentrations as blood (i.e., isotonic), and induce no measurable alterations in plasma electrolytes or muscle water (Bergstrom & Hultman, 1966).

Other than plasma volume reduction and diminished cardiovascular function, the mechanism(s) of diuretic action on performance are not well defined. However, the authors of the investigation (Armstrong et al., 1985) acknowledged four possible non-cardiovascular effects

of diuretic use on performance. First, because blood lactic acid accumulation was lower in the dehydration trials at distances of 5000 m and 10,000 m (5468 and 10,936 yd), either anaerobic production or clearance of lactic acid may have been altered by diuretic use. This phenomenon also may occur because furosemide either (a) induces metabolic alkalosis (i.e., increased pH due to K^+ loss, Cl^- loss, or contraction of plasma volume; Hinchcliff & Muir, 1991) in arterial and mixed venous blood (Carlson & Jones, 1999) or (b) promotes a smaller contribution of anaerobic metabolism to the total energy requirement, thereby reducing lactate production (Hinchcliff et al., 1996). The phenomenon was observed initially by Caldwell and colleagues in a human laboratory study conducted in 1984. Second, reduced sweating and skin blood flow (i.e., secondary to dehydration and reduced cardiac output) may have induced hyperthermia during the dehydration trials, even though the ambient temperature was only 16 °C. Thus, the two longer competitive distances may have exhibited a greater decrement in performance because of longer heat storage times. Third, the interaction of several factors (i.e., elevated body temperature, body water loss, reduced cardiac output) may have potentiated an increase in perceived exertion during the dehydration trials, causing slowing running velocities. Fourth, the act of ingesting a diuretic tablet and losing a large quantity of urine in a brief period of time may have negatively affected the mood state or competitive intensity of these runners. Although no study has evaluated such psychological effects to date, mental determination is obviously vital to successful athletic performance.

Because of the important role that muscular power and anaerobic metabolism play in their sport, wrestlers rely on $\dot{V}O_2$max and aerobic metabolism less than endurance athletes. However, we have insufficient research evidence to conclude that diuretic use reduces strength and power performance, simply because few studies have been conducted. But this does not mean that the athletes experience no performance decrements. One investigation, for example, showed that wrestlers lost upper-body strength after exercise-induced dehydration (Webster et al., 1990). Logically, diuretic-induced dehydration should have similar effects.

In general, the scientific literature indicates that water losses of 2% or 3% of body weight, when induced by techniques other than diuretics, mark the threshold beyond which endurance performance is impaired. Power and strength deficits become evident at a body weight loss of 4% to 5% (Armstrong, 1992). However, because the magnitude of plasma volume decrease is greater following diuretic dehydration than other forms of dehydration (table 10.2), the potential effect on cardiovascular function is greater. Also, because psychological perception of effort is greatly affected by circulatory stress, perceived exertion may be affected more by diuretic dehydration

Table 10.2 The Effect of Dehydration Technique on the Relative Contribution of Plasma Volume and Total Body Water[1]

Technique	Ratio of % plasma volume change to % body weight change[2]
Diuretic-induced dehydration (cool environment) with no exercise	6:1
Resting in a hot environment (sweat and urine loss)	4.5:1
Exercise-induced sweating in a cool environment	3.5:1
Exercise-induced sweating in a hot environment	2.5:1
Moderate exercise plus withholding fluids and food from wrestlers for 48 hours	1:1

[1]Revised from Hubbard & Armstrong, 1988.

[2]Note: A large ratio (versus a small one) means that a greater relative proportion of the total body water loss was derived from the blood plasma.

than other types. Regarding the method of dehydration, evidence indicates that a 24-hr diuretic-induced weight reduction protocol has a greater impact on physiological responses than a 4% weight loss over a 48-hr period (Caldwell et al., 1984).

Contrary to the research showing a decline in many aspects of performance with diuretic use (table 10.1), the study by Viitasalo and colleagues (1987) indicates that rapid, diuretic-induced weight loss results in improved vertical jump performance, probably due to the reduced body mass lifted during this task. This suggests that weight loss might improve other types of explosive, anaerobic performance, and the issue deserves further study.

In contrast to healthy individuals, patients with symptoms of cardiac or pulmonary diseases seem to be exceptions to the observations reported in table 10.1 in that their exercise responses improve with diuretic use. A rapid diuresis reduces blood volume, unloads the failing heart muscle, and improves hemodynamic function, angina symptoms, electrical function of the heart (Bhatia et al., 1969; Caldwell, 1987), and treadmill walking endurance time (Eterno et al., 1998). In fact, the adult recreational enthusiast with hypertension is the primary legitimate user of diuretics (Eichner, 1984).

Side Effects

The general side effects resulting from diuretic use include fatigue, drowsiness, muscle cramps or soreness,

and sensations of numbness, tingling, or prickling. It is likely that these are related to alterations of the resting electrical potentials of nerve and muscle membranes and their subsequent effects on the conduction of neuromuscular impulses (Kaplan, 1984). In addition, the material safety data sheet lists these possible adverse effects in some individuals: nausea or vomiting, diarrhea, mood or mental changes, blurred vision, and increased skin sensitivity to light (U.S. Pharmacopeial Convention, 1997). It is likely that these side effects are due to either allergic responses or sensitivity to the specific diuretic drug type.

Although low blood levels of Na^+, Ca^{++}, Mg^{++}, and K^+ have been reported with prolonged diuretic therapy, the neuromuscular side effects most often result from hypokalemia (discussed earlier in the chapter). The prevalence and symptoms of hypokalemia are determined by the dose and type of diuretic, the original blood K^+ level, and the extent of the deficit. For example, the average decrease in serum K^+ concentration is 0.62 mmol/L for thiazides and only 0.30 mmol/L for the loop diuretic furosemide. Of course, the decline in the blood K^+ concentration reflects a whole-body deficit; each 0.3 mmol/L decrease in serum concentration reflects a 100 mmol K^+ deficiency (Caldwell, 1987). Thus, it is not surprising that the serum K^+ concentration is related to clinical symptoms (table 10.3).

Table 10.3 Side Effects of Diuretic Use That Are Related to Potassium Levels[1]

Serum K^+ concentration (mmol/L)	Complex of symptoms
>3.5	Normal
3.0-3.5	Discomfort, uneasiness; fatigue, weakness
3.0-2.6	Tenderness or pain in muscles; occasional cramps
<2.5	Paralysis, muscle breakdown
<2.0	Muscle cell death, appearance of myoglobin in urine

Other side effects related to hypokalemia[2]

Muscle irritability

Diminished local muscle blood flow

Rhabdomyolysis

Paralysis

Elevated cholesterol low-density lipoprotein and triglycerides

Diminished glucose tolerance

[1]Revised from Caldwell, 1987.

[2]Particularly the thiazide and loop diuretics.

Metabolism also may be affected by hypokalemia. For example, glycogen synthesis is curtailed and the resynthesis of muscle glycogen may be blocked (Blackley et al., 1973). A decrease in glucose tolerance is a well-known side effect of thiazide diuretic use (Boone, 1986), as is increased glucose concentration in blood. Further, several studies have demonstrated unfavorable shifts in blood lipid profiles following thiazide use (Ames & Peacock, 1984). Although the mechanisms of these shifts have not been fully described, the shifts serve as important markers of increased cardiovascular disease risk. Hypokalemia also raises concerns about inducing potentially lethal cardiac arrhythmias or irregular heartbeats (Caldwell, 1987). Although few studies have measured the effects of chronic diuretic use on either exercise metabolism or health, the metabolic changes just discussed are likely to have a negative effect on physical performance due to the alterations in muscle glycogen resynthesis, glucose tolerance, and fat metabolism.

Certain medical conditions may be aggravated by furosemide exposure. These include active alcoholism, diabetes mellitus, gout, hearing impairment, liver function impairment, acute heart disease, pancreatitis, and lupus erythematosus. The use of furosemide during pregnancy is not recommended.

An Important Drug Interaction

Numerous drugs interact with furosemide, but perhaps the most important interaction for athletes involves nonsteroidal anti-inflammatory drugs (NSAIDs) including aspirin. Certain pain relievers/anti-inflammatory agents in the NSAID family reduce the effectiveness of furosemide. This occurs because both compounds act on the nephron's loop of Henle (figure 10.1).

Furosemide acts by directly stimulating production of the chemical prostaglandin E_2 (PE_2) in the thick ascending limb of the loop. In turn, PE_2 inhibits Na^+ and Cl^- reabsorption and causes rapid, large water and salt losses. Nonsteroidal anti-inflammatory drugs prevent the furosemide-induced increase in PE_2 (Hinchcliff & Muir, 1991). Thus, when an athlete utilizes furosemide and a prostaglandin-blocking NSAID concurrently, diuresis and the loss of electrolytes are greatly diminished.

Other commonly used drugs and herbs that interact negatively with furosemide include ginseng, activated charcoal, cortisone, digoxin, hydrocortisone, lithium, neomycin, propranolol, and streptomycin.

Overdose Precautions

The complications of an acute, large overdose of a diuretic formulation such as furosemide involve possible eye, skin, gastrointestinal, and respiratory tract irritation. Chronic overdosing of Lasix may result in fluid and electrolyte imbalances as already described, hepatitis, and irreversible or reversible deafness (Caldwell, 1987; Reents, 2000). The exact amount of furosemide that constitutes an overdose in humans has not been reported, but the U.S. Food and Drug Administration limits daily intake to 600 mg. In rats, a dose of 2600 mg/kg body weight results in the deaths of half of the test animals (U.S. Pharmacopeial Convention, 1997).

Conclusion

Diuretics, pharmacological agents that affect the kidneys, are effective because a large volume of water and electrolytes are excreted within 2 to 4 hrs of use. Diuretics are used when (a) athletes choose to reduce body weight to qualify for an established weight class; (b) gymnasts and ballet dancers emphasize appearance and slender body types; (c) bodybuilders want to achieve greater muscle definition; (d) jockeys strive to reduce the load that racing horses carry; and (e) athletes attempt to dilute the urine to mask the presence of performance-enhancing drugs. Diuretics negatively affect athletic performance by reducing cardiorespiratory endurance and muscular strength. They also increase whole-body heat storage during exercise by reducing sweating and skin blood flow. These physiological effects, coupled with the potential for electrolyte (e.g., potassium) depletion, demonstrate that diuretic use is counterproductive and sometimes deleterious to health. Finally, because diuretics are banned by the IOC, USOC, and NCAA, their use by athletes should not be accepted or ignored.

References

Ames, R.P., & Peacock, P.B. (1984). Serum cholesterol during treatment of hypertension with diuretic drugs. Archives of Internal Medicine, 144, 710-714.

Anonymous. (1998). Wrestlers' deaths prompt new discussions. Athletic Management, 10(3), 6-9.

Armstrong, L.E. (1992). The Effects of Heat, Humidity, and Dehydration on Athletic Performance, Strength, and Endurance. Colorado Springs, CO: U.S. Olympic Committee.

Armstrong, L.E., Costill, D.L., & Fink, W.J. (1985). Influence of diuretic-induced dehydration on competitive running performance. Medicine and Science in Sports and Exercise, 17(4), 456-461.

Associated Press. (2000). Two banned for drugs. Hartford Courant, September 20, sect. C, p. 10.

Associated Press. (2001). Russian ski jumper banned for two years. New York Times, February 7, sect. D, p. 7.

Baum, K., Ebfeld, D., & Stefeman, J. (1986). The influence of furosemide on heart rate and oxygen uptake in exercising man. European Journal of Applied Physiology, 55, 619-623.

Benzi, G. (1994). Pharmacoepidemiology of the drugs used in sports as doping agents. Pharmacology Research, 29, 13-26.

Bergstrom, J., & Hultman, E. (1966). The effect of thiazides, chlorthalidone, and furosemide on muscle electrolytes and muscle glycogen in normal subjects. Acta Medica Scandinavica, 180(3), 363-376.

Bhatia, R.W., Singh, I., Manchanda, S.C., Khanna, P.K., & Roy, S.B. (1969). Effects of furosemide on pulmonary blood volume. British Medical Journal, 2, 551-552.

Blackley, J., Knochel, J.P., & Long, J. (1973). Impaired muscle glycogen synthesis and prevention of muscle glycogen supercompensation by potassium deficiency. Clinical Research, 22, 517A.

Boone, T. (1986). Exercise prescription for cardiac patients. Sports Medicine, 3, 157-164.

Caldwell, J.E. (1987). Diuretic therapy and exercise performance. Sports Medicine, 4, 290-304.

Caldwell, J.E., Ahonen, E., & Nousiainen, U. (1984). Differential effects of sauna-, diuretic-, and exercise-induced hypohydration. Journal of Applied Physiology, 57(4), 1018-1023.

Carlson, G.P., & Jones, J.H. (1999). Effects of furosemide on electrolyte and acid-base balance during exercise. Equine Veterinary Journal Supplement, 30, 370-374.

Claremont, A.D., Costill, D.L., Fink, W.J., & Van Handel, P.J. (1976). Heat tolerance following diuretic-induced dehydration. Medicine and Science in Sports, 8(4), 239-243.

Di Pasquale, M.G. (1984). Diuretics. In Drug Use and Detection in Amateur Sports (pp. 79-82). Warkworth, ON, Canada: M.G.D. Press.

Eichner, E.R. (1984). The exercise hypothesis—an updated review. In L.J. Krakauer (Ed.), 1984 Yearbook of Sports Medicine. Chicago: Year Book Medical.

Eterno, F.T., de Oliveira-Junior, M.T., & Barretto, A.C. (1998). Diuretics improve functional capacity in patients with congestive heart failure [Portuguese]. Archives of Brazilian Cardiology, 70(5), 315-320.

Freis, E.D. (1983). How diuretics lower blood pressure. American Heart Journal, 106, 185-187.

Guyton, A.C., & Hall, J.E. (1996). Textbook of Medical Physiology, 9th edition (pp. 315-330). Philadelphia: Saunders.

Hickson, J.F., Johnson, T.E., Lee, W., & Sidor, R.J. (1990). Nutrition and the precontest preparations of a male bodybuilder. Journal of the American Dietetic Association, 90(2), 264-267.

Hinchcliff, K.W., McKeever, K.H., Muir, W.W., & Sams, R.A. (1996). Furosemide reduces accumulated oxygen deficit in horses during brief intense exertion. Journal of Applied Physiology, 81, 1550-1554.

Hinchcliff, K.W., & Muir, W.W. (1991). Pharmacology of furosemide in the horse: a review. Journal of Veterinary Internal Medicine, 5(4), 211-218.

Hubbard, R.W., & Armstrong, L.E. (1988). The heat illnesses: biochemical, ultrastructural, and fluid-electrolyte considerations. In K.B. Pandolf, M.N. Sawka, & R.R. Gonzalez (Eds.), Human Performance Physiology and Environmental Medicine at Terrestrial Extremes (pp. 305-359). Indianapolis: Benchmark Press.

Kaplan, N.M. (1984). Our appropriate concern about hypokalemia. American Journal of Medicine, 77, 1-4.

Martin, M., Schlabach, G., & Shibinski, K. (1998). The use of nonprescription weight loss products among female basketball, softball, and volleyball athletes from NCAA Division I institutions: issues and concerns. Journal of Athletic Training, 33, 41-44.

Nadel, E.R., Fortney, S.M., & Wenger, C.B. (1980). Effect of hydration state on circulatory and thermal regulations. Journal of Applied Physiology, 49(4), 715-721.

Patterson, P. (1981). Diuretics in sport. What price to be paid? Science Periodical on Research and Technology in Sport, February, 1-4.

Reents, S. (2000). Sport and Exercise Pharmacology (pp. 47-69). Champaign, IL: Human Kinetics.

Robinson, J.J. (1974). Problems in weight control in jockeys. Twentieth World Congress of Sports Medicine: Congress proceedings (pp. 345-346). Carlton, Australia: University of Melbourne.

U.S. Pharmacopeial Convention. (1997). Material Safety Data Sheet: Furosemide (pp. 1-3). Rockville, MD: Author.

Vest, D.W. (1993). Wrestling looks to body building. Wrestling USA, 29(5), 91-92.

Viitasalo, J.T., Kyrolainen, H., Bosco, C., & Alen, M. (1987). Effects of rapid weight reduction on force production and vertical jumping height. International Journal of Sports Medicine, 8(4), 281-285.

Webster, S., Rutt, R., & Weltman, A. (1990). Physiologic effects of a weight loss regimen practiced by college wrestlers. Medicine and Science in Sports and Exercise, 22, 229-234.

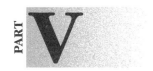
Narcotic and Non-Narcotic Analgesics and Depressants

 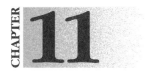
Narcotic Analgesics and Athletic Performance

Dean F. Connors, MD, PhD

John Sudkamp, MD

Every day in the United States alone, hundreds of thousands of American take medications with the intent of relieving pain. These medications range from nonsteroidal anti-inflammatory drugs (NSAIDs) to potent narcotics and their derivatives. Some of these medications are available over the counter while others require a physician's prescription. Many are also taken with the intent of improving athletic performance. The purpose of this chapter is twofold: to discuss narcotics in general and to discuss the effect of narcotics on athletic performance.

Narcotic Analgesics: An Overview

Currently, the term *narcotic* is used to describe opium, opium derivates, or substances that mimic the effects of morphine in vivo. Opium and its derivatives interact with specific receptors in the central nervous system. The use of the poppy seed and its derivative opium dates back to the third century B.C. Opium itself is derived from the juice of the poppy, *Papaver somniferum*. Over time, the medical community gradually began to realize the tremendous abuse potential associated with these substances. Accordingly, the search was on to find substances that would provide the analgesic effect of morphine without the concomitant physical dependence. As a by-product of these efforts, derivatives of morphine were developed. The term *opioid* is used to refer to all

exogenous substances, natural and synthetic, that bind to any of the subpopulations of opioid receptors and produce at least some agonist effects (4). While this chapter is not intended to serve as the definitive reference on opiates and narcotic analgesics, it should serve as a useful review of the basic pharmacology of opiates, including pharmacokinetics (the effect of the body on the drug), mechanism of action, and pharmacodynamics (the effect of the drug on the body). For an in-depth discussion of these topics, the reader is referred to more extensive resources (9, 17, 20). What follows here is a brief overview of these very complex topics.

Pharmacokinetics

As just noted, the term *pharmacokinetics* describes the absorption, distribution, and elimination of a given agent or drug. With the notable exception of remifentanil, all of the opiates are metabolized to a major extent in the liver. The degree of hepatic metabolism varies between agents. In addition, some of the opiates (e.g., morphine) are also modified in the kidney. Some opiates also have active metabolites that continue to exert physiologic effects. For example, morphine has two main metabolites: morphine-3-glucuronide, which is metabolically inactive, and morphine-6-glucuronide, which continues to exert pharmacologic effects such as analgesia and respiratory depression (18). The speed of degradation and elimination is modified in the presence of hepatic disease (e.g., cirrhosis) and renal insufficiency/renal failure. Respiratory depression has been observed in patients with renal failure and is thought to be due to the buildup of active metabolites (9).

The method of administration is directly related to the desired speed of onset. Opiates have been administered intravenously, intrathecally, intramuscularly, orally, rectally, subcutaneously, and transdermally. Opiate effects are observed soonest with intravenous and intrathecal administration and in a more delayed fashion with administration by the transdermal route. The absorption of opiates orally and rectally is variable dependent on significant first-pass metabolism. The distribution and uptake of the opiates are beyond the scope of the chapter. It is reasonable to say, however, that the uptake and distribution of the opiates in general are closely related to the complex interplay between protein binding, lipid solubility, hepatic breakdown, and renal excretion.

Mechanism of Action

The opiate receptors are located in both the central nervous system and the periphery (17). In general, the opioid receptors are members of the G-protein-coupled receptor family. It is currently felt that the G-protein receptor family mediates many of the physiologic effects of neurotransmitters and hormones. The analgesic actions of the opiates are mediated by G-protein inhibition of calcium channels, activation of potassium channels, and reductions in cyclic adenosine monophosphate (3, 13). The opiate receptors have been further classified into mu (1 and 2), kappa, and delta. The mu receptor (mu 1) is thought to be primarily responsible for the analgesic action of the pure opiate morphine. Concurrent binding of the mu 2 receptor is felt to be responsible for many of the side effects associated with mu receptor binding including respiratory depression, nausea, bradycardia, and physical dependence. The endogenous opioids can be grouped based on receptor binding.

Pharmacodynamics

The opiates have many physiologic effects in addition to their analgesic actions. A good way to understand these effects is to examine the effects of opiates (primarily morphine, which is a pure mu agonist) on various physiologic systems. The systems most commonly affected by the opiates include the central nervous system, the respiratory system, the gastrointestinal system, and the cardiovascular system (17).

Central Nervous System

Opiate binding in the central nervous system is responsible for analgesia. As noted earlier, this binding occurs at the mu receptor. The analgesic effect of opiates on patients in pain is achieved with relatively small amounts of agent. Associated with the analgesic effect is a decrease in anxiety, relief of tension (5, 16), and respiratory depression (21). The analgesia associated with morphine administration is possibly due to many factors, including a decrease in the perception of pain and painful stimulus, the euphoria and sleep that occur, and an elevation in the pain threshold.

When opiates are administered to individuals who are not in pain, a dysphoric effect may be noted. In addition, mental clouding, drowsiness, lethargy, an inability to concentrate, and sedation may result. In addition, after the administration of opiates, the pupils become miotic (small and pinpoint). In addition to miosis, morphine administration is associated with nausea and vomiting. This side effect is primarily related to stimulation of the chemoreceptor trigger zone (18). High-dose administration of opiates (morphine and short-acting opiates such as fentanyl) is also associated with abdominal and chest wall rigidity. This rigidity is attenuated by the depolarizing muscle relaxant succinylcholine (18).

Respiratory System

Morphine administration is associated with respiratory depression. Respiratory depression is a consequence of decreased sensitivity to $PaCO_2$ at the level of the brainstem (21). These changes in respiration are dose dependent and are thought to be mediated through opiate binding at the mu 2 receptor (18). Changes in respiration are characterized by prolonged pauses between breaths and periodic breathing (18). With high doses of opiates, the patient may very well remain awake and be able to initiate breaths in response to command. In the event of opioid overdose, death is typically due to respiratory arrest.

Gastrointestinal System

Opiate administration is associated with a host of gastrointestinal effects. These effects include delayed peristalsis, constipation, and biliary colic. The effects are reversible with the administration of the pure opioid antagonist naloxone (21). These gastrointestinal effects appear to be specific for the opiates in that they are not observed after administration of other analgesics such as acetaminophen and other NSAIDs.

Cardiovascular System

Generally, the opiates have minimal direct effects on the heart and vascular system. That is, they have no direct cardiac depressant properties. Accordingly, these medications (in particular the short-acting agents such as fentanyl, sufentanyl, and remifentanyl) are used extensively in patients with compromised cardiovascular systems. They are used primarily either as a main anesthetic agent or as an adjunct to anesthesia. There are some cardiovascular effects associated with opiates; these include vagally mediated bradycardia and hypotension. The bradycardia is probably mediated via the vagal nerve exerting an effect at the level of the vagal nuclei in the medulla. Hypotension is observed after the administration of opiates. This hypotension is either related to vasodilation associated with histamine release or with removal of sympathetic tone in severely compromised patients who have become dependent on increased sympathetic tone to maintain blood pressure (10).

Specific Agents

Many opiates have been isolated and are available on the market today. It must be stressed that to varying degrees, all of these agents have physical dependence and abuse potential. The reader is referred to more in-depth resources for detailed discussions of these agents. A brief summary

of the pure opioid agonists and mixed agonist/antagonists is displayed in table 11.1 and table 11.2. However, some of these medications warrant brief discussion.

Pure Opiate Agonists

These agents act exclusively at the mu receptor. The pharmacologic actions and side effects were noted earlier. They provide analgesia that is frequently accompanied by sedation, respiratory depression, and dysphoria. They have abuse and dependence potential that restrict their availability on an over-the-counter basis.

Morphine

Morphine is a pure mu agonist. The effects of morphine are mediated through both the mu 1 and mu 2 receptors. Morphine administration is associated with analgesia, sedation, and diminished ability to concentrate (18). Its side effects include nausea, vomiting, respiratory depression, and a feeling of chest and extremity heaviness.

Table 11.1 Opioid (mu) Agonists

Agent	Preferred route	Time to onset (min)	Duration of action (hr) (19, 20)	Relative potency (19)
Morphine	IV, IM	20-30	3-4	10
Meperidine	IV, IM	20-30	2-4	1
Codeine	IV, oral	15-60	3-4	1
Methadone	IV, oral	30-60	4-6	10
Oxymorphone	Oral	20-30	4-5	1
Hydromorphine	IM, oral	20-30	4-5	1.5
Oxycodone	Oral	20-30	4-5	10
Fentanyl	IV	5	0.5	100 mcg
Sufentanyl	IV	5	0.5	15 mcg
Alfentanyl	IV	5	0.25	750 mcg
Remifentanyl	IV*			

*Remifentanyl given in continuous infusion. It has a very rapid onset, and because it is metabolized so quickly by plasma esterases, it has a very rapid offset. It is felt to be 15 to 20 times more potent than alfentanyl (19).

Table 11.2 Opioid Agonists/Antagonists

Agent	Preferred route	Time to onset (min)	Duration of action (hr) (19, 20)	Relative potency (19)
Pentazocine	IV, oral	20-30	3	20-30
Butorphanol	IV, IM	20-30	3	20-30
Nalbuphine	IV, IM	20-30	3-6	1
Buprenorphine	IM	30	8	300

Adapted, by permission, from M. Wood, 1990, Opioid agonists and antagonists. In *Drugs and anesthesia, pharmacology for anesthesiologists*, 2nd ed. edited by M. Wood and J.J. Wood (Baltimore: Lippincott, Williams, and Wilkins), 136. Modification of table by permission of M. Wood.

Codeine

Codeine is classified as a relatively mild analgesic. It is frequently used clinically in combination with other analgesics (such as acetaminophen) and as a cough suppressant. Codeine is not associated with significant respiratory depression.

Meperidine

Meperidine is a synthetic opiate with morphine-like actions. It is roughly one-tenth as potent as morphine and has a similar side-effect profile. It has multiple derivatives that include fentanyl, alfentanyl, sufentanyl, and the recently developed remifentanyl. The analgesic effect of meperidine lasts for 2 to 4 hr (21), whereas its derivatives have much shorter durations of action.

Methadone

Methadone is a synthetic opioid that was originally developed as a substitute for morphine (9). Its side-effect profile is similar to that of morphine. It is very effective when taken orally. It differs from morphine in that it has a longer half-life. Accordingly, methadone tends to accumulate systemically over time. Because of its longer half-life, methadone is frequently used as an adjunct to opiate withdrawal.

Hydromorphone, Oxycodone, and Oxymorphone

Hydromorphone and oxycodone are semisynthetic derivatives of morphine, while oxymorphone is a derivative of oxycodone. These agents are used for the treatment of mild to moderate pain. They are commonly taken orally, although hydromorphone is effective intravenously.

Fentanyl, Sufentanyl, Alfentanyl, and Remifentanyl

These agents are extremely potent ultra-short-acting derivatives of meperidine. They all have a relatively quick onset of analgesic effect. Remifentanyl (18) is unique in that it is metabolized by plasma esterases. Accordingly, it is usually administered by continuous infusion. Fentanyl deserves particular mention in that in addition to being administered intravenously, it is frequently administered by the transdermal route for the treatment of chronic pain (9). These agents are frequently used perioperatively in patients whose cardiovascular stability is tenuous.

Mixed Agonist-Antagonists

Another group of agents are classified as mixed agonist-antagonists. They exert a physiologic effect through binding to the mu receptor; they also exhibit binding to the other opiate receptors. These agents provide analgesia without associated respiratory depression. They are felt to have less abuse/dependence potential when contrasted with the pure mu receptor agonists. They are antagonistic in that they diminish the effect of subsequent agonist administration. In addition, when these agents are administered after a pure mu agonist, they have been shown to precipitate a withdrawal syndrome (17, 18). These agents undergo significant first-pass metabolism. Accordingly, they are administered parenterally. Additionally, the agonist-antagonist agents are unique in that they have a "ceiling effect." That is, there is a graduation in ventilatory depression up to a given dose. Thereafter, analgesia occurs with increasing dosages without the accompanying respiratory depression.

Pentazocine

Pentazocine possesses both agonist and antagonist activity. Its antagonist activity is felt to be weak (21). When administered parenterally, it is sufficient to precipitate a withdrawal syndrome. It has poor oral bioavailability. It is typically used for the treatment of moderate pain. Even though pentazocine is a mixed agonist-antagonist, its side-effect profile is similar to that of morphine.

Butorphanol

Structurally, butorphanol is similar to pentazocine. Its agonist and antagonist effects are significantly greater than those of pentazocine. Because it is available only in the parenteral form and its elimination half-life is comparatively short, it is used primarily for the treatment of acute pain.

Nalbuphine

Nalbuphine is structurally similar to oxymorphone and naloxone. As with the other opiates, it is primarily metabolized in the liver. The most common side effect is sedation. The incidence of dysphoria is less than that observed with pentazocine and butorphanol.

Buprenorphine

Buprenorphine is an extremely potent mixed agonist-antagonist agent (18). It is estimated to be greater than 30 times more potent than morphine. Its primary route of administration is intramuscular with a duration of analgesic action of at least 8 hr.

Antagonists

Opiate antagonists differ from the agents mentioned thus far in that they are devoid of analgesic activity. The side effects associated with opiate administration are also avoided. Indeed, these agents are used primarily to reverse the ventilatory depression associated with opiate overdose. They bind at the mu receptor. The primary opiate antagonist in use clinically is naloxone.

Naloxone

Naloxone is used for the reversal of opiate-induced ventilatory depression. It is also used in the emergency treatment of deliberate opioid overdose and for evaluation of suspected opiate dependence (18). Administration of naloxone is associated with abrupt reversal of analgesia in addition to the reversal of respiratory depression. Naloxone administration is also associated with nausea, vomiting, and pulmonary edema. Other opioid antagonists include naltrexone, nalmefene, and methylnaltrexone (21).

Narcotics and Human Performance

For the athlete (professional, amateur, and recreational), the use of narcotics is usually limited to the relief of pain (analgesia) (table 11.3). The side effects of these agents (nausea, euphoria, and constipation) are usually tolerated to achieve continued performance. Very little is known about how these medications enhance or limit athletic performance. A limited number of studies have been performed on healthy volunteers. Fewer studies have been done on cancer patients receiving orally administered opioids. A few investigators have looked at the effect of opioids on exercise performance in patients with chronic obstructive pulmonary disease (COPD).

All studies that have addressed the effects of opiates on human performance (either in the healthy population or in the subject population with underlying disease) monitored such vital signs as heart rate, noninvasive blood pressure, and noninvasive blood oxygen saturation by pulse oxymetry. In addition, the presence of miosis (papillary constriction) was assessed to ensure that an opiate effect was in fact present physiologically.

Multiple tests are available to assess psychomotor performance in healthy volunteers. These tests include the Maddox-Wing (MW) test, the auditory reaction time (ART) test, eye-hand coordination, and the digital symbol substitution test (DSST). In the pharmacologic arena, Hannington-Kiff (2) used a modification of the MW to evaluate patients after they had received general anesthesia. The MW assesses the degree of ocular divergence. This divergence is secondary to a decrease in the general muscle tone of the ocular muscles. This test has been shown to be a sensitive indicator of psychomotor impairment. Manner (8) extended the results of Hannington-Kiff to include psychomotor impairment secondary to opiate administration.

The ART is a derivative visual reactive test (12). In the visual reactive test, the subject responds as soon as possible (by pressing the space key on a computer keyboard) to the random appearance of a letter in the

Table 11.3 Trade Names of Various Analgesics and Indications

Generic name	Brand name (19, 20)	Clinical use
Morphine		Moderate to severe pain
Meperidine	Demerol	Severe pain
Codeine		Mild to moderate pain
Methadone	Dolophine	Moderate to severe pain
Oxymorphone	Numorphan	Moderate to severe pain
Hydromorphone	Dilaudid	Moderate to severe pain
Oxycodone	Percodan	Moderate to severe pain
Fentanyl	Sublimaze	Severe pain IV anesthetic
Sufentanyl	Sufenta	Severe pain IV anesthetic
Alfentanyl	Alfenta	IV anesthetic
Remifentanyl	Ultiva	IV anesthetic
Pentazocine	Talwin	Severe pain
Butorphanol	Stadol	Severe pain
Nalbuphine	Nubain	Moderate to severe pain
Buprenorphine	Buprenex	Moderate to severe pain

middle of the computer screen. The ART differs from the visual reactive test in that the patient responds to a "beep" instead of to the appearance of a letter on the screen.

Nuotto and Kortilla (11) also used a computer screen to assess eye-hand coordination. In this test, subjects track a randomly moving target on a computer screen with a small cross for 1 min.

The DSST is a pencil-and-paper test that relies on the patient's ability to replace symbols with numbers. In this test, subjects are required to pair digits to symbols correctly for 2 min. This test evaluates the ability of the patient to perform information-processing tasks and to concentrate.

Typically, the studies that have been performed on healthy volunteers also examine the patient's subjective feelings (16). Multiple questionnaires are used to assess the patient's ability to concentrate. The Addiction Research Center Inventory, one such test (27), is a true-false test designed to evaluate ability to concentrate. It is typically given before drug administration and at periodic intervals after administration. This test has five scales that deal with such subjective effects of medications as sedation, intellectual efficiency and energy, somatic and dysphoric effects, and euphoria.

A visual analog scale (VAS) is also used, allowing patients to qualitate how they feel (e.g., "light-headed, dizzy, spaced-out . . .") (27). This scale is a subjective measure of how subjects estimate their degree of overall performance, mental acuity (assessed as mental slowness), physical coordination (assessed as clumsiness), and body stability (assessed as dizziness). The scale ranges from "none" to "extreme." Other instruments are frequently used that assess the somatic and subjective effects of opiates from the mu class (27). Additionally, a questionnaire (Drug Effects/Liking Questionnaire) evaluates the degree to which the subject felt a drug effect (27).

Zancy (23-26) has investigated the effects of the pure mu agonist morphine on human performance. Zancy (24) administered morphine in varying amounts to his subject population (10 males and 2 females) and demonstrated a dose-response relationship between morphine dose and subjective feelings of being "dizzy," "fuzzy-headed," mentally slow, and "dreamy." There also appeared to be a dose-response relationship between opiate dose and the subjective effects of morphine. Regarding the psychomotor effects of morphine, Zancy found that subjects' performance on the tests requiring rapid speed, the DSST and the ART tests, was impaired by morphine whereas performance on the test not requiring speed, the eye-hand coordination test, was unaffected. Physiologic monitoring revealed changes in systolic and diastolic blood pressure, heart rate, and respiration.

Zancy (23) has also looked at the effect of the pure mu agonist meperidine on mood and psychomotor performance. In this investigation of 10 healthy volunteers, Zancy found that psychomotor performance (as evidenced by changes in hand-eye coordination) was impaired. Using a "drug liking" questionnaire, he observed that many of the drug's subjective effects persisted for up to 5 hr after drug administration. Interestingly, only eye-hand coordination was affected significantly. The MW test, the ART, and the DSST were all relatively unaffected.

Fentanyl has also been evaluated by Zancy (28). In a study design similar to the one just described, 13 subjects were administered increasing doses of fentanyl and thereafter administered multiple tests of cognitive and psychomotor performance. Zancy found impairment in some aspects of psychomotor performance, for example on the eye-hand coordination test. This effect was transient. Interestingly, the same subjects reported feelings of dysphoria 3 hr after fentanyl injection.

The findings of psychomotor impairment are not limited to the pure mu agonist. Various investigators have shown that mixed agonist-antagonists also elicit decrements in psychomotor performance. Butorphanol (27) and nalbuphine (24) have both been shown to decrease psychomotor performance. Interestingly, equianalgesic doses of butorphanol elicited decrements in psychomotor performance as measured by the MW test, the eye-hand coordination test, and the DSST, while morphine did not elicit these impairments. These findings led the investigators to propose that the clinically relevant dose of butorphanol produces a different profile of subjective effects and greater psychomotor impairment. In equianalgesic doses, nalbuphine has been shown to lead to similar psychomotor performance when compared with morphine. Pentazocine has also been found to induce psychomotor impairment in a dose-dependent fashion similar to that seen with morphine (26). At higher doses (i.e., 30 mg intravenously), the subjects experienced more dysphoria than observed at equianalgesic doses of morphine.

Other investigators have evaluated the effect of opioids on reaction times in a subject population that may have some degree of tolerance. That is, Banning (1) and others (15,19) have evaluated the effect of parenterally administered morphine in cancer patients. Subjects using opioids for the control of cancer pain were matched with subjects who were not using opioids for pain control. Cerebral performance was assessed using a cerebral reaction time (CRT). Headphones were applied to each subject, and the subject was then given a series of auditory stimuli. The time from stimulus to response (pressing a button with the dominant hand) was recorded. Banning et al. (1) found that CRT values were prolonged in cancer patients treated with long-term opiates. These findings are consistent with those of Sjogren et al. (15), who observed that reaction time was longer in subjects taking long-term opiates for the control of cancer pain when contrasted with healthy controls. Vainio et al. (19) studied the effect of morphine on driving ability in cancer patients. There was no statistically significant difference in psychomotor performance in cancer patients taking opiates for the control of pain versus cancer patients not taking morphine. Noteworthy, however, was a decrement in the processing of information in the morphine group when contrasted with the nonmorphine group.

The effect of morphine on exercise tolerance has been investigated by Light et al. (6, 7). In one study, morphine alone or in conjunction with promethazine or prochlorperazine was administered to patients with COPD (7). In this crossover study, Light found that exercise performance was significantly improved in the patient population receiving morphine and promethazine while mental capabilities remained unimpaired. In another investigation, Light (6) found that morphine administration had the effect of increasing the maximal work performed to exhaustion in patients with COPD. In these subjects performing aerobic work, Light et al. (6) felt that the improved exercise tolerance may be related to a higher $PaCO_2$ that resulted in lower ventilatory requirements for a given workload. The ventilatory requirement may be lower because opiates decrease hypoxic and hypercapnic responses and are associated with an increase in $PaCO_2$ at rest and at any given exercise intensity. Accordingly, if the subject has a higher $PaCO_2$, she will require a lower minute ventilation to achieve the same $\dot{V}CO_2$. The authors also hypothesized that the observed improvement in exercise capacity may be at least partially attributable to reduced perception of breathlessness for a given level of ventilation.

Woodcock et al. (22) also demonstrated increased exercise tolerance in patients with COPD who were administered dihydrocodeine. Increased exercise tolerance was accompanied by reduced feelings of "breathlessness" by the subject population. These patients also demonstrated a reduction in minute ventilation and oxygen consumption at submaximal workloads without change in spirometric volume. The mechanism behind the improvement in exercise tolerance is unclear.

Santiago et al. (14) have demonstrated that morphine administration brings about decreased resting ventilation in subjects with COPD. This reduction in ventilation is associated with an increase in exercise capacity. These findings are consistent with the findings of Woodcock (22). Additionally, Santiago found that the metabolic cost for any given level of aerobic exercise was lower in this patient population with morphine.

Conclusion

The opiates are a large group of analgesic medications that have been used for the treatment of chronic and acute pain for many years. While these medications have a demonstrated role in the treatment of pain, they are associated with a host of side effects that limit their use. These side effects include gastrointestinal, respiratory, cardiovascular, and central nervous system effects. In addition, there is a very high abuse potential.

There are very few studies on the effect of opiates on human performance. These investigations are limited to the effects of the various opiates on psychomotor performance, mood, and coordination. A compelling body of literature supports the deleterious effect of opiates on psychomotor performance. Some studies suggest that opiates improve aerobic exercise performance in patients with COPD; however this is clearly a subject population with abnormal physiology. The effect of opiates on exercise performance in the healthy subject population is unknown. Opiates may have a role in helping athletes recover from injury. These medications may provide analgesia that will allow the athlete to continue to train and thus minimize deconditioning. However, these medications may predispose the athlete to further injury by blunting or removing the sensory modality of pain.

References

1. Banning, A., P. Sjogren, and F. Kaiser. Reaction time in cancer patients receiving peripherally acting analgesics alone or in combination with opioids. Acta Anaesthesiologica Scandinavica 36: 480-482, 1992.

2. Hannington-Kiff, J.C. Measurement of recovery from outpatient general anesthesia with a simple ocular test. British Medical Journal 3: 132-135, 1970.

3. Hemmings, H.C. Cell signaling. In Foundations of Anesthesia; Basic and Clinical Sciences, 1st ed. Edited by H.C. Hemmings and P. Hopkins. Philadelphia: Mosby Publishing, pp. 21-36, 2000.

4. Jaffe, J.H., and W.R. Martin. Opiod analgesics and antagonists. In The Pharmacologic Basis of Therapeutics, 7th ed. Edited by A.G. Goodman, L.S. Goodman, T.W. Rall, and F. Murad. New York: Macmillan, pp. 491-582, 1985.

5. Lasagna, L., J.M. Felsinger, and J.K. Beecher. Drug induced mood changes in man. Journal of the American Medical Association 157: 1006-1020, 1955.

6. Light, R.W., J.R. Muro, R.I. Sato, D.W. Stansbury, C.E. Fischer, and S.E. Brown. Effects of oral morphine on breathlessness and exercise tolerance in patients with chronic obstructive pulmonary disease. American Review of Respiratory Disease 139: 126-133, 1989.

7. Light, R.W., D.W. Stansbury, and J.S. Webster. Effect of 30 mg of morphine alone or with promethazine or prochlorperazine on the exercise capacity of patients with COPD. Chest 109: 975-981, 1996.

8. Manner, T., J. Kanto, and M. Salomen. Simple devices in differentiating the effects of buprenorphine and fentanyl in healthy volunteers. European Journal of Clinical Pharmacology 31: 673-676, 1987.

9. Raj, P.R. (Ed.). Practical Management of Pain. Philadelphia: Mosby, 2000.

10. Morgan, G.E., and M.S. Mikhail. Clinical Anesthesiology, 2nd ed. New York: Appleton and Lange, pp. 128-149, 1996.

11. Nuotto, E.J., and K.T. Korttila. Evaluation of a new computerized psychomotor test battery: effects of alcohol. Pharmacology and Toxicology 68: 360-365, 1991.

12. Nuotto, E.J., K.T. Korttila, J.L. Lichtor, P.L. Ostman, and G. Rupani. Sedation and recovery of psychomotor function after intravenous administration of various doses of midazolam and diazepam. Anesthesia and Analgesia 74: 265-271, 1992.

13. Pasternak, G.W. Opioids. In Foundations of Anesthesia; Basic and Clinical Sciences, 1st ed. Edited by H.C. Hemmings and P. Hopkins. Philadelphia: Mosby, pp. 275-292, 2000.

14. Santiago, T.V., J. Johnson, D.J. Riley, and N.H. Edelman. Effects of morphine on ventilatory response to exercise. Journal of Applied Physiology 47(1): 112-118, 1979.

15. Sjoren, P., A.K. Olsen, A.B. Thomsen, and J. Dalberg. Neuropsychological performance in cancer patients: the role of oral opioids, pain and performance status. Pain 86: 237-245, 2000.

16. Smith, G.M., and H.K. Beecher. Measurement of "mental clouding" and other subjective effects of morphine. Journal of Pharmacology and Experimental Therapeutics 129: 50-62, 1959.

17. Stein, C. The control of pain in peripheral tissues by opioids. New England Journal of Medicine 332: 1685-1690, 1995.

18. Stoelting, R.K. Opioid agonists and antagonists. In Pharmacology and Physiology in Anesthetic Practice, 3rd ed. Philadelphia: Lippincott, Williams & Wilkins, 1999.

19. Vainio, V.J., Anneli, J. Ollila, E. Matikainen, P. Rosenberg, and E. Kalso. Driving ability in cancer patients receiving long-term morphine analgesia. Lancet 346: 667-670, 1995.

20. Wechler, D. The Measurement and Appraisal of Adult Intelligence. Baltimore: Williams & Wilkins, 1958.

21. Wood, M. Opioid agonists and antagonists. In Drugs and Anesthesia; Pharmacology for Anesthesiologists, 2nd ed. Edited by M. Wood and A.J.J. Wood. Philadelphia: Williams & Wilkins, pp. 129-178, 1982.

22. Woodcock, A.A., E.R. Gross, A. Gellert, S. Shah, M. Johnson, and D.M. Geddes. Effects of dihydrocodeine, alcohol, and caffeine on breathlessness and exercise tolerance in patients with chronic obstructive lung disease and normal blood gases. New England Journal of Medicine 305: 1611-1616, 1981.

23. Zancy, J.P., J.L. Lichtor, W. Binstock, D.W. Coalson, T. Cutter, D.C. Flemming, and B. Glosten. Subjective, behavioral and physiological responses to intravenous meperidine in health volunteers. Psychopharmacology 111: 306-314, 1993.

24. Zancy, J.P., K. Conley, and S. Marks. Comparing the subjective, psychomotor and physiological effects of intravenous nalbuphine and morphine in healthy volunteers. Journal of Pharmacology and Experimental Therapeutics 280(3): 1159-1169, 1997.

25. Zancy J.P., J.L. Lichtor, D. Flemming, D.W. Coalson, and W.K. Thompson. A dose-response analysis of the subjective, psychomotor and physiological effects of intravenous morphine in healthy volunteers. Journal of Pharmacology and Experimental Therapeutics 268(1): 1-9, 1994.

26. Zancy, J.P., J.L. Hill, M.L. Black, and P. Sadeghi. Comparing the subjective, psychomotor and physiological effects of intravenous pentazocine and morphine in normal volunteers. Journal of Pharmacology and Experimental Therapeutics 286(3): 1197-1998, 1998.

27. Zancy, J.P., J.R. Lichtor, P. Thapur, D.W. Coalson, D. Flemming, and W.K. Thompson. Comparing the subjective, psychomotor and physiological effects of intravenous butorphanol and morphine in healthy volunteers. Journal of Pharmacology and Experimental Therapeutics 270(2): 570-588, 1994.

28. Zancy, J.P., J.L. Lichtor, J.G. Zaragoza, and H. De Wit. Subjective and behavioral responses to intravenous fentanyl in healthy volunteers. Psychopharmacology 107: 319-326, 1992.

12

Nonsteroidal Anti-Inflammatory Drugs and Corticosteroids

Louis C. Almekinders, MD

Athletic activities can place tremendous mechanical stresses on the musculoskeletal system. Bones, joint cartilage, ligaments, muscles, and tendons all have to withstand these stresses in order for the athlete to train and compete successfully. Breakdown of this musculoskeletal system is, to some degree, inevitable during regular athletic activities. Acute injuries are, of course, obvious examples of breakdown in the musculoskeletal system. However, most of the breakdown is less obvious. Each strenuous exercise session most likely causes a mild degree of breakdown on a microscopic level (Leadbetter 1990b). Fortunately, in most instances the body is able to heal this type of microtrauma before the next exercise session is started (Leadbetter 1990b). In addition, the musculoskeletal system is able to adapt to the mechanical demands by becoming stronger and minimizing any breakdown that occurs. Not only muscle hypertrophy and increased bone density but also increased ligament strength have been well documented as normal responses (Cabaud 1980).

Any breakdown that occurs can be accompanied by pain. In addition, an inflammatory response following the breakdown is common and augments the pain and disability. Pain and swelling following acute injuries are often obvious. In chronic injuries these responses are often more subtle but can still be disabling for the athlete. One of the most commonly used pharmaceutical interventions for the pain and disability accompanying musculoskeletal problems is anti-inflammatory drugs. There are two types of anti-inflammatory medications: corticosteroids and nonsteroidal anti-inflammatory drugs or NSAIDs. These drugs have become extremely popular with athletes as well as health care professionals for acute and chronic musculoskeletal pain as well as several other pain syndromes (Metropolitan Insurance Company 1992). Corticosteroids are mainly used in chronic musculoskeletal conditions. Corticosteroids are associated with many possible adverse effects, some of which are more likely to occur in acute injuries than in chronic injuries. Therefore, corticosteroids are rarely used in acute injuries. This chapter reviews the biochemistry, pharmacology, indications, usage, and side effects of corticosteroids and NSAIDs. It focuses on their effects in the musculoskeletal system, as this represents their most common indication and it is these effects that are most widely studied.

Nonsteroidal Anti-Inflammatory Drugs

The most original form of an NSAID is acetylsalicylic acid (ASA) or aspirin, which was first synthesized and marketed by Bayer in Germany. It was quickly noted that ASA had remarkable analgesic, anti-inflammatory, and antipyretic (fever lowering) effect. Although ASA was widely used for those reasons, its exact mechanism was not known until the 1970s. In a landmark study, Sir John Vane was the first to determine that ASA was capable of inhibiting the production of prostaglandins (Vane 1971). Prostaglandins are generally considered to be mediators of the inflammatory response and as such contribute to pain, swelling, and fever in inflammatory processes. They are derived from phospholipids from the cell membrane in situations in which cell damage occurs. The cell damage can be the result of mechanical trauma, chemical irritation, or intrinsic diseases. The liberated phospholipids can be converted into arachidonic acid. Through the enzyme cyclooxygenase (COX), arachidonic acid can be metabolized into prostaglandins (figure 12.1). Prostaglandins can have numerous effects, many directly related to the inflammatory response. They contribute to vasodilatation, increased capillary permeability, and attraction of inflammatory cells and produce pain through direct effects on nerve endings (Belch 1989). The primary action of ASA and other NSAIDs is through inhibition of COX. The decreased production of prostaglandins as a result of COX inhibition results in a decrease in the inflammatory response.

Although many of the clinical effects of NSAIDs can be explained through COX inhibition, other effects have been reported. Direct effects on leukocyte and macrophage function, which also can affect the inflammatory response, appear possible (Ceuppens 1982; Wahl 1977). In addition, direct effects of NSAIDs on the central nervous system have been reported (McCormack 1991). It seems likely that NSAIDs can produce analgesia through this system without necessarily exerting a measurable anti-inflammatory effect. This could explain

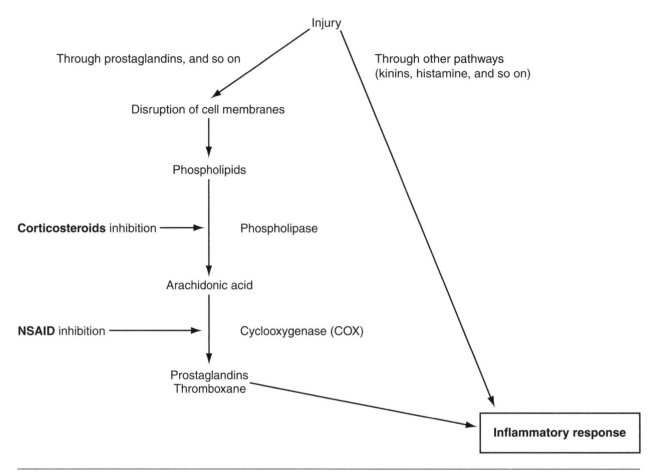

Figure 12.1 Inflammatory cascade involving prostaglandin production through complement system, kinins, histamine, and so on.

the clinical finding that low doses of NSAIDs may be sufficient to have an analgesic effect whereas higher doses are needed to obtain an anti-inflammatory effect as well. Finally, it may be important to note that other inflammatory mediators like leukotrienes, histamine, kinins, and the complement system are not inhibited by NSAIDs (figure 12.1). Therefore, the net anti-inflammatory effect of NSAIDs is still relatively small as these other substances can continue to act as pro-inflammatory mediators.

During the past 40 years, many different NSAIDs have been developed. All NSAIDs have the same basic feature of COX inhibition. The chemical structure of NSAIDs is quite diverse, although some have a comparable structure and therefore can be categorized on a chemical basis. Table 12.1 lists the currently available NSAIDs in the United States by chemical category, both generic NSAIDs and the most commonly used brand names. Most NSAIDs are weak acids and well absorbed through the gastrointestinal tract. Apart from ASA or aspirin, several NSAIDs are available as over-the-counter (OTC) medication (table 12.1). The approved OTC drugs

are not different from the original prescription drugs except that they are generally marketed in a lower dose than is used in a prescription drug.

Clinical Use of Nonsteroidal Anti-Inflammatory Drugs

Most of our knowledge regarding the effects of NSAIDs comes from studies on their use in patients rather than healthy athletes. Therefore, a brief review of their clinical use appears here. As explained in the previous section, NSAIDs are most commonly used for musculoskeletal conditions in which prostaglandin-mediated inflammation produces pain, swelling, and other symptoms. These conditions can be divided into acute and chronic conditions. Arthritis is the most common chronic condition for which NSAIDs are prescribed. The most common form of arthritis is osteoarthritis or degenerative arthritis. It is not unusual to see early osteoarthritis in competitive athletes. The condition is generally considered a wear-and-tear phenomenon. Years of use or repeated injury to a joint can lead to cartilage

Table 12.1 Commonly Used Nonsteroidal Anti-Inflammatory Drugs

Generic name (brand name)	Average daily dose
Salicylates	
Acetylsalicylic acid, i.e., aspirin	325-650 mg four times
Diflunisal (Dolobid)	500 mg twice
Salsalate (Disalcid)	1500 mg twice
Propionic acids	
Ibuprofen (Nuprin, Advil, Motrin)	200-800 mg three to four times
Naproxen (Aleve, Naprosyn, Anaprox)	220-500 mg twice
Flurbiprofen (Ansaid)	100 mg two to three times
Ketoprofen (Orudis)	50-75 mg three to four times
Oxaprozin (Daypro)	600-1200 mg once
Fenoprofen (Nalfon)	200 mg four times
Indole/indene acetic acids	
Indomethacin (Indocin)	25-50 mg four times
Sulindac (Clinoril)	200 mg twice
Etodolac (Lodine)	200-400 mg three to four times
Aryl acetic acids	
Diclofenac (Voltaren, Cataflam)	50-75 mg three to four times

degeneration and symptoms of osteoarthritis with joint pain and stiffness. Although inflammation is not a primary feature of osteoarthritis, NSAIDs still can offer pain relief in many athletes with mild to moderate osteoarthritis who continue to pursue their athletic careers. Many other chronic conditions in athletes are often treated with NSAIDs in spite of the fact that a clear inflammatory component may not always be present. Tendinitis and bursitis are frequently diagnosed as chronic painful conditions in athletes. Although their names imply the presence of an inflammatory response, many studies have shown a non-inflammatory, degenerative lesion as the primary pathology (Almekinders 1998). In addition, the efficacy of anti-inflammatory medication for these conditions is not conclusively proven (Astrom 1992). Nevertheless NSAIDs are frequently used. Other common examples of chronic and subacute conditions in athletes are headaches, fibromyalgia, menstrual pains, and flu-like symptoms. It is possible that NSAIDs are somewhat effective in these conditions merely because they have analgesic effects similar to those of acetaminophen (Tylenol) and other mild analgesics (McCormack 1991).

Acute conditions in which NSAIDs are used include most acute musculoskeletal injuries. Fractures, ligament tears or sprains, and muscle-tendon tears or strains are acute athletic injuries that clearly evoke an inflammatory response. Pain, swelling, redness, and impaired function are the classic symptoms of acute inflammation and can be found in most fractures, sprains, and strains.

Nonsteroidal anti-inflammatory drugs certainly can ameliorate the symptoms of the inflammatory response with less pain and improved function for the involved athlete. Most studies indicate that NSAIDs cannot fully abolish the inflammatory response in these acute conditions (Almekinders 1986). In addition, it is possible that a marked decrease of the inflammatory response in an acute athletic injury is not a desired effect. The inflammatory response appears to be a physiologic way for the body to clear away injured cells and tissue and initiate a regenerative, healing response. At this point it does not appear that NSAIDs can have such a dramatic anti-inflammatory effect that the healing response is markedly impaired.

Nonsteroidal anti-inflammatory drugs are routinely used as oral medication, as the absorption in the gastrointestinal tract is good. Other forms of administration are possible. Ketorolac is a NSAID that is available in an injectable form. It is mostly used for its analgesic effects rather than its anti-inflammatory effects. The injectable form allows it to be used in the postoperative period as an analgesic when the patient is unable to tolerate oral medication. Nonsteroidal anti-inflammatory drugs can also be applied in topical form. Methyl and trolamine salicylate are available in OTC preparations (e.g., Ben-Gay, Aspercreme) in the United States. These salicylate preparations have been mainly studied in arthritic conditions and were found to have similar analgesic effects when compared to oral salicylates

(Shamszad 1986). Topical nonsalicylate NSAID preparations have not been routinely available in the United States but have been used extensively in Europe. Again, in clinical studies they appear to have analgesic effects similar to those of oral agents (Moore 1998; Vanderstraeten 1990). There are no studies available that document the effects of topical agents in athletes who continue to train and compete. Anecdotally, there have been suggestions that athletes prepare their own topical drugs. Oral NSAIDs are crushed and mixed with a vehicle such as dimethyl sulfoxide (DMSO), which is well absorbed through the skin and is capable of driving medication into the deeper layers underneath the skin. No controlled studies are available that document the efficacy of this method of administration.

The commonly used dosage for each oral NSAID is listed in table 12.1. The listed higher dosage is generally considered an anti-inflammatory dose. Lower doses can still result in significant analgesic effects, but it appears that the anti-inflammatory effect significantly diminishes at the lower doses. Doses are generally not adjusted for age or gender.

Nonsteroidal Anti-Inflammatory Drug Use in Sport and Exercise

As acute and chronic musculoskeletal pain is common in athletes, NSAIDs are frequently used by athletes. They are used not only during rehabilitation for injuries and other musculoskeletal problems but also during regular training and competition. In these athletes they may be started to treat emerging and mild problems that are not severe enough to warrant interruption of training or competition. Anecdotally, there are also athletes who take NSAIDs in a prophylactic manner for anticipated pain or injuries.

Little is known about the incidence of NSAID use in athletes. Most epidemiological studies focus on older patients and the use of NSAIDs for chronic conditions such as arthritis. Millions of NSAID prescriptions are written each year (Metropolitan Insurance Company 1992). With the increased availability of OTC NSAIDs it has become more difficult to estimate the use of NSAIDs in the athletic population. From anecdotal reports, however, it seems safe to say that NSAID use is widespread among athletes.

Only a few of the effects of NSAIDs in the athletic population have been studied. One of the most often studied issues in relation to NSAID use is delayed onset muscle soreness or DOMS, a well-known phenomenon of muscle soreness that peaks approximately 48 hr after an intense bout of eccentric exercise. Eccentric exercise is characterized by lengthening contractions of the involved muscle groups. Particularly if the athlete is not accustomed to eccentric exercise, lengthening contractions evoke a mild inflammatory response within two to three days after the exercise. The athlete experiences pain, stiffness, and decreased strength in the involved muscles. Nonsteroidal anti-inflammatory drugs seem a logical choice to avoid or treat DOMS. The studies on the use of NSAIDs in DOMS have yielded conflicting results. Some have shown a mild improvement of the symptoms and/or the chemical parameters of DOMS (Dudley 1997; Lecomte 1998). Others have not been able to show significant differences over placebo treatment (Bourgeois 1999; Pizza 1999). It seems safe to assume that NSAIDs have, at best, only a small beneficial effect on DOMS. In elite athletes, however, DOMS is generally not considered to be a major problem. The soreness as a consequence of eccentric exercise has a distinct tendency to decrease or even disappear after repeated bouts of eccentric exercise. The year-round training used by many elite athletes generally keeps them accustomed to eccentric exercise, and therefore DOMS is generally not a concern for these athletes.

The majority of athletes who use NSAIDs do so to combat the pain of injuries, acute and/or chronic. Muscle activation is inhibited in the presence of pain (Herbison 1979). This phenomenon is thought to be a physiologic adaptation mechanism. The limited muscle activation results in a decreased use of the painful structure, thus protecting it from further injury. Athletes and coaches often want to override this pain inhibition in order to maintain athletic performance. As NSAIDs have analgesic properties and are allowed during athletic competition, they are a popular choice of athletes and coaches as well as sports medicine health professionals.

As discussed previously, the anti-inflammatory and analgesic effects of NSAIDs are well recognized. How much these effects can improve athletic performance is not known. There are no controlled studies available in which the performance in athletes using NSAIDs for a painful condition was compared to that with placebo treatment. If the results of the DOMS studies can be extrapolated to other painful conditions, it appears that the beneficial effect on muscle performance is small at best. However, in elite athletes even a small improvement can make a major difference during competition. In clinical studies, the analgesic effects of NSAIDs in acute and chronic athletic injuries also appear limited (Almekinders 1990, 1993, 1999). Therefore, it is unlikely that NSAID use in athletes with a painful condition will result in a significant improvement of their performance. Conversely, there is no evidence that the analgesic effect of NSAIDs will put the athlete at significant risk by abolishing the protective pain inhibition mechanism. The analgesic effect of NSAIDs does not appear strong enough to make this a realistic concern, although actual data on this issue are not available. As mentioned before, some athletes use NSAIDs in a prophylactic manner either for DOMS or for other expected aches or pains. No study is available on the effects of NSAIDs on athletic performance in otherwise asymptomatic athletes. However, there is no theoretical advantage of NSAIDs with respect to either pulmonary, cardiac, or muscular performance in normal athletes. In fact, there are some potential disadvantages to the use of NSAIDs for these athletes, as discussed in the following section.

Clinical Pharmacology

Nonsteroidal anti-inflammatory drugs are inhibitors of COX. This results in an inhibition of the conversion of arachidonic acid into prostaglandins. Besides the conversion into prostaglandins, COX also allows conversion of arachidonic acid into thromboxane. Thromboxane A2 is needed in platelet aggregation, and its inhibition has an antithrombotic effect. The elongation of the bleeding time as a result of NSAIDs is used therapeutically in patients at risk for strokes or myocardial infarction. Low-dose aspirin has traditionally been used for this purpose. Bleeding, however, can be a problem during surgery on patients who are taking NSAIDs. Aspirin binds covalently to the active site of COX. This results in an irreversible inhibition of the platelet over the lifetime of the platelet. Other NSAIDs do not bind covalently, and their effect on bleeding time is reversible when the drug is withdrawn.

Recently, it has become clear that at least two isoforms of COX exist (Seibert 1997). Cyclooxygenase-1 is the constitutive enzyme. It is present and active in several tissues, performing a normal, protective function. In the gastric mucosa COX-1 is essential in maintaining the integrity of the mucosal barrier. Cyclooxygenase inhibition makes the gastric mucosa susceptible to breakdown leading to ulceration. As will be discussed later, gastrointestinal adverse effects are among the most common problems with NSAIDs. In inflammatory disease or injury states, the isoform COX-2 is induced. The prostaglandins produced by the inducible COX-2 generally lead to symptoms. Cyclooxygenase-2 allows production of prostaglandins that regulate vasomotor responses, pain generation, inflammatory cell migration, edema production, and other pathologic reactions. Inhibition of COX-2 has been shown to result in decreased pain and less swelling. Aspirin (ASA) and the vast majority of NSAIDs are nonselective COX inhibitors. Nonselectivity indicates simultaneous COX-1 and COX-2 inhibition at the commonly used clinical dosage. Although these drugs are effective in diminishing the symptoms associated with COX-2 induction, they are also associated with adverse effects. Many adverse effects are associated with COX-1 inhibition. Recently, selective COX-2 inhibitors have become available for clinical use

(table 12.1). Use of these selective inhibitors has been shown to have significantly fewer adverse effects (Simon 1996). Their overall efficacy in treatment of both acute and chronic conditions appears similar to that of nonselective inhibitors.

Contraindications

Many of the contraindications of NSAIDs are directly related to their side effects (Gardner 1991). As mentioned before, the COX-1 inhibition in the gastric mucosa by many NSAIDs leads to decreased protection of the mucosa with the possibility of ulceration. Athletes with a known history of gastric ulcers or other gastrointestinal bleeding disorders are generally advised not to take NSAIDs. The selective COX-2 inhibitors could be considered in these athletes, as their gastrointestinal side effects are much reduced (Silverstein 2000). Patients scheduled to undergo surgery or dental procedures should also avoid NSAIDs because of their platelet inhibition. The platelet inhibition leads to an increased bleeding tendency that can be a problem under such circumstances. Some NSAIDs such as nabumetone and selective COX-2 inhibitors do not have a significant effect on platelet function and can be used preoperatively. Any athlete with a known impaired renal function also should use NSAIDs with extreme care. The renal circulation is in part maintained by locally produced prostaglandins. Inhibition of the prostaglandins can lead to worsening of the renal function. Many NSAIDs have a mild hepatotoxic effect. Prolonged NSAID use can lead to altered liver function, although major hepatotoxicity is uncommon. Checking liver function is recommended after continuous use for six to eight weeks of some NSAIDs like diclofenac (Banks 1995).

True allergy to aspirin or other NSAIDs is an absolute contraindication to the use of those or other NSAIDs. Severe allergy can manifest itself as acute respiratory distress that can be life threatening. Milder reactions include rashes and hives. Selective COX-2 inhibitors can cause the same allergic response and should be avoided in these patients as well.

Adverse Reactions

The most common adverse reactions have been described in the section on contraindications. Gastrointestinal pain and even bleeding are the most commonly feared adverse reactions with the use of NSAIDs. Epidemiological studies have suggested a high incidence of gastrointestinal reactions (Scheiman 1996). However, virtually all studies have been done in the general population with many elderly patients using NSAIDs for prolonged periods of time. It is well known from these studies that associated medical conditions significantly increase the chance of adverse reactions. This situation does not necessarily apply to the otherwise healthy athlete who uses a NSAID for a short period of time to treat a temporary pain from an injury. Although no specific studies have been done in this regard, it seems reasonable to assume that the overall incidence of adverse reactions, gastrointestinal or otherwise, is much lower in athletes. One exception can be the use of ketorolac. Ketorolac is often used for its analgesic properties rather than its anti-inflammatory effects. It has the added advantage that it is available in oral and injectable form. Although it appears to have good analgesic efficacy, it also has an increased adverse-effect profile. Gastrointestinal adverse effects are possible even with short-term use. The recommendation is not to use ketorolac for more than five consecutive days (Reinhart 2000).

Impairments of renal and hepatic function are possible adverse reactions associated with NSAID use (Rodriguez 1994; Whelon 1991). Again, these reactions are more likely to occur in patients who already have compromised kidney and liver function and use NSAIDs chronically. They are not a major concern in athletes who use NSAIDs for relatively short periods of time. One study showed that ibuprofen decreased the glomerular filtration rate of the kidney in healthy athletes, but the magnitude of change was minor (Farquhar 1999). In another study, no significant renal effects were found with NSAIDs in healthy subjects (Olsen 1999).

Exercise in itself may have adverse effects on gastrointestinal permeability, and NSAIDs can possibly worsen this (Brouns 1993). Increased permeability could result in loss of body fluids and dehydration. This could affect performance particularly for endurance athletes. Controlled studies have suggested that a mild increase in permeability can occur with selected NSAIDs (Ryan 1996; Smetanka 1999). It does not appear to be a dramatic adverse reaction, but NSAIDs should be used with some caution before and during competitive endurance events.

A rebound effect or noticeable worsening of the pain and inflammation after the NSAIDs are stopped has not been reported. This rebound effect seems possible after corticosteroid use but does not appear to be a problem with NSAIDs. It is possible that NSAIDs are not potent enough in their anti-inflammatory action to make a rebound effect noticeable.

Overdosage

Overdosage of NSAIDs is a relatively rare problem. Some of the reported problems with overdosage have been related to the adverse effects on the gastrointestinal system such as bleeding and ulceration (Smolinske 1990). Neurologic symptoms such as drowsiness or coma can result from an overdosage. Convulsions are rare but can occur with all NSAIDs. Finally, a metabolic acidosis can result, as most NSAIDs are weak acids.

Regulations

Nonsteroidal anti-inflammatory drugs are available as OTC drugs as well as through prescription. Their use is permitted by the governing bodies in collegiate, professional, and international competition. Neither the National Collegiate Athletic Association (NCAA) nor the U.S. Olympic Committee (USOC) limits the use of NSAIDs in athletes.

Corticosteroids

Corticosteroids are drugs with a basic sterol structure similar to that of cortisol. Cortisol is a hormone produced in the adrenal glands. It has numerous effects but is mainly considered a stress hormone. Cortisol is released during periods of psychological and/or physical stress. Among its most important effects are the elevation of blood sugar by mobilization of energy stores, anti-inflammatory effects though stabilization of cell membranes, and direct inhibitory effects on inflammatory cells. Originally corticosteroids were extracted and purified from live sources. However, the currently used corticosteroids are synthesized in laboratories and have potency that can vastly exceed that of cortisol. Some of the most commonly used synthetic corticosteroids are listed in table 12.2. The anti-inflammatory effect of corticosteroids is one of the main reasons for their use in sports medicine. This effect is thought to relate to the inhibition of phospholipid breakdown during and after cell injury. The cell membrane largely consists of phospholipids. These can be converted into arachidonic acid and subsequently into numerous inflammatory mediators (see figure 12.1). Corticosteroids appear capable of inhibiting this response. In addition there can be direct inhibitory effects on inflammatory cells. The overall anti-inflammatory effects can be dramatic and generally much more pronounced than with the use of NSAIDs. Although this can be associated with beneficial effects such as decreased pain and swelling, it also means an increased chance of certain adverse reactions, as discussed in a later section.

Corticosteroids can be administered in various ways. Oral administration is common when corticosteroids are used for a generalized problem or disease. Examples of oral use for systemic problems or diseases are the use of corticosteroids as an anti-inflammatory drug for severe rheumatoid arthritis, as an anti-rejection drug following organ transplantation, and as an anti-allergy drug for a systemic allergic reaction. Although effective, oral administration of corticosteroids also carries the risks of systemic adverse effects. These adverse effects can be significant, as will be discussed later. To avoid systemic adverse effects, corticosteroids are often administered locally. Local injection is a commonly used method in

Table 12.2 Commonly Used Injectable, Synthetic Corticosteroid Preparations

Generic name (brand name)	Recommended dose per injection
Triamcinolone acetonide (Aristocort)	5-40 mg
Triamcinolone hexacetonide (Aristospan)	2-20 mg
Betamethasone acetate (Celestone Soluspan)	2-6 mg
Methylprednisolon acetate (Depo-Medrol)	10-80 mg
Dexamethasone acetate (Decadron)	4-16 mg

isolated musculoskeletal problems. Corticosteroids can be injected in joints, around tendons and ligaments, and in bursae. The agent will exert its strong anti-inflammatory effect with relatively few systemic adverse effects (Leadbetter 1990a). The steroids are usually contained within a suspension that is active locally and is only slowly absorbed in the systemic circulation. Finally, corticosteroids can be administered topically. The topical use is almost exclusively for dermatological and ophthalmological purposes. Rashes, pruritus, and local allergic reaction of the skin and eyes can be treated in this manner. Over-the-counter corticosteroid creams are available for dermatologic use, and stronger preparations can be obtained as prescription drugs. Eye drops containing corticosteroids are available only through prescriptions.

The dosage of corticosteroids is largely dependent on the type of corticosteroid to be used, the severity of the problem, and the size of the area to be treated. Synthetic corticosteroids have varying degrees of anti-inflammatory potency and can be ranked in this regard. The dosage is directly related to this potency. For severe problems, high doses may have to be used initially that can be gradually tapered as the problems resolve or respond. The dosage for local injection is largely dependent on the size of the joint or tendon to be injected. Examples of commonly used dosages are given in table 12.2.

Use in Sport and Exercise

There are no studies available that determine the prevalence of corticosteroid use in athletes. Use of corticosteroids appears largely restricted to the treatment of chronic painful musculoskeletal injuries in athletes (Cox 1984). Common examples include tendinitis, bursitis, and arthritis. Tennis elbow, rotator cuff, and Achilles tendon problems are among the most frequent

musculoskeletal problems treated with corticosteroids if NSAIDs have not been successful (Stanley 1998). If corticosteroids are used for these conditions, many health professionals prefer local administration through injection in and around the affected structure and avoid the systemic adverse effects of oral corticosteroids (Stanley 1998). The anti-inflammatory and cell membrane-stabilizing effects of corticosteroids can result in a marked and rapid improvement of the symptoms associated with some of these conditions (Fredberg 1997). However, as will be discussed in the following section, corticosteroids can actually adversely affect the healing process. This means that these athletes will often feel markedly improved following an injection while healing of their problem is actually retarded or even halted. This places the athlete at potential risk of additional injury to this area as the pain feedback mechanism is lost and the athlete is unable to discern additional injury (Ljungqvist 1968). Dramatic additional injury such as complete tendon rupture is a potential risk. For example, the possibility of Achilles tendon rupture following steroid injection for Achilles tendinitis is frequently mentioned in the sports medicine literature (Ljungqvist 1968). The majority of data on the negative effects on musculoskeletal tissues come from animal studies (Kennedy 1976). No human studies are available that allow us to determine the exact risk of steroid injections in athletes. In an attempt to avoid these types of additional injuries, athletes should be counseled regarding this problem and probably be kept out of competition and vigorous training for at least several weeks following local administration of the corticosteroids (Fredberg 1997).

Limited data are available on the direct effect of corticosteroids on athletic performance in healthy athletes. A study by Soetens (1995) showed no significant effect on exercise performance with the use of adrenocorticotropic hormone or ACTH. Adrenocorticotropic hormone stimulates the adrenal glands to release increased amounts of cortisol. The increased circulating levels of cortisol could theoretically enhance performance as energy stores are mobilized and blood sugar levels are elevated. However, many other negative effects of corticosteroids can probably negate this possible positive effect. Several studies have investigated exercise tolerance in patients with systemic illnesses requiring the systemic use of corticosteroids (Danneskiold-Samsoe 1986; Lampert 1996; Renlund 1996). In these studies it is difficult to separate the effects of the disease and the corticosteroids. The data suggest that both beneficial and negative effects can be seen. The beneficial effects are largely derived from the treatment effects of the corticosteroids. For instance, as corticosteroids improve the symptoms of the arthritis or asthma, exercise tolerance improves. Similarly, it seems reasonable to assume that treatment of a painful condition with corticosteroid in a healthy athlete can improve the individual's performance as a direct result of the decrease in symptoms. Negative effects may be related to effects of corticosteroids on muscle tissue. It has been long known that myopathy is one of the adverse effects of chronic systemic corticosteroid use. This can adversely affect athletic performance. It seems unlikely that this a major concern when steroids are used locally through injection or topical preparation.

Several studies have addressed the effect of corticosteroids on exercise-induced leukocyte and lymphocyte changes (Ratge 1988; Singh 1996). Normally, strenuous exercise can affect the number and type of circulating inflammatory cells. Although corticosteroids have pronounced effects on the immune system, the studies indicate that corticosteroids have no significant effect on these exercise-induced changes.

Little is known about the psychological effects of corticosteroids in healthy athletes, since most studies involve the effects of steroids in patients with illnesses (Milgrom 1993). Patients with systemic illnesses requiring oral corticosteroid treatment can be subject to psychological changes, which can range from euphoria to frank hallucinations. Steroid psychosis is a well-described complication of systemic steroid use. It can take the form of a severe mental illness, but usually resolves once the steroids are withdrawn. Short-term or local corticosteroid use has not been associated with this adverse effect.

Clinical Pharmacology

As mentioned earlier, corticosteroids have strong anti-inflammatory effects. A part of the anti-inflammatory effect is related to the inhibition of the enzyme phospholipase. Phospholipase promotes the production of precursors for inflammatory mediators from cell membrane phospholipids. In addition, corticosteroids have direct inhibitory effects on inflammatory cells. This combined action results in the strong anti-inflammatory effects of corticosteroids. Many systemic problems and illnesses are mediated through the immune system. Allergies, many forms of inflammatory arthritis, the rejection of transplanted organs, and inflammatory bowel disease are all examples of inflammatory cell reaction mediated through the immune system. Corticosteroids are used in many of these patients, often with marked improvement of their symptoms. The inflammation of arthritic joints subsides, organ rejection reaction dissipates, and allergic reactions such as asthma and skin changes are controlled with corticosteroids. Similarly, local effects on tendinitis and bursitis include disappearance of the pain and swelling. Corticosteroids can also produce these effects in acute injuries like muscle strains and ligament sprains. However, in an animal model, corticosteroids clearly had negative effects on the healing of an acute muscle injury (Beiner 1999). Initially, the corticosteroid-treated muscles had less inflammation, but later in the postinjury period the muscles showed evidence of poor healing of the injured segment. Because of the marked adverse effects in acute injuries, corticosteroids are not recommended for acute sprains and strains.

Contraindications

There are several conditions in which corticosteroids are contraindicated (Truhan 1989). Active infection as well as dormant infection is a clear contraindication for corticosteroid use. Corticosteroids have a strong inhibitory effect on the immune system. In the presence of an infection, either bacterial or viral, the body may be unable to fight the infection as a result of corticosteroid use. Lethal infections with concurrent corticosteroid use have been reported even from bacteria or viruses that are normally not lethal (Ahmed 1982).

The presence of diabetes mellitus is a relative contraindication for the use of corticosteroids (Bialas 1998). Corticosteroids elevate blood sugar level and as such increase insulin requirements. Blood sugars should be monitored carefully if corticosteroids are used in people with diabetes.

Adverse Reactions

Unlike the anabolic steroids, corticosteroids can be considered to act as a catabolic hormone. The adverse reactions associated with systemically administered corticosteroids are numerous and can be profound (Gray 1986). As mentioned before, they have a distinct effect on the glucose metabolism. Energy stores are mobilized. Corticosteroids elevate blood glucose levels and in fact counteract the effects of insulin. Development of diabetes mellitus is possible with chronic corticosteroid use, and existing diabetes can be markedly worsened by corticosteroid use (Bialas 1998). Corticosteroids are therefore also often designated as glucocorticoids. As part of the disturbance of the energy metabolism, corticosteroids tend to mobilize and redistribute fat stores. The typical pattern is a disappearance of the subcutaneous fat stores in the extremities and redistribution to the torso and face. The "buffalo hump" and "moon face" are characteristic findings in patients who use systemic steroids chronically.

Some corticosteroids have a structure and effects similar to those of the hormone aldosterone. Aldosterone also has a sterol structure and has direct effects on the kidney, resulting in fluid and sodium retention. Steroids with aldosterone-like effects are generally designated mineralocorticoids. Most clinically used anti-inflammatory corticosteroids have minimal mineralo-corticoid action, but some fluid retention is possible (Truhan 1989).

The exogenous administration of systemic corticosteroids also suppresses the normal production of cortisol by the adrenal glands. If increased cortisol levels are needed, the chronically suppressed adrenal glands may not be able to respond. Cortisol is generally considered a stress hormone. During periods of physical or emotional stress the adrenal glands normally produce increased amounts of cortisol. The resultant increased level of blood glucose and mobilization of fat stores are physiologic effects that allow the body to respond to the stress. After chronic systemic corticosteroid use, the adrenal glands may be irreversibly suppressed, resulting in an inability to deal with the stress. This is generally described as an Addisonian crisis and can be occasionally seen in patients undergoing major surgery while using corticosteroids chronically for their disease (Truhan 1989). Additional corticosteroid administration is often recommended to avoid an Addisonian crisis.

Corticosteroids can disturb bone metabolism. Bone production is inhibited, and chronic corticosteroid use can lead to pronounced osteoporosis (Bialas 1998). Pathologic fractures of the hip, spine, and wrist are typically the result of steroid-induced osteoporosis.

Local injection or topical use of corticosteroids generally avoids the adverse reactions just outlined. However, even local use produces adverse reactions that should be recognized and that are probably more common in athletes, as they are more likely candidates for local use. Locally, corticosteroids can cause significant atrophy of the tissues. This can occur at several levels. Most superficially, corticosteroids can thin the skin and eliminate the subcutaneous fat. The resulting skin can look like cigarette paper and has poor healing properties. These changes are seen after topical use as well as after injection directly under the skin. In addition, the corticosteroids can cause depigmentation of the skin, which is often permanent. Combined with the atrophy this can leave a cosmetically very unappealing skin lesion, particularly in dark-skinned individuals or in facial areas. These chronic skin changes also are a concern if trauma or surgery causes skin disruption in the area. Poor healing and increased infection rates have been reported in areas of steroid use (Howes 1950).

Deeper tissues are similarly affected. Atrophy of tendons and ligaments has been described in animal models (Kennedy 1976) as well as human specimens (Ferretti 1983). As mentioned before, this effect has led to a concern of catastrophic rupture during athletic activities. Tendons and ligamentous structure appear to be able to recover mechanically from this effect after some time. Therefore, a period of restricted athletic activity is generally recommended following local administration of corticosteroids around ligaments or tendons. In addition, most authors recommend that the steroid preparation be injected around the tendon or ligament and not in its substance. Animal research has suggested that intratendinous or intraligamentous injection is more harmful (Kennedy 1976).

Overdosage

No studies are available that document the effects of corticosteroid overdosage.

Regulations

Corticosteroids are available for topical use as both OTC and prescription preparations. Oral corticosteroids are available by prescription only. As they have no proven performance-enhancing or anabolic effects like the androgenic steroids, they are permitted under certain conditions by the governing bodies. The NCAA places no restrictions on the use of corticosteroids at all. The USOC has a different policy. It bans intravenous, intramuscular, rectal, and oral use but allows topical use for skin, eye, and ear problems. However, with prior written permission from the USOC, the USOC will allow inhaled corticosteroids for respiratory problems like asthma and local, intra-articular use for musculoskeletal problems. There are no reported adverse effects of corticosteroids use on testosterone test results when one is judging anabolic steroid abuse.

References

Ahmed AR, Moy R. Death in pemphigus. J Am Acad Derm 7: 221-228, 1982.

Almekinders, LC. Anti-inflammatory treatment of muscular injuries in sports. An update on recent studies. Sports Med 28: 383-388, 1999.

Almekinders, LC. Etiology, diagnosis and treatment of tendonitis: an analysis of the literature. Med Sci Sports Exerc 30: 1183-1190, 1998.

Almekinders, LC. Anti-inflammatory treatment of muscular injuries in sports. Sports Med 15: 139-145, 1993.

Almekinders, LC. The efficacy of nonsteroidal anti-inflammatory drugs in the treatment of ligament injuries. Sports Med 9: 137-142, 1990.

Almekinders LC, Gilbert JA. Healing of experimental muscle strains and the effects of nonsteroidal antiinflammatory medication. Am J Sports Med 14: 303-308, 1986.

Astrom M, Westlin N. No effect of piroxicam on Achilles tendinopathy: a randomized study of 70 patients. Acta Orthop Scand 63: 631-634, 1992.

Banks AT, Zimmerman HJ, Ishak KG, Harter JG. Diclofenac-associated hepatotoxicity: analysis of 180 cases reported to the Food and Drug Administration as adverse reactions. Hepatology 22: 820-827, 1995.

Bialas MC, Routledge PA. Adverse effects of corticosteroids. Adv Drug React Toxic Rev 17: 227-235, 1998.

Beiner JM, Jokl P, Cholewicki J, Panjabi MM. The effect of anabolic steroids and corticosteroids on the healing of a muscle injury. Am J Sports Med 27: 2-9, 1999.

Belch JJF. Eicosanoids and rheumatology: inflammatory and vascular aspects. Prostag Leukotr Ess Fatty Acids 36: 219-234, 1989.

Bourgeois J, MacDougall D, MacDonald J, Tarnopolsky M. Naproxen does not alter indices of muscle damage in resistance-exercise trained men. Med Sci Sports Exerc 31: 4-9, 1999.

Brouns F, Beckers E. Is the gut an athletic organ? Digestion, absorption and exercise. Sports Med 15: 242-257, 1993.

Cabaud HE, Chatty A, Gildengorin V, Feltman RY. Exercise effects on the strength of the anterior cruciate ligament. Am J Sports Med 8: 79-86, 1980.

Ceuppens JL, Rodriguez MA, Godwin JS. Non-steroidal anti-inflammatory agents inhibit synthesis of IgM rheumatoid factor in vitro. Lancet 1 (8271): 528-531, 1982.

Cox JS. Current concepts in the role of steroids in the treatment of sprains and strains. Med Sci Sports Exerc 16: 216-218, 1984.

Danneskiold-Samsoe B, Grimby G. The relationship between the leg muscle strength and physical capacity in patients with rheumatoid arthritis, with reference to the influence of corticosteroids. Clin Rheumat 5: 468-474, 1986.

Dudley GA, Czerkawski J, Meinrod A, Gillis G, Baldwin A, Scarpone M. Efficacy of naproxen sodium for exercise-induced dysfunction muscle injury and soreness. Clin J Sports Med 7: 3-10, 1997.

Farquhar WB, Morgan AL, Zambraski EJ, Kenney WL. Effects of acetaminophen and ibuprofen on renal function in the stressed kidney. J Appl Phys 86: 598-604, 1999.

Ferretti A, Ippolito E, Mariani P, Puddu G. Jumper's knee. Am J Sports Med 11: 58-62, 1983.

Fredberg U. Local corticosteroid injection in sport: review of the literature and guidelines for treatment. Scand J Med Sci Sports 7: 131-139, 1997.

Gardner GC, Simkin PA. Adverse effects of NSAID's. Pharmacy Therap 16: 750-754, 1991.

Gray ES, Doherty SM, Galloway EA. Oral glucocorticoids and their complications. J Am Acad Dermatol 14: 61-177, 1986.

Herbison GJ, Jaweed MM, Ditunno JF. Muscle atrophy in rats following denervation, casting, inflammation and tenotomy. Arch Phys Med Rehabil 60: 401-404, 1979.

Howes EL, Plotz CM, Blunt JW, Ragan C. Retardation of wound healing by cortisone. Surgery 28: 177-181, 1950.

Kennedy JC, Willis RB. The effects of local steroid injections on tendons: a biomechanical and microscopic correlative study. Am J Sports Med 4: 11-21, 1976.

Lampert E, Mettauer B, Hoppeler H, Charloux A, Charpentier A, Lonsdorfer J. Structure of skeletal muscle in heart transplant patients. J Am Coll Card 28: 980-984, 1996.

Leadbetter WB. Corticosteroid injection therapy in sports injuries. In: Sports-induced inflammation. Leadbetter WB, Buckwalter JA, Gordon SL (eds). Am Acad Orthop Surgeons, Park Ridge IL, 527-545, 1990a.

Leadbetter WB. An introduction in sports-induced soft tissue inflammation. In: Sports-induced inflammation. Leadbetter WB, Buckwalter JA, Gordon SL (eds). Am Acad Orthop Surgeons, Park Ridge IL, 3-23, 1990b.

Lecomte JM, Lacroix VJ, Montgomery DL. A randomized controlled trial of the effect of naproxen on delayed onset muscle soreness and muscle strength. Clin J Sports Med 8: 82-87, 1998.

Ljungqvist R. Subcutaneous partial rupture of the Achilles tendon. Acta Orthop Scand 113S: 1-86, 1968.

McCormack K, Brune K. Dissociation between antinociceptive and anti-inflammatory effects of non-steroidal anti-inflammatory drugs: a survey of their analgesic efficacy. Drugs 41: 533-547, 1991.

Metropolitan Insurance Company. Anti-arthritic medication usage: United States, 1991. Stat Bull Metropol Insur Co 73: 25-34, 1992.

Milgrom H, Bender BG. Psychologic side effects of therapy with corticosteroids. Am Rev Respir Dis 147: 471-473, 1993.

Moore RA, Tramer MR, Carroll D. Quantitative systematic review of topically applied non-steroidal anti-inflammatory drugs. Br Med J 316: 333-338, 1998.

Olsen NV, Jensen NG, Hansen JM, Christensen NJ, Fogh-Andersen N, Kanstrup IL. Non-steroidal anti-inflammatory drugs and the renal response to exercise: a comparison of indomethacin and nabumetone. Clin Sci 97: 457-465, 1999.

Pizza FX, Cavender D, Stockard A, Baylies H, Beighle A. Anti-inflammatory doses of ibuprofen: effect on neutrophils and exercise-induced muscle injury. Int J Sports Med 20: 98-102, 1999.

Ratge D, Wiedemann A, Kohse KP, Wisser H. Alterations in beta-adrenoceptors on human leucocyte subsets induced by dynamic exercise: effect of prednisone. Clin Exp Pharm Phys 15: 43-53, 1988.

Reinhart DI. Minimising the adverse effects of ketorolac. Drug Safety 22: 487-497, 2000.

Renlund DG, Taylor DO, Ensley RD, O'Connell JB, Gilbert EM, Bristow MR, Ma H, Yanowitz FG. Exercise capacity after heart transplantation: influence of donor and recipient characteristics. J Heart Lung Transpl 15: 16-24, 1996.

Rodriguez LAG, William R, Derby LE. Acute liver injury associated with nonsteroidal antiinflammatory drugs and the role of risk factors. Arch Intern Med 154: 311-316, 1994.

Ryan AJ, Chang RT, Gisolfi CV. Gastrointestinal permeability following aspirin intake and prolonged running. Med Sci Sports Exerc 28: 698-705, 1996.

Scheiman JM. NSAIDS: gastrointestinal injury and cytoprotection. Gastrenterol Clin Am 25: 279-298, 1996.

Seibert K, Zhang Y, Leahy K, Hauser S, Masferrer J, Isakson P. Distribution of COX-1 and COX-2 in normal and inflamed tissues. Adv Exper Med Biol 400A: 167-170, 1997.

Shamszad M, Perkal M, Golden EL. Two double-blind comparisons of a topically applied salicylate cream and orally ingested aspirin in the relief of chronic musculoskeletal pain. Curr Therap Res 39: 470-479, 1986.

Silverstein FE, Faich G, Goldstein JL, Simon LS, Pincus T, Whelton A, Makuch R, Eisen G, Agrawal NM, Stenson WF, Burr A, Zhao WW, Kent J, Lefkowith JB, Verburg KM, Geis GS. Gastrointestinal toxicity with celecoxib vs nonsteroidal anti-inflammatory drugs for osteoarthritis and rheumatoid arthritis: a randomized controlled trial. JAMA 284: 1247-1255, 2000.

Simon LS. Nonsteroidal anti-inflammatory drugs and their effects: the importance of COX selectivity. J Clin Rheumat 2: 135-140, 1996.

Singh A, Zelazowska EB, Petrides JS, Raybourne RB, Sternberg EM, Gold PW, Deuster PA. Lymphocyte subset responses to exercise and glucocorticoid suppression in healthy men. Med Sci Sports Exerc 28: 822-828, 1996.

Smetanka RD, Lambert GP, Murray R, Eddy D, Horn M, Gisolfi CV. Intestinal permeability in runners in the 1996 Chicago marathon. Int J Sport Nutr 9: 426-433, 1999.

Smolinske SC, Hall AH, Vandenberg SA, Spoerke DG, McBride PV. Toxic effects of nonsteroidal anti-inflammatory drugs in overdose. Drug Safety 5: 252-274, 1990.

Soetens E, Demeirleir K, Hueting JE. No influence of ACTH on maximal performance. Psychopharmacology 118: 260-266, 1995.

Stanley KL, Weaver JE. The pharmacologic management of pain and inflammation in athletes. Clin Sports Med 17: 375-392, 1998.

Truhan AP, Ahmed AR. Corticosteroids: a review with emphasis on complications of prolonged systemic therapy. Ann Allergy 62: 375-391, 1989.

Vanderstraeten G, Schuermans P. Study on the effects of etofenamate 10% cream in comparison with an oral NSAID in strains and sprains due to sports injuries. Acta Belg Med Phys 13: 139-141, 1990.

Vane JR. Inhibition of prostaglandin synthesis as a mechanism of action of aspirin-like drugs. Nature New Biol 231: 232-235, 1971.

Wahl LM, Olsen CE, Sandberg LE, Margen Ragen SE. Prostaglandin regulation of macrophage collagenase production. Proc Nat Acad Sci 74: 4955-4958, 1977.

Whelon A, Hamilton CW. Nonsteroidal antiinflammatory drugs: effects on kidney function. J Clin Pharmacol 31: 588-598, 1991.

CHAPTER 13

Hypnotics, Anxiolytics, and Neuroleptics

Michel Bourin, MD, PharmD

Danièle Bentué-Ferrer, PhD

Hervé Allain, MD

Pierre Rochcongar, MD

The goal of this chapter is to review the impact of the various psychotropic drugs on performance in sport and exercise. Theoretically, an athlete or sport amateur is no different from a qualified healthy volunteer or a patient taking a psychotropic agent; so, for the drugs we discuss here, our objective could be limited to establishing the list of the main adverse effects reported from clinical trials (development phase in healthy volunteers or in patients) or recorded in drug monitoring and pharmacoepidemiological data (Kaufman and Shapiro, 2000). Nevertheless, it is intuitively impelling to look at the sport population as a specific subpopulation—like infants, women, or elderly persons—in which targeted studies would be useful. We can identify six elements that specifically distinguish the sport population: (1) the prerequisite for "zero" physical and psychic risk; (2) the temptation to use psychotropic drugs to enhance performance, with the inherent risk of misuse and doping; (3) demand for the use of drugs to correct for states or symptoms induced by training, the preparation phase before competition, or the competition itself (e.g., "performance" anxiety; stress; reactional or sport-induced insomnia, fatigue, or sagging motivation; clinically evidenced overtraining expressed by a declining performance level despite intense training [Kentta and Hassmen, 1998]); (4) the necessary reevaluation of size-effect data from healthy volunteers— that is, a deleterious effect that may be considered irrelevant for therapeutic applications (minimal reduction in psychomotor reaction time) could have a catastrophic consequence for the competitive athlete since the principal evaluation criterion (the term used in human pharmacology!) is measured in thousandths of seconds; (5) the evidence that even an athlete can develop signs or symptoms of a psychiatric disorder requiring the prescription of psychotropic drugs, given that all psychiatric disorders are associated with altered performance and cerebral function (most specifically memory, cognitive and executive performance); and (6) the frequent exposure to jet lag (international championships) with the subsequent disruption of circadian cycles and the necessary adaptation to different climates (Shephard, 1999).

These few preliminary remarks announce a series of difficulties resulting from the fact that drug development and new drug approval (NDA) procedures applied in the pharmaceutical industry are largely designed around therapeutic management of clearly identified signs and symptoms (for psychotropic drugs, see the list of psychiatric disorders in the *Diagnostic Statistical Manual* [DSM-V]). Drug development (from screening to NDA) has to comply with ethical and regulatory standards, generally harmonized on an international level (International Conference of Harmonization), that do not require preapproval studies in athletes. The summaries presented in drug reference lists used in various countries (e.g., *Physician's Desk Reference, Dictionnaire Vidal, Rote Buch*) do not mention the use of psychotropic drugs in sport and exercise, and there is no item for "athlete" or "sport activity" in drug monitoring databases. Moreover, very few studies include sport activity among inclusion criteria (see later). This situation is a classic one in clinical pharmacology in which decision making, by the prescriber and user alike, is based more on irrational belief than on evidence-based medicine, with the consequent risks of over- or underdosing, inappropriate timing, misuse, and so on. At the same time, intensified anti-doping programs have encountered complex situations because certain disease states can mimic the undesirable effects of psychotropic drugs (in their instructive work reported in 1997, Dawson and Reid demonstrated that sleep deprivation induces the same psychomotor consequences as alcohol intake!).

Pharmacologists have responded scientifically, focusing their rigorously prepared reports on phase I and II trials in healthy young adults in full compliance with good clinical practices. The final output from these neuropsychopharmacology studies in humans, based on quantified electroencephalography and computer-assisted psychometrics, provides a comparative description of the precise impact of psychotropic drugs on cognition and psychomotor functions (cognitive mapping). This new dimension in pharmacology has been applied to several drugs in the development phase (monoamine oxidase A inhibitors, anti-anxiety drugs, antipsychotic drugs), constantly relying on the same tests (see Patat, 1998 and 2000 for review). The potential for addiction can also be explored with these same methods (e.g., our study on the anti-appetite effect of mefenorex compared with amphetamine and placebo; Patat et al., 1996). Our selection among the abundant literature was therefore guided by a search for descriptions of the effects of psychotropic drugs on physical, cognitive, and psychic performance in sport and exercise. But it is most noteworthy that certain other functions, for example, motivation, desire to win, and decision making, remain to be studied; some remarks could be applied to unexplored symptomatology such as fatigue (Allain et al., 1999) or procedural and skill memories (Thomas et al., 1996), which a priori are important factors contributing to athletes' performances.

Sedatives

Hypnotic agents, or "sleeping pills," are used to induce sleep, prolong its duration, and reduce the number of nocturnal awakenings. The ideal hypnotic would not modify the physiological architecture of sleep, would not produce residual effects after awakening, would have no addictive effect, and would not induce sleep rebound after interruption (Bonin and François, 1995). Most sedatives, like most anti-anxiety agents, are benzodiazepines, or, in the case of the two most commonly prescribed agents—zolpidem and zopiclone—belong to two other drug families, the imidazopyridines and cyclopyrrolones.

Stress caused by overexertion, an upcoming competition, or change in environment can provoke insomnia the night or nights preceding the event (Gremion et al., 1992). In addition, the effects of jet lag may contribute to impaired sleep when the event occurs in a geographically distant location (French, 1995). Many studies have demonstrated that even partial loss of sleep can hinder performance, particularly if the sport activity requires high-performance psychomotricity. Mougin et al. (1991, 1992) investigated this question in high-level athletes, assessing the consequences of perturbed sleep on physiological adaptation of the body to exercise. The authors demonstrated a modification of the ventilatory and metabolic capacity of athletes the day after a poor night's sleep. A sedative drug may be indicated in such cases. It is essential, however, to carefully evaluate the risk/benefit ratio to ensure that the drug has no negative impact on sport performance the next day. In other words, a daytime hangover effect following hypnotic administration must not cancel any performance

improvements that may result from improved nocturnal sleep (Roth et al., 1980).

Hypnotic Drugs

Hypnotic drugs constitute a pharmacological class of compounds that aim at restoring a normal sleep in insomniac patients. This chapter deals with a richness of products, from plant products to the more recent chemical products. Only the most recent drugs have been extensively studied as far as cognition and psychomotor performance are concerned. The use of hypnotic drugs implies a sound knowledge of sleep disorders and of the basis in pharmacology.

Benzodiazepine Hypnotics

All drugs belonging to the benzodiazepine family have common anticonvulsant, sedative, myorelaxing, and anxiolytic properties. They also have the same mechanism of action, a modification of GABAergic neurotransmission. Gamma-aminobutyric acid (GABA) is the major inhibitory neurotransmitter in the central nervous system (CNS). It interacts with three types of receptors on neuronal membranes, called A, B, and C receptors. The GABAA receptor is an heteroligomeric receptor whose subunits form an anionic, chloride-selective channel. It is coupled to calcium or potassium ion channels via Guanosine-5-triphosphate-binding protein. The binding of GABA regulates GABAA receptor gating of the chloride ion channel, allowing passage of chloride down the neuron electrochemical gradient, resulting in membrane hyperpolarization. Benzodiazepines bind to the GABAA receptor macromolecular complex (the α-subunit). Binding causes an allosteric modulation of GABA linkage to its receptor, increasing chloride flow by increasing the frequency of channel opening; benzodiazepines thus potentate the effects of GABA throughout the CNS. The GABAA receptor is also the target of other interesting compounds (barbiturates, certain anesthetics, alcohol, anticonvulsants, and certain steroid metabolites) (Bentué-Ferrer et al., 1996; Hobbs et al., 1998; Chebib and Johnston, 1999; Doble, 1999; Kardos, 1999; Mehta and Ticku, 1999; Bormann, 2000).

Benzodiazepines administered for their anti-anxiety or hypnotic effect have specific pharmacokinetic properties. In particular, their rapid resorption is a key factor for classification, the sedative effect being related to the time required to reach peak plasma concentration. The rate of elimination is also an important factor, since a short half-life would reduce the risk of accumulating residual effects and, inversely, increase the risk of undesirable nocturnal awakenings. The distinction between anti-anxiety and hypnotic benzodiazepines is not, however, clear-cut because of the dose-effect relationship and the variability resulting from the intrinsic activity of each compound. All these compounds are metabolized in the liver. Active metabolites and their respective half-lives must also be taken into consideration.

Sleep is an active, circadian, physiological depression of consciousness. It is characterized by cyclical electroencephalographic (EEG) and eye movement changes, measures of which are used to describe sleep stages that are correlated with the fundamental physiological changes in the main central neurotransmitters. Normal sleep is of two kinds: NREM (nonrapid eye movement) orthodox, forebrain, or slow-wave EEG sleep, and REM (rapid eye movement) paradoxical, hindbrain, or fast EEG sleep. A normal night begins with a sleep latency period; an initial NREM sleep is followed by about 20 min of REM sleep, after which cycles of NREM sleep abruptly alternate with REM sleep for the rest of the night. This architecture (stages I to IV and paradoxical sleep), best observed and analyzed by polysomnography, may be modified by CNS diseases, environmental factors (i.e., light), or jet lag. Sleep disorders are classified according to an international classification and frequently require pharmacological intervention (Hajak, 2000), notably because of the diurnal consequences of insomnia.

Benzodiazepines modify the architecture of sleep and do not induce physiological sleep. Phase II sleep lasts longer, accounting for the supplementary duration of sleep induced by administration of a hypnotic benzodiazepine. Benzodiazepines also reduce the duration of deep, slow sleep, especially phase IV, and paradoxical sleep (Ashton, 1994). The principal hypnotic benzodiazepines and a few of their characteristics are listed in table 13.1.

The most commonly described adverse effects include morning hangover, decreased wakefulness, muscle hypotonia, anterograde amnesia, reduced libido, and paradoxical psychiatric reactions.

Non-Benzodiazepinic Hypnotics

Currently available barbiturates no longer satisfy the criteria of a good hypnotic and should be used only in exceptional circumstances. Drugs belonging to other families can be proposed for psychiatric care, including sedative neuroleptics or sedative antidepressants. These drugs should not, however, be used to improve sleep in athletes. Certain H1 antihistamines (alimemazine, promethazine, aceprometazine, doxylamine, niaprazine) have hypnotic properties, but are generally reserved for children. We should also mention the large number of phytotherapy or homeopathy formulations, for which pharmacological assessment is still lacking (Colin, 2000). In practice, and particularly in sports medicine, the choice of a sedative should be limited to hypnotic benzodiazepines and two similar compounds: zolpidem and zopiclone.

Zolpidem (Langtry and Benfield, 1990; Salvà and Costa, 1995; Holm and Goa, 2000) is an imidazopyridine with characteristic sedative properties and minimal anxiolytic, myorelaxing, and anticonvulsant effects. The usual dose is 10 mg once a day in adults. A lower dose is recommended in persons who are elderly and in cases of liver impairment. Like benzodiazepines, zolpidem acts on the GABA receptor of the CNS. It specifically binds to the α1-subunit. It does not interfere with α2-subunit-mediated muscle coordination. Its main therapeutic contribution is to reduce the delay to sleep onset and to lengthen total sleep duration. It is logically prescribed for insomnia or anesthesia premedication. Sleep-recording studies have demonstrated that administration of zolpidem increases the duration of phase II, III, and IV sleep. Paradoxical sleep is not modified, except for dosages above 20 mg.

Peak plasma concentration is reached about 2 hr after administration, and the mean half-life is 2.5 hr in healthy volunteers. Half-life is longer in people who are elderly and in cases of liver impairment.

Table 13.1 Hypnotic Benzodiazepines

DCI	T_{max} (hr)	$T_{1/2}$ (hr)	Recommended dose (mg)	Metabolites ($T_{1/2}$ hr)
Estazolam	1 to 1.5	10 to 30	2	
Flunitrazepam	1 to 1.5	15 to 30	0.5-1	Desmethylflunitrazepam, active (23-33)
Loprazolam	1 to 2	8 to 10	1	
Lormetazepam	1 to 3	10 to 12	1-2	Lorazepam, active (10-20)
Nitrazepam	1 to 3	16 to 48	5-10	Several, inactive
Temazepam	1 to 4	5 to 8	10-20	Oxazepam (5%), active (8)
Triazolam	0.5 to 4	1 to 4	0.125-0.250	Hydroxylated metabolite

Occasional administration produces few side effects. The most commonly cited effects are nausea, dizziness, and drowsiness. In case of repeated use, there is a risk of developing dependence, withdrawal syndrome, and insomnia rebound at sudden discontinuation; but there is little evidence of such problems when the drug is given at the recommended dose. Because of its pharmacokinetic properties and its recognized "flexibility," zolpidem can now be recommended on an "as-needed" basis of prescription (Allain, Lebreton, et al., 2000; Allain, Arbus, et al., 2001; Hajak et al., 2001); this characteristic would justify choosing this drug over others in cases of transient or recurrent episodes of insomnia.

Zopiclone (Wadworth and McTavish, 1993; Noble et al., 1998) belongs to the cyclopyrrolone family. The usual dosage, 7.5 mg once daily, can be increased to 15 mg if necessary. Elderly patients or patients with renal or hepatic dysfunction should be given a lower dose initially. Although not structurally related to benzodiazepines, zopiclone has the same mechanism of action and pharmacological properties. However, at the usual dose, the EEG pattern associated with its use is different from that of benzodiazepines. Zopiclone reduces phase I sleep, prolongs phase II, and has little effect on deep and paradoxical sleep. The hypnotic effects of zopiclone, such as reduced sleep onset latency, increased total sleep time, and reduction in the number of nighttime awakenings, have been demonstrated in numerous studies in healthy volunteers and patients with insomnia.

Peak plasma concentrations are reached 1 hr 30 min to 2 hr after administration. The half-life is about 5 hr. The drug is metabolized in the liver.

A bitter, metallic aftertaste is generally the most common adverse event. As for other hypnotics, dependence is a risk in cases of long-term use.

Effect of Hypnotics on Performance

A question that has been debated for years is whether a single or repeated dose of a sedative will lead to early-morning hangover and perturb psychomotor performance (Amado-Boccara et al., 1992; Hindmarch and Fairweather, 1994). The answer is crucial for deciding which drugs can be prescribed in certain categories of persons. For athletes, particularly when the sport requires precision (shooting sports) or speed, as well as for pilots or drivers, even a minimal risk of reduced wakefulness would be unacceptable.

Classically, several tests have been used to assess psychomotor performances (figure 13.1). The critical flicker fusion frequency test (CFF) is a means of measuring the ability to distinguish discrete units of sensory data and is taken as an index of overall CNS activity. Subjects are required to detect flicker in a set of four light-emitting diodes in foveal fixation of 1 m according to the psychophysiological method of limits for ascending and descending thresholds. The choice reaction time (CRT) is a measure of basic sensorimotor performance. Subjects are required to scan an array of small lights that are illuminated on a random basis. They are asked to touch the appropriate response button to extinguish the light as soon as they detect it. Saccadic eye movement has also proved to be a rapid and sensitive marker of drug-induced sedation or stimulation in humans. Volunteers are instructed to follow the

Psychomotor performance	**Memory**
Actual car driving, simulated car driving	Continuous memory task, short-term memory
Psychomotor speed	**Sensory skills**
Choice reaction time, simple reaction time	Vigilance task
Sensorimotor coordination	Attention task, continuous attention task, simulated assembly line task
Adaptive tracking, critical tracking, continuous tracking, pursuit rotor, simulated car tracking, visuomotor coordination	Dynamic visual acuity
	Spatial perception
Central nervous system arousal, information processing	**Motor ability**
Critical flicker fusion	Dexterity test, finger tapping, glass bead picking test, pegboard
Digit symbol substitution task, letter cancellation, visual search task	
Grammatical/logical reasoning, mental arithmetic	
Stroop color test	

Figure 13.1   Main assessment criteria used for "cognitive mapping" of drugs.

Adapted from Shamsi and Hindmarch, 2000.

movements of a target presented to them on a television monitor, and a recording of the resulting electrooculogram is used to monitor the movements of the eyes. The digit symbol substitution test (DSST), a subtest of the Weschsler Adult Intelligence Schedule, is used to check memorizing and learning, which could interfere by themselves with performance assessment.

Studies Conducted in Healthy Volunteers

Most of the data available on the effects of hypnotics on cognitive and/or psychomotor performance, more rarely physical performance, have been obtained with healthy volunteers. We describe here the principal findings, presenting a few studies in some detail.

The sedative, amnestic, and performance-disruptive effects of triazolam (0.25 and 0.5 mg), zolpidem (10 and 20 mg), and placebo were studied in 23 healthy subjects (17 men and 6 women, 26.8 ± 1.0 years). Compounds were administered at bedtime. During an awakening 90 min later (at approximate peak concentration of each drug), a 30-min performance battery, which included memory, vigilance, and psychomotor tasks, was completed. Each drug and dose impaired memory, vigilance, and psychomotor performance relative to placebo. The next morning, delayed recall (anterograde amnesia) was also impaired by all drugs and doses (Roehrs et al., 1994).

Berlin et al. (1993) assessed the effects of zolpidem (10 mg) on memory and psychomotor performances in 18 healthy male subjects (20-31 years) and compared them with those of triazolam (0.25 mg) and placebo. Both drugs decreased psychomotor performance, impaired memory, and increased postural sway, the maximal effect occurring 1.5 hr after intake. No subsequent alterations were found 6 and 8 hr after drug intake. Another double-blind, placebo-controlled study (Richens et al., 1993), conducted with 12 healthy male volunteers (20-30 years), also demonstrated that zolpidem at 5, 10, and 20 mg significantly and dose-dependently depressed peak saccade velocity during the 1.5 hr after a single administration; but the next morning this parameter had returned toward pretreatment levels. In this study, nitrazepam (10 mg) also statistically significantly depressed peak saccade velocity, but the effect was maintained the following morning. The absence of residual effects with zolpidem (10 or 15 mg) was also confirmed, 4 hr after administration, by Wilkinson (1995) in 24 male subjects (21-40 years) assessed with a battery of four tests (divided attention test, visual backward masking test, Stenberg test, vigilance test).

Stanley et al. (1987) investigated the relative effects on morning psychomotor performance of temazepam (10 mg), flunitrazepam (1 mg), and nitrazepam (2.5 mg).

The double-blind, randomized study included six men and six women (18-36 years). Results showed that no drug significantly affected psychomotor performance (five tests performed: CRT, DSST, time estimation, digit span, simple and complex card sorting) after single or repeated (seven nights) administration.

In 20 subjects (22-58 years), Hindmarch (1979) studied the acute and chronic effects of nitrazepam (5 mg) and temazepam (15 and 30 mg) on subjective appraisal of sleep and early-morning behavior and on laboratory-assessed psychomotor performance the morning after overnight medication. Subjects reported improved sleep with nitrazepam and temazepam at 30 mg, but there was evidence of impaired performance the next day with temazepam at 30 mg. The effects of six nightly doses of temazepam (20 mg), nitrazepam (10 mg), and placebo on saccadic eye movements, CFF, and CRT and on subjective feelings were also studied by Tedeschi et al. (1985) in a double-blind, crossover study in eight male volunteers. Nitrazepam, but not temazepam, produced a residual performance impairment at 7 hr, but not at 10 hr, the morning after the first night.

In a comparative bedtime study (Allain et al., 1995), zolpidem (10 mg), zopiclone (7.5 mg), and flunitrazepam (1 mg) similarly impaired psychomotor performance and memory for 4 hr after intake; some impairment was still found at 7 hr. In elderly volunteers, when compared with zopiclone (3.75 mg), lormetazepam (1 mg), and placebo, zolpidem did not induce increased body sway and had minimal effect on next-day memory (Allain, Gandon, et al., 2001).

Residual effects of zolpidem (10 mg), zopiclone (7.5 mg), and flunitrazepam (1 mg) on driving performance and ocular saccades were simultaneously assessed in 16 subjects (9 men, 7 women). Bocca et al. (1999) concluded that zopiclone and flunitrazepam had residual effects in the first part of the morning, whereas zolpidem had no residual effects.

Mattila et al. (1998) conducted a placebo-controlled, randomized, double-blind, crossover study to compare the psychomotor and cognitive effects of 15 mg zolpidem, 30 mg oxazepam, and 7.5 mg zopiclone given to 12 subjects (five women, seven men, 21-28 years). Four psychomotor tests were done at 1, 3.5, and 5 hr after intake (CFF, DSST, body sway, simulated driving). Zolpidem impaired coordinative, reactive, and cognitive skills at 1 and 3.5 hr more clearly than the other agents did, with the most sensitive performance remaining impaired by zolpidem at 5 hr.

In a recent trial, Nakajima et al. (2000) compared the effects of zolpidem and zopiclone on nocturnal sleep and sleep latency in the morning during a crossover study in nine healthy young male subjects during nine-night sessions. The authors concluded that zolpidem showed a striking superiority. Another recent study compared insomniacs' preferences between two hypnotics, zolpidem (10 mg) and a new compound (zaleplon, 10 mg) and concluded in favor of zolpidem (Allain, Gandon, et al., 2001).

Elsewhere, the positive residual effects of lormetazepam (Deijen et al., 1991) and temazepam (Bourin et al., 1987) on motor control or memory and vigilance in healthy volunteers have also been described.

Studies Conducted in Athletes

Few studies have specifically examined the effect of hypnotics on physical performance in sport activities. Gremion et al. (1992) compared temazepam, zolpidem, and placebo in a double-blind, randomized study in 26 regional-level long-distance male runners (35.3 ± 7 years). Psychomotor performance (CFF and Tracing Test Series) was assessed the day after drug administration, between 8 and 10 A.M. A maximal treadmill exercise test and determination of maximal isokinetic work of the quadriceps were also administered. The results of this study showed that none of the tests of physical or psychomotor performance were modified by administration of the sedatives. The authors concluded that hypnotics do not improve performance level per se but also do not decrease it, and can help avoid the risk of performance impairment due to the lack of sufficient sleep.

Another double-blind, crossover study (Tafti et al., 1992) evaluated eight male volleyball players (22-29 years) and showed a residual effect with zopiclone at 7.5 mg, administered at 11 P.M., on a battery of psychomotor and physical performance tests (CRT, CFF, eye-hand coordination test, standing jump test, running time test) done at 8 A.M. and 1 and 6 P.M. the next day. A questionnaire was also used to determine the players' subjective assessment of morning awakening. There was no significant difference in the performance between treated players and controls. There was a slight deterioration in subjective assessment at 8 A.M., and a slight improvement at 1 and 8 P.M., for subjects taking verum. The duration of sleep was slightly longer in the group treated with zopiclone.

To determine the effects of sedative hypnotics on psychomotor and physical performance in 12 athletes (10 males, 2 females, 22.75 ± 2.53 years, various sports), a double-blind, placebo-controlled crossover trial compared zopiclone (7.5 mg) to loprazolam (2 mg). Eye-hand coordination tests, a 30-m (32.8 yd) sprint test, an agility test, and a graded treadmill run to exhaustion for determination of $\dot{V}O_2$max were performed 10 hr after drug administration. Following the ingestion of loprazolam, subjects experienced a significant hangover effect and altered reaction time, whereas the ingestion of zopiclone did not significantly impair either psychomotor or physical performance in the tests (Grobler et al., 2000).

Nitrazepam (10 mg) and temazepam (30 mg) were compared with placebo in 27 physical education students (14 males, 13 females, 18-22 years). Medication was given for nine nights, with measurements (quality of sleep, psychomotor performance, and lung function) made after the second and ninth nights. The drugs were equally efficient in providing good-quality sleep. The psychomotor tests (CRT, CFF) did not show any marked difference between treatments, but the specific airway conductance values were consistently lower with nitrazepam (Charles et al., 1987).

Studies Conducted in Other Populations

Specific populations other than athletes who need hypnotics are also concerned about the problem of secondary early-morning effects. Civilian or military pilots must cope with jet lag and the requirement for recuperating sleep while perfectly maintaining their capacity when they return to work.

A controlled, double-blind, crossover study evaluated zolpidem (10 mg), flunitrazepam (1 mg), and placebo on daytime wakefulness in ground air force personnel (Group 1, 12 subjects) and navy fighter plane pilots (Group 2, 12 subjects). With both hypnotics there was a subjective improvement in the quality of sleep without any objective modification of psychomotor performance for Group 1 or, in flight simulations, for Group 2. Spectral analysis of the electroencephalograms (EEG) confirmed the absence of daytime residual effects with zolpidem. In contrast, subjective daytime sedative effects observed in Group 1 subjects after flunitrazepam intake were supported by modifications of their EEG (Sicard et al., 1993).

Ramsey and McGlohn (1997) collected data on hypnotics used by the U.S. Air Force for on-duty military personnel. The objective of the drug treatment was to allow personnel to sleep in inappropriate conditions and environments with the assurance the medication would not cause residual memory, reaction time, or judgment impairments. Temazepam, with a long half-life, required 12 hr before its effects disappeared. Triazolam exhibited a short 6-hr grounding period, but sometimes caused rebound insomnia, even after a single dose. Zolpidem appeared to cause less global impairment than benzodiazepines and to be free of persistent performance decrement or hangover effect. These studies suggest a benefit of effective sleep produced by hypnotics on next-day performance compared with sleep of questionable quality without medication.

Drug Dependence and Misuse

Benzodiazepines and related compounds can induce tolerance (leading to increasing dosages) and psychic and physical dependence. This state of dependence can lead to weaning difficulties at treatment withdrawal (e.g., headache, anxiety, myalgia), as well as rebound insomnia. Generally, at usual dosages, there is no risk of pharmacodependence except after long-term use. The incidence of misuse and dependence is generally considered to be low with conventional use. The risk is, however, quite real in subjects with a history of alcohol or multiple drug abuse.

Zolpidem appears to have a low potential for abuse. Several studies of up to six months duration showed no evidence of development of tolerance to the hypnotic effects of this compound. Likewise, zopiclone does not appear to have a high potential to cause dependence in nonabusing patients; where case reports of dependence have emerged, these have involved patients with a history of drug abuse or psychiatric illness (Hajak, 1999). Rebound insomnia has occasionally been detected (Lader, 1997).

Conclusion

The capacity of hypnotics to induce and maintain sleep is well proven. The results reviewed here of the effects of hypnotic use on physical and cognitive performance lead to converging and reassuring conclusions. It is undeniable that different hypnotics provoke some psychomotor and memory impairment within hours of intake. When they are used as recommended, this period occurs while the subject is sleeping, so the perturbations have no deleterious effect. After a variable delay, however (the half-life of hypnotics being directly related to the duration of residual effects on daytime performance), there are no notable residual effects that would hinder performance the next day (Roth et al., 1980). The largest numbers of studies have been conducted with zolpidem, which has a short half-life. Mougin et al. (1991) compared the effect of a single dose of a short-half-life hypnotic in eight male high-level athletes (24.0 ± 2.4 years), examining the respective consequences of perturbed nighttime sleep with sleep induced by a single dose of a short-half-life hypnotic; they concluded that physiological adaptations and ability to perform maximal exercise are affected by a partial sleep loss, but not by a single ingestion of a sedative prior to sleep. In a review, Unden and Schechter (1996) analyzed the scientific literature for potential next-day residual effects of zolpidem, based on more than 30 international clinical trials involving more than 2600 subjects. They concluded that at the recommended dose (10 mg), at single or repeated dosing, this compound appears to induce minimal residual effects. Nevertheless, even an effect considered to be very minimal can be unacceptable during a championship competition. Unfortunately no studies have been conducted in this setting.

Anxiolytics

Anxiety disorders are schematically categorized into five different diseases, according to the DSM-V: panic disorders, generalized anxiety disorder, social phobia, obsessive-compulsive disorder, and posttraumatic stress disorder. Allgulander (1999) has recently reviewed the use of anti-anxiety agents in common practice. While most of the drugs at our disposal are efficient, their side-effects profile is highly divergent. Such knowledge is important whenever anxiolytics are to be prescribed for active young adults and more particularly athletes, who have a risk of developing anxiety disorders (i.e., performance anxiety). The currently marketed anxiolytics are classified into several chemical families (table 13.2), but the most widely prescribed drugs belong to the benzodiazepine family. Nonhypnotic benzodiazepines possess the same pharmacodynamic properties and, roughly speaking, induce the same side effects as hypnotic benzodiazepines.

Effects of Anxiolytics on Performance

In a double-blind, crossover study in 20 students (7 males, 13 females, mean age 21 years), impaired performance and sedation were demonstrated after a single dose of lorazepam (1 or 2.5 mg). Lorazepam impaired reaction time, verbal learning, number cancellation, symbol copying, and performance in the DSST, with maximum impairment 4 hr after drug administration (File and Bond, 1979).

O'Neill et al. (1995), using 12 healthy volunteers (3 males, 9 females, 30-50 years) demonstrated in a randomized, controlled trial that lorazepam (2 mg) produced a marked slowing on both the simple and the choice reaction time throughout the 6-hr testing period. Performance on digit vigilance tasks, memory scanning tests, word recall, and word and picture recognition tasks showed a clear disruption with lorazepam.

Table 13.2 Anxiolytic Drugs

Chemical family	Compounds
1,4-benzodiazepines	Alprazolam, bromazepam, clotiazepam, diazepam, desmethyldiazepam, loflazepate, lorazepam, nordazepam, oxazepam, prazepam
1,5-benzodiazepines	Clobazam
Carbamates	Meprobamate
Hydroxyzine	Hydroxyzine
Azapirone	Buspirone

Acute behavioral effects of three doses of alprazolam (0.25, 0.5, 1 mg) were studied in healthy volunteers. Performance tasks included DSST, a repeated-acquisition of response sequence task, a differential reinforcement of low-response-rate task designed to monitor time estimation, a number recognition task, and a second-order repeated-acquisition of response sequences task. The data indicate that the risk of adverse performance effects following use of alprazolam is related to dose, with risks increasing at doses at or above 0.5 mg (Kelly et al., 1997).

Hindmarch et al. (1990) compared the actions of five benzodiazepines—alprazolam (1 or 2 mg), bromazepam (3 or 6 mg), clobazam (10 or 20 mg), oxazepam (30 or 50 mg), and lorazepam (1 or 2 mg)—on psychomotor performance (CFF, CRT). The study included 28 female volunteers (21-45 years) and was based on a double-blind, placebo-controlled crossover design. The CFF was shown to be significantly lowered by chronic administration of oxazepam alone, and CRT was variously affected by higher doses of oxazepam, alprazolam, lorazepam, and bromazepam. On the other hand, clobazam and bromazepam at 3 mg were clearly differentiated from the other compounds and had no significant effects on any of the measures of psychological function. The absence of a negative effect with the clobazam was confirmed by Nicholson, who in 1979 had shown that 1,5-benzodiazepines have minimal immediate effects on performance; and Hindmarch (1979) even demonstrated that clobazam improves early-morning performance on CRT. Likewise, it has been demonstrated that low-dose alprazolam or lorazepam in healthy volunteers produces significant improvement in cognitive functions and psychomotor performances (Bourin et al., 1994, 1995, 1998).

Neuroleptics

Neuroleptics, or antipsychotics, include a group of compounds defined by common pharmacological properties: all neuroleptics are more or less active antagonists of type D2 dopaminergic receptors. Neuroleptics are indicated almost exclusively for drug treatment of psychotic disorders, especially schizophrenia. These drugs are given for their sedative, reductive, or de-inhibitory antipsychotic properties, depending on the situation, or their anti-deficit action. These compounds can cause serious adverse effects, particularly neurological effects, prohibiting their use outside specific indications (Petit et al., 1995). We do not discuss this family of psychotropic drugs in detail since their prescription has little pertinence in high-level sport practice; in addition, there has been no study of their potential action on sport performance. Most published work has focused on assessing the effect of neuroleptic

administration on performance in schizophrenic patients in order to compare the reduced level of performance caused by the disease with possible improvement provided by drug therapy. Different classifications have been proposed, using clinical or chemical criteria. Most researchers also distinguish atypical neuroleptics, clozapine for example, which have clinical effects and neurobiological mechanisms of action that differentiate them from classical neuroleptics. Unlike their classical counterparts, atypical neuroleptics used at recommended doses have no or few extra-pyramidal adverse effects (and are unable to produce catalepsy in animal models). They may also be distinguished on the basis of the lower dopamine D2 and higher serotonin (5-HT2A) affinities. Drugs currently available are presented in table 13.3.

Effect of Neuroleptics on Performance

A few clinical research trials have been conducted in healthy volunteers to determine the effects of various neuroleptics on cognitive and psychomotor function. We review the principal trials, but any generalization is greatly hindered by pharmacotherapeutic variations among the compounds.

Using a randomized, double-blind, crossover design, visuomotor performance was assessed in 12 male subjects (20-34 years) receiving 300 mg of sulpiride or placebo. Subjectively, the volunteers were not able to differentiate whether they received placebo or sulpiride, but some time reactions were prolonged under medication (Meyer-Lindenberg et al., 1997). In a double-blind design, either 3 mg haloperidol, 150 mg remoxipride, or placebo was administered to 36 male volunteers (19-39 years).

Table 13.3 Neuroleptic Drugs

Chemical family	Compounds
Phenothiazines	Chlorpromazine, thioproperazine, thioridazine, fluphenazine, propericiazine, levomepromazine, pipotiazine, cyamemazine, trifluoperazine, perphenazine
Butyrophenones	Pipamperone, droperidol, haloperidol, penfluridol
Benzamides	Sulpiride, sultopride, tiapride, amisulpride
Thioxanthenes	Zuclopenthixol, flupentixol
Dibenzo-diazepines	Clozapine, olanzapine
Dibenzo-oxazepines	Loxapine, risperidone
Diphenylpiperidine	Pimozide

Performances were assessed using time estimation, CFF, and CRT. The findings reveal that haloperidol caused more severe alteration in cognitive functioning, cortical arousal, and psychomotor performance than the clinically equipotent dose of remoxipride (Rammsayer and Gallhoffer, 1995). The effects of single oral doses of chlorpromazine (50 mg) and risperidone (2 mg), relative to placebo, were investigated using seven psychomotor function tests. Objective assessment mirrored the subjective reports, demonstrating that impairment in volunteers treated with risperidone was greater in extent and magnitude than with chlorpromazine (Hughes et al., 1999). Dosages used may be a critical factor in all these studies as exemplified by risperidone (Zaudig, 2000), which at optimum dosage is devoid of any deleterious effects on cognition.

The same results have been validated, and the same remarks hold true for a benzamide, tiapride, which in contradistinction to lorazepam did not induce any modification of vigilance, body sway, or memory in elderly healthy volunteers. This study, moreover, exemplified the predictivity of such laboratory data insofar as in a phase III randomized clinical trial, tiapride (150 mg/day) was proven to be devoid of deleterious effects on cognitive functions (Allain et al., 2000).

Legal Aspects

At the end of the year 2000, none of the drugs discussed in this chapter are on the list of prohibited substances and methods, and none are subject to restricted use by the anti-doping regulations established by the French Ministry of Youth and Sports (France is the only country that has adopted legislation on the protection of athletes) or the International Olympic Committee.

This fact can be explained by the present review, which demonstrates that the main risk of the psychotropics discussed is a decrease of psychomotor performance; the opposite (enhancement of performances) would have led to the possibility of misuse and dependence. Pharmacoepidemiology studies, not restricted to athletes, confirm that hypnotics, anxiolytics, or neuroleptics are not illegally consumed in healthy populations. On the other hand, in cases of pathology such drugs can be legally prescribed, always in full accordance with the indications summarized in the NDA and the official guidelines; under these conditions, the risk of altering psychomotor performance is minimized in athletes who have to be pharmacologically treated anyway if ill. The emergence of sport competition for athletes with disabilities (i.e., Olympic games for persons who are disabled) presumes that those persons—because of their handicap—may receive psychotropics or compounds acting on CNS, hence capable of modifying performance.

Perspectives

Several key points emerge from the present review. (1) Data from studies carried out in laboratory settings in healthy volunteers are the best guidelines for prescription of psychotropics in athletes and sportspersons; (2) obtaining an exact definition of the impact of psychotropics on human cognition and psychomotor performance should be a compulsory step in drug development, as this "cognitive mapping" possesses a reliable predictive value for the prescriber; (3) debate should not be restricted to sedatives but rather should be extended to antidepressants (Allain et al., 1992) and psychostimulants that carry the risk of misuse and probably dependence (e.g., caffeine [Patat et al., 2000]); (4) prescribers and consumers of drugs, at the least, should not forget that many non-CNS drugs may have an impact on the brain and as a consequence modify intellectual and psychomotor functions (i.e., anti-allergics, antibiotics [quinolones], and the like). Phase I and II studies thus appear more and more as a prerequisite whenever a drug has to be prescribed in a target population such as athletes or individuals involved in sport competition, whatever their basal health status (psychiatric condition, disability, or handicap) and the type or duration of competition (sport involves not only muscles!).

Conclusion

The present review is devoted to analysis of the effects of two main classes of psychotropics (hypnotics and tranquilizers) on cognition and psychomotor performance in athletes. The issue is important because sportpersons and athletes appear today as a specific target population for whom even slight deleterious consequences of such psychotropics on brain functions are unacceptable. It appears that at the right dosage and adequate duration of treatment, some compounds are preferable whenever the goal is to avoid cognitive side effects (e.g., zolpidem is preferable to benzodiazepines in the treatment of sleep disorders; non-benzodiazepine compounds are preferable for treating anxiety disorders). Such reports should be extended to any class of drugs acting on the CNS, including antidepressant and psychostimulants (e.g., caffeine), with the understanding that in this case, misuse and doping are the main concern.

References

Allain H. Pharmacologie de la cognition **www.med.univ-rennes1.fr/etud/pharmaco**.

Allain H, Arbus L, Schück S and the Zolpidem Study Group. Efficacy and safety of zolpidem administered "as needed" in primary insomnia; results of a double blind, placebo controlled study. Clin Drug Invest 2001, 21 (in press).

Allain H, Bentué-Ferrer D, Rochcongar P, Schuck S. Fatigue: from biology to pharmacology. BVS Europe 1999, 10, 6-12.

Allain H, Dautzenberg K, Maurer K, Schuck S, Bonhomme D, Gerard D. Double blind study of tiapride versus haloperidol and placebo in agitation and aggressiveness in elderly patients with cognitive impairment. Psychopharmacology 2000, 148, 361-366.

Allain H, Gandon JM, Kleinermans D, Schweich C, Soubrane C. Effects of a single dose of zolpidem (5 mg), zopiclone (3,5 mg) and lormetazepam (1 mg) on postural sway and memory functions in elderly subjects. Sleep 2001, 24, A336 (abstract).

Allain H, Lebreton S, Mauduit N, Schuck S, Kleinermans D, Lavoisy J, Gandon JM. Assessment of patients preferences between two hypnotics, zolpidem (10 mg) vs zaleplon (10 mg). J Sleep Res 2000, 9 (Suppl 1) (abstract).

Allain H, Lieury A, Brunet-Bourgin F, Miraband C, Trebon P, Le Coz F, and Gandon. Antidepressants and cognition: comparative effects of moclobemide, viloxazine and maprotiline. Psychopharmacology 1992, 106, S56-S61.

Allain H, Patat A, Lieury A, Le Coz F, Janus C, Menard G, Gandon JM. Comparative study of the effects of zopiclone, zolpidem, flunitrazepam and a placebo on nocturnal cognitive performance in healthy subjects, in relation to pharmacokinetics. Eur Psychiatry 1995, 10 (Suppl 3), 129 S-135 S.

Allain H, Schuck S, Mauduit N, Djemai M. Comparative effects of pharmacotherapy on the maintenance of cognition function. Eur Psychiatry 2000, 16 (Suppl 1), 35S-41S.

Allgulander C. Anti-anxiety agents: a pharmacoepidemiological review. Hum Psychopharmacol Clin Exp 1999, 14, 149-160.

Amado-Boccara I, Galinowski A, Poirier MF, Loo H. Influence des psychotropes sur la vigilance et les performances motrices. Presse Méd 1992, 21, 899-902.

Ashton H. Guidelines for the rational use of benzodiazepines. When and what to use. Drugs 1994, 48, 25-40.

Bentué-Ferrer D, Bureau M, Patat A, Allain H. Flumazenil. CNS Drug Reviews 1996, 2, 390-414.

Berlin I, Warot D, Hergueta T, Molinier P, Bagot C, Puech AJ. Comparison of the effects of zolpidem and triazolam on memory functions, psychomotor performances, and postural sway in healthy subjects. J Clin Psychopharmacol 1993, 13, 100-106.

Bocca ML, Le Doze F, Etard O, Pottier M, L'Hoste J, Denise P. Residual effects of zolpidem 10 mg and zopiclone 7.5 mg versus flunitrazepam 1 mg and placebo on driving performance and ocular saccades. Psychopharmacology 1999, 143, 373-379.

Bonin B, François T. Hypnotiques. In: Thérapeutique psychiatrique, Senon JL, Sechter D, Richard D eds, Paris, Hermann, 1995, 369-422.

Bormann J. The "ABC" of GABA receptors. TIPS 2000, 21, 16-19.

Bourin M, Colombel MC, Guitton B. Alprazolam 0.125 mg twice a day improves aspects of psychometric performance in healthy volunteers. J Clin Psychopharmacol 1998, 18, 364-372.

Bourin M, Colombel MC, Malinge M. Lorazepam 0.25 mg twice a day improves aspects of psychometric performance in healthy volunteers. J Psychopharmacol 1995, 9, 251-257.

Bourin M, Couetoux du Tertre A, Colombel MC, Auget JL. Effects of low doses of lorazepam on psychometric tests in healthy volunteers. Int Clin Psychopharmacol 1994, 9, 83-88.

Bourin M, Hubert C, Colombel MC, Larousse C. Residual effects of temazepam versus nitrazepam on memory and vigilance in the normal subject. Hum Psychopharmacol 1987, 2, 185-189.

Charles RB, Kirkham AJT, Guyatt AR, Parker SP. Psychomotor, pulmonary and exercise responses to sleep medication. Br J Clin Pharmac 1987, 24, 191-197.

Chebib M, Johnston GA. The "ABC" of GABA receptors: a brief review. Clin Exp Pharmacol Physiol 1999, 26, 937-940.

Colin P. An epidemiological study of a homeopathic practice. Br Homeopath J 2000, 89, 116-121.

Comité International Olympique Classes de substances interdites et méthodes interdites. **http://www.olympic.org/ioc/f/org/medcom/pdf/prohibited_subst_0004_f.pdf**.

Dawson D, Reid K. Fatigue, alcohol and performance impairment. Nature 1997, 388, 235.

Deijen J, Heemastia ML, Orlebeke JF. Residual effects of lormetazepam on mood and performance in healthy elderly volunteers. Eur J Clin Pharmacol 1991, 40, 267-271.

Doble A. New insights into the mechanism of action of hypnotics. J Psychopharmacol 1999, 13 (Suppl 1), S11-S20.

File SE, Bond AJ. Impaired performance and sedation after a single dose of lorazepam. Psychopharmacology 1979, 66, 309-313.

French J. Circadian rhythms, jet-lag and the athlete. In: Current therapy in sport medicine, Torg J, Shephard RJ eds, Philadelphia, Mosby, 1995, pp. 596-600.

Gremion G, Sutter-Weyrich C, Rostan A, Forster A. Performance physique et sédation: étude comparative des effets d'une benzodiazépine (temazepam) et d'un hypnotique non benzodiazépinique (zolpidem). Schweiz-Ztschr Sport Med 1992, 40, 113-118.

Grobler LA, Schwellnus MP, Trichard C, Calder S, Noakes TD, Derman WE. Comparative effects of zopiclone and loprazolam on psychomotor and physical performance in active individuals. Clin J Sport Med 2000, 10, 123-128.

Hajak G. A comparative assessment of the risks and benefits of zopiclone. A review of 15 years' clinical experience. Drug Saf 1999, 21, 457-469.

Hajak G. Insomnia in primary care. Sleep 2000, 23 (Suppl 3), S54-S63.

Hajak G, Cluydts R, Allain H et al. The challenge of chronic insomnia: is non-nightly hypnotic treatment a feasible alternative. Eur Psychiatry 2001 (in press).

Hindmarch I. Effects of hypnotic and sleep-inducing drugs on objective assessments of human psychomotor performance and subjective appraisals of sleep and early morning behaviour. Br J Clin Pharmacol 1979, 8, 43S-46S.

Hindmarch I, Fairweather DB. Assessing the residual effects of hypnotics. Acta Psychiat Belg 1994, 94, 88-95.

Hindmarch I, Haller J, Sherwood N, Kerr JS. Comparison of five anxiolytic benzodiazepines on measures of psychomotor performance and sleep. Neuropsychobiology 1990-91, 24, 84-89.

Hobbs WR, Rall TW, Verdoorn TA. Hypnotiques et sédatifs; alcool. In: Les bases pharmacologiques de l'utilisation des medicaments, Hardman JG, Limbird LE eds, New York, McGraw-Hill, 1998, 367-402.

Holm KJ, Goa KL. Zolpidem. An update of its pharmacology, therapeutic efficacy and tolerability in the treatment of insomnia. Drugs 2000, 59, 865-889.

Hughes AM, Lynch P, Rhodes J, Ervine CM, Yates RA. Electroencephalographic and psychomotor effects of chlorpromazine and risperidone relative to placebo in normal healthy volunteers. Br J Clin Pharmacol 1999, 48, 323-330.

Kardos J. Recent advances in GABA research. Neurochem Int 1999, 34, 353-358.

Kaufman DW, Shapiro S. Epidemiological assessment of drug-induced disease. Lancet 2000, 356, 1339-1343.

Kelly TH, Foltin RW, Serpick E, Fischman MW. Behavioral effects of alprazolam in humans. Behav Pharmacol 1997, 8, 47-57.

Kentta G, Hassmen P. Overtraining and recovery: a conceptual model. Sports Med 1998, 26, 1-16.

Lader M. Zopiclone: is there any dependence and abuse potential? J Neurol 1997, 244 (Suppl 1), S18-S22.

Langtry HD, Benfield P. Zolpidem. A review of its pharmacodynamic and pharmacokinetic properties and therapeutic potential. Drugs 1990, 40, 291-313.

Mattila MJ, Vanakoski J, Kalska H, Seppala T. Effects of alcohol, zolpidem and some other sedatives and hypnotics on human performance and memory. Pharmacol Biochem Behav 1998, 59, 917-923.

Mehta AK, Ticku MK. An update on GABAA receptors. Brain Res Rev 1999, 29, 196-217.

Meyer-Lindenberg A, Rammsayer T, Ulferts J, Gallhofer B. The effects of sulpiride on psychomotor performance and subjective tolerance. Eur Neuropsychopharmacol 1997, 7, 219-223.

Ministère de la Jeunesse et des Sports Lutte anti-dopage: produits et méthodes interdits. **http://www.jeunesse-sports.gouv.fr/francais//mjsdopliste3.htm**.

Mougin F, Simon-Rigaud ML, Davenne D, Bourdin H, Guilland JC, Kantelip JP, Magnin P. Tolérance à l'effort après réduction de sommeil et après prise d'un hypnotique: le zolpidem. Arch Int Physiol Biochim Biophys 1992, 100, 255-262.

Mougin F, Simon-Rigaud ML, Davenne D, Renaud A, Garnier A, Kantelip JP, Magnin P. Effects of sleep disturbances on subsequent physical performance. Eur J Appl Physiol 1991, 63, 77-82.

Nakajima T, Sasaki T, Nakagome K, Takagawa S, Ikebuchi I, Ito Y. Comparison of the effects of zolpidem and zopiclone on nocturnal sleep and sleep latency in the morning. A cross-over study in healthy young volunteers. Life Sci 2000, 67, 81-90.

Nicholson AN. Differential effects of the 1,4 and 1,5 benzodiazepines on performance in healthy man. Br J Clin Pharmac 1979, 7, 83S-84S.

Noble S, Langtry HD, Lamb HM. Zopiclone. An update of its pharmacology, clinical efficacy and tolerability in the treatment of insomnia. Drugs 1998, 55, 277-302.

O'Neill WM, Hanks GW, White L, Simpson P, Wesnes K. The cognitive and psychomotor effects of opioid analgesics. I. A randomized controlled trial of single doses of dextropropoxyphene, lorazepam and placebo in healthy subjects. Eur J Clin Pharmacol 1995, 48, 447-453.

Patat A. Driving, drug research and the pharmaceutical industry. Hum Psychopharmacol Clin Exp 1998, 13, 5124-5132.

Patat A. Clinical pharmacology of psychotropic drugs. Hum Psychopharmacol Clin Exp 2000, 15, 361-387.

Patat A, Cercle M, Trocherie S, Peytavin E, Potin C, Allain H, and Gandon JM. Lack of amphetamine-like effects after administration of mefenorex in normal young subjects. Hum Psychopharmacol Clin Exp 1996, 11, 321-335.

Patat A, Rosenzweig P, Enslen M, Trocherie S, Miget N, Bozon MC, Allain H, and Gandon JM. Effects of a new slow release formulation of caffeine on EEG, psychomotor and cognitive functions in sleep-deprived subjects. Hum Psychopharmacol Clin Exp 2000, 15, 153-170.

Petit M, Dollfus S, Langlois S, Moity F. Neuroleptiques. In: Thérapeutique psychiatrique, Senon JL, Sechter D, Richard D eds, Paris, Hermann, 1995, 369-422.

Rammsayer T, Gallhofer B. Remoxipride versus haloperidol in healthy volunteers: psychometric performance and subjective tolerance profiles. Int Clin Psychopharmacol 1995, 10, 31-37.

Ramsey CS, McGlohn SE. Zolpidem as a fatigue counter measure. Aviat Space Environ Med 1997, 68, 926-931.

Richens A, Mercer AJ, Jones DM, Griffiths A, Marshall RW. Effects of zolpidem on saccadic eye movements and psychomotor performance: a double-blind, placebo controlled study in healthy volunteers. Br J Clin Pharmac 1993, 36, 61-65.

Roehrs T, Merlotti L, Zorick F, Roth T. Sedative, memory, and performance effects of hypnotics. Psychopharmacology 1994, 116, 130-134.

Roth T, Hartse KM, Zorich FJ, Kaffeman ME. The differential effects of short- and long-acting benzodiazepines upon nocturnal sleep and daytime performance. Arzneim-Forsch Drug Res 1980, 30, 891-894.

Salvà P, Costa J. Clinical pharmacokinetics and pharmacodynamics of zolpidem—therapeutic implications. Clin Pharmacokinet 1995, 29, 142-153.

Senon JL, Richard D. Anxiolytiques. In: Thérapeutique psychiatrique, Senon JL, Sechter D, Richard D eds, Paris, Hermann, 1995, 369-422.

Shamsi Z, Hindmarch I. Sedation and antihistamines: a review of inter-drug differences using proportional impairment ratios. Hum Psychopharmacol Clin Exp 2000, 15, S3-S30.

Shephard RJ. Minimizing the practical problems of worldwide soccer competition: management of heat exposure and a shift in circadian rhythms. Science Sport 1999, 14, 248-253.

Sicard BA, Trocherie S, Moreau J, Vieillefond H, Court LA. Evaluation of zolpidem on alertness and psychomotor abilities among aviation ground personnel and pilots. Aviat Space Environ Med 1993, 64, 371-375.

Stanley RO, Tiller JWG, Adrian J. The psychomotor effects of single and repeated doses of hypnotic benzodiazepines. Int Clin Psychopharmacol 1987, 2, 317-323.

Tafti M, Besset A, Billiard M. Effects of zopiclone on subjective evaluation of sleep and daytime alertness and on psychomotor and physical performance tests in athletes. Prog Neuro-Psychopharmacol Biol Psychiat 1992, 16, 55-63.

Tedeschi G, Griffiths AN, Smith AT, Richens A. The effect of repeated doses of temazepam and nitrazepam on human psychomotor performance. Br J Clin Pharmacol 1985, 20, 361-367.

Thomas V, Reymann JM, Lieury A, Allain H. Assessment of procedural memory in Parkinson's disease. Prog Neuro-Psychopharmacol Biol Psychiatry 1996, 20, 641-650.

Unden M, Schechter BR. Next day effects after nighttime treatment with zolpidem: a review. Eur Psychiatry 1996, 11 (Suppl 1), 21S-30S.

Wadworth AN, McTavish D. Zopiclone. A review of its pharmacological properties and therapeutic efficacy. Drugs Aging 1993, 3, 441-459.

Wilkinson CJ. The acute effects of zolpidem, administered alone and with alcohol, on cognitive and psychomotor function. J Clin Psychiatry 1995, 56, 309-318.

Zaudig M. A risk-benefit assessment of risperidone for the treatment of behavioural and psychological symptoms in dementia. Drug Saf 2000, 23, 183-195.

14

Beta-Adrenergic Antagonists

Kurt A. Mossberg, PT, PhD

Claire Peel, PT, PhD

Beta-adrenergic antagonists are pharmacologic agents that have been developed to bind to cell surface receptors for epinephrine and norepinephrine (figure 14.1) (Hoffman and Lefkowitz, 1996). These adrenergic receptors exist in a multitude of tissues, and four subtypes (β1, β2, β3, and β4) have been identified (for review see Kaumann, 1997; Nagatomo and Koike, 2000). A thorough review of the literature indicates that the β1-receptor predominates in the heart (Lefkowitz, Hoffman and Taylor, 1996); and it is the binding of the antagonist to this receptor that brings about the major clinical and therapeutic effects on the cardiovascular system. The "therapeutic" or enhancing effects seen in sport and other physical performance activities can be attributed to the multiple receptor types and the wide array of agents available (Nagatomo and Koike, 2000).

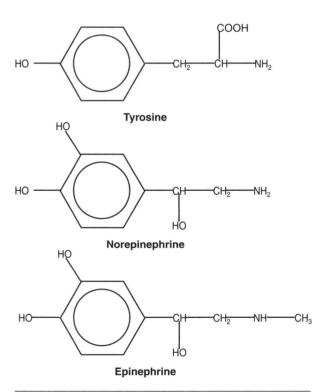

Figure 14.1   Epinephrine and norepinephrine are synthesized in vivo from the essential amino acid tyrosine (Stryer, 1995).

Beta blockers are classified as nonselective or selective, depending on their affinity for the various receptors (Molinoff, 1992; Kaumann, 1997). Table 14.1 lists the more common β-receptor antagonists that are on the market, and from figure 14.2 one can see the similarities and differences between two of these agents. The nonselective versus selective designation is based on the response brought about through binding to β1, β2, or both receptors (Hoffman and Lefkowitz, 1996). These agents have been called β-receptor antagonists, adrenergic antagonists, β-adrenoreceptor antagonists, sympatholytics, or simply beta blockers—and even "anti-cats" because of their ability to blunt the cardiovascular effects of the catecholamines. New agents are continuously being developed as new therapeutic and clinical uses for these compounds are demonstrated.

Indications for Use in Clinical Medicine

The use of β-adrenergic antagonists in clinical practice is extensive (Hoffman and Lefkowitz, 1996), with the primary therapeutic benefit being derived by individuals with impairments of the cardiovascular system. Because of the ubiquitous nature of the β-adrenergic receptor, other noncardiac problems have been treated successfully. These include prophylaxis of migraine, glaucoma, hyperthyroidism, and situational anxiety resulting in social phobias (Molinoff, 1992). The many indications for use of β-adrenergic antagonists are probably due to the variety of agents available; their affinity for the various receptors, not only β- but also α-adrenergic receptors; lipid solubility and their capacity to cross the blood-brain barrier; and whether or not they have agonist characteristics (intrinsic sympathomimetic activity) (Hoffman and Lefkowitz, 1996; Lefkowitz, Hoffman and Taylor, 1996). The mechanism of action is better understood in patients with cardiac disease than it is in those who are diagnosed with other clinical impairments (Molinoff, 1992).

Beta blockers were originally developed for the treatment of chest pain associated with myocardial ischemia (Opie, Sonnenblick, Frishman and Thadani, 1997). The strategy was to develop a drug that would

Table 14.1 Common Beta-Adrenergic Blocking Agents

| | Name | | |
	Generic	Trade/Brand/Proprietary	Action/Characteristic
Nonselective	Propranolol	Inderal	Cardiac deceleration and force of contraction
	Sotalol	Betapace	(decreased myocardial oxygen consumption),
	Penbutolol	Levatol	inhibition of peripheral vasodilation, inhibition
	Nadolol	Corgard	of bronchodilation, metabolic effects
Selective β1	Acebutolol	Sectral	Cardiac deceleration and force of contraction
	Metoprolol	Lopressor	(decreased myocardial oxygen consumption)
	Atenolol	Tenormin	
	Bisoprolol	Zebeta	

Physician's Desk Reference, 2001.

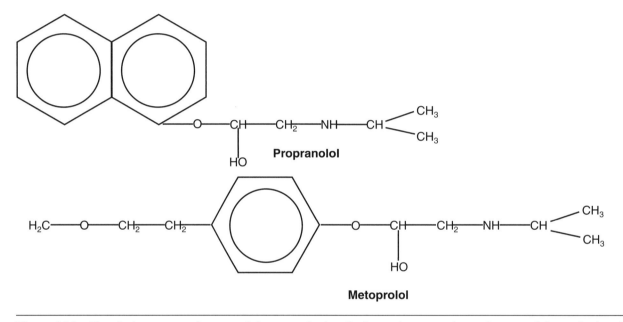

Figure 14.2 Chemical structure of propranolol, a nonselective β-adrenergic antagonist, and metoprolol, a selective, β1-antagonist.

counteract the effects of adrenergic stimulation and diminish the accompanying increases in myocardial oxygen demand. When successful blockade is achieved, the fight-or-flight response of the organism is therefore blunted. The cardiovascular inhibition results from a decreased heart rate via slowing of conduction through the atria and atrioventricular node (negative chronotropy) and decreased contractility of cardiac myocytes (negative inotropy and a decrease in systolic blood pressure). Because of the decrease in heart rate, these agents also increase end-diastolic volume, resulting in an increase in ventricular wall tension (Robertson and Robertson, 1996). This effect results in an increase in myocardial oxygen consumption acting in opposition to the beneficial effects of the lower heart rate and systolic blood pressure (i.e.,

lower rate-pressure product). However, the net effect is an improvement in the relationship between myocardial oxygen supply and demand at rest and under conditions of stress. By improving this relationship, beta blockers are considered standard therapy for all types of angina, with the exception of Prinzmetal's vasospastic angina (Robertson, Wood, Vaughn and Robertson, 1982). Beta-antagonists are potentially harmful in vasospastic angina because of the possibility of increasing spasm due to unopposed α-receptor activity (Robertson, Wood, Vaughn and Robertson, 1982).

A major benefit for the patient with cardiac disease is the increase in physical activity allowed with the use of a β-receptor antagonist (Eriksson, Osvik and Dedichen, 1977; Ling and Groel, 1979). For a given level of exertion, it is well known that patients taking beta blockers for angina are able to exercise at higher workloads and/or for a longer duration (Eriksson, Osvik and Dedichen, 1977; Ling and Groel, 1979). In a double-blind study comparing atenolol to placebo in persons with stable angina, 16 of 19 subjects demonstrated an increase in bicycle exercise performance when taking atenolol (Eriksson, Osvik and Dedichen, 1977). In a large, multisite study involving over 500 subjects with angina, nadolol was compared to propranolol (Ling and Groel, 1979). Compared to values during a baseline placebo period, there was an increase in physical performance for both drugs, as well as a decrease in the frequency of anginal attacks and in nitroglycerin requirements. These studies illustrate that beta blockers can increase exercise capacity in persons with limitations imposed by myocardial ischemia.

In addition to improving the anginal threshold, adrenergic antagonists have been designated by the Joint National Committee as one of two preferred first-line therapies for hypertension (National Institutes of Health, 1997). The mechanism of action for the antihypertensive effects are not well understood (Opie, Sonnenblick, Frishman and Thadani, 1997). The initial response to beta blockers is a decrease in cardiac output with a reflex increase in peripheral resistance, which occurs during the first 24 hr of treatment. After one to two days of treatment, peripheral resistance begins to fall and arterial pressure decreases. Studies suggest that the decrease in peripheral resistance may result from inhibition of presynaptic receptors that act to increase the release of norepinephrine, from a decrease in adrenergic outflow from the central nervous system, or from a decrease in activity of the renin-angiotensin system (Opie, Sonnenblick, Frishman and Thadani, 1997).

Beta-1 receptor antagonists have also been shown to control supraventricular and ventricular arrhythmias (Mason, 1993). They act by slowing conduction through the atrioventricular node and decreasing the ventricular response rate. They are particularly effective in the management of arrhythmias caused by increased circulating catecholamines, which occur in conditions such as acute myocardial infarction (MI), anxiety, and the postoperative period. These agents also have been found to be effective in treating ventricular tachycardia and fibrillation and mitral valve prolapse (Opie, Sonnenblick, Frishman and Thadani, 1997).

Beta-adrenergic antagonists are used in the management of acute MI and for secondary prevention of recurrences after an initial MI. For acute MI, optimal time for administration is during the initial 4 hr when the risk of ventricular fibrillation is high (Opie, Sonnenblick, Frishman and Thadani, 1997). Several trials have shown that intravenous administration of beta blockers during the early phases post-MI may reduce mortality by 10%

(Hoffman and Lefkowitz, 1996). In the postinfarction period, these agents have been shown to decrease the mortality rate when started within several weeks post-MI (Frishman and Lazar, 1990). The benefits appear to be greatest during the first year postinfarction and for persons with large infarctions (Frishman and Lazar, 1990).

For many years, beta blockers were considered contraindicated for heart failure (Cruickshank, 2000). However, recent clinical trials have shown that the addition of β-receptor antagonists to standard therapy provides a significant benefit (Squire and Barnett, 2000). Beta blocker therapy is associated with improved mortality and morbidity in terms of progression of heart failure and numbers of hospitalizations (Squire and Barnett, 2000). The desired therapeutic effect is to decrease the enhanced adrenergic tone that occurs with heart failure.

Other cardiac conditions in which β-receptor blocking agents are used include hypertrophic obstructive cardiomyopathy and acute dissecting aortic aneurysm (Hoffman and Lefkowitz, 1996). In patients with hypertrophic obstructive cardiomyopathy, beta blockers are used to relieve angina, palpitations, and syncope (Hoffman and Lefkowitz, 1996). In persons with acute dissecting aortic aneurysm, β-adrenergic blockade decreases both the force of myocardial contraction and the rate of force development (Hoffman and Lefkowitz, 1996). Additionally, long-term administration of a beta blocker may slow the progression of aortic dilation in patients with Marfan's syndrome (Shores, Berger, Murphy and Pyeritz, 1994).

As one would expect, given the variety of β-adrenergic antagonists available and the variety of clinical problems treated, administration and dosages can be quite varied. Most of these drugs are given orally, with the dosing schedule based on the half-life of the drug (*Physician's Desk Reference,* 2001). Some agents are available in sustained-release forms. There are products available in liquid form (*Physician's Desk Reference,* 2001) that can be given intravenously for acute conditions such as immediately post-MI. Beta blockers that are used for glaucoma are administered directly to the eye. The specific agent and the condition being treated determine the dose. When these drugs are used to enhance sport performance, they are given orally on the day of competition. An example of a protocol is 50 mg of metoprolol on the morning of the competition with a second dose of 100 mg 1 hr prior to the competition (Kruse, Ladefoged, Nielsen, Paulev and Sorensen, 1986).

History of Use of Substance in Sport and Exercise

In contrast to their primary use in clinical practice to manage cardiovascular conditions, the β-antagonists are used in sport to decrease anxiety. Competing in sport events creates anxiety, which is associated with increased activity of the sympathetic nervous system and increased blood levels of catecholamines. The result is increased heart rate, nervousness, and skeletal muscle tremor. Beta-antagonists block this response, preventing an increase in heart rate and allowing greater control of skeletal muscle. Theoretically, both a lower heart rate and greater control of skeletal muscle could contribute to improved performance in activities requiring precision and accuracy.

To Improve Performance in Activities Requiring Precision and Accuracy

Investigations into the enhancement of sport performance by beta blockers have been limited, and published reports have been directed to those activities requiring precision and accuracy (Kruse, Ladefoged, Nielsen, Paulev and Sorensen, 1986; Schmid, 1990). From a true sporting perspective, one of the first studies compared metoprolol to placebo in 33 amateur marksmen (Kruse, Ladefoged, Nielsen, Paulev and Sorensen, 1986). In this double-blind, crossover trial, subjects participated in two competitions that were scheduled one week apart. Subjects received either 100 mg of metoprolol or placebo 2 hr prior to shooting. Shooting scores were significantly improved with metoprolol. The enhancement in shooting performance was not correlated with changes in heart rate or systolic blood pressure. The results suggest that the improved performance resulted from decreased hand tremor. A second study reported improved performance in bobsled and sport shooting during beta blockade (Schmid, 1990).

Researchers have also investigated the effects of β-adrenoreceptor antagonists on other performance activities requiring precision and accuracy that many have not considered typical sporting events. Beta blockers have been used for many years by performing artists to reduce "stage fright" by decreasing anxiety and tremor (Cirigliano and Lynn, 1992). Stage fright is defined as somatic anxiety caused by sympathetic stimulation (Brantigan, Brantigan and Joseph, 1982). Emotion or stress produces an increase in sympathetic nervous system activity and in the release of catecholamines. The result is tachycardia, muscle tremor, and anxiety. In a double-blind, crossover trial, the effect of oxprenolol on musical performance was assessed (James, Griffith, Pearson and Newbury, 1977). Twenty-four string players received 40 mg of oxprenolol 90 min prior to a performance on one occasion, and a placebo on another occasion. Musical performance, as judged by two professional assessors, improved when the subjects received the oxprenolol

compared to the placebo. In a similar study, volunteers from a professional symphony orchestra were administered 50- and 100-mg doses of alprenolol and placebo tablets prior to performances (Liden and Gottfriess, 1974). Decreased symptoms of tremor and palpitation and increased muscle tone were reported during both the alprenolol and placebo trials. Although the finding was not statistically significant, the alprenolol trials did result in the greatest inhibition of symptoms. Brantigan and colleagues (Brantigan, Brantigan and Joseph, 1982) have also reported the effects of both β-receptor-stimulating and beta-blocking drugs in musicians. Situational anxiety symptoms were increased following the β-agonist administration and decreased with beta blocker administration. The quality of the musical performances was significantly improved as judged by experienced music critics. These studies provide evidence of improvement in performance with beta blockers and suggest a greater effect of the medication in subjects who are most affected by nervousness.

Researchers have recently reported the use of propranolol to decrease hand tremor and anxiety in surgical residents who were performing ocular microsurgery (Elman et al., 1998). This randomized, double-blind, crossover study compared 40 mg of propranolol to placebo administered 1 hr prior to surgery. As judged by the surgical resident, propranolol was effective in decreasing anxiety and surgical tremor. Whether decreased anxiety and tremor affected surgical outcome was not reported.

In the marksmanship study, Kruse and coworkers (Kruse, Ladefoged, Nielsen, Paulev and Sorensen, 1986) speculated that peripheral rather than central blockade of β1-receptors may have contributed to the beneficial effect of metoprolol on pistol shooting. Marsden and coworkers (Marsden, Foley, Owen and McAllister, 1967) reported that administering propranolol reduced and, in some cases, eliminated the increase in physiologic hand tremor (Halliday and Redfearn, 1956) brought about by β-receptor stimulation. The exact mechanism of action has not been studied in humans, but extrapolation from animal experiments suggests that β-receptors in or near the neuromuscular junction play a major role (Bowman and Raper, 1966; Molinoff, 1992). In addition, earlier evidence (Bowman and Zaimas, 1958) illustrated a differential effect of sympathomimetics (β-agonists) on slow-twitch fiber versus fast-twitch fiber and suggested that there is a dose-dependent response (Bowman and Zaimas, 1958). Type II muscle demonstrated increased submaximal tetanic contractions and enhanced fusion of twitch responses after sympathomimetic stimulation. From these data, one could speculate that high doses of β-agonists such as clenbuterol facilitate activation of type II fibers through a reduction in motor unit firing threshold and/or decreased calcium sequestration by the sarcoplasmic reticulum. On the other hand, β-receptor antagonists would effectively block these effects and reduce the frequency and magnitude of motor unit firing (Marsden, Foley, Owen and McAllister, 1967).

Another possible mechanism to explain the improvement in shooting performance with beta blockers is the effect on heart rate. Cardiac deceleration before a motor response has been associated with good performance in golf, shooting, and archery (Robazza, Bortoli and Nougier, 1999). Experienced shooters have slower heart rates during triggering compared to beginners (Helin, Sihvonen and Hanninen, 1987). Champion rifle shooters almost consistently fire during diastole and receive better scores (Helin, Sihvonen and Hanninen, 1987). Beginners who fire during diastole receive better scores than when they fire during systole (Helin, Sihvonen and Hanninen, 1987). During systole, the entire body makes a small jerk, which interferes with tasks that require careful aiming (Helin, Sihvonen and Hanninen, 1987).

Effects on Performance of Activities Requiring Increased Physical Work Capacity

As discussed previously, the major beneficial effects of beta blockers lie in their ability to decrease myocardial oxygen demands, resulting in an overall decrease in cardiac output. Numerous studies of individuals without cardiac limitations during acute exercise generally have concluded that administration of a β-receptor antagonist does not enhance, but reduces, maximal exercise capacity (Kaiser, Hylander, Eliasson and Kaijser, 1985; Gordon and Duncan, 1991; Cruickshank, 2000). However, several factors that affect the acute response must be taken into account, including the specific characteristics of the agent, the level of physical conditioning, and the dosage (Gordon and Duncan, 1991; Loefsjoegaard-Nilsson, Atmer, Gunolf and Krug-Gourley, 1992).

In both normotensive persons and individuals with uncomplicated hypertension, nonselective beta blockers decrease maximal exercise capacity in a dose-dependent manner (Kaiser, Hylander, Eliasson and Kaijser, 1985; Cruickshank, 2000). Beta-1 selective agents have less of an effect on maximal exercise capacity compared to nonselective agents (Gordon and Duncan, 1991). Cohen-Solal and colleagues (Cohen-Solal, Baleynaud, Laperche, Sebag and Gourgon, 1993) reported no effect on maximal oxygen consumption, or on duration of exercise, in untrained persons with hypertension who were taking a β1 selective agent. A similar study showed minimal effects on exercise performance in well-conditioned subjects who were taking carvedilol, a nonselective

beta blocker with α-receptor-blocking properties (Loefsjoegaard-Nilsson, Atmer, Gunolf and Krug-Gourley, 1992). With β-adrenergic blockade, there appears to be an increase in stroke volume and arteriovenous oxygen difference that compensates for the decreased heart rate (van Baak, 1988).

In contrast to the acute responses, long-term cardiovascular adaptations to exercise training appear to occur both in asymptomatic persons and in coronary artery disease patients with beta blockade (Gordon, Kruger, Hons and Cilliers, 1983; Savin, Gordon, Kaplan, Hewitt, Harrison and Haskell, 1985). However, improvements with training appear to be less than these occurring in subjects taking a placebo (Stewart, Effron, Valenti and Kelemen, 1990; Gordon and Duncan, 1991). Additionally, β-antagonists do not seem to interfere with training-induced improvements in muscle strength (Stewart, Effron, Valenti and Kelemen, 1990).

The studies cited (Kaiser, Hylander, Eliasson and Kaijser, 1985; Gordon and Duncan, 1991; Loefsjoegaard-Nilsson, Atmer, Gunolf and Krug-Gourley, 1992; Cohen-Solal, Baleynaud, Laperche, Sebag and Gourgon, 1993; Cruickshank, 2000), as well as another study (Thadani, Davidson, Singleton and Taylor, 1979), suggest that the only consistent improvement in exercise capacity and physical work performance occurs in the individual with cardiac disease under beta blockade. Aerobic exercise and circuit weight training are key components of well-designed cardiac rehabilitation programs. Often patients as well as the members of the health care team consider some of the physical rehabilitation activities to be athletic events. However, the element of competition should be minimized because of its inherent, and often counterproductive, increase in sympathetic activity.

Clinical Pharmacology

As previously discussed, β-receptor antagonists have a variety of effects on the cardiovascular system. In addition, they can have significant effects on the pulmonary system; they impact both glucose and fat metabolism; and they have been shown to induce clinically significant changes in temperature regulation (Gordon, Myburgh, Schwellnus and Van Rensburg, 1987). This broad range of effects can be attributed to the extensive distribution of β-receptors throughout the body (Nagatomo and Koike, 2000).

In addition to the aforementioned effects on the heart and its pumping ability, the cardiovascular system can be affected by blockade of β2-receptors that reside on smooth muscle cells in the periphery (Molinoff, 1992). Stimulation of β2-receptors by epinephrine or norepinephrine results in vasodilation. Binding of a β2-receptor antagonist results in an inhibition of smooth muscle relaxation and higher total peripheral resistance (afterload on the heart) (Oates, 1996). Likewise, in the lung, β2-receptor antagonists inhibit smooth muscle relaxation in pulmonary bronchioles (Hoffman and Lefkowitz, 1996). The result is an increase in bronchoconstriction and narrowing of the airways. Inhibition of liver receptor sites results in decreased glycogenolysis and the potential for hypoglycemia (Molinoff, 1992). Lypolysis and the mobilization of free fatty acids can also be affected by β-receptor inhibition (Molinoff, 1992; Hoffman and Lefkowitz, 1996).

Contraindications and Warnings

Although some benefit has been derived by individuals who have congestive heart failure (Squire and Barnett, 2000), this has only recently been demonstrated, and these patients and their health care providers should use extreme caution concerning use of a beta blocker. Persons with either first- or second-degree heart block should not take beta blockers (Taboulet, Cariou, Berdeaux and Bismuth, 1993; Hoffman and Lefkowitz, 1996). Furthermore, antagonists with high lipid solubility and anti-arrhythmic characteristics (e.g., propranolol, oxprenolol) are extremely lethal (Ellenhorn and Barceloux, 1988). Administration of nonselective beta blockers and successful inhibition of the β2-receptor sites in the pulmonary bronchioles could induce bronchospasm in the individual with asthma (Hoffman and Lefkowitz, 1996). Metabolic changes, especially in blood glucose levels, could have severe consequences for the type I or insulin-dependent diabetic (Molinoff, 1992).

Toxicity, Adverse Reactions, and Overdosage

The most common clinical characteristics suggesting an adverse reaction to ingestion of a beta-blocking agent are bradycardia (heart rate <60 bpm), orthostatic hypotension (a drop in blood pressure), and life-threatening arrhythmias (Love, 1994). In a review of the literature, Love (1994) found that the most common signs and symptoms occurring with overdosage of beta-blocking agents were hypotension and bradycardia. The agent most frequently found to be responsible was propranolol. This finding is more than likely attributable to the fact that propranolol is the prototypical beta blocker, having first been developed in the early 1960s, and that Love reviewed studies conducted between 1963 and 1993. Adverse reactions are also accentuated with ingestion of alcohol (Taboulet, Cariou, Berdeaux and Bismuth, 1993; Love, 1994). As mentioned previously, these effects depend on the selectivity of the agent; but usually at an overdose level, even a cardioselective agent (β1 selective) will successfully compete for β2- and other adrenergic receptor sites (Ellenhorn and Barceloux, 1988; Taboulet, Cariou, Berdeaux and Bismuth, 1993).

Precautions

When we think of an athlete, the typical image is generally one of a relatively young and very healthy individual. The athlete competing in a sport that requires a very steady hand and little physical exertion (e.g., a marksman) does not necessarily fit this stereotype and could be older and/or under the care of a physician for a significant medical problem. For those individuals discussed earlier who participate in sporting events that require accuracy and precision, concern should arise when β-adrenergic antagonists are taken without medical supervision.

Other populations of athletes, particularly those with lower-extremity impairments, enjoy the competition of archery, riflery, and pistol shooting. Use of β-antagonist drugs should be a concern, especially for those with a spinal cord injury above T4-T6. Individuals with this level of injury may already have compromised sympathetic nervous systems, and administration must be done with caution. In particular, temperature control and the potential inhibition of vasodilation of skin vessels could lead to hyperthermia if environmental conditions are not optimal (Hoffman, 1986). Some evidence exists for an increase in body temperature in cardiac patients, who typically have an intact sympathetic nervous system (Gordon, Myburgh, Schwellnus and Van Rensburg, 1987).

Participation in athletic events by individuals with significant medical problems has become more common as evidenced by the continuing success of the Paralympics. There is little concern for safety at this and larger events because of the close monitoring of athletes that already occurs. We suggest that organizers of even small sporting events do a screening to determine whether participants have any of the medical conditions we have discussed in the chapter. One should be especially concerned about newcomers who happen to be cognizant of the calming effects of anti-catecholamines. After all, first-time performers in an event usually experience the greatest anxiety levels.

Legal Versus Banned Beta-Adrenergic Antagonists

Beta-adrenergic antagonists are legal and are used primarily in the treatment of hypertension and cardiac impairments, and they should be considered therapeutic. However, beta blockers were added to the list of prohibited substances in 1986 by the National Collegiate Athletic Association (Wagner, 1987) when it was documented that their use resulted in improved shooting scores. Through association, they have also been prohibited in archery, ski jumping, freestyle skiing, sailing, synchronized swimming, diving, and the pentathlon (Catlin and Murray, 1996). Use of adrenergic antagonists is considered a serious offense, and few excuses are accepted by the International Olympic Committee. Persons being treated with beta blockers for a cardiac condition can participate in shooting competitions only with special permission (Kruse, Ladefoged, Nielsen, Paulev and Sorensen, 1986).

As a substitute for beta blockers, athletes may take herbal substances to decrease anxiety. Kava *(Piper methysticum)* preparations are used for nervous activity, insomnia, and restlessness (Murray and Pizzorno, 1998). In a double-blind study, subjects received either 300 mg/day of a 70% kavalactone extract or placebo for four weeks (Kinzler, Kromer and Lehmann, 1991). After four weeks, subjects who took the kava had a significant reduction in symptoms of anxiety including feelings of nervousness, heart palpitations, chest pain, headache, and dizziness. In comparison to benzodiazepines (valium) and alcohol, kava extract is not associated with depressed mental function or impairment in driving (Herberg, 1993; Munte, Heinze, Matzke and Steitz, 1993). Valerian, another herbal preparation used for insomnia and anxiety, is considered a second choice to kava (Murray, 1995). These two herbal preparations are not banned and may be used by athletes in an attempt to improve performance.

New agents are continuously being developed as new therapeutic uses for these compounds are demonstrated (Cruickshank, 2000; Squire and Barnett, 2000). The ability of sport governing bodies to identify these drugs through assays of blood or urine may be hampered because of the variety of compounds and their unique chemical structures. Given the rapid developments in molecular biology and receptor research, it is certain that future β-adrenergic antagonists will be developed that require examination and scrutiny by sport and competitive governing bodies if they are shown to enhance sport performance.

References

Bowman, W. and Raper, C. (1966). Effects of sympathomimetic amines on neuromuscular transmission. *Br J Pharmacol Chemother* 27: 313-331.

Bowman, W. and Zaimas, E. (1958). The effects of adrenaline, noradrenaline and isoprenaline on skeletal muscle contractions in the cat. *J Physiol* 144: 92-107.

Brantigan, C., Brantigan, T. and Joseph, N. (1982). Effect of beta blockade and beta stimulation on stage fright. *Am J Med* 72: 88-94.

Catlin, D. and Murray, T. (1996). Performance-enhancing drugs, fair competition, and Olympic sport. *JAMA* 276: 231-237.

Cirigliano, M. and Lynn, L. (1992). Diagnosis and treatment of stage fright. *Hosp Pract* 27(4A; Office Ed): 58-60, 62.

Cohen-Solal, A., Baleynaud, S., Laperche, T., Sebag, C. and Gourgon, R. (1993). Cardiopulmonary response during exercise of a β1 selective β-blocker (atenolol) and a calcium channel blocker (diltiazem) in untrained subjects with hypertension. *J Cardiovasc Pharmacol* 22(1): 33-38.

Cruickshank, J. (2000). Beta-blockers continue to surprise us. *Eur Heart J* 21: 354-364.

Ellenhorn, M. and Barceloux, D. (1988). Class II Drugs: Beta-Blockers. In Ellenhorn, M. and Barceloux, D. (Eds.) *Medical Toxicology. Diagnosis and Treatment of Human Poisoning.* New York, Elsevier.

Elman, M., Sugar, J., Fiscella, R., Deutsch, T., Noth, J., Nyberg, M., Packo, K. and Anderson, R. (1998). The effect of propranolol versus placebo on resident surgical performance. *Trans Am Ophthalmol Soc* 96: 283-291.

Eriksson, J., Osvik, K. and Dedichen, J. (1977). Atenolol in the treatment of angina pectoris. *Acta Medica Scand* 201(6): 579-584.

Frishman, W. and Lazar, E. (1990). Reduction of mortality, sudden death and non-fatal reinfarction with beta-adrenergic blockers in survivors of acute myocardial infarction: a new hypothesis regarding the cardioprotective action of beta-adrenergic blockade. *Am J Cardiol* 66: 66G-70G.

Gordon, N. and Duncan, J. (1991). Effect of beta blockers on exercise physiology: implications for exercise training. *Med Sci Sports Exerc* 23(6): 668-676.

Gordon, N., Kruger, P., Hons, B. and Cilliers, J. (1983). Improved exercise ventilatory responses after training in coronary heart disease during long-term beta-adrenergic blockade. *Am J Cardiol* 51: 755-758.

Gordon, N., Myburgh, D., Schwellnus, M. and Van Rensburg, J. (1987). Effect of β-blockade on exercise core temperature in coronary artery disease patients. *Med Sci Sports Exerc* 19(6): 591-596.

Halliday, A. and Redfearn, J. (1956). An analysis of the frequencies of finger tremor in healthy subjects. *J Physiol* 134: 600-611.

Helin, P., Sihvonen, T. and Hanninen, O. (1987). Timing of the triggering action of shooting in relation to the cardiac cycle. *Br J Sports Med* 21(1): 33-36.

Herberg, K. (1993). The influence of kava-special extract WS 1490 on safety-relevant performance alone and in combination with ethyl alcohol. *Blutalkohol* 30: 96-105.

Hoffman, B. and Lefkowitz, R. (1996). Catecholamines, sympathomimetic drugs, and adrenergic receptor antagonists. J. Hardman, L. Limbird, P. Molinoff and R. Ruddon. Goodman and Gilman's *The Pharmacological Basis of Therapeutics.* New York, McGraw-Hill, 199-248.

Hoffman, M. (1986). Cardiorespiratory fitness and training in quadriplegics and paraplegics. *Sports Med* 3: 312-330.

James, I., Griffith, D., Pearson, R. and Newbury, P. (1977). Effect of oxprenolol on stage-fright in musicians. *Lancet:* 952-954.

Kaiser, P., Hylander, B., Eliasson, K. and Kaijser, L. (1985). Effect of beta-sensitive and nonselective beta blockade on blood pressure relative to physical performance in men with systemic hypertension. *Am J Cardiol* 55: 79D-84D.

Kaumann, A. (1997). Four β-adrenoceptor subtypes in the mammalian heart. *Trends Pharmacol Sci* 18(3): 70-76.

Kinzler, E., Kromer, J. and Lehmann, E. (1991). Clinical efficacy of a kava extract in patients with anxiety syndrome: double-blind placebo controlled study over four weeks. *Arzneim Forsch* 41: 584-588.

Kruse, P., Ladefoged, J., Nielsen, U., Paulev, P. and Sorensen, J. (1986). Beta-blockade used in precision sports: effect on pistol shooting performance. *J Appl Physiol* 61: 417-420.

Lefkowitz, R., Hoffman, B. and Taylor, P. (1996). Neurotransmission: the autonomic and somatic motor nervous systems. J. Hardman, L. Limbird, P. Molinoff and R. Ruddon. Goodman and Gilman's *The Pharmacological Basis of Therapeutics.* New York, McGraw-Hill, 105-139.

Liden, S. and Gottfriess, C. (1974). Beta-blocking agents in the treatment of catecholamine-induced symptoms in musicians. *Lancet* 2: 529.

Ling, A. and Groel, J. (1979). Improved physical performance as a therapeutic objective in patients with angina. *Br J Clin Pharmacol* 7(Suppl 2): 161S-166S.

Loefsjoegaard-Nilsson, E., Atmer, B., Gunolf, M. and Krug-Gourley, S. (1992). Effects of carvedilol during exercise. *J Cardiovasc Pharmacol* 19(Suppl 1): S108-S113.

Love, J. (1994). Beta blocker toxicity after overdose: when do symptoms develop in adults? *J Emerg Med* 12(6): 799-802.

Marsden, C., Foley, T., Owen, D. and McAllister, R. (1967). Peripheral β-adrenergic receptors concerned with tremor. *Clin Sci Lond* 33: 53-65.

Mason, J.W. (1993). A comparison of seven antiarrhythmic drugs in patients with ventricular tachyarrhythmias. Electrophysiologic Study versus Electrocardiographic Monitoring Investigators. *N Eng J Med* 329: 452-458.

Molinoff, P. (1992). Evolving properties of β-adrenergic receptor antagonists. *Pharmacotherapy* 12(2): 144-153.

Munte, T., Heinze, H., Matzke, M. and Steitz, J. (1993). Effects of oxazepam and an extract of kava roots (piper methysticum) on event related potentials in a word recognition task. *Neuropsychobiology* 27: 46-53.

Murray, M. (1995). *The Healing Power of Herbs.* Rocklin, CA, Prima Health.

Murray, M. and Pizzorno, J. (1998). *Encyclopedia of Natural Medicine.* Rocklin, CA, Prima Health.

Nagatomo, T. and Koike, K. (2000). Recent advances in structure, binding sites with ligands and pharmacological function of β-adrenoceptors obtained by molecular biology and molecular modeling. *Life Sci* 66(25): 2419-2426.

National Institutes of Health (1997). The Sixth Report of the Joint National Committee on the Prevention, Detection and Treatment of High Blood Pressure. Washington, DC, U.S. Department of Health and Human Services.

Oates, J. (1996). Antihypertensive agents and the drug therapy of hypertension. J. Hardman, L. Limbird, P. Molinoff and R. Ruddon. Goodman and Gilman's *The Pharmacological Basis of Therapeutics.* New York, McGraw-Hill, 780-808.

Opie, L., Sonnenblick, E., Frishman, W. and Thadani, U. (1997). Beta-blocking agents. L. Opie. *Drugs for the Heart.* Philadelphia, Saunders, 1-30.

Physician's Desk Reference. (2001). Montvale, NJ, Medical Economics Co.

Robazza, C., Bortoli, L. and Nougier, V. (1999). Emotions, heart rate and performance in archery. *J Sports Med Phys Fitness* 39: 169-176.

Robertson, R. and Robertson, D., Eds. (1996). Drugs used in the treatment of myocardial ischemia. *The Pharmacological Basis of Therapeutics.* New York, McGraw-Hill.

Robertson, R., Wood, A., Vaughn, W. and Robertson, D. (1982). Exacerbation of vasotonic angina pectoris by propranolol. *Circulation* 65: 281-285.

Savin, W., Gordon, E., Kaplan, S., Hewitt, B., Harrison, D. and Haskell, W. (1985). Exercise training during long-term beta-blockade treatment in healthy subjects. *Am J Cardiol* 55: 101D-109D.

Schmid, P. (1990). Der einsatz von beta-rezeptoren-blockern im leistungssport. *Wiener Medizinische Wochenschrift* 140(6-7): 184-188.

Shores, J., Berger, K., Murphy, E. and Pyeritz, R. (1994). Progression of aortic dilation and the benefit of long term beta-adrenergic blockade in Marfan's syndrome. *N Eng J Med* 330: 1335-1341.

Squire, I. and Barnett, D. (2000). The rational use of beta-adrenoceptor blockers in the treatment of heart failure. The changing face of an old therapy. *Br J Clin Pharmacol* 49: 1-9.

Stewart, K., Effron, M., Valenti, S. and Kelemen, M. (1990). Effects of diltiazem or propranolol during exercise training of hypertensive men. *Med Sci Sports Exerc* 22: 171-177.

Stryer, L. (1995). *Biochemistry.* New York, Freeman.

Taboulet, P., Cariou, A., Berdeaux, A. and Bismuth, C. (1993). Pathophysiology and management of self-poisoning with beta-blockers. *J Toxicol Clin Toxicol* 31(4): 531-551.

Thadani, V., Davidson, C., Singleton, W. and Taylor, S. (1979). Comparison of the immediate effects of five beta-adrenoreceptor-blocking drugs with different ancillary properties in angina pectoris. *N Engl J Med* 300: 750-755.

van Baak, M. (1988). Beta-adrenergic blockade and exercise: An update. *Sports Med* 5: 209-225.

Wagner, J. (1987). Substance abuse policies and guidelines in amateur and professional athletics. *Am J Hosp Pharmacy* 44(2): 305-310.

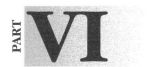

Nutritional Ergogenic Aids

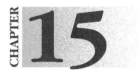

Macronutrients and Metabolic Intermediates

Ellen Coleman, RD, MA, MPH

Suzanne Nelson Steen, DSc, RD

Nutrition plays a key role in fitness and peak performance. Having the right fuel on board can improve daily training, enhance postexercise recovery, increase muscle mass, decrease body fat, help prevent injury, and maintain overall good health. Now more than ever, there is an increase in interest and demand for accurate sport nutrition information.

This chapter presents the role of carbohydrate, protein, and fat in exercise along with myths and facts about high-protein diets, amino acid supplements, fat loading, and medium-chain triglycerides. A discussion of the metabolic intermediates carnitine, pyruvate, and ribose follows.

Carbohydrate

It is well established that adequate carbohydrate stores (muscle and liver glycogen and blood glucose) are necessary for optimum athletic performance. Athletes are encouraged to consume a high-carbohydrate diet (7-10 g of carbohydrate/kg/day) to meet the energy demands of training (table 15.1). Consuming adequate carbohydrate prior to endurance exercise can reduce the risk of early fatigue during exercise. Carbohydrate intake during endurance exercise can improve performance by maintaining blood glucose levels and carbohydrate oxidation. After exercise, a high carbohydrate intake is necessary to replenish muscle and liver glycogen stores.

Carbohydrate Availability During Exercise

Muscle glycogen represents the major source of carbohydrate in the body (300-400 g or 1200-1600 calories), followed by liver glycogen (75-100 g or 300-400 calories) and, lastly, blood glucose (25 g or 100 calories).

Exercise energetics dictate that carbohydrate is the preferred fuel for exercise intensities at and above 65% of $\dot{V}O_2$max—the levels at which most athletes train and compete. Fat oxidation cannot supply adenosine triphosphate (ATP) rapidly enough to support such high-intensity exercise. While it is possible to exercise at light to moderate levels (<60% of $\dot{V}O_2$max) with low levels of muscle glycogen and blood glucose, it is impossible to meet the ATP requirements required for heavy exercise when these fuels are depleted. The utilization of muscle glycogen is most rapid during the early stages of exercise and is exponentially related to exercise intensity. Although muscle glycogen is the primary source of carbohydrate during exercise intensities above 65% of $\dot{V}O_2$max, blood glucose becomes an increasingly important source of carbohydrate as muscle glycogen stores decline (Frail and Burke, 1994).

Consuming Carbohydrates Before Exercise

Consuming carbohydrate several hours prior to morning exercise helps to restore suboptimal liver glycogen stores,

Table 15.1 High-Carbohydrate Foods

Food group	Calories	Carbohydrates (grams)	Food group	Calories	Carbohydrates (grams)
Milk			**Vegetables**		
Low-fat (2%) milk (1 cup)	121	12	Corn (1/2 cup)	89	21
Skim milk (1 cup)	86	12	Lima beans (1/2 cup)	108	20
Chocolate milk (1 cup)	208	26	Peas, green (1/2 cup)	63	12
Pudding, any flavor (1/2 cup)	161	30	Potato (1 large)	220	50
Frozen yogurt, low-fat (1 cup)	220	34	Sweet potato (1 large)	118	28
Fruit-flavored low-fat yogurt					
(1 cup)	225	42	**Grains**		
			Bagel (1)	165	31
Beans			Biscuit (1)	103	13
Blackeye peas (1/2 cup)	134	22	White bread (1 slice)	61	12
Pinto beans (1 cup)	235	44	Whole wheat bread		
Navy beans (1 cup)	259	48	(1 slice)	55	11
Refried beans (1/2 cup)	142	26	Breadsticks (2 sticks)	77	15
Garbanzo beans (chick peas)			Cornbread (1 square)	178	23
(1 cup)	269	45	Cereal, ready-to-eat (1 cup)	110	24
White beans (1 cup)	249	45	Oatmeal (1/2 cup)	66	12
			Cream of rice (3/4 cup)	95	21
Fruits			Cream of wheat (3/4 cup)	96	20
Apple (1 medium)	81	21	Flavored oatmeal, Quaker		
Apple juice (1 cup)	111	28	instant (1 packet)	110	25
Applesauce (1 cup)	232	60	Graham crackers (2 squares)	60	11
Banana (1)	105	27	Saltines (5 crackers)	60	10
Canteloupe (1 cup)	57	14	Triscuit crackers (3 crackers)	60	10
Dates, dried (10)	228	61	Pancake (4-in. diameter)	61	9
Fruit Roll-Ups (1 roll)	50	12	Waffles (2, 3.5 by 5.5 in.)	130	17
Grapes (1 cup)	114	28	Rice (1 cup)	223	50
Grape juice (1 cup)	96	23	Rice, brown (1 cup)	232	50
Orange (1)	65	16	Hamburger bun (1)	119	21
Orange juice (1 cup)	112	26	Hot dog bun (1)	119	21
Pear (1)	98	25	Noodles, spaghetti (1 cup)	159	34
Pineapple (1 cup)	77	19	Flour tortilla (1)	85	15
Prunes, dried (10)	201	53	Oatmeal raisin cookie	62	9
Raisins (2/3 cup)	302	79	Pizza (cheese, 1 slice)	290	39
Raspberries (1 cup)	61	14	Popcorn, plain (1 cup,		
Strawberries (1 cup)	45	11	popped)	26	6
Watermelon (1 cup)	50	12	English muffin	130	25
			Fig bar (1)	50	10
Vegetables			Granola bar (honey		
Three-bean salad (1/2 cup)	90	20	and oats, 1 oz)	125	19
Carrots (1 medium)	31	8	Pretzels (1 oz)	106	21

From: Coleman, E., Steen, S.N. *Ultimate Sports Nutrition,* 2nd ed. Bull Publishing: Palo Alto, CA, 2000.

which will aid events that rely heavily on blood glucose (figure 15.1). If muscle glycogen stores are also low, consuming carbohydrate 2 to 4 hr before exercise can help to increase them as well. The pre-exercise meal also helps prevent athletes from feeling hungry, which in itself may be distracting and impair performance (Coggan and Swanson, 1992).

Research by Sherman and colleagues suggests that the pre-exercise meal contain 1 to 4.5 g of carbohydrate/kg, consumed 1 to 4 hr prior to exercise (Sherman et al.,

1989, 1991). To avoid potential gastrointestinal distress, the carbohydrate and calorie content of the meal should be reduced the closer to exercise the meal is consumed. For example, a carbohydrate feeding of 1 g/kg is appropriate an hour before exercise, whereas 4.5 g/kg can be consumed 4 hr before exercise.

Examples of solid high-carbohydrate foods for pre-exercise meals include fruit and grain products such as cereal, breads, and pasta. Some lean protein can also be included in the meal, such as low-fat/nonfat yogurt,

Breakfast	Lunch/dinner
Waffles with strawberries	Turkey sandwich with tomato on whole wheat roll
Low-fat yogurt	Fresh fruit salad
Banana	Oatmeal raisin cookie
Orange juice	Low-fat frozen yogurt
	Sport drink
Cornflakes	
Low-fat milk	Pasta with tomato sauce
English muffin with jam	Mixed green salad
Cranberry juice	Italian bread
	Sherbet
Scrambled eggs	Low-fat milk
Bagel with jam	
Orange juice	Thick crust cheese pizza
	Fresh fruit salad
	Breadsticks
	Lemonade

Figure 15.1   Examples of pre-event meals. Serving sizes depend on the weight of the athlete and the length of time before an event.

chicken, turkey, and low-fat cheese. Adequate fluids from fruit juices, sport drinks, milk, and water are important to promote hydration. The athlete may also incorporate liquid meals or high-carbohydrate liquid supplements.

Liquid Meals

Liquid meals such as the Gatorade Nutrition Shake, Nutrament, and Go! may be considered if gastric emptying is a concern. These can be consumed closer to competition than regular meals because of their shorter gastric emptying time. This may help to avoid precompetition nausea for athletes who are tense and who have an associated delay in gastric emptying. Liquid meals are also convenient for athletes competing in daylong competitions, tournaments, and multiple events (table 15.2).

Glycemic Index

The glycemic index (GI) provides a way to rank carbohydrate-rich foods according to the blood glucose response following their intake. Generally, foods are divided into those that have a high GI (glucose, bread, potatoes, breakfast cereal, sport drinks), a moderate GI (sucrose, soft drinks, oats, tropical fruits such as bananas and mangos), or a low GI (fructose, milk, yogurt, lentils, pasta, cold-climate fruits such as apples and oranges) (figure 15.2). Tables of the GI of a large number of foods have been published internationally (Foster-Powell and Brand Miller, 1995).

Some practitioners have recommended manipulating the GI of foods and meals to enhance carbohydrate availability and improve athletic performance. For example, low-GI foods are often recommended before exercise to promote sustained carbohydrate availability. Moderate- to high-GI foods are recommended during exercise to promote carbohydrate oxidation and following exercise to promote glycogen repletion.

Thomas and colleagues initially raised interest in the use of GI in sport by manipulating the glycemic response to pre-exercise meals (Thomas et al., 1991). They reported that the consumption of 1 g of carbohydrate/kg from a low-GI food (lentils) 1 hr prior to cycling at 67% of $\dot{V}O_2$max increased endurance compared to an equal amount of carbohydrate from a high-GI food (potatoes). The low-GI lentils promoted lower postprandial blood glucose and insulin responses and more stable blood glucose levels during exercise compared with the high-GI potatoes.

In a second study, Thomas and associates provided 1 g of carbohydrate/kg from two low-GI meals and two high-GI meals (powdered foods and breakfast cereals) 1 hr prior to cycling to exhaustion at 70% of $\dot{V}O_2$max (Thomas et al., 1994). The low-GI meals were associated with higher blood glucose levels after 90 min of exercise compared to the high-GI meals and appeared to provide a sustained source of carbohydrate throughout exercise. However, there were no differences in time to exhaustion between the low-GI meals and high-GI meals, and there was no correlation between exercise time and meal GI.

There is insufficient evidence to support the recommendation that all athletes consume low-GI index foods before exercise. A low-GI pre-exercise meal may be beneficial for athletes who react negatively to high-GI pre-exercise meals (early fatigue or hypoglycemia) and for endurance events in which consuming carbohydrate is not practical or possible (Burke et al., 1998).

Table 15.2 Nutrition Beverages

Beverage	Flavors	Calories per 8-oz serving	Carbohydrate (grams)	Protein (grams)	Fat (grams)
GatorPro Sports Nutrition Supplement (Gatorade Company)	Chocolate, vanilla	360	58	16	7
Sport Shake (Mid-America Farms)	Chocolate, vanilla, strawberry	310	45	11	10
Endura Optimizer (Unipro, Inc.)	Chocolate, vanilla, orange	260	57	11	Less than 1
Protein Repair Formula (PurePower Sports Nutrition)	Vanilla	200	26	20	1.5
Metabolol II (Champion Nutrition)	Plain	260	40	20	2
Ensure (Ross Laboratories)	Chocolate, vanilla, strawberry	254	35	9	9
Nutrament (Mead Johnson Nutritionals)	Chocolate, banana, vanilla, strawberry, coconut	240	34	6.5	11
Sustacal (Mead Johnson Nutritionals)	Chocolate, vanilla, strawberry, eggnog	240	33	5.5	14.5
Go!	Vanilla, chocolate, strawberry, banana, orange cream	235	40	14	3

From: Coleman, E., Steen, S.N. *Ultimate Sports Nutrition,* 2nd ed. Bull Publishing, Palo Alto, CA, 2000.

Athletes who react negatively to high-GI foods can choose from several strategies (Coleman, 1998). These are (1) to consume a low GI carbohydrate before exercise, (2) to take in carbohydrate a few minutes before exercise, or (3) to wait until exercising to consume carbohydrate. The exercise-induced rise in the hormones epinephrine, norepinephrine, and growth hormone inhibits the release of insulin and so counters insulin's effect in lowering blood glucose.

Carbohydrate Intake During Exercise

Carbohydrate feedings during exercise lasting an hour or longer may enhance performance by providing glucose at a time when muscle glycogen stores are diminished. Thus, carbohydrate utilization (and therefore ATP production) can continue at a high rate and performance is enhanced. Coyle and colleagues have demonstrated that consuming carbohydrate during cycling exercise at 70% of $\dot{V}O_2$max can delay fatigue by 30 to 60 min (Coyle et al., 1983; Coyle et al., 1986). Practically speaking, athletes can exercise longer and/or sprint harder at the end of exercise.

Coyle and colleagues compared the effects of carbohydrate feedings on the onset of fatigue and decrease in work capacity of cyclists (Coyle et al., 1983). The carbohydrate feedings enabled the cyclists to exercise an average of 33 min longer (159 min compared to 126 min) before reaching the point of fatigue. The carbohydrate feedings maintained blood glucose at higher levels, thereby increasing the utilization of blood glucose for energy.

Coyle and associates also measured performance during strenuous prolonged bicycling with and without carbohydrate feedings (Coyle et al., 1986). During the ride without carbohydrate feedings, fatigue occurred after 3 hr and was preceded by a drop in blood glucose. During the ride in which the cyclists were fed carbohydrate, blood glucose levels were maintained and the cyclists were able to ride an additional hour before reaching the point of fatigue. The two groups utilized muscle glycogen at the same rate, indicating that endurance was improved through the maintenance of blood glucose levels rather than through glycogen sparing.

Carbohydrate feedings may also improve performance in sports such as football, soccer, and basketball that require repeated bouts of high-intensity, short-duration effort. Davis and colleagues evaluated the effect of carbohydrate feedings on performance during intermittent, high-intensity cycling (Davis et al., 1997). The subjects performed repeated 1-min sprints at 120% to 130% of $\dot{V}O_2$max, separated by 3 min of rest, until fatigue. Before the exercise and every 20 min during

High Glycemic Index Foods (GI > 85)

Breads/Cereals/Grains

White bread, whole wheat bread, rye flour bread, barley flour bread, plain bagel, cornmeal, cornflakes, couscous, millet, Cheerios, cream of wheat, Mueslix, corn bran cereal, Crispix cereal, Rice Krispies, Corn Chex cereal, Grape-Nuts, shredded wheat, Total cereal, oatmeal, brown rice, rice cakes, soda crackers, melba toast, muffins, waffles, cheese pizza

Vegetables/Fruits

Raisins, watermelon, carrots, potatoes

Desserts/Snacks

Angel food cake, cake doughnut, croissant, corn chips, ice cream

Beverages

Sport drinks, soft drinks

Simple sugars

Sucrose, glucose, hard candy, maltose, molasses, honey/syrups

Moderate Glycemic Index Foods (GI = 60-85)

Breads/Cereals/Grains

Oat bran bread, rye kernel bread, white pita bread, bulgar bread, mixed grain bread, all-bran cereal, Bran Chex cereal, oat bran cereal, Special K cereal, cracked barley, buckwheat, bulgur, white rice, basmati rice, par-boiled rice, wild rice, spaghetti, linguine

Vegetables/Fruits

Banana, fruit cocktail, grapefruit juice, grapes, kiwi, mango, papaya, orange, sweet potatoes/yams, sweet corn

Desserts/Snacks

Sponge cake, pastry, popcorn, low-fat ice cream

Low Glycemic Index Foods (GI < 60)

Breads/Cereals/Grains

Barley kernel bread, barley, rice bran, wheat kernels, spaghetti

Vegetables/Fruits

Tomato soup, apples, dried apricots, cherries, grapefruit, fresh peaches, fresh pears, plums, beans (all types), lentils, dried peas

Beverages

Milk

Desserts/Snacks

Peanuts, yogurt

Simple sugars

Fructose

Figure 15.2   The glycemic index for some foods. White bread was used as the reference food.

Adapted from Foster-Powell K, Miller JB. International tables of glycemic indices. *Am J. Clin Nutr,* 62:871S-93S, 1995.

exercise, the subjects drank a placebo or a 6% carbohydrate-electrolyte drink that provided 47 g of carbohydrate per hour. The average time to fatigue in the carbohydrate trial was 89 min (21 sprints) compared to 58 min (14 sprints) for the placebo trial. The results of this study suggest that the benefits of carbohydrate feedings are not limited to prolonged endurance exercise.

The performance benefits of a pre-exercise carbohydrate feeding appear to be additive to those of consuming carbohydrate during exercise. In a study by

Wright and colleagues (Wright et al., 1991), cyclists who received carbohydrate both 3 hr before and during exercise were able to exercise longer (289 min) than when receiving carbohydrate either before exercise (236 min) or during exercise (266 min) compared to placebo (201 min).

Combining carbohydrate feedings improved performance more than either feeding alone. However, the improvement in performance with pre-exercise carbohydrate feedings was less than when smaller quantities of carbohydrate were consumed during exercise. If the goal is to provide a continuous supply of glucose during exercise, the athlete should consume carbohydrate during exercise.

Coyle and Montain suggest that athletes take in 30 to 60 g (120-240 kcal) of carbohydrate every hour to improve performance (Coyle and Montain, 1992). This amount can be obtained through either carbohydrate-rich foods or fluids. Consuming small amounts at frequent intervals (every 30 to 60 min) helps to promote hydration, maintain blood glucose levels, and prevent gastrointestinal upset.

Although it makes sense for athletes to consume carbohydrate sources that are rapidly digested and absorbed to promote carbohydrate oxidation, the glycemic response to carbohydrate feedings during exercise has not been systematically studied. However, most athletes choose carbohydrate-rich foods (sport bars and gels) and fluids (sport drinks) that would be classified as having a moderate to high GI (Burke et al., 1998).

Liquid Versus Solid Carbohydrate

The benefits of consuming beverages containing carbohydrate during exercise are well established. However, endurance athletes often consume high-carbohydrate foods such as sport bars, fig bars, cookies, and fruit. The protein and fat found in many high-carbohydrate foods can delay gastric emptying. Despite this, liquid and solid carbohydrate feedings are equally effective in increasing blood glucose levels and improving performance.

Lugo and colleagues evaluated the metabolic effects of consuming liquid carbohydrate, solid carbohydrate, or both during 2 hr of cycling at 70% of $\dot{V}O_2$ followed by a time trial (Lugo et al., 1993). The liquid was a 7% carbohydrate-electrolyte beverage, and the solid carbohydrate was a sport bar that provided 76% of calories from carbohydrate, 18% from protein, and 6% from fat. Each feeding provided 0.4 g of carbohydrate/kg (an average of 28 g per feeding and 56 g per hour) and was consumed immediately before and every 30 min during the first 120 min of exercise.

Although the caloric content of the treatments varied, they were isoenergetic with respect to carbohydrate. Carbohydrate availability and time trial performance were similar when equal amounts of carbohydrate were consumed as liquid, solid, or in combination. Regardless of carbohydrate form, there were no differences in blood glucose, insulin, or total carbohydrate oxidized during 120 min of cycling at 70% of $\dot{V}O_2$max.

Each carbohydrate form (liquid vs. solid) holds certain advantages for the athlete (Coleman, 1994). Sport drinks and other liquids encourage the consumption of water needed to maintain hydration during exercise. Also, carbohydrate must be in a liquid or semiliquid state before leaving the stomach. Drinking 5 to 10 oz (150-300 ml) of a sport drink (6-8% carbohydrate concentration) every 15 to 20 min can provide the proper amount of carbohydrate and fluid for energy and hydration. For example, hourly drinking of 20 oz (600 ml) of a sport drink that contains 6% carbohydrate provides 36 g of carbohydrate.

High-carbohydrate foods are easy to carry during exercise and provide both variety and satiety. Eating one banana (30 g), one Power Bar (47 g), two gels (about 50 g), or three large graham crackers (66 g) every hour also supplies an adequate amount of carbohydrate. Athletes should drink plenty of fluids when they eat solid food to avoid gastrointestinal distress. In addition to aiding digestion, drinking water while one eats solid foods promotes proper hydration.

Fructose

Fructose causes a lower blood glucose and insulin response than glucose, which has led some athletes to believe erroneously that it is an energy source superior to glucose.

Murray compared the physiological, sensory, and exercise performance responses to the ingestion of 6% glucose, 6% sucrose, and 6% fructose solutions during cycling exercise (Murray et al., 1989). Blood insulin levels were lower with fructose, as expected. However, fructose was associated with greater gastrointestinal distress, higher perceived exertion ratings, and higher serum cortisol levels (indicating greater physiological stress) than glucose or sucrose. Cycling performance times were also significantly better with sucrose and glucose than with fructose.

Fructose metabolism occurs primarily in the liver, where it is converted to liver glycogen. Fructose probably cannot be converted to glucose and released fast enough to provide adequate energy for the exercising muscles. In contrast, blood glucose is maintained or elevated by feedings of glucose, sucrose, or glucose polymers. These have been shown to enhance performance and are the predominant carbohydrates in sport drinks.

The greater incidence of gastrointestinal distress often reported with high fructose intakes may be due to the slower intestinal absorption of fructose compared to glucose. This usually does not occur when a small amount of fructose is used in combination with other carbohydrates (glucose, sucrose, glucose polymers) in a sport drink.

Carbohydrate Intake After Exercise

The restoration of glycogen stores following strenuous training is important in order to minimize fatigue associated with repeated days of heavy training. Athletes need to consume 7 to 10 g of carbohydrate/kg and adequate calories to replace their muscle glycogen stores during consecutive days of hard workouts.

The time period in which carbohydrate is consumed following exercise is also important for glycogen repletion. Ivy and colleagues evaluated glycogen repletion following 2 hr of hard cycling exercise that depleted muscle glycogen (Ivy et al., 1988b). When 2 g of carbohydrate/kg was consumed immediately after exercise, muscle glycogen synthesis was 15 mmol/kg. When the same carbohydrate feeding was delayed for 2 hr, muscle glycogen synthesis was cut by 66% to 5 mmol/kg. By 4 hr after exercise, total muscle glycogen synthesis for the delayed feeding was still 45% less than for the feeding given immediately after exercise.

Delaying carbohydrate intake for too long after exercise may reduce muscle glycogen storage and impair recovery. Athletes who are not hungry after exercising can consume a high-carbohydrate drink (e.g., sport drink, fruit juice, or a commercial high-carbohydrate beverage). This will also aid in rehydration.

Athletes who exercise hard for 90 min or more daily should consume 1.5 g of carbohydrate/kg immediately after exercise, followed by an additional 1.5 g of carbohydrate/kg feeding 2 hr later (Ivy et al., 1988a). The first carbohydrate feeding can be a high-carbohydrate beverage followed by a high-carbohydrate meal. Replenishing muscle glycogen stores after exercise is particularly beneficial for athletes who train hard more than once during the day. This will enable them to get the most out of their second workout.

Glycogen repletion occurs faster following exercise for several reasons. The blood flow to the muscles is much greater immediately after exercise, and the muscle cell is more likely to take up glucose at this time. Also, the muscle cells are more sensitive to the effects of insulin during this time period, which promotes glycogen synthesis.

Glucose and sucrose are twice as effective as fructose in restoring muscle glycogen after exercise (Blom, et al., 1987). Most fructose is converted to liver glycogen, whereas glucose appears to bypass the liver and is stored as muscle glycogen.

The most rapid increase in muscle glycogen content during the first 24 hr of recovery may be achieved through consumption of foods with a high GI. Burke and associates investigated the effect of GI on muscle glycogen repletion following exercise (Burke et al., 1993). The subjects cycled for 2 hr at 75% of $\dot{V}O_2$max to deplete muscle glycogen, then consumed foods with either a high GI or a low GI. The total carbohydrate feeding over 24 hr was 10 g of carbohydrate/kg, evenly distributed at meals eaten at 0, 4, 8, and 21 hr after exercise. The increase in muscle glycogen content after 24 hr was greater with the high-glycemic diet (106 mmol/kg) than with the low-glycemic diet (71.5 mmol/kg). Burke and colleagues note, however, that the total amount of carbohydrate consumed is the most important consideration for glycogen repletion. They recommend an intake of 7 to 10 g of carbohydrate/kg for maximum daily glycogen restoration.

Athletes may have impaired muscle glycogen synthesis following unaccustomed exercise that results in muscle damage and delayed-onset muscle soreness. The muscular responses to such damaging exercise appear to decrease both the rate of muscle glycogen synthesis and the total muscle glycogen content. While a diet providing 7 to 10 g of carbohydrate/kg usually replaces muscle glycogen stores within 24 hr, the damaging effects of unaccustomed exercise result in significant delays to muscle glycogen repletion. Also, Sherman notes that even the normalization of muscle glycogen stores does not guarantee normal muscle function after unaccustomed exercise (Sherman, 1992).

Protein

Many athletes believe that they require large amounts of protein to perform at an optimum level. Bodybuilders and power athletes typically focus on a high-protein diet and supplement plan in an effort to enhance muscle mass and strength (table 15.3). Endurance athletes may consume specific amino acids to delay the onset of fatigue during endurance exercise.

Factors That Influence Protein Requirements

Amino acids enter the free amino acid pool located in body tissues and blood after digestion and absorption or as a result of tissue degradation. Once in the free amino acid pool, amino acids have two fates—they can be used to synthesize body tissue or they can be burned (oxidized) for energy (Lemon, 1998).

Research on protein requirements suggests that athletes need more protein than sedentary people. The factors that influence protein requirements include exercise type (endurance vs. strength), exercise intensity, carbohydrate availability, training state, energy balance, gender, and age (Lemon, 1998).

Table 15.3 Protein Content in Some Common Foods

Food	Amount	Protein content (grams)
Meat, fish, poultry		
Lean beef	1 oz	8
Chicken	1 oz	8
Turkey breast	1 oz	8
Fish	1 oz	7
Eggs	1	6
Beans, nuts		
Kidney beans	½ cup	9
Navy beans	½ cup	7
Garbanzo beans (chick peas)	½ cup	6
Tofu	2 oz	5
Peanut butter	1 tbsp	4
Dairy		
Low-fat cottage cheese	½ cup	13
Milk, whole, skim	1 cup	8
Yogurt	1 cup	8
Cheddar cheese	1 oz	7
Ice cream	½ cup	4
Frozen yogurt	½ cup	4
American cheese	1 oz	3
Breads, cereals, grains		
Macaroni and cheese	½ cup	9
Spaghetti	1 cup cooked	8
Bagel	2 oz	6
Raisin bran	1 oz (⅔ cup)	3
Rice	1 cup cooked	3
Bread	1 slice	2
Vegetables		
Baked potato	1 large	4
Peas, green	½ cup	4
Corn	½ cup	2
Lettuce	¼ head	1
Carrot	1 large	1
Fruits		
Banana, orange	1 medium	1
Apple	1 medium	1

From: Coleman, E., Steen, S.N. *Ultimate Sports Nutrition,* 2nd ed. Bull Publishing, Palo Alto, CA, 2000.

Exercise Type

During endurance exercise, there is an increased oxidation of branched-chain amino acids (leucine, isoleucine, and valine) that is proportional to exercise intensity. The hormonal changes that occur with endurance exercise—increased epinephrine and norepinephrine and decreased insulin—promote increased protein breakdown. Following endurance exercise, protein synthesis is increased to minimize or repair any muscle damage that has occurred. Endurance athletes require about 1.2 to 1.4 g of protein/kg/day, or 150% to 175% of the RDA for protein (Lemon, 1998).

In contrast to endurance exercise, strength exercise does not increase amino acid oxidation relative to rest (Lemon, 1998). The anaerobic nature of strength exercise minimizes the contribution of amino acids to fuel needs. Carbohydrate appears to be the major fuel burned during strength exercise. However, increased protein is required during strength training to support the higher rates of muscle synthesis induced by this type of exercise. Strength athletes need about 1.6 to 1.7 g of protein/kg/day, or 200% to 212% of the RDA (Lemon, 1998).

Carbohydrate Availability

When muscle glycogen stores are low as a consequence of prolonged exercise or a low-carbohydrate diet, protein may contribute as much as 15% of the energy during exercise. When glycogen stores are high, protein utilization decreases to about 5% (Williams, 1999). Consuming a high-carbohydrate diet during repeated days of heavy training helps maintain glycogen stores and provides a significant protein-sparing effect (Lemon, 1998).

Training State

Increased protein intake may be more important during the initiation of strength training than later in the training program. Strength athletes need more protein to support increases in muscle mass—the existing muscle fibers become larger (hypertrophy). Although more protein may be necessary to build muscle than to maintain it, further research is required to determine whether chronic strength training reduces the increased need observed with the initiation of training (Lemon, 1998).

Chronic endurance training appears to increase the oxidation of branched-chain amino acids (leucine, isoleucine, and valine) both at rest and during exercise. Also, when endurance training begins, athletes need more protein to support increases in myoglobin (an oxygen carrier in muscle similar to hemoglobin), aerobic enzymes in the muscle, and red blood cell formation (Lemon, 1998).

Gender

Men excrete more nitrogen in their urine than women following endurance exercise, suggesting that there may be exercise-gender-protein interactions. The differences may be caused by gender-specific hormonal responses that favor fat metabolism in women and carbohydrate-protein metabolism in men. Additional research is needed to confirm this theory (Lemon, 1998).

Energy Balance

The recommendation of 1.2 to 1.7 g of protein/kg/day assumes that the athlete is consuming sufficient calories (energy). There is an inverse relationship between energy intake and protein need. Some athletes may not consume adequate calories and therefore don't consume enough protein in relation to their high energy expenditures (rowing, swimming, football); others don't consume enough because of caloric restriction for low-body weight sports (wrestling, gymnastics, figure skating, ballet). Either situation increases the athlete's protein requirement because the protein is used for energy rather than for muscle growth and repair. Female athletes are more likely to consume insufficient calories than male athletes (Lemon, 1998).

Total energy intake is more important than elevated protein intake when one is attempting to increase muscle mass (Lemon, 1998). Since 1 lb of muscle (454 g) contains about 3500 calories, the athlete must increase calorie intake by about 500 calories per day to gain 1 lb in a week. Many athletes mistakenly emphasize protein intake over caloric intake when trying to "bulk up." Athletes who have difficulty gaining weight probably are not consuming enough calories.

Age

Some research suggests that older individuals need more protein than younger people. Since strength training increases muscle protein synthesis in older as well as in younger individuals, the muscle size and strength of older people may be positively influenced by protein intake. Although there is little research on children and adolescents, the greater protein requirements associated with growth may further increase the protein requirements of physically active youngsters (Lemon, 1998). A diet supplying 1.2 to 1.7 g of protein/kg/day should meet the needs of most children and adolescents in sport (Williams, 1999).

Protein Intake for Recovery

The type of exercise (endurance vs. strength training) alters the magnitude of both protein synthesis and protein breakdown. Although the precise time course is still unclear, small changes in either could have significant effects on muscle growth (Lemon, 1998).

The powerful anabolic stimulus of strength training may be further enhanced by either carbohydrate ingestion or amino acid infusion/ingestion immediately after exercise, due to insulin-mediated increases in muscle amino acid uptake and protein synthesis. Such a response may also be beneficial following endurance exercise through minimizing or enhancing repair of exercise-induced muscle damage. Similarly, the timing of subsequent strength or endurance training sessions could enhance or retard muscle growth/repair.

Consuming 1.0 g of carbohydrate/kg immediately after resistance exercise may enhance muscle protein synthesis as well as muscle glycogen repletion as a consequence of the associated insulin response (Roy et al., 1997). Infusing amino acids intravenously following strength training may also enhance amino acid uptake, but this strategy is not practical (Biolo, 1997).

Tipton and colleagues examined the effect of orally administered amino acids (1-quart [1 L] solution with 40 g of amino acids) following resistance exercise on muscle protein synthesis (Tipton et al., 1999). The researchers found that net muscle protein synthesis from amino acid ingestion was similar to that seen after amino acid infusion. Since amino acid availability can be increased as effectively with oral intake as with infusion, consuming a source of amino acids following resistance exercise (food or a supplement) should promote muscle anabolism.

Resting levels of the anabolic hormone testosterone were shown to be the greatest when the ratio of dietary protein to carbohydrate was 1:4 during strength training (Volek et al., 1997). Anything that increased the ratio of protein to carbohydrate (e.g., increased protein intake and/or decreased carbohydrate intake) reduced testosterone levels.

The theoretical potentiating effects of nutrient intake and subsequent exercise on muscle growth require much more study before specific recommendations are possible (Lemon, 1998).

Protein in Food

Athletes can easily meet their protein requirements with diet. The average American consumes about 100 g of protein per day (most from animal sources that contain all the essential amino acids), for a total protein intake of about 1.4 g/kg of body weight. Athletes also consume more protein when their caloric intake increases as a result of training (Williams, 1999).

Since muscle is composed of about 70% water and 22% protein, 1 lb (454 g) of muscle contains only about 100 g of protein. To gain 1 lb of muscle a week represents an additional 14 g of protein a day. This is easily supplied by 1 cup of nonfat milk and 1 oz of chicken (15 g total).

Good sources of complete proteins are meat, poultry, fish, dairy products, and eggs. An ounce of meat, poultry, or cheese, or one egg, supplies about 7 g of protein containing all the essential amino acids. Milk and yogurt are also excellent protein sources, with 8 oz supplying about 8 g of protein. Legumes and nuts are also quality sources of protein. To reduce dietary fat, athletes should emphasize chicken or turkey without the skin, lean meat, fish, and nonfat/low-fat dairy products.

Athletes can obtain 1.2 to 1.7 g of protein/kg when their diet provides 12% to 15% of calories as protein (Williams, 1999). This amount of protein is consistent with dietary recommendations for athletes and the Dietary Guidelines for Americans.

High-Protein Diets

Tarnopolsky and colleagues reported that increasing protein intake to 2.4 g/kg/day did not increase protein synthesis more than a protein intake of 1.4 g/kg/day (Tarnopolsky et al., 1992). However, the larger intake of protein did increase amino acid oxidation. Thus, the extra dietary protein was burned for energy rather than being incorporated into more muscle protein. Using protein for energy is expensive and wasteful. Carbohydrates provide energy more efficiently and at less cost.

Currently, the research does not support a protein intake above 2 g/kg/day to increase muscle mass. Athletes who consume adequate calories and have reasonably balanced diets generally meet or exceed their protein requirements.

Supplemental amino acid or protein intake increases the production of urea, which may increase the risk of dehydration. The kidneys require more water to eliminate the extra nitrogen load imposed by the excess protein. Athletes should monitor their body weight daily and drink sufficient water to match increased losses (Lemon, 1998).

Patients with impaired kidney function should not consume large amounts of protein because the added nitrogen excretion increases the kidney's workload. However, there is no persuasive evidence that the normal kidney cannot handle this extra workload (Lemon, 1998).

There is a concern that high-protein diets may increase calcium loss from the body, thereby increasing the risk of osteoporosis. Fortunately, the calcium loss that is observed with purified proteins may be prevented by the increased phosphate intake that occurs with most food proteins (Lemon, 1998).

A diet that provides the amount of protein recommended for athletes (1.2-1.7 g/kg/day) will probably not contain an amount of fat that is harmful for cardiovascular health (Lemon, 1998). Athletes can choose concentrated protein sources that are low in saturated fat (nonfat dry milk powder, tuna canned in water, and soy protein powder).

Ketogenic diets are currently popular among many bodybuilders and weight lifters. Such diets are high in saturated fat and may increase the risk of coronary heart disease and stroke. Consuming a high-protein, high-fat ketogenic diet after strenuous exercise will cause slow or incomplete replacement of muscle glycogen and so impair performance. This type of diet also takes a long time to digest. By comparison, a high-carbohydrate diet promotes rapid repletion of muscle glycogen and is readily digested.

Amino Acid Supplements

Amino acid supplements containing one or more amino acids are fashionable among bodybuilders and weight lifters. Arginine and ornithine are particularly popular since they supposedly stimulate the secretion of growth hormone—resulting in increased muscle mass and decreased body fat. Although injecting large amounts of arginine and ornithine may cause a temporary rise in growth hormone levels, there is no evidence that the small amounts of these amino acids contained in supplements have any effect on growth hormone levels or body composition (Lemon, 1991). Exercise itself raises growth hormone far more than injecting arginine or ornithine. Combining the supplements with exercise does not increase growth hormone levels above what is seen with exercise (Lemon, 1991; Lambert et al., 1993).

Amino acid supplements usually contain 500 mg per capsule, while 1 oz of beef, chicken, or fish supplies 7 g of protein—7000 mg of amino acids! It is useful to compare 1 cup of a low-fat fruited yogurt that contains 10 g of high-quality protein, 18 different amino acids (including 300 mg of arginine), carbohydrate, calcium, magnesium, and potassium to one tasteless 500-mg arginine supplement (Clarkson, 1998).

With the exception of the eosinophilia-myalgia syndrome (due to contaminated tryptophan), there have not been significant problems with the ingestion of single amino acids. However, large intakes of some single amino acids may interfere with absorption and lead to metabolic imbalances. Ornithine ingestion may cause mild to severe stomach cramping and diarrhea. Other amino acids may alter brain neurotransmitter activity; and some, such as methionine, are very toxic (Lemon, 1991). It seems prudent to avoid a large intake of any single amino acid until its safety is determined (Lemon, 1991, 1998).

Dry milk powder (casein) is a high-quality, inexpensive protein supplement (1/4 cup provides 11 g protein) that provides all of the necessary amino acids at less than half the cost of the "high-tech" protein supplements marketed to athletes. The majority of "high-tech" protein supplements do provide additional energy and protein. Although some protein supplements contain a variety of ingredients (e.g., whey protein, enzymes) purported to boost weight gain, no research is available to support the claims made for these products (Clarkson, 1998).

Branched-Chain Amino Acids

The central fatigue hypothesis suggests that increased concentrations of brain serotonin can impair central nervous system function during prolonged endurance exercise and thereby cause a deterioration in performance. An increase in serotonin synthesis occurs when the brain receives elevated levels of bloodborne tryptophan, an amino acid precursor to serotonin (Davis, 1995).

Most of the tryptophan in blood plasma circulates loosely bound to albumin. Unbound, or free, tryptophan, however, is transported across the blood-brain barrier. Tryptophan shares this transport mechanism with other large neutral amino acids, especially branched-chain amino acids (BCAA)—leucine, isoleucine, and valine (Davis, 1995).

The BCAA compete with and limit plasma free tryptophan entry into the brain. However, plasma BCAA levels decrease during endurance exercise because they are oxidized for energy by the working muscles. The BCAA are important nitrogen sources for alanine, which may be converted to glucose for fuel via the alanine-glucose cycle. The fall in plasma BCAA during prolonged exercise facilitates the transport of plasma free tryptophan into the brain. Also, an increase in plasma free fatty acids during exercise causes a proportional increase in plasma free tryptophan. Free fatty acids displace tryptophan from its usual binding sites on albumin (Davis, 1995).

According to the central fatigue hypothesis, high levels of plasma free tryptophan combined with low levels of BCAA (a high free tryptophan:BCAA ratio) increase brain serotonin and cause fatigue during prolonged endurance exercise (Davis, 1995).

Some research suggests that BCAA supplementation may help to maintain a normal free tryptophan:BCAA ratio during prolonged exercise. Although there appears to be a logical theoretical basis to support BCAA as an ergogenic aid for endurance exercise, the available scientific data are limited and equivocal. Additional research is warranted with both acute and chronic BCAA supplementation before BCAA supplement recommendations can be established (Williams, 1999). Furthermore, the large amounts of BCAA required to make physiologically relevant changes in the plasma free tryptophan:BCAA ratio can increase plasma ammonia, which may be toxic to the brain and impair muscle metabolism. Consuming large doses of BCAA during exercise can also slow water absorption from the gut and cause gastrointestinal disturbances. Since BCAA supplements may be not be safe or effective, and since it is easy to obtain sufficient quantities from food, BCAA supplements are not recommended at the present time (Davis, 1995; Williams, 1999).

Carbohydrate feedings, on the other hand, are associated with dramatic reductions in the plasma free tryptophan:BCAA ratio. Carbohydrate feedings lower plasma free tryptophan by suppressing the rise in free fatty acids that compete with tryptophan for binding sites

on albumin (Davis, 1995). Davis and associates evaluated the ingestion of a 6% carbohydrate-electrolyte drink, a 12% carbohydrate-electrolyte drink, and water placebo on prolonged cycling to fatigue at 70% of $\dot{V}O_2$max (Davis et al., 1995). When subjects drank the water placebo, plasma free tryptophan increased sevenfold. When subjects drank either the 6% or 12% carbohydrate-electrolyte drink, the increase in plasma free tryptophan was greatly reduced and fatigue was delayed by approximately 1 hr.

It is not possible to determine whether the benefits of carbohydrate feedings are attributable to decreased central fatigue in the brain or decreased peripheral fatigue in the exercising muscles. However, unlike BCAA supplementation, carbohydrate feedings during exercise can be recommended because their safety, performance, and cost benefits are well established (Davis, 1995; Williams, 1999).

Glutamine

Glutamine is the most abundant free amino acid in human muscle and plasma. Skeletal muscle synthesizes, stores, and releases glutamine at a high rate. Glutamine is a major fuel source for lymphocytes, macrophages, and gut enterocytes. Glutamine is also a precursor to the synthesis of proteins, a nitrogen donator for the synthesis of nucleotides, a nitrogen transporter between various tissues, and a substrate for the production of urea (Lacey and Wilmore, 1990).

Although classified as a nonessential amino acid, glutamine appears to be conditionally essential during times of metabolic stress and critical illness. Skeletal and plasma glutamine levels are lowered by infection, surgery, trauma, acidosis, and burns. Prolonged endurance exercise, such as the marathon, may also reduce plasma glutamine concentration. All of these catabolic stresses are associated with increases in the plasma concentrations of cortisol and glucagon and with a greater tissue requirement of glutamine for gluconeogenesis (Walsh et al., 1998).

The increased gluconeogenesis and accompanying increases in hepatic, gut, and renal glutamine uptake may cause the depletion of plasma glutamine concentration that is observed in prolonged exercise and other catabolic states (Walsh et al., 1998). Since glutamine is critical for optimal functioning of the immune system, a decreased plasma glutamine concentration may impair immune function and increase the risk of infection. In theory, glutamine supplementation may enhance immune function and decrease the risk of infection.

The benefits of glutamine supplementation for hospital patients during periods of major physiological stress are well established. Oral or parenteral glutamine supplementation after major trauma or surgery has helped to maintain muscular glutamine concentration, improve nitrogen balance, increase protein synthesis, decrease 3-methylhistidine excretion (a marker of muscle catabolism), prevent intestinal atrophy, improve weight gain, and decrease length of stay (Lacey and Wilmore, 1990).

The benefits of glutamine supplementation for athletes during periods of heavy training, however, are not well established. Castell and colleagues investigated the effects of feeding glutamine to middle-distance, marathon, and ultramarathon runners and to elite rowers during training and competition (Castell et al., 1996). The researchers provided a drink containing either glutamine (72 subjects) or a placebo (79 subjects) to athletes immediately after heavy exercise and 2 hr after exhaustive exercise. The athletes completed questionnaires about the incidence of infections during the seven days following the exercise. The percentage of athletes reporting no infections was significantly higher in the glutamine-supplemented group (81%) than in the placebo group (49%). The incidence of infection was lowest in middle-distance runners and highest in runners after a full marathon or ultramarathon and in elite rowers after intensive training. In a later study, however, Castell and associates reported that glutamine supplementation did not appear to have an effect on immune function (as assessed by lymphocyte distribution) following completion of the Brussels marathon (Castell et al., 1997).

Plasma glutamine concentration may fall after periods of intense training that result in muscle glycogen depletion. However, an adequate daily intake of carbohydrate and energy may help to prevent muscle glycogen depletion and overtraining as well as help to maintain normal glutamine status. Although some preliminary research suggests that glutamine supplementation may reduce the incidence of respiratory infections in athletes, further research is required to provide supporting data (Williams, 1999).

Fat

Fat is a necessary component of the diet—providing energy, essential fatty acids, and associated nutrients such as vitamins E, A, and D. Athletes, like most Americans, typically eat about 34% of their calories as fat. Most U.S. health agencies recommend that people consume no more than 30% of calories from fat and less than 10% of calories from saturated fat (Krauss et al., 2000; U.S. Department of Agriculture, 2000). Athletes should follow these general recommendations and also ensure that their fat intakes are not excessively low (American College of Sports Medicine, 2000).

A high-fat diet increases the risk of cardiovascular disease (heart attack and stroke) and certain cancers (U.S. Department of Agriculture, 2000). A high-fat diet also contributes to obesity, which is associated with a wide range of health problems (National Heart, Lung, and Blood Institute, 1998).

Energy Available From Fat

Whereas the total glycogen stores (in muscle and liver) amount to only about 2000 kcal, every pound of fat supplies 3500 calories. The amount of energy stored as fat is about 110,000 calories for a 176-lb (80 kg) man and about 135,000 calories for a 132-lb (60 kg) woman with average body composition (Jeukendrup and Saris, 1998).

Fat Metabolism During Exercise

The hormonal environment generated by exercise (increased epinephrine and decreased insulin) promotes lipolysis and mobilization of fatty acids from intramuscular triglycerides and adipose tissue. The concentration of free fatty acids then rises in the blood. Fat oxidation increases as the exercise duration increases. Relative fat oxidation is maximal at low to moderate intensities, whereas during high intensities, carbohydrate is the major fuel (Jeukendrup and Saris, 1998).

Per unit of time, more ATP can be generated from carbohydrate than from the oxidation of fat. When bloodborne fatty acids are oxidized, the maximum rate of ATP formation is ~0.40 mol/min, whereas the aerobic or anaerobic breakdown of endogenous glycogen can generate ~1.0 to 2.0 mol/min, respectively. At higher exercise intensities, the rate of ATP breakdown is too high to be matched by the rate of ATP formation from free fatty acids. This is the major reason carbohydrate is the essential fuel for high-intensity exercise (Jeukendrup and Saris, 1998).

Fat Loading

Nutritional strategies to improve endurance usually focus on increasing muscle glycogen stores prior to exercise. However, several popularized studies have led some endurance athletes to try "fat loading" in place of carbohydrate loading (Phinney et al., 1983; Munio et al., 1994; Lambert et al., 1994).

A 1983 study by Phinney evaluated the influence of a high-fat diet on cycling time to exhaustion and muscle glycogen utilization (Phinney et al., 1983). The cyclists ate an average American diet (50% carbohydrate) for one week and then exercised to exhaustion at 63% of $\dot{V}O_2$max. Then they ate a high-fat diet (85% of calories), which was also low in carbohydrate (less than 20 g of carbohydrate). After four weeks on this diet, they again exercised to exhaustion at 63% of $\dot{V}O_2$max.

The exercise time to exhaustion was not significantly different on the two diets (147 min and 152 min, respectively). After adaptation to the high-fat diet, muscle glycogen utilization dropped fourfold and glucose utilization dropped threefold on the ride to exhaustion. Fat utilization rose to make up the difference. This study indicated that while fat loading improved fat oxidation, it did not improve performance.

The study can be faulted because it did not include comparison of a high-carbohydrate diet (8-10 g of carbohydrate/kg) to the high-fat diet. A high-carbohydrate diet would provide higher muscle glycogen stores than the 50% carbohydrate diet used in the study, and thus would result in a longer cycling time to exhaustion. Also, the cyclists rode to exhaustion at an exercise intensity low enough (63% of $\dot{V}O_2$max) to be fueled by fat and not limited by muscle glycogen depletion. If the rides had been conducted at an exercise intensity known to be limited by muscle glycogen depletion (e.g., above 70% of $\dot{V}O_2$max), impaired endurance would have been expected.

The results of a study by Lambert and colleagues on dietary fat and performance continue to promote the notion that high-fat diets will enhance endurance. The authors investigated the effects of two weeks of either a high-fat (70% fat, 7% carbohydrate) or a high-carbohydrate (74% carbohydrate, 12% fat) diet on exercise performance in trained cyclists (Lambert et al., 1994). The subjects did three consecutive cycle tasks with 30 min of rest between each test: a Wingate test of peak muscle power, cycling to exhaustion at 90% of $\dot{V}O_2$max (HI), and cycling to exhaustion at 60% of $\dot{V}O_2$max (MOD).

The maximal power output for the Wingate test was the same with the two diets. Although starting muscle glycogen content was lower on the high-fat diet (68.1 mmol/kg) versus the high-carbohydrate diet (120.6 mmol/kg), the exercise time to exhaustion during HI was not significantly different. However, the exercise time to exhaustion during the subsequent MOD was significantly longer on the high-fat diet (79.7 min) compared to the high-carbohydrate diet (42.5 min) despite a lower muscle glycogen content at the onset of MOD (32 mmol/kg vs. 73 mmol/kg).

While the respiratory exchange ratios support the assertion that the high-fat diet improved fat burning and performance time, the calculated amount of fat and carbohydrate oxidized (grams per minute) and the blood free fatty acid and glycerol responses were not consistent with the notion that the high-fat diet increased fat oxidation study (Sherman and Leenders, 1995). This weakens the study's findings. Also, the Lambert study, like the Phinney study, used a relatively low intensity (60% of $\dot{V}O_2$max) compared to the intensities that most endurance athletes perform in training and competition. Whether these findings can apply to actual endurance events remains uncertain.

Munio and colleagues investigated the effect of a moderate-fat diet on running performance (Munio et al.,

1994). Diets were assigned for seven days in the order of normal diet (2789 kcal, 61% carbohydrate, 24% fat), high-fat diet (3500 calories, 50% carbohydrate, and 38% fat), and high-carbohydrate diet (3500 calories, 73% carbohydrate, and 15% fat). The run time to exhaustion at 75% to 85% $\dot{V}O_2$max was significantly longer following the high-fat diet (91 min) compared to the normal diet (69 min) and high-carbohydrate (76 min) diet.

Although this study suggests that a seven-day, 38% fat diet improves endurance performance, there were major flaws in the study (Sherman and Leenders, 1995). The order of the diets was not randomly administered. Also, certain metabolic responses were not consistent with increased fat utilization and so did not support the concept that the high-fat diet produced the improvement in performance. Blood glycerol fell (it should have risen if more fat was burned) and the respiratory exchange ratio was unchanged (it should have decreased if more fat was burned), considerably weakening the results of the study.

There is no convincing evidence that a high-fat diet improves performance. Furthermore, the potential adverse effects on health are too risky to warrant consuming a high-fat diet during endurance training.

Medium-Chain Triglycerides

Medium-chain triglycerides (MCTs) are 6- to 12-carbon compounds that yield 8 calories/g. They are water soluble and readily absorbed into the hepatic system via the portal vein. Medium-chain triglycerides have been used in clinical applications for many years to treat fat malabsorption, defects in lipid absorption due to major intestinal resection, and defective lipid transport (Berning, 1996).

It is generally accepted that an increased oxidation of free fatty acids decreases muscle glycogen utilization. Since MCTs are oxidized as quickly as glucose, they could theoretically enhance performance by sparing muscle glycogen during exercise (Berning, 1996). On the basis of this theory, proponents claim that MCTs increase energy, extend endurance, enhance fat metabolism, decrease body fat, and increase lean tissue.

Jeukendrup and colleagues evaluated the oxidation rate of oral MCT feedings in eight well-trained athletes during four different 3-hr bouts of exercise at 50% of maximal work rate (Jeukendrup et al., 1995). The subjects consumed either carbohydrate (CHO), MCTs, a combination of CHO + MCTs, or placebo. During the second hour of exercise, 72% of the MCTs ingested in the CHO + MCTs trial were oxidized. By comparison, only 33% of the MCTs ingested in the MCTs trial were oxidized during the same time period. Thus, the MCTs were oxidized at a higher rate when combined with CHO. Furthermore, the amount of MCTs that could be tolerated by the gastrointestinal tract was small (30 g), which further limited the contribution of MCTs to the total energy expenditure.

In a later study, Jeukendrup and associates investigated whether increasing the amount of MCTs from 30 g to 85 g would enhance fat oxidation and improve performance during 60% of maximal work rate for 2 hr (Jeukendrup et al., 1998). The subjects consumed either CHO, MCTs, a combination of CHO + MCTs, or a placebo. The CHO and the CHO + MCT feedings had no effect on performance or fat metabolism. When the subjects received only MCTs, performance was decreased compared to that in the placebo trial. The negative effect of the MCTs was attributed to gastrointestinal distress.

Van Zyl and colleagues evaluated the effect of MCT + CHO feedings on fat oxidation and performance during 2-hr exercise bouts at 60% of maximal work rate plus a 40-km (25 miles) time trial (Van Zyl et al., 1996). Endurance-trained cyclists consumed a CHO + MCT formulation containing 86 g of MCT. The MCT feeding was associated with a small increase in fat oxidation and improved time trial performance, suggesting a glycogen-sparing effect. The subjects did not report any gastrointestinal distress.

Although one study (Van Zyl et al., 1996) indicates that CHO + MCT feedings may improve endurance performance lasting 2 hr or more, more research is needed to replicate these findings. The majority of research does not support an ergogenic effect for MCTs. Even if MCTs do improve performance, the fact that large amounts cause gastrointestinal distress limits their potential usefulness as an ergogenic aid.

Metabolic Intermediates

Metabolic intermediates are compounds that are involved in the production of energy from protein, carbohydrate, and fat. These compounds are often marketed with claims that they will enhance athletic performance by having a positive influence on energy production. In theory, L-carnitine increases fatty acid oxidation, pyruvate increases glucose extraction and utilization, and ribose increases the synthesis and regeneration of ATP.

Carnitine

L-carnitine is synthesized in the body from the amino acids lysine and methionine and is found in animal foods (particularly meat and dairy products) and, to a much lesser extent, in plant foods. It is a short-chained carboxylic acid and contains nitrogen. About 90% of the body's supply of carnitine is located in muscle tissues (Williams, 1999).

In theory, supplementation of L-carnitine would increase fatty acid oxidation by facilitating the transport of long-chain fatty acids into the mitochondria. L-carnitine may also facilitate the oxidation of pyruvate, which would enhance glucose utilization and reduce lactic acid production during exercise (Williams, 1999).

The results of studies on L-carnitine supplementation do not support an ergogenic effect. Trappe and colleagues evaluated the effect of L-carnitine supplementation in swimmers to determine whether carnitine would improve performance by reducing lactic acid accumulation (Trappe et al., 1994). The subjects were 20 male college varsity swimmers who had been training for 16 weeks prior to the study. The subjects completed five repeat 100-yd (91 m) swims, with a 2-min recovery between intervals, before and after one week of carnitine supplementation. The supplement group received a 236-ml (7.9 oz) citrus drink containing 4 g of L-carnitine in the morning and afternoon. The placebo group received the same amount of the citrus drink without carnitine. There were no differences between the supplement group and the placebo group with regard to lactic acid, blood pH, or swim velocity in the final swim interval, indicating that carnitine did not improve performance (Trappe et al., 1994).

Greig and colleagues examined L-carnitine supplementation and its effect on maximum and submaximum exercise capacity (Greig et al., 1987). In two separate trials, two groups of untrained subjects received either 2 g of L-carnitine a day or placebo for two weeks. Exercise capacity was assessed using continuous progressive cycle ergometry. There was a small improvement in submaximal performance at 50% of $\dot{V}O_2$max in the carnitine trial. However, heart rate was not significantly lower at any exercise intensity during the maximal exercise test in the carnitine trial. The researchers concluded that carnitine supplementation was of little or no benefit to exercise performance.

The studies on L-carnitine supplementation have largely produced results showing no ergogenic benefits, though further research is warranted. While L-carnitine appears to be a safe supplement, there is a concern that L-carnitine supplements may be adulterated and contain D-carnitine. D-carnitine may be toxic, as it can deplete L-carnitine and lead to a carnitine deficiency (Williams, 1999).

Pyruvate

Pyruvate is a three-carbon ketoacid produced in the end stages of glycolysis. Pyruvate supplements are sold for weight loss and to enhance training and performance.

The claim of improved endurance is supported by only two studies by Stanko and colleagues using untrained male subjects. The first study evaluated the effects of seven days of pyruvate and dihydroxyacetone (DHA) supplementation on arm ergometry exercise to exhaustion at 60% of $\dot{V}O_2$max (see Stanko et al., 1990a). The 10 subjects consumed diets that provided 35 calories/kg (55% carbohydrate, 15% protein, and 30% fat) and either 100 g of polycose (placebo) or 75 g DHA and 25 g pyruvate (triose treatment) substituted for a portion of the carbohydrate. Arm endurance was significantly improved by 20% (160 min) for the triose-supplemented group compared to the placebo group (133 min). The triose group had greater pre-exercise triceps glycogen stores (130 mmol/kg) compared to the placebo group (88 mmol/kg). The authors noted that pyruvate and DHA supplementation increased arm muscle glucose extraction, thereby enhancing endurance capacity.

The second study evaluated the effects of seven days of a pyruvate and DHA supplementation diet on leg cycle exercise to exhaustion at 70% of $\dot{V}O_2$max (see Stanko et al., 1990b). The eight subjects consumed diets that provided 35 calories/kg (70% carbohydrate, 18% protein, and 12% fat) and either 100 g of polycose (placebo) or 75 g DHA and 25 g pyruvate (triose treatment) substituted for a portion of the carbohydrate. Leg endurance was significantly improved by 20% (79 min) for the triose-supplemented group compared to the placebo group (66 min). Muscle glycogen at rest and exhaustion did not differ between the treatment and placebo groups. The authors note that pyruvate and DHA supplementation in conjunction with a high-carbohydrate diet increased leg muscle glucose extraction, thereby enhancing endurance capacity.

These studies appear valid, as an appropriate experimental design (randomized, crossover, placebo controlled, double blind) was utilized. However, Sukala suggests that one should consider several points before taking pyruvate supplements to improve performance (Sukala, 1998). (1) The results have not been reproduced by other researchers in other labs; (2) the subjects were untrained, so the results cannot be applied to trained individuals or elite athletes; (3) the triose-supplemented subjects experienced side effects in the form of intestinal gas, flatus, and diarrhea; (4) performance benefits were observed with 75 g DHA and 25 g pyruvate, but commercial pyruvate preparations contain only 500 mg to 1 g of pyruvate and may not contain DHA; and (5) the Dietary Supplement and Health Education Act of 1994 allows products to be marketed without proof of safety, efficacy, purity, or potency, so there is no guarantee of consistent dosage.

Stanko and colleagues have also conducted several studies to evaluate the effect of pyruvate and DHA supplementation, in conjunction with hypocaloric feedings for 21 days, on weight loss and body composition in obese women in a metabolic ward. In one study (see Stanko et al., 1992a), 13 subjects consumed either a 500-calorie placebo diet (60% carbohydrate, 40% protein) or a 500-calorie treatment diet (a 28-g mixture of pyruvate and DHA was isocalorically substituted for glucose). The triose-treated subjects lost 16% (2 lb or 0.9 kg) more body weight and 18% (1.8 lb or 0.8 kg) more body fat than the placebo group.

In another study (see Stanko et al., 1992b), 14 subjects consumed a 1000-calorie placebo diet (68% carbohydrate, 22% protein, 10% fat) or a 1000-calorie treatment diet (22 g of pyruvate was isocalorically substituted for glucose) for 21 days. The pyruvate-supplemented subjects lost 37% (3.5 lb or 1.6 kg) more body weight and 48% (2.9 lb or 1.3 kg) more fat than the placebo group.

These studies suggest that substitution of pyruvate and DHA for glucose in a hypocaloric diet will increase weight and fat loss. However, Sukala notes that the following points should be considered before supplemental pyruvate is recommended for weight loss (Sukala, 1998). (1) Again, the results have not been reproduced; (2) the subjects were obese and completely sedentary, so the results cannot be applied to a lean, active population; (3) the population at large doesn't live in a metabolic ward and subsist on a hypocaloric diet providing 500 to 1000 calories; (4) the differences in body weight loss and fat loss were statistically significant, but such a small change (about 2.2-3.3 lb [1-1.5 kg]) is physiologically insignificant and difficult to measure accurately; and (5) weight loss was observed with a 28-g triose mixture and with 22 g pyruvate, but, as noted above, commercial pyruvate preparations contain minuscule doses and the potency of the preparation is questionable.

At the present time, the best course is to discourage pyruvate supplementation since product potency is questionable and there is not adequate research available to support performance and weight loss claims.

Ribose

Ribose is a five-carbon sugar that is formed from the conversion of glucose via the pentose phosphate pathway. Ribose is a necessary substrate for the formation of 5-phosphororibosyl-1-pyrophosphate (PRPP), which is used in the de novo synthesis of nucleotides such as adenosine, ATP, and inosine. The ribose-containing PRPP is also essential for metabolic pathways that salvage adenosine to regenerate stores of ATP. Nucleotides, including ATP, are essential energy sources for energy transfer and metabolic reactions and play important roles in protein, glycogen, and nucleic acid (RNA and DNA) synthesis.

Hellsten-Westing and colleagues found that one week of high-intensity exercise significantly reduced ATP levels by 23% and total adenine nucleotides by 24% in human skeletal muscle (Hellsten-Westing et al., 1993). These levels had not recovered even after 72 hr of rest, presumably due to reduced PRPP availability and subsequent decreased recovery of adenine nucleotides by the de novo synthesis and salvage pathways.

Since ribose is a precursor to adenosine, ribose supplementation could theoretically increase the de novo synthesis and regeneration of ATP by improving PRPP availability. Tullson and Terjung conducted an in vitro study on de novo synthesis of adenine nucleotides using an isolated perfused rat hindquarter preparation. Supplementing the perfusate with 5 mM ribose increased the rate of adenine nucleotide de novo synthesis by three- to fourfold (Tullson and Terjung, 1991). In another study, Brault and Terjung found that supplementing the rat hindquarter perfusate with 5 mM ribose increased the rate of adenine nucleotide salvage by three- to sixfold (see Brault and Terjung, 1999).

Ribose has also been studied as a treatment for myocardial ischemia, which causes a substantial decrease in myocardial ATP content and an associated depression of cardiac function. Pliml and colleagues (Pliml et al., 1992) evaluated the effects of ribose supplementation on exercise tolerance and exercise-induced cardiac ischemia in patients with stable coronary heart disease (CHD). Twenty male patients with documented severe CHD underwent two symptom-limited treadmill exercise tests on two consecutive days. Ten patients received a placebo (glucose) for three days, and 10 received ribose dissolved in water (60 g daily in four divided doses). On day 5, exercise testing was repeated, and treadmill walking time until 1-mm ST-segment depression was significantly greater in the ribose group (276 sec) than in the placebo group (223 sec). Compared to baseline, the time to both ST-segment depression and onset of moderate angina was also significantly longer in the ribose group but not the placebo group. The researchers concluded that three days of ribose supplementation improved the heart's tolerance to ischemia by stimulating ATP synthesis and improving cardiac function.

While there is preliminary evidence that supplemental ribose improves exercise tolerance in patients with CHD, the purported ergogenic effects of ribose have yet to be convincingly demonstrated in healthy athletes. At the present time, no research has been published in peer-reviewed journals indicating that ribose supplementation improves athletic performance. Only one unpublished study by Trappe on four athletic subjects is cited in the reference section on the ribose Web page (**www.ribose.com/research7.htm**) to support an ergogenic benefit (Trappe, 1999).

Conclusion

Choosing the proper fuel is as important to athletic success as having a state-of-the-art training program. To gain a competitive advantage, athletes should focus on fueling the body with energy from a carbohydrate-rich, moderate-protein, low-fat diet. Dietary supplements such as amino acids or ribose, or dietary plans that are high in protein or high in fat, may appear to be a simple solution for improved performance—but they are not. All the supplements in the world are worthless if athletes don't cover the basics (Coleman and Steen, 2000).

References

American College of Sports Medicine, American Dietetic Association, and Dietitians of Canada. Joint position statement: Nutrition and athletic performance. Med Sci Sports Exerc 32:2130-2145, 2000.

Berning JR. The role of medium chain-triglycerides in exercise. Int J Sport Nutr 6:121-133, 1996.

Biolo G. An abundant supply of amino acids enhances the metabolic effect of exercise on muscle protein. Am J Physiol 273:E122, 1997.

Blom PCS et al. Effect of different post-exercise sugar diets on the rate of muscle glycogen synthesis. Med Sci Sports Exerc 19:491, 1987.

Brault JJ, Terjung RL. Purine salvage rates differ among skeletal muscle fiber types and are limited by ribose supply. Med Sci Sports Exerc 31(5 Suppl):S1365(abstract), 1999.

Burke LM, Collier GR, Hargreaves M. Muscle glycogen storage after prolonged exercise: Effect of glycemic index. J Appl Physiol 75:1019-1023, 1993.

Burke LM, Collier GR, Hargreaves M. The glycemic index—a new tool in sport nutrition? Int J Sport Nutr 8:401-415, 1998.

Castell LM et al. Does glutamine have a role in reducing infections in athletes? Eur J Appl Physiol 73:488-490, 1996.

Castell LM et al. Some aspects of the acute phase response after a marathon race, and the effects of glutamine supplementation. Eur J Appl Physiol 75:47-53, 1997.

Clarkson PM. Nutritional supplements for weight gain. Sport Sci Exch 11(1):1, 1998.

Coggan AR, Swanson SC. Nutritional manipulations before and during exercise: Effects on performance. Med Sci Sports Exerc 24(Suppl):S331, 1992.

Coleman E. Update on carbohydrate: Solid versus liquid. Int J Sport Nutr 4:80-88, 1994.

Coleman E. Carbohydrate—the master fuel. In: Nutrition for sport and exercise, ed. Berning JR, Steen SN. 2nd ed. Aspen, 1998.

Coleman E, Steen SN. Ultimate sports nutrition. 2nd ed. Bull, Palo Alto, CA, 2000.

Coyle EF et al. Carbohydrate feedings during prolonged strenuous exercise can delay fatigue. J Appl Physiol 55:230, 1983.

Coyle EF et al. Muscle glycogen utilization during prolonged strenuous exercise when fed carbohydrate. J Appl Physiol 61:165, 1986.

Coyle EF, Montain SJ. Benefits of fluid replacement with carbohydrate during exercise. Med Sci Sports Exerc 24(Suppl): S324, 1992.

Davis JM. Carbohydrates, branched-chain amino acids, and endurance: The central fatigue hypothesis. Int J Sport Nutr 5(Suppl):S29, 1995.

Davis JM et al. Effects of carbohydrate feedings on plasma free tryptophan and branched-chain amino acids during prolonged cycling. Eur J Appl Physiol 65:513(Suppl 5):S29, 1995.

Davis JM et al. Carbohydrate drinks delay fatigue during intermittent high intensity cycling in active men and women. Int J Sport Nutr 7:261, 1997.

Foster-Powell K, Brand Miller J. International tables of glycemic index. Am J Clin Nutr 62(Suppl): S871-S893, 1995.

Frail H, Burke L. Carbohydrate needs for training. In: Clinical sports nutrition, ed. Burke L, Deakin V, pp. 151-173, McGraw-Hill, Roseville, Australia, 1994.

Greig C, Finch KM, Jones DA, Cooper M, Sargeant AJ, Forte CA. The effect of oral supplementation with L-carnitine on maximum and submaximum exercise capacity. Eur J Appl Physiol 56:457-460, 1987.

Hellsten-Westing Y, Norman B, Balsom PD, Sjodin B. Decreased resting levels of adenine nucleotides in human skeletal muscle after high-intensity training. J Appl Physiol 74(5):2523-2528, 1993.

Ivy JL et al. Muscle glycogen storage after different amounts of carbohydrate ingestion. J Appl Physiol 65:2018, 1988a.

Ivy JL et al. Muscle glycogen synthesis after exercise: Effect of time of carbohydrate ingestion. J Appl Physiol 64:1480, 1988b.

Jeukendrup AE, Saris WHM. Fat as a fuel during exercise. In: Nutrition for sport and exercise, ed. Berning JR, Steen SN. 2nd ed. Aspen, 1998.

Jeukendrup AE, Saris WHM, Schrauwen P, Brouns R, Wagenmakers AJM. Metabolic availability of medium-chain triglycerides coingested with carbohydrates during prolonged exercise. J Appl Physiol 79:736-762, 1995.

Jeukendrup AE, Thielen JHC, Wagenmakers AJM, Brouns F, Saris AE. Effect of medium-chain triglycerol and carbohydrate ingestion during exercise on substrate utilization and subsequent cycling performance. Amer J Clin Nutr 67:397-404, 1998.

Krauss RM, Eckel RH, Howard B et al. AHA dietary guidelines revision 2000: A statement for healthcare professionals from the Nutrition Committee of the American Heart Association. Circulation 102:2296-2311, 2000.

Lacey JM, Wilmore DW. Is glutamine a conditionally essential amino acid? Nutr Rev 48:297-309, 1990.

Lambert EV et al. Enhanced endurance in trained cyclists during moderate intensity exercise following 2 weeks adaptation to a high fat diet. Eur J Appl Physiol 69:287, 1994.

Lambert MI et al. Failure of commercial oral amino acid supplements to increase serum growth hormone concentrations in male body builders. Int J Sport Nutr 3:290, 1993.

Lemon PRW. Protein and amino acid needs of the strength athlete. Int J Sport Nutr 1:127, 1991.

Lemon PWR. Effects of exercise on dietary protein requirements. Int J Sport Nutr 8(4):426-447, 1998.

Lugo M, Sherman WM, Wimer GS, Garleb K. Metabolic responses when different forms of carbohydrate energy are consumed during cycling. Int J Sport Nutr 3:398, 1993.

Munio DM et al. Effect of dietary fat on metabolic adjustments to maximal VO_2 and endurance in runners. Med Sci Sports Exerc 26:81, 1994.

Murray et al. The effects of glucose, fructose, and sucrose ingestion during exercise. Med Sci Sports Exerc 21:275, 1989.

National Heart, Lung, and Blood Institute. Clinical guidelines on the identification, evaluation, and treatment of overweight and obesity in adults. NIH Publication No. 98-4083, 1998.

Phinney SD et al. The human metabolic response to chronic ketosis without caloric restriction: Preservation of submaximal exercise capacity with reduced carbohydrate oxidation. Metabolism 32:769, 1983.

Pliml W, von Arnim T, Stablein A, Hofmann H, Zimmer HG, Erdmann E. Effects of ribose on exercise-induced ischaemia in stable coronary artery disease. Lancet 340(8818):507-510, 1992.

Roy et al. Effect of glucose supplement timing on protein metabolism after resistance training. J Appl Physiol 82:1882, 1997.

Sherman WM. Recovery from endurance exercise. Med Sci Sports Exerc 24(Suppl): S336, 1992.

Sherman WM, Leenders N. Fat loading: The next magic bullet? Int J Sport Nutr 5(Suppl): S1, 1995.

Sherman WM et al. Carbohydrate feedings 1 hr before exercise improves cycling performance. Am J Clin Nutr 54:866, 1991.

Sherman WM et al. Effects of 4 hr preexercise carbohydrate feedings on cycling performance. Med Sci Sports Exerc 12:598, 1989.

Stanko RT et al. Enhancement of arm exercise endurance capacity with dihydroxyacetone and pyruvate. J Appl Physiol 68(1):119-124, 1990a.

Stanko RT et al. Enhancement of leg exercise endurance with a high-carbohydrate diet and dihydroxyacetone and pyruvate. J Appl Physiol 69(5):1651-1656, 1990b.

Stanko RT et al. Body composition, energy utilization, and nitrogen metabolism with a severely restricted diet supplemented with dihydroxyacetone and pyruvate. Am J Clin Nutr 55(4):771-776, 1992a.

Stanko RT et al. Body composition, energy utilization, and nitrogen metabolism with a 4.25 MJ/d low-energy diet supplemented with pyruvate. Am J Clin Nutr 56(4):630-635, 1992b.

Sukala W. Pyruvate: Beyond the marketing hype. Int J Sport Nutr 8:241-249, 1998.

Tarnopolsky MA et al. Evaluation of protein requirements for strength trained athletes. J Appl Physiol 73:1986, 1992.

Tipton KD, Ferrando AA, Phillips SM et al. Postexercise net protein synthesis in human muscle from orally administered amino acids. Am J Physiol 276(4 Pt 1):E628-E634, 1999.

Thomas DE, Brotherhood JR, Brand JC. Carbohydrate feeding before exercise: Effect of glycemic index. Int J Sport Med 12:180-186, 1991.

Thomas DE, Brotherhood JR, Brand Miller, J. Plasma glucose levels after prolonged strenuous exercise correlate inversely with glycemic response to food consumed before exercise. Int J Sport Nutr 4:361-373, 1994.

Trappe S. Effect of ribose supplementation on nucleotide depletion following high-intensity exercise in human skeletal muscle. Data on file at Bioenergy, Inc., 13840 Johnson St. NE, Minneapolis, MN 55304, 1999.

Trappe SW, Costill DL, Goodpaster B, Vukovich MD, Fink WJ. The effects of L-carnitine supplementation on performance during interval swimming. Int J Sport Med 15:181-185, 1994.

Tullson PC, Terjung RL. Adenine nucleotide synthesis in exercising and endurance-trained skeletal muscle. Am J Physiol 261(2 Pt 1):C342-C347, 1991.

U.S. Department of Agriculture and U.S. Department of Health and Human Services. Nutrition and your health: Dietary guidelines for Americans. 5th ed. Home and Garden Bulletin No. 232, 2000.

Van Zyl CG, Lambert EV, Hawley JA, Noakes TD, Dennis SC. Effects of medium-chain triglyceride ingestion on fuel metabolism and cycling performance. J Appl Physiol 80:2217-2225, 1996.

Volek J et al. Testosterone and cortisol in relationship to dietary nutrients and resistance exercise. J Appl Physiol 82:49, 1997.

Walsh NP et al. Glutamine, exercise, and immune function: Links and possible mechanisms. Sports Med 26:177-191, 1998.

Wright et al. Carbohydrate feedings before, during, or in combination improves cycling performance. J Appl Physiol 71:1082, 1991.

Williams MH. Nutrition for health, fitness, and sport. 5th ed. WCB/McGraw-Hill, Dubuque, IA, 1999.

16

Creatine As an Ergogenic Supplement

J. David Branch, PhD, FACSM

Melvin H. Williams, PhD, FACSM

Creatine is one of the most popular dietary supplements in the world (Strauss and Mihoces, 1998). Although creatine was isolated in 1832, its ergogenic potential was extensively studied beginning in the early 1990s (Balsom et al., 1994). Since then, a considerable body of knowledge has come into existence on the efficacy of creatine in increasing body mass and performance in high-intensity, short-duration exercise tasks (Williams et al., 1999). This chapter is divided into several sections. Creatine biochemistry, endogenous biosynthesis, dietary sources, and the role of creatine in energy metabolism are discussed in the first section of this chapter, followed by sections on the use of creatine in clinical medicine, methods of creatine supplementation, and a brief history of creatine use in sport. The main body of this chapter summarizes the research on the efficacy of creatine supplementation in improving anaerobic power, anaerobic endurance, and aerobic endurance performance, as well as its effects on body composition. Health issues related to creatine use and legality of creatine use are discussed next, followed by a chapter summary.

Creatine Biochemistry and Metabolism

Creatine (methylguanidine acetic acid) is an amino acid derivative that is both endogenously synthesized and consumed as part of an omnivorous diet (Balsom et al., 1994; Walker, 1979). De novo biosynthesis of creatine involves the amino acids glycine, arginine, and methionine in a two-reaction pathway. The first reaction, catalyzed by glycine amidinotransferase, consists of the reversible transfer of the amidine group from arginine to glycine to form guanidinoacetate and ornithine. The second irreversible reaction catalyzed by S-adenosylmethionine:guanidinoacetate N-methyltransferase involves the methylation of guanidinoacetate by S-adenosylmethionine to form methylguanidine acetic acid (creatine) and S-adenosylhomocysteine (Balsom et al., 1994; Walker, 1979). Dietary sources of creatine include beef (4.5 g/kg), pork (5 g/kg), and cold-water fish such as tuna, salmon, and cod (1.5-2.0 g/kg). A typical daily diet with 1 to 2 g of animal protein/kg body mass includes 0.1 to 0.7 g of creatine. For example, a 4-oz (114 g) raw steak includes approximately 0.5 g of creatine. However, food preparation is known to degrade some of the dietary creatine, so the actual dietary intake of creatine is less than the amount contained in the unprepared food (Balsom et al., 1994; Greenhaff, 1997). Since virtually no creatine is present in plant products, strict vegetarians must rely on endogenous creatine biosynthesis for their creatine needs. Creatine is nonenzymatically degraded in the muscle to creatinine, which is eventually excreted in urine (Walker, 1979).

Dietary creatine is absorbed intact by the intestine and enters the bloodstream where it is transported into muscle, brain, and testicular tissue via a sodium-dependent transport mechanism that appears to be facilitated by insulin (Greenhaff, 1997; Green et al., 1996A, 1996B). Total muscle creatine concentration ([TCr]) is approximately 120 mmol/kg dry mass in the average 154-lb (70 kg) male (Greenhaff et al., 1994). Most (~95%) creatine is found in skeletal muscle, with 60% to 70% in the form of phosphocreatine (PCr) that is trapped in the cell (Balsom et al., 1994).

There are several important roles for creatine in cellular function. Creatine is an important cellular energy source for rapid resynthesis of adenosine triphosphate (ATP). In a reversible reaction catalyzed by creatine phosphokinase (CPK), creatine rapidly undergoes phosphorylation to generate PCr and dephosphorylation to resynthesize ATP from adenosine diphosphate (ADP) as follows: $PCr + ADP + H^+ \leftrightarrow Cr + ATP$. Although the mechanisms are not completely understood, creatine and PCr are possibly linked to cellular respiration and may serve as messengers in a "phosphate shuttle" between the cytosol and mitochondria. At the sarcomere, the enzyme kinetics of the MM (myofibril)-CPK isoform facilitates ATP formation. Creatine formed from this reaction crosses the outer mitochondrial membrane to the matrix where the MI (mitochondrial)-CPK isoform facilitates the formation of PCr, which then diffuses to the cytosol (Ma et al., 1996). There is also evidence that PCr may buffer acidity produced during high-intensity exercise (Walker, 1979).

Use of Creatine in Clinical Medicine

Creatine supplementation has been reported to improve skeletal muscle function in various clinical conditions such as congestive heart failure (CHF) (Andrews et al., 1998; Gordon et al., 1995), gyrate atrophy (Sipilä et al., 1981), mitochondrial cytopathies (Tarnopolsky et al., 1997), and guanidinoacetate methyltransferase deficiency (Stöckler et al., 1997). Gyrate atrophy patients who were supplemented with creatine reported increases in strength, body mass, and type II fiber diameter (Sipilä et al., 1981). Improved performance was later shown by Casey et al. (1996) to be related to PCr availability and ATP resynthesis in type II fibers.

Method, Dosage, and Administration of Creatine Supplementation

Creatine monohydrate, the most commonly supplemented form of creatine, is commercially available as powder, tablets, gel, liquid, gum, and candy (Williams et al., 1999). Creatine phosphate is also commercially available, but it is no more effective than creatine monohydrate since it is broken down to creatine and phosphate by intestinal and blood phosphatase activity (Saks and Strumia, 1993). Most of the research on creatine involves short-term supplementation of 20 to 30 g of creatine monohydrate per day for ≤14 days. In biopsy studies, [TCr] has consistently increased by 17% to 24% following a supplementation regimen of 20 g/day for five to seven days (Balsom et al., 1995; Casey et al., 1996; Gordon et al., 1995; Green et al., 1996A; Greenhaff et al., 1994; Harris et al., 1992; Hultman et al., 1996; McKenna et al., 1999; Snow et al., 1998; Volek et al., 1999). As illustrated in figure 16.1, Hultman et al. (1996) demonstrated that muscle [TCr] could be maintained following this five- to

seven-day "loading" phase with a "maintenance" ingestion of 2 g/day. Creatine is commonly ingested in four daily doses of 5 to 6 g in ~250 ml (~8 oz) warm fluid containing carbohydrate. There is some evidence that creatine uptake is greater in subjects with low baseline [TCr] (Greenhaff et al., 1994), although Green et al. (1996A) showed that ingestion of creatine with an 18.5% (mass/volume) warm carbohydrate solution resulted in greater muscle creatine uptake (27%) compared to that with sugar-free orange juice (17%). This finding suggests the presence of an insulin-mediated mechanism for muscle uptake of creatine. It has been shown that muscle [TCr] returns to baseline approximately four weeks following cessation of supplementation (Vandenberghe et al., 1997).

Brief History of Creatine Use in Sport and Exercise

The following is a summary of the history of creatine from its discovery to the present day as discussed by Williams et al. (1999) and Balsom et al. (1994). Briefly, in 1832 the French scientist Michel Eugene Chevreul discovered a metabolite in meat that he named creatine. Fifteen years later, the existence of creatine in meat was confirmed by Justus von Liebig, who reported that wild foxes had much greater concentrations of creatine than captive animals. In the 1880s, creatinine was discovered in urine and was identified as a marker for both muscle creatine storage and total muscle mass. Chanutin (1926) reported that supplemented creatine was absorbed intact by the intestine, with a portion retained by the body, and that increased creatine ingestion was associated with

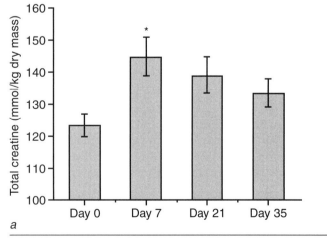

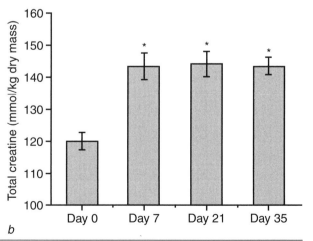

Figure 16.1 (a) Effects of creatine supplementation (20 g/day for 6 days) on muscle [TCr]. Muscle [TCr] declined to baseline levels over the next 28 days. (b) Effects of creatine loading (20 g/day for 6 days) followed by maintenance supplementation (2 g/day for the next 28 days). Muscle [TCr] remains elevated above baseline with maintenance supplementation. Data are from healthy and active, but not highly trained, males.

Reprinted, by permission, from E. Hultman et al., 1996, "Muscle creatine loading in men," *Journal of Applied Physiology* 81 232-237.

increased urinary [creatinine]. As described by Balsom et al. (1994), Fiske and Subbarow discovered PCr in 1927. Their observation that [PCr] decreased during electrical stimulation of muscle and increased during recovery established its role in energy metabolism. In recent years, creatine has become a popular dietary supplement for many strength-power athletes. Amid much publicity, major league baseball players Mark McGwire and Sammy Sosa used creatine in their race during the 1998 season to break the single-season home run record.

Prevalence and Incidence of Creatine Use

Creatine is one of the most popular dietary supplements worldwide. The acknowledged use of creatine by several prominent professional athletes has contributed to its popularity. Creatine users are primarily young males who are involved in resistance training (Johnson, 1998; Sheppard et al., 2000). Annual sales of creatine in the United States alone are well over $100 million (Strauss and Mihoces, 1998). Prevalence estimates of creatine use range from 28% in National Collegiate Athletic Association athletes (LaBotz and Smith, 1999), to 29% and 57% in military and civilian health club members, respectively (Sheppard et al., 2000), and 45% in power athletes (Ronsen et al., 1999).

Research on Creatine Usage and Efficacy of Supplementation in Sport and Exercise

Although creatine was first isolated in 1832, essentially all research on the ergogenic potential of creatine has been conducted in the 1990s. The reader is referred to several reviews of this literature (Balsom et al., 1994; Demant and Rhodes, 1999; Juhn and Tarnopolsky, 1998A; Kraemer and Volek, 1999; Mujika and Padilla, 1997), as well as a comprehensive monograph on creatine supplementation (Williams et al., 1999). The following sections summarize the results of over 80 published studies of the effects of creatine supplementation on performance and body composition. Short-term creatine supplementation was defined as ≤30 g/day for ≤14 days, and long-term supplementation was defined as any dose taken for >14 days.

Anaerobic Power Tasks

The dominant energy system for high-intensity, short-duration tasks (≤30 sec) is ATP-PCr. According to the principle of training specificity, it is logical to hypothesize that much of the research on creatine supplementation would focus on high-intensity, short-duration tasks. There is considerable research on the effects of creatine on

performance tasks of ≤30-sec duration such as arm and leg ergometry, isokinetic torque production, isometric force production, isotonic strength, jumping, running, and swimming performance. Indeed, most of the support for the efficacy of creatine supplementation is related to tasks of anaerobic power. A summary of the effects of creatine supplementation on anaerobic power performance tasks is presented in figure 16.2. The relative change was calculated as $[(creatine_{post} - creatine_{pre}) \div creatine_{pre} \times 100]$ for each dependent variable in these studies. Graphed values are $\bar{x} \pm SE$ for change in variables for which a significant effect was reported (■) or for which there was no significant effect of creatine (□). For the sake of consistency, the absolute values of the mean relative changes are graphed for swimming and running variables.

Ergometer Performance

One of the most commonly used exercise protocols to evaluate the efficacy of creatine supplementation is ergometry. Ergometer protocols include single and repetitive bouts of cycling sprints with measurement of such variables as power (W), work (kJ), and revolutions per minute (rev/min). In the studies described here, ergometer performance following creatine supplementation was examined.

Studies reporting improvement following short-term creatine supplementation   We are aware of only one study of the effect of creatine supplementation on upper-body work and power production as measured by arm ergometry. Grindstaff et al. (1997) measured arm swim ergometer performance (3 × 20-sec sprints) in 18 male and female elite swimmers before and following creatine or placebo supplementation. Work performed and peak power in the first sprint were greater following creatine supplementation compared to baseline. No group differences in performance in either the second or third sprints were observed following supplementation.

Many studies have addressed the effect of creatine supplementation on cycle (leg) ergometer performance. Significant improvements in performance have been reported in 12 studies (Balsom et al., 1993A, 1995; Birch et al., 1994; Casey et al., 1996; Dawson et al., 1995; Earnest et al., 1995; Kamber et al., 1999; Kirksey et al., 1999; Kreider et al., 1998; Prevost et al., 1997; Schneider et al., 1997; Shomrat et al., 2000; Vandebuerie et al., 1998). Balsom et al. (1993A) examined the effect of creatine supplementation on rev/min during 10 × 6-sec sprints at 880 W in 16 healthy males. Ergometer rev/min were measured for 0-2 sec, 2-4 sec, and 4-6 sec for each sprint. Following creatine supplementation, significantly greater rev/min were observed for 4-6 sec of the last four sprints. The creatine group also had lower postexercise blood lactate ([HLa]) and [hypoxanthine] (a marker of

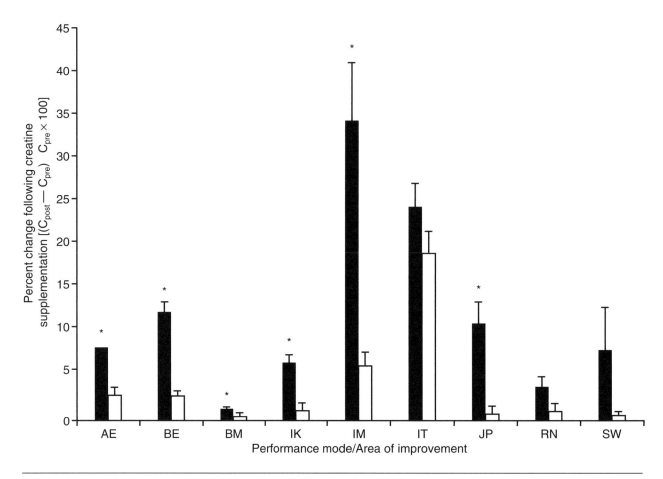

Figure 16.2 Percent improvement in various modes of anaerobic power and body mass following creatine supplementation. Values are $\bar{x} \pm SE$ for relative improvement from baseline for each dependent variable calculated as $[(creatine_{post} - creatine_{pre})] \div creatine_{pre} \times 100$.

For all groups receiving creatine supplementation, ■ = variables for which a significant change was reported, □ = variables for which no change was reported, * = significant difference within area (■ > □, p ≤ 0.05).

AE = arm ergometry (1 study); BE = bicycle ergometry (21 studies); BM = body mass (55 studies); IK = isokinetic torque production (10 studies); IM = isometric force production (8 studies); IT = isotonic strength (13 studies); JP = jumping performance (6 studies); RN = sprint running (5 studies), SW = sprint swimming (3 studies).

protein degradation) following supplementation despite having accomplished more work. In a later study of seven physically active males, Balsom et al. (1995) examined rev/min in a 10-sec sprint that followed 5 × 6-sec sprints with a 30-sec rest between sprints. The percent decline in rev/min following creatine supplementation was significantly less than before supplementation. In contrast to findings in their earlier study (Balsom et al., 1993A), however, the researchers reported increased [HLa] following supplementation.

Birch et al. (1994) randomly assigned 14 healthy but not highly trained males to either a creatine or placebo group. Subjects completed three sets of 30-sec isokinetic cycling at 80 rev/min with 4-min rest between sets. Increases in peak and mean power output and total work were observed following creatine supplementation. Postexercise plasma ammonia concentration ($[NH_3]$)

was lower following creatine supplementation, but no difference was observed between groups in [HLa] response. Using similar methodology, Casey et al. (1996) examined the effects of creatine supplementation on total work performed by nine healthy males during 2 × 30-sec maximal isokinetic cycle sprints (80 rev/min) with 4-min rest between sprints. Increases in total work were observed for both sprints following supplementation. The increase in total work was significantly correlated with muscle [TCr] (r = 0.7). The investigators attributed their findings to increased ATP resynthesis in type II fibers during recovery due to uptake of supplemented creatine.

Dawson et al. (1995) randomly assigned 22 healthy active males to creatine or placebo groups. Exercise consisted of 6 × 6-sec sprints with a 24-sec rest interval during which peak power and total work were recorded.

Supplementation improved peak power and total work in all sprints. Postexercise [HLa] was higher for both groups following supplementation, with no difference between the groups.

Earnest et al. (1995) examined the effect of creatine supplementation or placebo on Wingate test performance (3 × 30-sec tests with 5-min rest between tests) in weight-trained males. Compared to placebo, creatine supplementation resulted in improvements in total work for all three tests.

Kamber et al. (1999) measured mean rev/min at 0-2, 2-4, and 4-6 sec of 10 × 6-sec sprints in 10 well-trained males. In a counterbalanced crossover design with a two-month washout, creatine supplementation significantly increased muscle [TCr] and [PCr]/[ATP] ratio (as reported by Kreis et al., 1999) and resulted in a 3.5% improvement in rev/min across all 10 sprints. In addition, [HLa] after sprints 5, 7, and 10 and at 2 min postexercise was lower in the creatine group compared to presupplementation.

Prevost et al. (1997) assigned physically active male and female college students to either creatine supplementation or placebo groups. Following supplementation, increases in time to exhaustion of 62% and 100%, respectively, were observed for two sessions at 150% of $\dot{V}O_2$max consisting of work/rest intervals of 20 sec/40 sec and 10 sec/20 sec. Postexercise [HLa] was also lower in creatine group following supplementation. No change was observed in the placebo group for any variable.

Using a single-blind ordered design with placebo preceding creatine supplementation, Schneider et al. (1997) measured sprint cycle performance (5 × 15-sec maximal sprints with 60-sec rest) in nine untrained males. Creatine supplementation resulted in an increase in total work across the five sprints as well as increased work in each individual sprint. There was no difference between creatine and placebo trials in [HLa] measured 4 min after the last sprint.

Shomrat et al. (2000) compared vegetarians and meat eaters consuming creatine to a placebo group of meat eaters. Subjects were administered three modified (20 sec) Wingate tests separated by 4 min of recovery prior to and following supplementation. Compared to values in the placebo group, increases in mean power were observed in both creatine groups for all three Wingate tests. In addition, postsupplementation peak power production was greater in the group of creatine meat eaters compared to the placebo group. A significant reduction of rate of fatigue was observed in the vegetarian group in the second Wingate test following supplementation.

Following an exhaustive 2-hr bout of exercise at progressive work rates equivalent to [HLa] of 1, 2, 3, and 4 mmol/L, 12 well-trained amateur cyclists completed 5 × 10-sec maximal sprints with a 2-min rest interval between sprints (Vandebuerie et al., 1998). The effects of creatine supplementation and creatine supplementation plus acute creatine ingestion during exercise were compared to those of a placebo condition in a counterbalanced crossover design. Creatine supplementation increased peak and mean power production in all five sprints compared to placebo. However, the consumption of additional creatine during exercise following creatine supplementation did not improve peak or mean power production compared to placebo. Rate of fatigue was unaffected by creatine supplementation or consumption of creatine during exercise.

Studies reporting no improvement following short-term creatine supplementation Ten studies (Barnett et al., 1996; Burke et al., 1996; Cooke and Barnes, 1997; Cooke et al., 1995; Dawson et al., 1995; Ledford and Branch, 1999; McKenna et al., 1999; Odland et al., 1997; Snow et al., 1998; Vogel et al., 2000) indicated no improvement in ergometer performance following supplementation. Barnett reported no change in peak or mean power production during 7 × 10-sec sprints in recreationally active males following creatine supplementation. In addition, there were no postsupplementation group differences in postexercise [HLa], pH, or oxygen consumption. In a study of elite male and female swimmers, Burke et al. (1996) reported no difference between creatine and placebo supplementation groups in cycle sprint mean peak power, mean total work, or mean time to peak power in 2 × 10-sec maximal sprints with 10-min rest between sprints. Cooke et al. (1995) reported no effect of creatine compared to placebo on peak power, time to peak power, total work, or rate of fatigue in 12 untrained males during 2 × 15-sec sprints with 111.8 N of resistance. In a later study, Cooke and Barnes (1997) assigned 80 healthy active males to either placebo or creatine and 30, 60, 90, or 120 sec of recovery between two maximal sprints to fatigue. Within each recovery time, there was no effect of creatine on peak power production or time to fatigue.

In a separate group of 18 active males reported in the same paper (Dawson et al., 1995), there were no effects of creatine supplementation on peak power, time to peak power, total work, or work during a single 10-sec maximal sprint test. McKenna et al. (1999) assigned 13 healthy male and female subjects to either creatine supplementation or placebo groups. Subjects completed 5 × 10-sec maximal sprints with 180-, 50-, 20-, and 20-sec rest between sprints. No changes in peak power, total work, or rate of fatigue were observed immediately, two weeks, or four weeks following supplementation.

In a counterbalanced crossover design with three-month washout, Ledford and Branch (1999) reported no effect of creatine supplementation on peak power or total work during three Wingate tests in nine trained females. In another counterbalanced crossover design with only a 14-day washout, Odland et al. (1997) reported no effect of creatine supplementation on power, rate of fatigue, or [HLa] in nine males during and following a single Wingate test. In a third crossover study with trials separated by four weeks, Snow et al. (1998) also reported no effect of creatine supplementation on peak or mean power production, time to peak power, decrement in power production, [HLa], [NH$_3$], or [hypoxanthine] during a 20-sec sprint test in eight untrained males.

Vogel et al. (2000) provided creatine or placebo to 16 recreationally active males who completed 5 × 5-sec sprints prior to and during hyperthermic exercise. There was no effect of creatine on power production or total work immediately following supplementation or at 75 min and 150 min of hyperthermic exercise designed to induce hypohydration.

Studies reporting improvement following long-term creatine supplementation and training Kirksey et al. (1999) compared the effects of placebo and long-term creatine supplementation (0.3 g/kg body mass/day [22 g/day] for 42 days) on sprint performance (5 × 10-sec) in 35 male and female athletes who were also undergoing preseason conditioning. Compared to the placebo group, the creatine group showed greater increases in peak and mean power, work, and initial power rate for all five sprints following supplementation. In another study of long-term supplementation (15.75 g/day for 28 days) combined with resistance training, Kreider et al. (1998) reported that creatine supplementation resulted in increases of 11% to 15% in work performed in the first five of 12 × 6-sec sprints compared to values in the placebo group.

Studies reporting no improvement following long-term creatine supplementation and training Stone et al. (1999) randomly assigned 42 football players to placebo, creatine (0.22 g/kg body mass/day [~20 g/day]), creatine + pyruvate (0.09 g creatine/kg body mass/day [~8 g/day]), or calcium pyruvate supplementation groups. Subjects completed 15 × 5-sec maximal sprints before and after five weeks of supplementation combined with resistance training. There were no group differences in average peak power production, average total work, rate of perceived exertion, or [HLa].

Summary Among ergometer variables for which significant improvements were reported following creatine supplementation, the average improvement was ($\bar{x} \pm$ SE) 11.7 ± 1.7%. In contrast, the change in ergometer variables that did not significantly increase following creatine supplementation was 2.5 ± 0.5% (p < 0.05, figure 16.2). Creatine supplementation has consistently

been reported to improve performance in single and repetitive high-intensity, short-duration ergometry tasks.

Isokinetic Torque Production

Another commonly used exercise protocol in creatine supplementation research is isokinetic torque production (Nm) and work (J) at various angular velocities. Isokinetic performance following creatine supplementation was examined in the following studies.

Studies reporting improvement following short-term or long-term creatine supplementation Six published studies have shown significant increases in isokinetic torque production following creatine supplementation (Greenhaff et al., 1993; Rawson et al., 1999; Rawson and Clarkson, 1999; Vandenberghe et al., 1996, 1997, 1999). Greenhaff et al. (1993) assigned 12 physically active, nonvegetarian males and females to short-term creatine or placebo groups. Subjects performed five sets of 30 maximal isokinetic knee extensions before and following supplementation. Total peak torque production was increased by 5.5% and 5.0% in sets 2 and 3, respectively, with a trend toward increased torque in set 4 (p = 0.056). Plasma [NH$_3$] was decreased following creatine supplementation compared to placebo, a finding that may be related to increased [PCr] to maintain ATP without nucleotide deamination. There was no difference between groups in [HLa] response.

There is evidence that creatine supplementation may increase isokinetic torque production in older subjects. Rawson et al. (1999) assigned 20 older (67 ± 7 years of age) males to either a placebo or creatine (30 days of supplementation) group. Subjects performed five sets of 30 knee extensions at 180°/sec. The sum of peak knee extension torque for each repetition was greater following 10 days and 30 days of supplementation. In a second study using the same methodology (Rawson and Clarkson, 1999), a small but significant increase was observed in the sum of peak torque values for all contractions in set 3.

Three studies by Vandenberghe and colleagues demonstrate improvement in isokinetic torque following creatine supplementation. In the first study (Vandenberghe et al. 1996), nine physically active males received in counterbalanced order each of the following treatments for six days: 40 g creatine/day, creatine + 5 mg caffeine/kg/day, and placebo. Subjects performed the following knee extension exercise: three sets × 30 dynamic contractions, four sets × 20 dynamic contractions, and five sets × 10 dynamic contractions. Torque production increased by 10% to 23% following creatine supplementation. Although caffeine + creatine resulted in increased muscle [creatine], the ergogenic effect was counteracted by the addition of caffeine, which suggests that caffeine impairs ATP resynthesis in some manner. In another short-term study, Vandenberghe et al. (1999) examined the effects of two and five days of creatine supplementation (20 g/day) on 5 × 30 knee extension contractions of the right leg at 180°/sec in nine healthy males. Significant increases in knee extension torque were observed in sets 2 through 5 after two days of supplementation and in the first three sets after five days of supplementation. In a third study, on the effects of short-term and long-term supplementation, Vandenberghe et al. (1997) assigned 19 untrained females to either a placebo group or a long-term creatine (74 day) group. Following the four-day loading phase (20 g/day), both groups began a progressive resistance training program including 5 g of supplementation/day for 70 days. Isokinetic torque production (5 × 30 maximal arm flexion contractions with 2-min rest between sets) was measured at baseline, 5 weeks of training, and 10 weeks of training. Isokinetic torque production was unchanged following the loading phase. During training, however, the creatine group had a greater increase in mean power output for all five sets than the placebo group. Torque production remained elevated in a subgroup of subjects who continued supplementation during 10 weeks of detraining.

Studies reporting no improvement following short-term or long-term creatine supplementation Gilliam et al. (2000) reported no effect of short-term supplementation on peak torque in five sets of 30 maximal voluntary contractions performed by untrained males. In a crossover study designed to examine the effect of creatine supplementation during loss of body mass, Ööpik et al. (1998) reported that peak knee extension torque and total work at 1.57, 3.14, and 4.71 rad/sec declined at similar rates in placebo and creatine-supplemented hypohydration conditions. In one of two studies of long-term creatine supplementation, Brenner et al. (2000) reported no change in total isokinetic work (five sets × 30 knee extensions at 180°/sec with 1-min rest between sets), fatigue index, [HLa], blood urea nitrogen (BUN), or serum glutamyltransferase activity in 16 female college lacrosse players following creatine supplementation (20 g/day for 7 days, then 2 g/day for 28 days). Pearson et al. (1999) also reported no change in peak flexion or extension torque at 1.05 rad/sec in college football players engaged in resistance training who were assigned to placebo or creatine (5 g/day for 70 days) supplementation groups.

Summary Among isokinetic variables for which significant improvements were reported following creatine supplementation, the average improvement was ($\bar{x} \pm$ SE) $5.9 \pm 0.9\%$. In contrast, the change in isokinetic variables that did not significantly increase following creatine supplementation was $1.6 \pm 0.9\%$ (p < 0.05,

figure 16.2). Creatine supplementation may improve torque and work accomplished in single and repetitive high-intensity, short-duration isokinetic tasks.

Isometric Force Production

The effect of creatine supplementation on static force production has been investigated in several studies. Commonly measured variables are force (N) and time to exhaustion at various percentages of maximal voluntary contraction (MVC).

Studies reporting improvement following short-term creatine supplementation Three studies indicate improvement in isometric force production following creatine supplementation (Andrews et al., 1998; Maganaris and Maughan, 1998; Urbanski et al., 1999). Andrews et al. (1998) reported that congestive heart failure (CHF) patients who consumed 20 g creatine for five days improved handgrip performance and had lower postexercise [NH_3] and [HLa] compared to placebo patients. Maganaris and Maughan (1998) compared creatine and placebo supplementation in 10 trained males using a crossover design with no washout. Knee extension force in both the dominant and nondominant legs was improved following creatine supplementation. Moreover, force remained elevated in the subjects receiving the placebo treatment last, due in part to inadequate creatine washout. The authors also reported increased time to exhaustion at 80% of MVC in the dominant leg and improvements in time to exhaustion at 80% of MVC in 10 bouts in the nondominant leg. Urbanski et al. (1999) compared large (3 × submaximal knee extension exercise at 67% of MVC) and small (three sets of handgrip exercise at 67% of MVC) muscle group fatigue in 10 males who received both creatine and placebo supplements. Time to fatigue was increased in the last two bouts of both small and large muscle group exercise. The investigators also reported improvement in maximal isometric work for large but not small muscle groups.

Studies reporting no improvement following short-term or long-term creatine supplementation Two studies of short-term supplementation show no effect on isometric force production. In their crossover study comparing creatine, creatine + caffeine, and placebo treatments, Vandenberghe et al. (1996) tested nine physically active males at 95°, 120°, and 145° of knee extension. Compared with placebo, short-term supplementation with creatine (40 g/day for 6 days) or creatine + caffeine did not increase force production at any joint angle. Van Leemputte et al. (1999) reported that creatine supplementation significantly reduced mean muscle relaxation time following 12 maximal isometric elbow flexion contractions at 110° angle in 16 male physical education students; but there was no effect of creatine on maximal torque, maximal contraction time, muscle activation time, or deactivation time (derived from electromyogram data).

Three studies of creatine supplementation in older subjects indicate no effect on isometric force production. Bermon et al. (1998) assigned 32 elderly (74 ± 2 years of age) male and female subjects to sedentary-placebo, sedentary-creatine, training-placebo, or training-creatine groups. Creatine supplementation consisted of 20 g/day for five days followed by 3 g/day for 47 days. Within each training condition, there were no effects of creatine on leg press, chest press, or leg extension peak force. Rawson et al. (1999) reported no effect of creatine supplementation (20 g/day for 10 days, then 4 g/day for 20 days) on mean arm flexor isometric force in 20 healthy males (67 ± 6 years) following 10 days or 30 days of supplementation. In a follow-up study, Rawson and Clarkson (1999) found no effect of short-term supplementation (20 g/day for 5 days) on maximal elbow flexion force kg at 90° joint angle.

Summary Among variables of isometric force production for which significant improvements were reported after creatine supplementation, the average improvement was ($\bar{x} \pm$ SE) 34.4 ± 6.6% compared to 5.7 ± 1.7% improvement in variables that did not significantly increase with creatine supplementation (p < 0.05, figure 16.2). The literature is equivocal regarding the effect of creatine supplementation on isometric force production. Moreover, creatine supplementation does not appear to improve isometric force production in older subjects.

Isotonic Strength

In applied settings, the most common system of resistance training is dynamic constant resistance, which is also known as isotonic training. Commonly measured variables for an isotonic resistance exercise include one-repetition maximum (1-RM), lifting volume (calculated as resistance multiplied by repetitions), and number of repetitions at a given percentage of 1-RM. The following studies examined changes in isotonic strength following short-term or long-term creatine supplementation with or without resistance training.

Studies reporting improvement in males following short-term creatine supplementation Two studies investigated the effect of short-term creatine supplementation on isotonic strength (Earnest et al., 1995; Volek et al., 1997). Earnest et al. (1995) reported increases in number of bench press repetitions at 70% of 1-RM, absolute total strength, and relative strength in male subjects following short-term creatine supplementation compared to placebo. Volek et al. (1997) randomly assigned 14 active males to short-term creatine or placebo supplementation groups. They also reported that creatine

supplementation resulted in significant increases in five sets of bench press 10-RM to exhaustion and five sets of jump squat 1-RM compared to values in the placebo group. Following supplementation, a higher post-bench press [HLa] and a trend toward a lower post-squat [HLa] response were observed.

Studies reporting improvement in males following long-term creatine supplementation Several studies indicate significant improvements following long-term creatine supplementation combined with resistance training (Becque et al., 2000; Brenner et al., 2000; Kelly and Jenkins, 1998; Kreider et al., 1998; Noonan et al., 1998; Pearson et al., 1999; Peeters et al., 1999; Stone et al., 1999; Vandenberghe et al., 1997; Volek et al., 1999). Becque et al. (2000) assigned 23 weight-trained males to either placebo or creatine (20 g/day for 5 days, then 2 g/day for 37 days) groups. During periodized training, the creatine group increased arm flexor 1-RM by 28% compared to 16% for the placebo group. Kelly and Jenkins (1998) provided 18 male power lifters with either placebo or creatine (20 g/day for 6 days, then 5 g/day for 21 days) supplementation. Creatine supplementation increased bench press 3-RM and total repetitions in five sets to fatigue at 70% of bench press 1-RM. Kreider et al. (1998) reported significantly greater increases in bench press lifting volume and total lifting volume (sum of bench press, squat, and power clean lifting volumes) in a group of creatine-supplemented (15.75 g/day for 28 days) football players following training compared to a training placebo group. Following short-term creatine loading (20 g/day for 5 days), Noonan et al. (1998) provided two training groups with 51 additional days of either 100 mg creatine/kg lean body mass (LBM)/day (~8 g/day) or 300 mg creatine/kg LBM/day (~26 g/day). Both creatine groups had a significantly greater improvement in bench press 1-RM than the placebo group. Pearson et al. (1999) examined the effect of long-term supplementation (70 days) with a lower dose (5 g/day) on strength in football players. Bench press, squat, and power clean 1-RM were increased following creatine supplementation compared to no change in the placebo group. Peeters et al. (1999) also reported increases in bench press 1-RM following either creatine monohydrate or creatine phosphate (20 g/day for 3 days, then 10 g/day for 39 days) supplementation. In two separate groups of football players engaged in five weeks of training and creatine supplementation (~8 and ~20 g/day), Stone et al. (1999) reported greater increases in bench press 1-RM than observed in the placebo group. Volek et al. (1999) assigned 19 resistance-trained males to either placebo or creatine (25 g/day for 5 days, then 5 g/day for 77 days) groups. Creatine supplementation resulted in greater increases in bench press 1-RM following both short-term loading and 12 weeks of training compared to the values in the placebo group. Significantly greater increases were also observed in the creatine group for peak power output during the last two sets of four sets of 10 jump squats at 30% of 1-RM.

Studies reporting improvement in females following long-term creatine supplementation Two studies demonstrated significant improvements following long-term creatine supplementation and resistance training in women (Brenner et al., 2000; Vandenberghe et al., 1997). Brenner et al. (2000) reported that female lacrosse players assigned to creatine (20 g/day for 7 days, then 2 g/day for 28 days) significantly increased bench press 1-RM compared to the placebo group. Vandenberghe et al. (1997) examined the effect of creatine supplementation on strength improvement in females during 10 weeks of resistance training. They reported significantly greater improvements in leg press, leg extension, and squat 1-RM following creatine supplementation (20 g/day for 4 days, then 5 g/day for 70 days) compared to values in the placebo training group.

Studies reporting no improvement in older subjects following long-term creatine supplementation In their study of creatine supplementation and training in older (74 ± 2 years of age) male and female subjects, Bermon et al. (1998) reported no effect of creatine supplementation (20 g/day for 5 days, then 3 g/day for 47 days) on leg press, leg extension, or chest press 1-RM or endurance compared to findings for a training placebo group. Creatine supplementation also did not improve isotonic strength or endurance in a separate sedentary treatment group compared to a sedentary placebo group.

Summary Most of the research and the significant results on isotonic strength have been reported in young, trained males. There is research support for the combination of creatine supplementation and resistance training to significantly improve isotonic strength compared to resistance training alone. As shown in figure 16.2, the average improvement among isotonic variables for which significant improvements were reported was ($\bar{x}$ ± SE) 23.9 ± 3.6%. The change in isotonic variables that did not significantly increase following creatine supplementation was 17.9 ± 2.6%. Two studies support the combination of creatine and resistance training to improve isotonic strength in females (Brenner et al., 2000; Vandenberghe et al., 1997). On the basis of one study (Bermon et al., 1998), creatine does not appear to improve isotonic strength in older subjects. More research is needed on the effects of creatine on isotonic strength improvement in women and older subjects.

Jumping Performance

The application of improved performance from the laboratory to the field setting is the logical objective of a purported ergogenic supplement. Jumping ability, an expression of power, is an asset in sports such as basketball, soccer, and various track and field events. The effects of creatine supplementation on vertical displacement (cm), force (N), and power (W) during jumping tasks were reported in the following studies.

Studies reporting improvement following creatine supplementation Three studies show significant improvements in jumping performance following short-term supplementation (Bosco et al., 1997) and long-term supplementation combined with resistance training (Kirksey et al., 1999; Stone et al., 1999). Bosco et al. (1997) assigned 14 sprinters and jumpers to either placebo or short-term supplementation groups. Following supplementation, the creatine group had a significantly greater mean rise in center of gravity for 0-15 sec and 16-30 sec of a 45-sec continuous jumping test. However, there was no effect of creatine on average jump height or average power (w/kg). Kirksey et al. (1999) reported significantly greater increases in countermovement vertical jump (CMVJ) performance in male and female athletes undergoing preseason conditioning and creatine supplementation (0.3 g/kg/day [~22 g/day] for 42 days) compared to a placebo group. However, there was no difference between groups in improvement in static movement vertical jump (SMVJ) distance or power index. Stone et al. (1999) compared the effects of two creatine doses (0.22 g/kg/day [~20 g/day] vs. 0.09 g/kg/day [~8 g creatine/day + pyruvate]) during five weeks of conditioning on SMVJ power, force, and rate of force development in football players. Compared to the placebo group, the low-dose creatine group showed significantly greater SMVJ power and force following supplementation, while the high-dose creatine group had significantly greater increases in all three SMVJ variables.

Studies reporting no improvement following creatine supplementation Three studies indicate no effect of creatine supplementation on jumping performance (Balsom et al., 1995; Mujika et al., 2000; Noonan et al., 1998). In a single-group ordered design, Balsom et al. (1995) reported no difference between placebo and short-term creatine supplementation in CMVJ or SMVJ displacement in seven physically active males. Short-term supplementation also failed to improve CMVJ performance (three maximal jumps with 30-sec rest) in highly trained soccer players (Mujika et al. 2000). In a study by Noonan et al. (1998), three groups of college athletes were assigned to either placebo or one of two creatine supplementation groups (20 g/day for 5 days, then 100 mg/kg LBM/day [~8 g/day] for 51 days; or 20 g/day for 5 days, then 300 mg/kg LBM/day [~26 g/day] for 51 days). Following supplementation, there were no group differences in vertical jump distance.

Summary Among jumping variables for which significant improvements were reported following creatine supplementation, the average improvement was ($\bar{x} \pm$ SE) 10.2 ± 2.9%. In contrast, the change in jumping variables that did not significantly increase following creatine supplementation was 0.8 ± 0.9% (p < 0.05, figure 16.2). The literature is equivocal regarding the effect of creatine supplementation on jumping performance.

Running Performance

Improved speed following creatine supplementation would be beneficial to athletes such as sprinters, basketball players, American football players, and soccer players. The following studies examined the effects of creatine supplementation on time to complete repetitive sprint bouts.

Studies reporting improvement following creatine supplementation Three studies indicate improved sprint running performance following creatine supplementation (Aaserud et al., 1998; Mujika et al., 2000; Noonan et al., 1998). Aaserud et al. (1998) examined the effects of short-term creatine supplementation on 8 × 40-m (44 yd) sprint performance in male handball players. Compared to baseline, the increase in time from the first to the last sprint was reduced following both the loading and maintenance phases of creatine supplementation. Mujika et al. (2000) reported decreased 5- and 15-m (5.5 and 16.4 yd) time during 6 × 15-m sprints in highly trained male soccer players following short-term creatine supplementation. [NH$_3$] and [HLa] were decreased in both placebo and creatine groups following supplementation, with no difference between groups. Noonan et al. (1998) observed a significant decrease in 40-yd (36.5 m) time in a group of male athletes receiving low-dose maintenance creatine (100 mg/kg LBM/day [~8 g/day] for 51 days) following loading (20 g/day for 5 days). No improvement was observed in a group receiving a higher maintenance dose (300 mg/kg LBM/day [~26 g/day] for 51 days).

Studies reporting no improvement following creatine supplementation Two studies report no effect of creatine supplementation on sprint running performance. In a study of moderately active males, Edwards et al. (2000) found no effect of short-term creatine supplementation on time to exhaustion following 4 × 15-sec sprint bouts (8 m/hr [214 m/min] up a 20% grade) on a treadmill. No differences were observed between creatine and placebo groups in [HLa], but lower [NH$_3$] was observed following creatine supplementation. Redondo et al. (1996) reported no effect of short-term creatine supplementation on 60-m (66 yd) sprint velocity in three zones (20-30, 30-40, 50-60 m) within each of three trials in male and female college athletes.

Summary As shown in figure 16.2, the average improvement was ($\bar{x} \pm$ SE) 3.6 ± 1.3% among studies reporting significant effects of creatine on various measures of sprint running performance compared to 1.49 ± 0.9% improvement in running variables that did not significantly increase with creatine supplementation. There is currently no consensus in the literature regarding improved sprint running performance following creatine supplementation. Depending on the type of activity, increased body mass associated with creatine supplementation may or may not be of benefit in athletic performance.

Swimming Performance

Improved swim performance would be a logical result of increased power of arm and leg action and a more explosive start off the blocks.

Swimming performance and creatine supplementation Only one study has indicated significant improvements in swimming performance following creatine supplementation. In a study of elite males, Peyrebrune et al. (1998) reported that compared to placebo, short-term creatine supplementation improved total sprint time and the last five sprint times of an 8 × 50-yd (45.7 m) interval session. There was no difference between creatine and placebo groups in postexercise [NH$_3$], [HLa], or pH. However, Burke et al. (1996) found that short-term creatine supplementation had no effect on 25-m (27.3 yd) and 50-m (55 yd) sprint times or postswim [HLa] in elite males and females. Leenders et al. (1999) also reported no effect of short-term creatine supplementation on 10 × 25-m swim interval performance in male and female college swimmers. In fact, Mujika et al. (1996) reported a trend for a slower 25-m time (p = 0.07) in competitive male and female swimmers following creatine supplementation (20 g/day for 5 days). It was speculated that this ergolytic trend may be related to increased drag secondary to increased body mass.

Summary As suggested in figure 16.2, the available research does not support the efficacy of creatine in improving swimming performance. Indeed, increased drag associated with increased body mass may explain the increase in swim times (0.55 ± 0.27%) observed in some studies following creatine supplementation (Burke et al., 1996; Mujika et al., 1996).

Anaerobic Endurance Tasks

Theoretically, increased muscle [PCr] following creatine supplementation could enhance prolonged (30-150 sec) anaerobic tasks via buffering of acidity by creatine and less reliance on anaerobic glycolysis. The following section summarizes research on ergometry, isokinetic torque production, isometric force production, isotonic strength, kayaking, jumping, running, and swimming anaerobic endurance performance following creatine supplementation.

Ergometry

The ability to mount a sustained sprint at the end of a race or to successfully break away from the peloton would be of ergogenic interest to the competitive cyclist or triathlete. The effect of creatine supplementation on high-intensity cycle sprinting during sustained ergometer exercise has been the focus of several studies.

Studies reporting improvement following short-term creatine supplementation Engelhardt et al. (1998) subjected 12 male triathletes to intense exercise including interval work at 7.5 W/kg body mass. Creatine supplementation improved the number of intervals completed compared to placebo. Jacobs et al. (1997) reported increased time to exhaustion and maximal accumulated oxygen deficit in 26 male and female recreational exercisers immediately and seven days following creatine supplementation. In another study, creatine supplementation resulted in significantly longer times to exhaustion for continuous cycling at 150% $\dot{V}O_2$max and 60-sec work/120-sec rest interval work, as well as lower [HLa] in physically active male and female college students (Prevost et al., 1997). Smith et al. (1998A) reported that creatine supplementation increased the time to exhaustion at 5 W/kg body mass in 15 untrained males and females. Stout et al. (1999) reported that creatine and creatine + carbohydrate supplementation increased anaerobic capacity in healthy male subjects.

Studies reporting no improvement following short-term creatine supplementation Febbraio et al. (1995) and Schneider et al. (1997) reported no effect of short-term creatine supplementation on high-intensity interval cycle ergometer performance tasks that rely primarily on anaerobic glycolysis.

Isokinetic Torque Production, Isometric Force Production, and Isotonic Strength

The following sections summarize the small body of published studies of the effects of creatine supplementation on anaerobic torque, force, and strength variables.

Isokinetic Torque Production

Ööpik et al. (1998) examined the effects of creatine and placebo supplementation with simultaneous loss of body mass (3%) on isokinetic work and power in six karate athletes. Following creatine supplementation, knee extension work during the last 2 min of a 3-min isokinetic

exercise bout was decreased in the hypohydrated condition compared to the euhydrated condition.

Isometric Force Production

Three studies have shown increased isometric force production following creatine supplementation. Maganaris and Maughan (1998) compared time to exhaustion following creatine and placebo supplementation in 10 trained males. Creatine supplementation resulted in increases in time to exhaustion in the stronger leg at 20%, 40%, and 60% of MVC, respectively. This effect remained in the placebo treatment for subjects who received the creatine treatment first because there was no washout period. Tarnopolsky et al. (1997) reported that creatine supplementation (10 g/day for 14 days, then 4 g/day for 7 days) increased ischemic handgrip and non-ischemic dorsiflexion torque in seven male and female patients with mitochondrial cytopathies. Urbanski et al. (1999) reported increased time to fatigue for the first of three submaximal contractions of large and small muscle groups (67% of knee extension and handgrip MVC) following short-term creatine supplementation.

Isotonic Strength

Bosco et al. (1995) and Smith et al. (1998B) reported improved leg extensor performance (power, total work, time to fatigue, number of repetitions to fatigue) in elite soccer players and physically active males and females, respectively, following short-term creatine supplementation. However, Bosco et al. (1995) also reported greater postexercise [HLa] following supplementation.

Jumping, Kayaking, and Running Performance

The effects of creatine supplementation on sustained anaerobic jumping, kayaking, and running performances are summarized in the following sections.

Jumping Performance

Bosco et al. (1997) reported increased power and vertical displacement in a 45-sec continuous jumping test in sprinters and jumpers following creatine supplementation. There was no difference between placebo and creatine groups in post-jump [HLa] following supplementation.

Kayaking Performance

McNaughton et al. (1998) reported that creatine supplementation increased work during 90-sec and 150-sec kayak tests in 16 elite kayakers (16% and 15%, respectively), but power was not affected. Compared to baseline, placebo, and washout 150-sec trials, postexercise [HLa] was higher following creatine supplementation.

Running Performance

Bosco et al. (1997) reported that sprinters and jumpers increased treadmill running time to exhaustion (20 km/hr up a 5% grade) following creatine supplementation. The creatine group had a higher [HLa] following supplementation compared to the presupplementation value. In a study of well-trained males (Earnest et al. 1997), total time to exhaustion in two treadmill running bouts was greater following creatine supplementation than in a placebo group. The creatine group also had a higher [HLa] at 3 and 7 min following each run. Viru et al. (1994) reported improved performance in 4 × 300-m (328 yd) interval runs in middle-distance runners following creatine supplementation. However, Terrillion et al. (1997) found no effect of creatine supplementation on run time for 2 × 700-m (766 yd) intervals or [HLa] in middle-distance runners.

Swimming Performance

As previously discussed, the available literature does not support an ergogenic effect of creatine on short-duration swimming performance. Nevertheless, several studies have investigated the effects of creatine supplementation on swimming performance of >30 sec in duration.

Studies reporting improvement following short-term and long-term creatine supplementation　Grindstaff et al. (1997) reported significant improvement in 3 × 50-m (55 yd) and 3 × 100-m (109 yd) swim interval work in young male and female competitive swimmers following short-term creatine supplementation. Leenders et al. (1999) reported significant improvement in mean swim velocity for 6 × 50-m interval work after 14 days of creatine in male but not female swimmers. In a study of long-term supplementation (25 g/day for 4 days, then 5 g/day for 56 days), Theodorou et al. (1999) reported that swim interval performance (10 × 50 m [55 yd], 8 × 100 m [109 yd], or 15 × 100 m) improved following the acute loading phase. However, maintenance supplementation had no effect on swim performance.

Studies reporting no improvement following short-term and long-term creatine supplementation　Three swim studies indicate no effect of creatine supplementation on swim performance. Burke et al. (1996) found no effect of short-term creatine supplementation on 100-m (109 yd) swim performance in males and females. Mujika et al. (1996) found that short-term creatine supplementation decreased post-swim [NH$_3$], but had no effect on 100-m time or post-50 m (55 yd) or post-100 m [HLa] in males and females. They also reported a trend for slower 50-m swim time (p = 0.05) following supplementation. Thompson et al. (1996) found no effect of creatine supplementation (2 g/day for 42 days) on 100-m (109 yd) swim times in females.

Summary　Although there are some reports of improved anaerobic endurance in some tasks (cycle ergometry, isotonic endurance) following creatine supplementation, the efficacy of creatine in improving performance in other tasks (isometric force and isokinetic torque production, jumping, running, swimming) is equivocal. In addition, consistent observations of increased [HLa] or no change in [HLa] following supplementation cast doubt on reduced reliance on anaerobic glycolysis as an ergogenic mechanism of creatine supplementation.

Aerobic Endurance

Although the research is limited, it has been proposed that creatine supplementation may modify substrate utilization in prolonged (>150 sec) exercise as measured by respiratory exchange ratio and $\dot{V}O_2$ (Stroud et al., 1994). The effect of creatine on performance in various tasks (cycle ergometry, isokinetic torque production, kayaking, rowing, running, swimming) that rely predominantly on oxida-tive phosphorylation has been examined in several studies.

Improved aerobic bicycle ergometer performances (power, time to exhaustion) have been reported following short-term creatine supplementation (Gordon et al., 1995; Rico-Sanz and Marco, 2000; Smith et al., 1998A; Stout et al., 2000). In addition, Rico-Sanz and Marco (2000) reported lower [HLa] and [NH$_3$] following supplementation. Other investigators have reported no effect of creatine on aerobic bicycle ergometer performance (Barnett et al., 1996; Engelhardt et al., 1998; Tarnopolosky et al., 1997; Vandebuerie et al., 1998).

Short-term creatine supplementation improved performance in a 4-min test of 100 knee extension isokinetic contractions at 180°/sec in CHF patients (Gordon et al., 1995), but did not improve time to fatigue in either single-knee extension exercise in physically active male and female subjects (Smith et al., 1999) or sustained dorsiflexion exercise in female swimmers (Thompson et al., 1996).

McNaughton et al. (1998) reported significantly greater work accomplished and higher postexercise [HLa], but no difference in peak power in a 300-sec kayak test following short-term creatine supplementation. In a study of elite rowers, short-term creatine supplementation improved total time as well as split times in a 1000-m (1094 yd) simulated rowing test (Rossiter et al., 1996).

Only one study has shown improved aerobic running performance following creatine supplementation. Viru et al. (1994) reported faster 4 × 1000-m (1094 yd) interval performance in male middle-distance runners following short-term supplementation. Others reported either no change (Stroud et al., 1994) or impairment

(Balsom et al., 1993B) in aerobic running performance after creatine supplementation.

In the only study of aerobic swimming performance, Thompson et al. (1996) reported no effect of six weeks of low-dose supplementation (2 g/day) on 400-m (437 yd) swim performance in females.

Summary

The small body of available literature suggests that creatine supplementation does not exert an ergogenic effect on aerobic performance. The ergogenic potential of creatine supplementation appears to decrease as performance duration increases. This is likely due in part to lack of energy system specificity with regard to aerobic exercise. In addition, the potential for increased body mass following creatine supplementation could be ergolytic in many endurance tasks (e.g., swimming, distance running).

Body Composition

Changes in body composition, especially body mass, have been consistently reported following creatine supplementation. Three mechanisms have been proposed to explain changes in body composition associated with creatine supplementation. The first mechanism relates to water retention. Since creatine is osmotically active, it has been proposed that increased intracellular [TCr] may also increase intracellular water content (Volek et al., 1997; Ziegenfuss et al., 1998). This would explain the consistently observed increase in body mass following short-term creatine supplementation. This hypothesis is supported by findings of decreased urinary output during short-term creatine loading, which is suggestive of increased retention of body water (Hultman et al., 1996). The second possible mechanism relates to training volume. Many individuals who consume creatine are also involved in resistance training. The ability to train at a higher volume following creatine supplementation may represent an indirect long-term mechanism leading to increases in body mass and LBM. The third mechanism relates to protein anabolism and/or catabolism. Studies of isolated cells have led to the suggestion that creatine may function at the transcriptional or translational level to stimulate contractile protein biosynthesis (Ingwall, 1976). It has been further suggested that increased cellular hydration may serve as a signal for increased protein synthesis and/or decreased protein degradation (Volek et al., 1997; Kreider et al., 1998; Ziegenfuss et al., 1998). More research is needed to examine all of these potential mechanisms. The following section summarizes results of studies that measured the effect of short-term (10-30 g/day for ≤14 days) and long-term (>14 days) creatine supplementation on body composition in various groups.

Body mass following short-term supplementation
There is considerable research on the effects of short-term creatine supplementation on body mass. Several studies report significant increases (~1.0-4.0%) in body mass in males following short-term creatine supplementation (Balsom et al., 1993A, 1993B, 1995; Cooke and Barnes, 1997; Dawson et al., 1995; Earnest et al., 1995; Gilliam et al., 2000; Green et al., 1996A, 1996B; Greenhaff et al., 1994; Kamber et al., 1999; Maganaris and Maughan, 1998; McNaughton et al., 1998; Mihic et al., 2000; Mujika et al., 2000; Rawson and Clarkson, 1999; Shomrat et al., 2000; Snow et al., 1998; Stroud et al., 1994; Viru et al., 1994; Volek et al., 1997, 2000). In addition, three studies of male and female subjects also showed slight but significant increases in body mass following short-term creatine supplementation (Jacobs et al., 1997; Mihic et al., 2000; Mujika et al., 1996). However, not all short-term creatine loading studies have resulted in significant gains in body mass (Barnett et al., 1996; Dawson et al., 1995 [a second group in the same study]; Earnest et al., 1997; Edwards et al., 2000; Francaux et al., 2000; Green et al., 1996B [a separate group in the same study]; Grindstaff et al., 1997; Ledford and Branch, 1999; Leenders et al., 1999; McKenna et al., 1999; Mihic et al., 2000; Prevost et al., 1997; Rico-Sanz and Marco, 2000; Schneider et al., 1997; Smith et al., 1998B, 1999; Stout et al., 1999, 2000; Terrillion et al., 1997; Urbanski et al., 1999). Furthermore, none of the studies that included females as a separate group showed an increase in body mass following short-term supplementation (Ledford and Branch, 1999; Leenders et al., 1999; Mihic et al., 2000; Stout et al., 2000).

Short-term creatine supplementation and internal loss of body mass Two studies are of particular interest regarding the effects of short-term creatine supplementation on attempts to lose body mass. In a counterbalanced crossover design, six well-trained male karate athletes attempted to decrease body mass following both placebo and creatine (20 g/day for 5 days) supplementation (Ööpik et al., 1998). The 3.1% body mass loss following creatine supplementation was significantly less than the 4.1% following the placebo treatment. Vogel et al. (2000) reported that short-term creatine supplementation increased body mass, but there was no difference between creatine and placebo groups in loss of body mass during 150 min of exercise designed to induce hypohydration. These findings have relevance for athletes such as power lifters, boxers, and wrestlers who compete by weight class. More research is needed to determine whether the purported benefits of creatine supplementation (increased strength/power) may be negated by increased body mass and/or inability to "make weight."

Body mass and composition in males following long-term supplementation Increases in body mass of up to 6% have been reported following long-term supplementation regimens (Becque et al., 2000; Kelly and Jenkins, 1998; Kirksey et al., 1999; Kreider et al., 1996, 1998; Noonan et al., 1998; Pearson et al., 1999; Peeters et al., 1999; Stone et al., 1999; Theodorou et al., 1999; Volek et al., 1999). Creatine supplementation was combined with resistance training in most of these studies. Becque et al. (2000) reported that creatine supplementation (20 g/day for 5 days followed by 2 g/day for 37 days) increased body mass and LBM in weight-trained males compared to a group of placebo subjects engaged in similar training. In another study, male power lifters who consumed creatine (20 g/day for 6 days followed by 5 g/day for 21 days) had an increase in LBM as determined from skinfold measurements compared to no change in a placebo group (Kelly and Jenkins, 1998). Kirksey et al. (1999) provided creatine (0.3 g/kg/day [~22 g/day] for 42 days) or placebo to 36 male and female track and field athletes who were also engaged in preseason conditioning. Creatine supplementation resulted in a greater increase in LBM as estimated from skinfold measurements than the placebo.

Kreider et al. (1998) reported that following creatine supplementation (15.75 g/day for 28 days), significantly greater gains in dual energy X-ray absorptiometry (DEXA)-measured body mass and LBM were observed in a group of college football players who were also engaged in resistance training as compared to a placebo training group. In a similar study of resistance-trained males, Kreider et al. (1996) also reported that the increase in LBM was significantly greater following 28 days of creatine supplementation (20 g/day) compared to both a placebo treatment and a high-carbohydrate supplement.

Noonan et al. (1998) compared the effects of two long-term doses of creatine on body mass in college athletes. Following a short-term loading phase of 20 g/day for five days, groups were given either 100 mg creatine/kg body mass/day (~8 g/day) or 300 mg creatine/kg body mass/day (~26 g/day) for an additional 51 days. Body mass and LBM increased in the 300 mg/kg/day group compared to the 100 mg/kg/day and placebo groups. Pearson et al. (1999) reported an increase in body mass compared to a decrease in the placebo group following a supplementation regimen consisting of 5 g creatine/day for 70 days. Peeters et al. (1999) reported that experienced male weight lifters who were engaged in training had similar improvements in body mass and LBM following creatine monohydrate and creatine phosphate supplementation (20 g/day for 3 days, then 10 g/day for 39 days) regimens.

Stone et al. (1999) reported similar results in college football players following five weeks of resistance training. Subjects were assigned to either a creatine group (~0.22 g/kg body mass/day [~20 g/day]), a creatine + pyruvate group (~0.09 g creatine/kg body mass/day [~8 g/day]), a calcium pyruvate group, or a placebo group. Similar increases in body mass were observed in the two creatine groups. Theodorou et al. (1999) randomly assigned 22 elite male and female swimmers to either a creatine group (25 g/day for 5 days, followed by 5 g/day for 56 days) or a placebo group. A small but significant increase was reported in the creatine group following supplementation. Volek et al. (1999) randomly assigned 19 resistance-trained males to either a placebo or creatine supplementation group. Supplementation consisted of an acute loading phase (20 g/day for 5 days) and a maintenance phase (5 g/day for 78 days [weeks 2-12]) during which periodized, progressive resistance training was also undertaken by both groups. Significant gains in body mass were reported for the creatine group following the short-term loading phase. Both groups increased body mass following training, but the increase in the creatine group was significantly greater than that of the placebo group.

Body mass and composition in females following long-term supplementation Two studies have examined the effects of training and creatine supplementation on body composition in females. In a study of female college lacrosse players, Brenner et al. (2000) reported that creatine supplementation (20 g/day for 7 days followed by 2 g/day for 28 days) decreased body fat percentage as estimated from skinfold measurements. There was no effect on LBM or on percent body fat as determined by hydrostatic weighing. Vandenberghe et al. (1997) assigned 19 healthy untrained females to either a placebo or creatine supplementation (20 g/day for 4 days followed by 5 g/day for 70 days) group in order to investigate the effects of resistance training and creatine supplementation on body composition. The increase in LBM at 5 and 10 weeks of training was greater in the creatine group than in the placebo group. There was no difference between groups in change in body mass or estimated body fat percentage.

Body mass in older individuals following creatine supplementation Most of the research data on creatine supplementation have been collected on young males ≤30 years of age. Few data are available on older populations. Rawson and Clarkson (1999) reported a small but significant increase in body mass in a group of older males (60-78 years of age) following ingestion of 20 g creatine/day for five days. In another study of older males (60-82 years of age), Rawson et al. (1999) reported that long-term supplementation (20 g/day for 10 days followed by 4 g/day for 20 days) did not increase body mass. In a study comparing young (31 ± 5 years) with older (58 ± 5 years) physically active male and female subjects, no increase in body mass was reported in either group following short-term supplementation (Smith et al., 1998B). Bermon et al. (1998) randomly assigned 32 elderly (74 ± 2 years) males and females to one of four groups: sedentary-placebo, sedentary-creatine, strength training-placebo, and strength training-creatine. Supplementation consisted of 20 g/day for five days followed by 3 g/day for an additional 47 days. There was no significant difference in body mass change between the two sedentary groups or the two training groups.

Creatine supplementation and body mass in vegans As previously discussed, vegans have no exogenous source of creatine in their diet and must rely on endogenous synthesis for their creatine needs. Shomrat et al. (2000) compared the effects of creatine supplementation (21 g/day for 6 days) in vegans and meat eaters to values in a third group of meat eaters assigned to a placebo treatment. In light of evidence that creatine uptake may be enhanced in individuals with muscle [TCr] ≤120 mmol/kg dry mass (Greenhaff et al., 1994) and that vegans have lower [TCr] (DeLanghe et al., 1989; Harris et al., 1992), it is logical to hypothesize that greater changes in body mass might be observed in vegans. However, the two creatine groups had similar and significant increases in body mass compared to the placebo group.

Effect of creatine supplementation on total body water Several research groups have estimated total body water following creatine supplementation using bioelectrical impedance methodology. Kreider et al. (1998) reported a significantly greater increase in total body water in a creatine supplementation (15.75 g/day for 28 days) training group (2.4%) compared to a placebo training group (0.9%). Ziegenfuss et al. (1998) also reported increases of 2% and 3%, respectively, in total body water (+0.86 L) and intracellular fluid (+0.57 L) in 10 aerobically trained males following creatine supplementation (0.35 g/kg LBM/day for 3 days). However, Rawson and Clarkson (1999) reported no effect of creatine supplementation (20 g/day for 5 days) on intracellular fluid, extracellular fluid, or total body water in healthy older males. More research is needed on mechanisms of change in body mass and composition associated with both short-term and long-term creatine supplementation. Future research should employ valid indicator dilution methods (e.g., labeled water [^3H_2O, D_2O, $H_2^{18}O$, NaBr]) to measure body water spaces.

Summary As illustrated in figure 16.2, there is considerable, but not unanimous, support for increased body mass ($\bar{x}$ ± SE = 1.76 ± 0.23%) following creatine supplementation. It has also been consistently reported that lean body mass increases (1.2 ± 0.35%) following creatine supplementation. The increase in body mass and LBM following short-term, loading supplementation can be augmented with the combination of long-term, low-dose maintenance supplementation and resistance training. These observations are seen predominantly in males. There is much less support for the efficacy of creatine to change body mass and composition in females and older subjects. One study has indicated that females may have greater endogenous [TCr] than males (Forsberg et al., 1991). The existence of a gender difference in baseline [TCr] and evidence of greater muscle creatine uptake in subjects with low [TCr] (Greenhaff et al., 1994) may be reasons for the decreased efficacy of creatine in females. More research on females and older subjects is needed.

Clinical Pharmacology: Health Effects

As previously stated, creatine supplementation may be beneficial to various clinical populations. Two studies offer support for the efficacy of creatine supplementation in CHF patients. Gordon et al. (1995) reported improved skeletal muscle function (knee extensor exercise) and cycle ergometer performance in CHF patients following short-term creatine supplementation. In a later study of CHF patients (Andrews et al., 1998), short-term creatine supplementation improved isometric handgrip performance (contractions at 75% of MVC) with a concurrent decrease in postexercise [NH_3] and [HLa]. Creatine supplementation has also improved function in patients with myophosphorylase deficiency (Vorgerd et al., 2000), Duchenne muscular dystrophy (Felber et al., 2000), gyrate atrophies (Sipilä et al., 1981), mitochondrial cytopathies (Tarnopolsky et al., 1997), and neuromuscular disease (Tarnopolsky and Martin, 1999). These studies provide preliminary support for a therapeutic role of creatine supplementation. Clearly, there is a need for continued research on the role of creatine in management of various cardiovascular and muscular diseases.

Contraindications and Adverse Reactions

Some clinicians have expressed concern about the effects of creatine on renal function. It was determined that creatine supplementation played no role in the 1998 deaths of three college wrestlers (Associated Press, 1998). Pritchard and Kaira (1998) reported a case study of renal dysfunction associated with creatine use in a soccer player, but their conclusion that creatine was responsible for the renal dysfunction is clouded by previous history of renal nephrotic syndrome that was stabilized by cyclosporine. It was unclear whether the observed improvement in renal function following creatine withdrawal was due to adverse effects of creatine itself, impurities in the creatine product, creatine/drug interactions, and/or other factors. In three small studies, no adverse effects of creatine on renal function were reported following either short-term (Poortmans et al., 1997; Ropero-Miller et al., 2000) or long-term supplementation of 2 to 30 g/day for up to five years (Poortmans and Francaux, 1999). There have also been anecdotal reports of dehydration, muscle cramping, and strains associated with creatine supplementation—symptoms that may be associated with increased intracellular water tension. In a survey of college athletes, Greenwood et al. (2000) reported that among creatine users, many of the 38% experiencing negative effects of creatine supplementation (gastrointestinal distress, cramping) were above recommended maintenance dosages (0.03 g/kg/day). In another survey of college athletes, LaBotz and Smith (1999) reported a muscle cramping prevalence rate of 11% among creatine users. Sheppard et al. (2000) reported no difference in perceived side effects between creatine users and users of creatine in combination with other supplements. Kreider et al. (1998) reported no adverse side effects in football players following creatine supplementation (15.75 g/day for 28 days). Juhn and Tarnopolsky (1998B) have written a review of potential side effects associated with creatine supplementation. However, few scientific data are available documenting adverse health effects of creatine supplementation; more research on possible health effects of creatine supplementation is needed. Moreover, the effects of excessive (>30 g/day) and/or long-term supplementation (>5 years) are unknown and remain to be investigated.

Approval or Disapproval of Creatine Use by Sport Governing Bodies

In 1998, the International Olympic Committee Medical Commission ruled that creatine is considered a food and not a banned substance. There is currently no upper limit for blood or urine [creatine] or [creatinine] as evidence of creatine supplementation. This is in contrast to the situation with caffeine, a dietary constituent that is regulated and for which there is an upper urine [caffeine] of 12 μg/ml as evidence of doping. It is important to point out, however, that creatine supplementation is not universally endorsed. Of the 71 teams responding to a 1998 *USA Today* survey of 115 professional sport franchises, 16 teams approved of creatine use by their athletes, 24 provided creatine to their athletes, and 21 disapproved of creatine use (Strauss, 1998). Part of the appeal of creatine is the perception that it is "safe" compared to other alternatives such as anabolic-androgenic steroids, insulin-like growth factor, and human growth hormone that are unsafe, expensive, and illegal. As has been pointed out, the fact that a compound such as creatine occurs naturally does not mean that supplementation with that compound is safe (Terjung et al., 2000). Although preliminary data suggest that creatine supplementation may not be harmful (Poortmans et al., 1997; Poortmans and Francaux, 1999), the use of creatine in excessive quantities, particularly by young athletes, is a source of concern among clinicians (Johnson and Landry, 1998). More research on the long-term health effects of creatine supplementation is needed.

Conclusion

Creatine is a naturally occurring amine that undergoes rapid phosphorylation and dephosphorylation as part of the ATP-PCr energy system. It is currently one of the most popular nutritional supplements in the world of sport. Although creatine was discovered over 150 years ago, it was not until the early 1990s that its ergogenic potential was first studied. There is now a considerable body of knowledge regarding creatine supplementation. Short-term supplementation (20-30 g/day for 5-7 days) has been reported to increase muscle [TCr] by ~20%. This increase can be maintained with a low-dose "maintenance" supplementation of 2 to 5 g/day. Most of the research has focused on young, trained males, the population most likely to use creatine. There is considerable, but not unanimous, support for the efficacy of creatine supplementation in improving high-intensity, short-duration (≤30 sec) single and repetitive cycle ergometer exercise, resistance exercise, and jumping tasks. Body mass has also been consistently reported to increase by ~2% following creatine supplementation. The increases in body mass and isotonic strength may be augmented when creatine supplementation is combined with resistance training. Creatine supplementation also has been shown to improve functioning in patients with gyrate atrophy, mitochondrial cytopathies, muscular dystrophies, and CHF. Creatine supplementation has been studied much less in females and older subjects, but the available evidence suggests that it is less effective in these populations. There are virtually no scientific data on creatine use in children and adolescents despite anecdotal reports of widespread use. Due in part to energy system specificity, the ergogenic effect of creatine diminishes as the duration of the performance task increases. Because creatine is a constituent of animal products, creatine use is not banned by sport governing bodies. There are anecdotal reports of cramping, dehydration, and muscle strains associated with creatine use. In addition, there are concerns about possible renal dysfunction. Although preliminary studies do not show renal problems during and following creatine supplementation, clinicians are concerned about the unknown effects of excessive and/or long-term chronic use. More research is needed on the ergogenic effects of creatine in young athletes, females, and older subjects as well as on the health effects of chronic supplementation. As is the case with any dietary supplement, the ethics of creatine supplementation are separate issues, discussion of which is beyond the scope of this chapter.

References

Aaserud, R., Gramvik, P., Olsen, S.R. and Jensen, J. 1998. Creatine supplementation delays onset of fatigue during repeated bouts of sprint running. Scandinavian Journal of Medicine and Science in Sports 8:247-251.

Andrews, R., Greenhaff, P., Curtis, S., Perry, A. and Cowley, A.J. 1998. The effect of dietary creatine supplementation on skeletal muscle metabolism in congestive heart failure. European Heart Journal 19:617-622.

Associated Press. 1998. FDA rejects creatine role in deaths, April 30.

Balsom, P.D., Ekblom, B., Söderlund, K., Sjödin, B. and Hultman, E. 1993A. Creatine supplementation and dynamic high-intensity intermittent exercise. Scandinavian Journal of Medicine and Science in Sports 3:143-149.

Balsom, P.D., Harridge, S.D.R., Söderlund, K., Sjödin, B. and Ekblom, B. 1993B. Creatine supplementation per se does not enhance endurance exercise performance. Acta Physiologica Scandinavica 149:521-523.

Balsom, P., Söderlund, K. and Ekblom, B. 1994. Creatine in humans with special reference to creatine supplementation. Sports Medicine 18:268-280.

Balsom, P., Söderlund, K., Sjodin, B. and Hultman, E. 1995. Skeletal muscle metabolism during short duration high-intensity exercise: Influence of creatine supplementation. Acta Physiologica Scandinavica 154:303-310.

Barnett, C., Hinds, M. and Jenkins, D.G. 1996. Effects of oral creatine supplementation on multiple sprint cycle performance. Australian Journal of Science and Medicine in Sports 28:35-39.

Becque, M.D., Lochmann, J.D. and Melrose, D.R. 2000. Effects of oral creatine supplementation on muscular strength and body composition. Medicine and Science in Sports and Exercise 32:654-658.

Bermon, S., Venembre, P., Sachet, C., Valour, S. and Dolisi, C. 1998. Effects of creatine monohydrate ingestion in sedentary and weight-trained older adults. Acta Physiologica Scandinavica 164:146-155.

Birch, R., Nobel, D. and Greenhaff, P. 1994. The influence of dietary creatine supplementation on performance during repeated bouts of maximal isokinetic cycling in man. European Journal of Applied Physiology 69:268-276.

Bosco, C., Tihanyi, J., Pucspk, J., Kovacs, I., Gabossy, A., Colli, R., Pulvirenti, G., Tranquilli, C., Foti, C., Viru, M. and Viru, A. 1997. Effect of oral creatine supplementation on jumping and running performance. International Journal of Sports Medicine 18:369-372.

Bosco, C., Tranquilli, C., Tihanyi, J., Colli, R., D'Ottavio, S. and Viru, A. 1995. Influence of oral supplementation with creatine monohydrate on physical capacity evaluated in laboratory and field tests. Medicina dello Sport 48:391-397.

Brenner, M., Rankin, J.W. and Sebolt, D. 2000. The effect of creatine supplementation during resistance training in women. Journal of Strength and Conditioning Research 14:207-213.

Burke, L., Pyne, L.D. and Telford, R. 1996. Effect of oral creatine supplementation on single-effort sprint performance in elite swimmers. International Journal of Sport Nutrition 6:222-233.

Casey, A., Constantin-Teodosiu, D., Howell, S., Hultman, E. and Greenhaff, P.L. 1996. Creatine ingestion favorably affects performance and muscle metabolism during maximal exercise in humans. American Journal of Physiology 271:E31-E37.

Chanutin, A. 1926. The fate of creatine when administered to man. Journal of Biological Chemistry 67:29-34.

Cooke, W. and Barnes, W.S. 1997. The influence of recovery duration on high-intensity exercise performance after oral creatine supplementation. Canadian Journal of Applied Physiology 22:454-467.

Cooke, W., Grandjean, P.W. and Barnes, W.S. 1995. Effect of oral creatine supplementation on power output and fatigue during bicycle ergometry. Journal of Applied Physiology 78:670-673.

Dawson, B., Cutler, M., Moody, A., Lawrence, S., Goodman, C. and Randall, N. 1995. Effects of oral creatine loading on single and repeated maximal short sprints. Australian Journal of Science and Medicine in Sports 27:56-61.

DeLanghe, J., De Slypere, J.P., De Buyzere, M., Robbrecht, J., Wieme, R. and Vermeulen, A. 1989. Normal reference values for creatine, creatinine, carnitine are lower in vegetarians. Clinical Chemistry 35:1802-1803.

Demant, T.W. and Rhodes, E.C. 1999. Effects of creatine supplementation on exercise performance. Sports Medicine 28:49-60.

Earnest, C.P., Almada, A.L. and Mitchell, T.L. 1997. Effects of creatine monohydrate ingestion on intermediate duration anaerobic treadmill running to exhaustion. Journal of Strength and Conditioning Research 11:234-238.

Earnest, C., Snell, P., Rodriguez, R., Almada, A.L. and Mitchell, T.L. 1995. The effect of creatine monohydrate ingestion on anaerobic power indices, muscular strength and body composition. Acta Physiologica Scandinavica 153:207-209.

Edwards, M.R., Rhodes, E.C., McKenzie, D.C. and Belcastro, A.N. 2000. The effect of creatine supplementation on anaerobic performance in moderately active men. Journal of Strength and Conditioning Research 14:75-79.

Engelhardt, M., Neumann, G., Berbalk, A. and Reuter, I. 1998. Creatine supplementation in endurance sports. Medicine and Science in Sports and Exercise 30:1123-1129.

Febbraio, M.A., Flanagan, T.R., Snow, R.J., Zhao, S. and Carey, M.F. 1995. Effect of creatine supplementation on intramuscular TCr, metabolism and performance during intermittent, supramaximal exercise in humans. Acta Physiologica Scandinavica 155:387-395.

Felber, S., Skladal, D., Wyss, M., Kresmer, C., Koller, A. and Sperl, W. 2000. Oral creatine supplementation in Duchenne muscular dystrophy: A clinical and 31P magnetic resonance spectroscopy study. Neurological Research 22:145-150.

Forsberg, A.M., Nilsson, E., Werneman, J., Bergström, J. and Hultman, E. 1991. Muscle composition in relation to age and sex. Clinical Science 81:249-256.

Francaux, M., Demeure, R., Goudemant, J.F. and Poortmans, J.R. 2000. Effect of exogenous creatine supplementation on muscle PCr metabolism. International Journal of Sports Medicine 21:139-145.

Gilliam, J.D., Hohzorn, C., Martin, D. and Trimble, M.H. 2000. Effect of oral creatine supplementation on isokinetic torque production. Medicine and Science in Sports and Exercise 32:993-996.

Gordon, A., Hultman, E., Kaijser, L., Kristjansson, S., Rolf, C.J., Nyquist, O. and Sylven, C. 1995. Creatine supplementation in chronic heart failure increases skeletal muscle creatine phosphate and muscle performance. Cardiovascular Research 30:413-438.

Green, A.L., Hultman, E., MacDonald, I.A., Sewell, D.A. and Greenhaff, P.L. 1996A. Carbohydrate feeding augments skeletal muscle creatine accumulation during creatine supplementation in humans. American Journal of Physiology 271:E821-E826.

Green, A.L., Simpson, E.J., Littlewood, J.J., MacDonald, I.A. and Greenhaff, P.L. 1996B. Carbohydrate ingestion augments creatine retention during creatine feeding in humans. Acta Physiologica Scandinavica 158:195-202.

Greenhaff, P.L. 1997. The nutritional biochemistry of creatine. Journal of Nutritional Biochemistry 11:610-618.

Greenhaff, P.L., Bodin, K., Söderlund, K. and Hultman, E. 1994. Effect of oral creatine supplementation on skeletal muscle phosphocreatine resynthesis. American Journal of Physiology 266:E725-E730.

Greenhaff, P.L., Casey, A., Short, A.H., Harris, R., Söderlund, K. and Hultman, E. 1993. Influence of oral creatine supplementation of [sic] muscle torque during repeated bouts of maximal voluntary exercise in man. Clinical Science 84:565-571.

Greenwood, M., Farris, J., Kreider, R., Greenwood, L. and Byars, A. 2000. Creatine supplementation patterns and perceived effects in select Division I college athletes. Clinical Journal of Sports Medicine 10:191-194.

Grindstaff, P.D., Kreider, R., Bishop, R., Wilson, M., Wood, L., Alexander, C. and Almada, A. 1997. Effects of creatine supplementation on repetitive sprint performance and body composition in competitive swimmers. International Journal of Sport Nutrition 7:330-346.

Harris, R.C., Söderlund, K. and Hultman, E. 1992. Elevation of creatine in resting and exercised muscle of normal subjects by creatine supplementation. Clinical Science 83:367-374.

Hultman, E., Söderland, K., Timmons, J.A., Cederblad, G. and Greenhaff, P.L. 1996. Muscle creatine loading in men. Journal of Applied Physiology 81:232-237.

Ingwall, J.S. 1976. Creatine and the control of muscle-specific protein synthesis in cardiac and skeletal muscle. Circulation Research 38:I-115-I-123.

Jacobs, I., Bleue, S. and Goodman, J. 1997. Creatine ingestion increases anaerobic capacity and maximal accumulated oxygen deficit. Canadian Journal of Applied Physiology 22:231-243.

Johnson, R. 1998. Demographics of creatine monohydrate users. Memorandum to Brett Hall. Experimental and Applied Sciences, July 30, 1998.

Johnson, W.A. and Landry, G.L. 1998. Nutritional supplements: Fact vs. fiction. Adolescent Medicine 9:501-513.

Juhn, M.S. and Tarnopolsky, M. 1998A. Oral creatine supplementation and athletic performance: A critical review. Clinical Journal of Sports Medicine 8:286-297.

Juhn, M.S. and Tarnopolsky, M. 1998B. Potential side effects of oral creatine supplementation: A critical review. Clinical Journal of Sports Medicine 8:298-304.

Kamber, M., Koster, M., Kreis, R., Walker, G., Boesch, C. and Hoppeler, H. 1999. Creatine supplementation—Part I: Performance, clinical chemistry, and muscle volume. Medicine and Science in Sports and Exercise 31:1763-1769.

Kelly, V.G. and Jenkins, D.G. 1998. Effect of oral creatine supplementation on near-maximal strength and repeated sets of high-intensity bench press exercise. Journal of Strength and Conditioning Research 12:109-115.

Kirksey, B., Stone, M.H., Warren, B.J., Johnson, R.L., Stone, M., Haff, G., Williams, F.E. and Prolux, C. 1999. The effects of 6 weeks of creatine monohydrate supplementation on performance measures and body composition in collegiate track and field athletes. Journal of Strength and Conditioning Research 13:148-156.

Kraemer, W.J. and Volek, J.S. 1999. Creatine supplementation. Its role in human performance. Clinics in Sports Medicine 18:651-666.

Kreider, R., Ferreira, M., Wilson, M., Grindstaff, P., Plisk, S., Reinhardy, J., Cantler, E. and Almada, A. 1998. Effects of creatine supplementation on body composition, strength, and sprint performance. Medicine and Science in Sports and Exercise 30:73-82.

Kreider, R.B., Klesges, R., Harmon, K., Grindstaff, P., Ramsey, L., Bullen, D., Wood, L., Li, Y. and Almada, A. 1996. Effects of ingesting supplements designed to promote lean tissue accretion on body composition during resistance training. International Journal of Sport Nutrition 6:234-246.

Kreis, R., Kamber, M., Koster, M., Felblinger, J., Slotboom, J., Hoppeler, H. and Boesch, C. 1999. Creatine supplementation—Part II: In vivo magnetic resonance spectroscopy. Medicine and Science in Sports and Exercise 31:1770-1777.

LaBotz, M. and Smith, B.W. 1999. Creatine supplement use in an NCAA Division I athletic program. Clinical Journal of Sports Medicine 9:167-169.

Ledford, A. and Branch, J.D. 1999. Creatine supplementation does not increase peak power production and work capacity during repetitive Wingate testing in women. Journal of Strength and Conditioning Research 13:394-399.

Leenders, N., Sherman, W.M., Lamb, D.R. and Nelson, T.E. 1999. Creatine supplementation and swimming performance. International Journal of Sport Nutrition 9:251-262.

Ma, T.M., Friedman, D.L. and Roberts, R. 1996. Creatine phosphate shuttle pathway in tissues with dynamic energy demand. In Conway, M.A., Clark, J.F. (Eds.), Creatine and creatine phosphate: Scientific and clinical perspectives. San Diego: Academic Press, pp. 17-32.

Maganaris, C.N. and Maughan, R.J. 1998. Creatine supplementation enhances maximum voluntary isometric force and endurance capacity in resistance trained men. Acta Physiologica Scandinavica 163:279-287.

McKenna, M., Morton, J., Selig, S.E. and Snow, R.J. 1999. Creatine supplementation increases muscle total creatine but not maximal intermittent exercise performance. Journal of Applied Physiology 87:2244-2252.

McNaughton, L.R., Dalton, B. and Tarr, J. 1998. The effects of creatine supplementation on high-intensity exercise performance in elite performers. European Journal of Applied Physiology 78:236-240.

Mihic, S., MacDonald, J.R., McKenzie, S. and Tarnopolsky, M.A. 2000. Acute creatine loading increases fat-free mass, but does not affect blood pressure, plasma creatinine, or CK activity in men and women. Medicine and Science in Sports and Exercise 32:291-296.

Mujika, I., Chatard, J.C., Lacoste, L., Barale, F. and Geyssant, A. 1996. Creatine supplementation does not improve sprint performance in competitive swimmers. Medicine and Science in Sports and Exercise 28:1435-1441.

Mujika, I. and Padilla, S. 1997. Creatine supplementation as an ergogenic aid for sports performance in highly trained athletes: A critical review. International Journal of Sports Medicine 18:491-496.

Mujika, I., Padilla, S., Ibanez, J., Izquierdo, M. and Gorostiaga, E. 2000. Creatine supplementation and sprint performance in soccer players. Medicine and Science in Sports and Exercise 32:518-525.

Noonan, D., Berg, K., Latin, R.W., Wagner, J.C. and Reimers, K. 1998. Effects of varying dosages of oral creatine relative to fat free body mass on strength and body composition. Journal of Strength and Conditioning Research 12:104-108.

Odland, L.M., MacDougall, J.D., Tarnopolsky, M., Borgmann, A. and Atkinson, S. 1997. Effect of oral creatine supplementation on muscle [PCr] and short-term maximum power output. Medicine and Science in Sports and Exercise 29:216-219.

Ööpik, V., Pääsuke, M., Timpmann, S., Medijainen, L., Ereline, J. and Smirnova, T. 1998. Effect of creatine supplementation during rapid body mass reduction on metabolism and isokinetic muscle performance capacity. European Journal of Applied Physiology 78:83-92.

Pearson, D.R., Hamby, D.G., Russel, W. and Harris, T. 1999. Long-term effects of creatine monohydrate on strength and power. Journal of Strength and Conditioning Research 13:187-192.

Peeters, B.M., Lantz, C.D. and Mayhew, J.L. 1999. Effect of oral creatine monohydrate and creatine phosphate supplementation on maximal strength indices, body composition, and blood pressure. Journal of Strength and Conditioning Research 13:3-9.

Peyrebrune, M.C., Nevill, M.E., Donaldson, F.J. and Cosford, D.J. 1998. The effects of oral creatine supplementation on performance in single and repeated sprint swimming. Journal of Sport Science 16:271-279.

Poortmans, J.R., Auquier, H., Renaut, V., Durussel, A., Saugy, M. and Brisson, G.R. 1997. Effect of short-term creatine supplementation on renal responses in men. European Journal of Applied Physiology 76:566-567.

Poortmans, J.R. and Francaux, M. 1999. Long-term oral creatine supplementation does not impair renal function in healthy athletes. Medicine and Science in Sports and Exercise 31:1108-1110.

Prevost, M.C., Nelson, A.G. and Morris, G.S. 1997. Creatine supplementation enhances intermittent work performance. Research Quarterly for Exercise and Sport 68:233-240.

Pritchard, N.R. and Kaira, P.A. 1998. Renal dysfunction accompanying oral supplements. Lancet 351:1252-1253.

Rawson, E.S. and Clarkson, P.M. 1999. Acute creatine supplementation in older men. International Journal of Sports Medicine 20:71-75.

Rawson, E.S., Wehnert, M.L. and Clarkson, P.M. 1999. Effects of 30 days of creatine ingestion in older men. European Journal of Applied Physiology 80:139-144.

Redondo, D., Dowling, E.A., Graham, B.L., Almada, A.J. and Williams, M.H. 1996. The effect of oral creatine monohydrate supplementation on running velocity. International Journal of Sport Nutrition 6:213-221.

Rico-Sanz, J. and Marco, M.T.M. 2000. Creatine enhances oxygen uptake and performance during intensity exercise. Medicine and Science in Sports and Exercise 32:379-385.

Ronsen, O., Sundgot-Borgen, J. and Maehlkm, S. 1999. Supplement use and nutritional habits in Norwegian elite athletes. Scandinavian Journal of Medicine and Science in Sports 9:28-35.

Ropero-Miller, J.D., Paget-Wilkes, H., Doering, P.L. and Goldberger, B.A. 2000. Effect of oral creatine supplementation on random urine creatinine, pH, and specific gravity measurements. Clinical Chemistry 46:295-297.

Rossiter, H.B., Cannel, T.R. and Jakeman, P.M. 1996. The effect of oral creatine supplementation on the 1000-m performance of competitive rowers. Journal of Sports Sciences 14:175-179.

Saks, V.A. and Strumia, E. 1993. Phosphocreatine: Molecular and cellular aspects of the mechanism of cardioprotective action. Current Therapeutic Research 53:565-598.

Schneider, D.A., McDonough, P.J., Fadel, P.J. and Berwick, J.P. 1997. Creatine supplementation and the total work performed during 15-s and 1-min bouts of maximal cycling. Australian Journal of Science and Medicine in Sports 29:65-68.

Sheppard, H.L., Raichada, S.M., Kouri, K.M., Stenson-Bar-Maor, L. and Branch, J.D. 2000. Use of creatine and other supplements by members of civilian and military health clubs: A cross-sectional survey. International Journal of Sport Nutrition and Exercise Metabolism 10:245-259.

Shomrat, A., Weinstein, Y. and Katz, A. 2000. Effect of creatine feeding on maximal exercise performance in vegetarians. European Journal of Applied Physiology 82:321-325.

Sipilä, I., Rapola, J., Simell, O. and Vannas, A. 1981. Supplementary creatine as a treatment for gyrate atrophy of the choroid and retina. New England Journal of Medicine 304:867-870.

Smith, J.C., Stephens, D.P., Hall, E.L., Jackson, A.W. and Earnest, C.P. 1998A. Effect of oral creatine ingestion on parameters of the work rate-time relationship and time to exhaustion in high-intensity cycling. European Journal of Applied Physiology 77:360-365.

Smith, S.A., Montain, S.J., Matott, R.P., Zientara, G.P., Jolesz, F.A. and Fielding, R.A. 1998B. Creatine supplementation and age influence muscle metabolism during exercise. Journal of Applied Physiology 85:1349-1356.

Smith, S.A., Montain, S.J., Matott, R.P., Zientara, G.P., Jolesz, F.A. and Fielding, R.A. 1999. Effects of creatine supplementation on the energy cost of muscle contraction: A 31P-MRS study. Journal of Applied Physiology 87:116-123.

Snow, R.J., McKenna, M.J., Selig, S.E., Kemp, J., Stathis, C.G. and Zhao, S. 1998. Effect of creatine supplementation on sprint exercise performance and muscle metabolism. Journal of Applied Physiology 84:1667-1673.

Stöckler, S., Marescau, B., De Deyn, P.P., Trijbels, J.M. and Hanefeld, F. 1997. Guanidino compounds in guanidinoacetate methyltransferase deficiency, a new inborn error of creatine synthesis. Metabolism 46:1189-1193.

Stone, M.H., Sanborn, K., Smith, L.L., O'Bryant, H.S., Hoke, T., Utter, A.C., Johnson, R.L., Boros, R., Hruby, J., Pierce, K.C., Stone, M.E. and Garner, B. 1999. Effect of in-season (5 weeks) creatine and pyruvate supplementation on anaerobic performance and body composition in American football players. International Journal of Sport Nutrition 9:146-165.

Stout, J., Eckerson, J., Ebersole, K., Moore, G., Perry, S., Housch, T., Bull, A., Cramer, J. and Batheja, A. 2000. Effect of creatine loading on neuromuscular fatigue threshold. Journal of Applied Physiology 88:109-112.

Stout, J.R., Eckerson, J.M., Housch, T.J. and Ebersole, K.T. 1999. The effects of creatine supplementation on anaerobic working capacity. Journal of Strength and Conditioning Research 13:135-138.

Strauss, G. 1998. 1 in 3 pro sports teams say "no" to creatine. USA Today, June 4, News, 1A.

Strauss, G. and Mihoces, G. 1998. Jury still out on creatine use. USA Today, June 4, C1-C2.

Stroud, M., Holliman, D., Bell, D., Green, A., Macdonald, I. and Greenhaff, P. 1994. Effect of oral creatine supplementation on respiratory gas exchange and blood lactate accumulation during steady-state incremental treadmill exercise and recovery in man. Clinical Science 87:707-710.

Tarnopolsky, M. and Martin, J. 1999. Creatine monohydrate increases strength in patients with neuromuscular disease. Neurology 52:854-857.

Tarnopolsky, M.A., Roy, B.D. and McDonald, J.R. 1997. A randomized, controlled trial of creatine monohydrate in patients with mitochondrial cytopathies. Muscle and Nerve 20:1502-1509.

Terjung, R.L., Clarkson, P., Eichner, E.R., Greenhaff, P.L., Hespel, P.J., Israel, R.G., Kraemer, W.J., Meyer, R.A., Spriet, L.L., Tarnopolsky, M.A., Wagenmakers, A.J.M. and Williams, M.H. 2000. American College of Sports MedicineSM Roundtable. The physiological and health effects of oral creatine supplementation. Medicine and Science in Sports and Exercise 32:706-717.

Terrillion, K.A., Kolkhorst, F.W., Dolgener, F.A. and Joslyn, S.J. 1997. The effect of creatine supplementation on two 700-m maximal running bouts. International Journal of Sport Nutrition 7:138-143.

Theodorou, A.S., Cooke, C.B., King, R.F.I.J., Hood, C., Denison, T., Wainwright, B.G. and Havenetidis, K. 1999. The effect of longer-tern creatine supplementation on elite swimming performance after an acute creatine loading. Journal of Sports Sciences 17:853-859.

Thompson, C.H., Kemp, G.J., Sanderson, A.J., Dixon, R.M., Styles, P., Taylor, D.J. and Radda, G.K. 1996. Effect of creatine on aerobic and anaerobic metabolism in skeletal muscle in swimmers. British Journal of Sports Medicine 30:222-225.

Urbanski, R.L., Loy, S.F., Vincent, W.J. and Yaspelkis, B.B. 1999. Creatine supplementation differentially affects maximal isometric strength and time to fatigue in large and small muscle groups. International Journal of Sport Nutrition 9:136-145.

Vandebuerie, F., Vanden Eynde, B., Vandenberghe, K. and Hespel, P. 1998. Effect of creatine loading on endurance capacity and sprint power in cyclists. International Journal of Sports Medicine 19:490-495.

Vandenberghe, K., Gillis, N., Van Leemputte, M., Van Hecke, P., Vanstapel, F. and Hespel, P. 1996. Caffeine counteracts the ergogenic action of muscle creatine loading. Journal of Applied Physiology 80:452-457.

Vandenberghe, K., Goris, M., Van Hecke, P., Van Leemputte, M., Van Gerven, L. and Hespel, P. 1997. Long-term creatine intake is beneficial to muscle performance during resistance training. Journal of Applied Physiology 83:2055-2063.

Vandenberghe, K., Van Hecke, P., Van Leemputte, M., Vanstapel, F. and Hespel, P. 1999. Phosphocreatine resynthesis is not affected by creatine loading. Medicine and Science in Sports and Exercise 31:236-242.

Van Leemputte, M., Vandenberghe, K. and Hespel, P. 1999. Shortening of muscle relaxation time after creatine loading. Journal of Applied Physiology 86:840-844.

Viru, M., Ööpik, V., Nurmekivi, A., Medijainen, L., Timpmann, S. and Viru, A. 1994. Effect of creatine intake on the performance capacity in middle-distance runners. Coaching and Sport Science Journal 1:31-36.

Vogel, R.A., Webster, M.J., Erdmann, L.D. and Clark, R.D. 2000. Creatine supplementation: Effect on supramaximal exercise performance at two levels of acute hypohydration. Journal of Strength and Conditioning Research 14:214-219.

Volek, J.S. 1997. Creatine supplementation and its possible role in improving physical performance. ACSM's Health and Fitness Journal 1(4):23-29.

Volek, J.S., Duncan, N.D., Mazzetti, S.A., Putukian, M., Gomez, A.L. and Kraemer, W.J. 2000. No effect of heavy resistance training and creatine supplementation on blood lipids. International Journal of Sport Nutrition and Exercise Metabolism 10:144-156.

Volek, J.S., Duncan, N.D., Mazzetti, S.A., Staron, R.S., Putukian, M., Gomez, A.L., Pearson, D.R., Fink, W.J. and Kraemer, W.J. 1999. Performance and muscle fiber adaptations to creatine supplementation and heavy resistance training. Medicine and Science in Sports and Exercise 31:1147-1156.

Volek, J.S., Kraemer, W.J., Bush, J.A., Boetes, M., Incledon, T., Clark, K.L., Lynch, J.M. and Knuttgen, K.G. 1997. Creatine supplementation enhances muscular performance during high-intensity resistance exercise. Journal of the American Dietetic Association 97:765-770.

Vorgerd, M., Grehl, T., Jäger, M., Müller, K., Freitag, G., Patzold, T., Bruns, N., Fabian, K., Tehenthoff, M., Mortier, W., Luttmann, A., Zange, J. and Malin, P. 2000. Creatine therapy in myophosphorylase deficiency (McArdle Disease). A placebo-controlled crossover trial. Archives of Neurology 57:956-963.

Walker, J.B. 1979. Creatine: Biosynthesis, regulation, and function. Advances in Enzymology 50:177-242.

Williams, M.H., Kreider, R.B. and Branch, J.D. 1999. Creatine: The power supplement. Champaign, IL: Human Kinetics.

Ziegenfuss, T.N., Lowery, L.M. and Lemon, P.W.R. 1998. Acute fluid volume changes in men during three days of creatine supplementation. Journal of Exercise Physiology$_{online}$ 1(3):1-9. **http://www.css.edu/users/tboone2/asep/jan3.htm**.

Sodium Bicarbonate

Michael J. Webster, PhD

With many proposed ergogenic nutritional supplements, there is typically an initial period during which they receive a great deal of attention and researchers form hypotheses, perform studies, and draw conclusions. Thereafter, interest gradually wanes; little more is said about the supplement and it fades into obscurity. In contrast, sodium bicarbonate first received attention as a proposed ergogenic aid in the late 1920s; a few studies were performed during the next 50 years, and then in the late 1970s and early 1980s the findings of new studies ignited a great deal of interest that continues today. This chapter briefly discusses the past and present literature as it relates to a number of topics: the role of acid-base balance in muscular fatigue; the effect of sodium bicarbonate administration on acid-base balance; the optimal dosage of sodium bicarbonate required to facilitate significant physiological changes; the possible side effects of sodium bicarbonate ingestion and ways of minimizing them; the timing of sodium bicarbonate ingestion prior to exercise; the possible impacts of exercise duration, intensity, and type on the effectiveness of bicarbonate loading; and the ethical implications of the use of sodium bicarbonate to enhance exercise performance. A final section of the chapter addresses conclusions that can be drawn from the nearly 75 years of research on this topic and presents suggestions for areas of future research.

The ability of an individual to maximize exercise performance is often dependent on the ability to delay the onset of fatigue [1, 2]. On an elementary level, the cause of fatigue appears to be relatively simple; however, it is also easily apparent that fatigue is a very complex phenomenon that is influenced by a variety of central and peripheral factors [3, 4].

One well-recognized cause of fatigue is disruption of the acid-base status of the plasma and tissues [5, 6]. Resting arterial pH is typically in the range of 7.35 to 7.45 [7] whereas muscle pH is approximately 7.0 to 7.1 [8]. During relatively intense physical exercise, a reliance on the nonoxidative metabolism of plasma glucose and muscle glycogen for the production of chemical energy results in the formation of lactic acid [8-10]. At physiological pH, greater than 99% of lactic acid will dissociate to a lactate anion (La$^-$) and a hydrogen cation (H$^+$). Any increase in the H$^+$ concentration ([H$^+$]) in the plasma and muscle results in a decrease in pH. Physical

activities demanding a high energy output and relying extensively on nonoxidative energy production can cause the pH to decrease to approximately 7.0 to 7.1 and 6.4 to 6.6 in the plasma and muscle, respectively [11].

Across the physiological range, there appears to be an inverse relationship between skeletal muscle pH and muscle fatigue [5, 6]. A decrease in pH has been shown to reduce adenosine triphosphatase (ATPase) activity, increase the binding of Ca^{2+} by the sarcoplasmic reticulum, and also decrease contractile protein interaction, all resulting in a decrease in the generation of muscle tension [6, 11-14]. A decrease in pH is also a known inhibitor of phosphofructokinase, which is considered the rate-limiting enzyme of glycolytic energy production [15-19]. From an exercise performance viewpoint, one may be inclined to view these inhibiting factors in a negative light. However, one has to keep in mind that they serve to preserve acid-base homeostasis. Through negative feedback mechanisms, an increase in acid accumulation resulting in a significant decrease in pH inhibits glycolytic energy production and muscle force production [15-19]. This reduces lactic acid formation and prevents any further decrease in pH, thereby maintaining the functional integrity of the cell.

The maintenance of acid-base balance occurs via chemical, respiratory, and renal mechanisms [7]. Both the chemical and respiratory mechanisms buffer acute acid-base changes, whereas the renal mechanisms buffer chronic changes [7]. Of the acute mechanisms, the chemical buffers are the primary line of defense in maintaining acid-base change [7]. The chemical buffers consist of bicarbonate, phosphate, and protein; and of these three, the most powerful extracellular buffer is bicarbonate [7]. Bicarbonate salt, primarily sodium bicarbonate (NaHCO$_3$), readily ionizes to form a bicarbonate ion (HCO$_3^-$) and a sodium ion (Na$^+$) [7]. HCO$_3^-$ rapidly buffers dissociated H$^+$ to form carbonic acid (H$_2$CO$_3$), which dissociates to carbon dioxide (CO$_2$) and water.

During physical exercise, energy formation is derived from both oxidative and nonoxidative sources [20]. The predominant source is determined largely by the exercise intensity. With an increase in exercise intensity, there is a shift away from oxidative sources and toward nonoxidative sources. A reliance on nonoxidative glucose and glycogen metabolism results in significant production and accumulation of lactic acid that decreases plasma and muscle pH and contributes to the onset of muscular fatigue.

To determine whether the decreases in pH associated with this type of exercise could be attenuated, researchers have posed questions regarding the potential effectiveness of alkaline salt administration on exercise performance and the onset of fatigue. One of the first studies to address this question indicated a significant improvement in running performance [21]. During the past 70 years, particularly the past 25 years, numerous studies have indicated that alkaline salt administration significantly alters resting and exercise acid-base status and improves exercise performance [11, 21-39].

The administration of alkaline salts in the form of sodium citrate, potassium bicarbonate, and $NaHCO_3$ has been evaluated, with $NaHCO_3$ receiving the most attention. $NaHCO_3$ administration, which is the focus of this review, is referred to as buffer boosting, soda loading, $NaHCO_3$ loading, and bicarbonate loading; the last term is the most commonly used. Even though the results of both field [21, 23, 30, 31, 41] and laboratory research [22, 24-29, 32, 34, 35, 39, 40, 42-48] are equivocal and there are no reported data indicating the prevalence of bicarbonate loading among athletes, personal communications and observations indicate that there is a great deal of interest in its use. This is especially noteworthy given that the practice is not specifically banned by sport governing bodies.

While many studies support the effectiveness of $NaHCO_3$ as an ergogenic aid [21-32], the contrasting findings of many other studies [40, 41, 44, 45, 47, 49-51] create considerable confusion regarding the efficacy of $NaHCO_3$ supplementation. Although methodological limitations often confound the direct comparison of studies, one likely factor relates to the training status of the subjects [30, 31, 41, 51]. Anaerobically trained subjects have been shown to have a higher muscle buffering capacity [52, 53] and a greater lactate accumulation [53] than do untrained subjects. However, muscle pH at exhaustion does not appear to be affected by training [53]. If muscle pH has an absolute "fatigue point," bicarbonate loading, in conjunction with the physiological adaptations with training noted earlier, should prolong the time to this fatigue point. Another factor related to training status concerns the difficulty of reproducing maximal physical efforts in untrained or moderately trained subjects [22, 39, 41, 54]. This may lead to large variations in performance and potentially mask statistically significant performance results. This is directly supported by Pfefferle and Wilkinson [39], who demonstrated that considerable performance variations between trained and untrained subjects could

account for the nonsignificant change reported in bicarbonate-loading studies.

Upon closer evaluation of the studies that show significant improvements in exercise performance, several additional commonalties appear: the dosage of $NaHCO_3$ administered; the timing of $NaHCO_3$ administration; and the duration, intensity, and mode of activity.

Dosage

The first question surrounding the practice of bicarbonate loading is "What dosage is required to elicit significant changes in the physiological acid-base status?" A significant alkaline shift has been reported with an acute $NaHCO_3$ dosage as small as 100 mg/kg body weight [23]; however, this is in conflict with the findings of McNaughton [26], who specifically attempted to determine the appropriate $NaHCO_3$ dosage. McNaughton [26] reported that the administration of 100 mg/kg of body weight did not significantly increase either plasma pH or HCO_3^-. However, the acid-base dosage response associated with a $NaHCO_3$ administration of 200 to 500 mg/kg body weight did significantly increase both plasma pH and HCO_3^-. It should be noted that significant changes in plasma pH are typically on the magnitude of 0.5 to 1.0 units above a resting value of 7.35 to 7.45, rarely resulting in a pH greater than 7.5, and do not show a strong positive correlation with dosage. The magnitude of the increase in plasma HCO_3^- is approximately 6 to 10 mEq/L above the resting value of 22 to 24 mEq/L and does show a strong positive correlation with dosage (i.e., the greater the $NaHCO_3$ dosage the greater the plasma HCO_3^- concentration) [26]. The most frequently administered $NaHCO_3$ dosage is 300 mg/kg.

Side Effects

Evaluation of the acid-base dosage relationship would seem to suggest that higher dosages would be more likely to exert a positive impact on exercise performance. However, individuals frequently report gastrointestinal distress with acute $NaHCO_3$ ingestion [24, 26, 30, 31, 47]. While several studies investigating the acute administration of $NaHCO_3$ supplementation have reported gastrointestinal problems with a dosage of 300 mg/kg body weight [24, 30, 47], virtually all studies using dosages of 400 to 500 mg/kg report these problems [26, 31]. These effects are likely due to the large sodium load that is imposed on the gut, with water drawn into the gastrointestinal tract to counter the increased osmotic load. At the same time there is also significant gas production. At dosages of up to 300 mg/kg, the consumption of a large volume of water appears to minimize gastrointestinal symptoms [47]. When contemplating these potential negative effects, one might eliminate 400 and 500 mg/kg dosages from consideration; however, it is necessary to consider when these negative side effects occur. Individuals reporting negative effects often do not experience these symptoms until after the exercise bout is completed, which negates any impact on performance. Because a greater rise in plasma HCO_3^- is observed with the higher dosages of $NaHCO_3$, the decision on dosage may actually be determined by the individual's perceived risk/benefit ratio (i.e., risk of potential discomfort/potential performance enhancement benefit). While many athletes would consider these side effects benign and manageable, it is worth noting that a potential lethal event, spontaneous gastric rupture, has been reported with bicarbonate administration [55], although never in an athlete.

Timing of Administration

A valid criticism of several of the earlier studies of alkaline salt administration is that the administered dosages were relatively small and that they were ingested in the days prior to exercise performance [21]. The mechanisms of acid-base regulation that occur over a period of days appear to be directed by the kidneys. These are different from the mechanisms that regulate acute acid-base balance (within hours of $NaHCO_3$ ingestion). Consequently, studies during the last 25 years have administered larger $NaHCO_3$ dosages 2 to 3 hr prior to exercise. Recent reports indicate that significant changes in both plasma pH and plasma bicarbonate occur within 30 min of $NaHCO_3$ ingestion. Maximal changes in these acid-base parameters occur approximately 90 to 120 min post-ingestion [40, 45, 47], suggesting this as the optimal timing of administration (figure 17.1).

Most researchers would suggest that a dosage of 300 mg/kg, with ad libitum fluid ingestion, might optimize buffering capacity and possibly aid in improving exercise performance [56, 57]. However, as mentioned previously, this dosage is associated with significant gastrointestinal problems. Consequently, a recent study has brought into question this protocol for the timing of $NaHCO_3$ administration [29]. A significantly larger dosage of 500 mg/kg was administered (well above that reported to elicit gastrointestinal distress); but rather than in a single bolus, it was administered in 125 mg/kg servings, four times each day for five consecutive days. Plasma pH and HCO_3^- were both significantly elevated at 24 hr and remained elevated over the following five days of supplementation. The magnitude of the increases in pH (0.05 units) and HCO_3^- (5.6 mEq/L) was very similar to that reported with acute dosages of 300 mg/kg; however, in contrast to what occurred in studies of acute administration, none of the subjects reported any negative gastrointestinal symptoms. Although this is the only

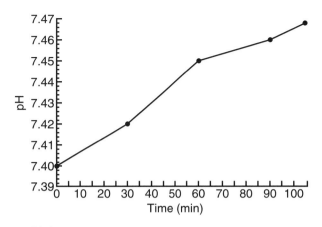

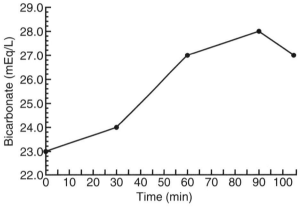

Figure 17.1 Time course of changes in pH and bicarbonate in response to bicarbonate loading with 300 mg/kg.

Figures are from data from Portington et al., *Med. Sci. Sports and Exerc.*, 30(4): 523-528, 1998 and from Webster et al., *Med. Sci. Sports and Exerc.*, 25(8): 960-965, 1993.

study that has used this administration protocol, the findings appear quite favorable and may suggest a viable alternative to the acute administration protocol that is presently accepted and practiced.

Duration and Intensity of Exercise

Bicarbonate-loading studies have used exercise protocols ranging from maximal-intensity activity lasting 10 sec to submaximal and maximal activities lasting 1 hr. The wide variety of exercise protocols employed in these studies makes the comparison of findings difficult. However, one can draw some conclusions by grouping studies according to similarities in experimental design and exercise protocol and then making comparisons within each grouping. For the purposes of this review the studies have been separated into the following four categories: (1) power, (2) anaerobic, (3) oxidative, and (4) interval. Although the interval category comprises exercise from one or more of the other three categories, the findings for repeated-bout exercise are often significantly different from those for a single exercise bout and warrant separate discussion.

Power

The power category consists of high-intensity activities that predominately emphasize the use of the phosphagen energy system for the formation of adenosine triphosphate (ATP) and that have a duration of approximately 3 to 30 sec. Very few studies have evaluated the effectiveness of bicarbonate loading during power-type exercise, and those that have done so present equivocal findings. One study indicated that total work performed during 10-sec and 30-sec maximal cycling sprints was not influenced by bicarbonate loading [25]. This is in agreement with two earlier studies indicating no improvements in peak power, mean power, and total work during 30-sec cycling sprints [44, 49]. In contrast, another study reported that bicarbonate loading resulted in a significantly greater power output throughout a 30-sec cycling sprint and improved performance in 11 of 13 subjects [42]. Although the majority of power studies indicate that bicarbonate loading is not warranted, there are data supporting its effectiveness.

No studies have evaluated the effect of bicarbonate loading on activities such as a single bench press, squat, or 40-m (43.7 yd) sprint; however, activities of this kind rely almost exclusively on the phosphagen energy system for the generation of ATP. There is really no logical biochemical rationale for suggesting that $NaHCO_3$

ingestion might enhance performance in these kinds of activities. Consequently, bicarbonate loading in these situations is not warranted.

Anaerobic

Exercise categorized as anaerobic consists of activities requiring approximately 100% maximal oxygen uptake ($\dot{V}O_2max$) and/or having a maximal duration of approximately 1 to 7 min. Exercise of this type places a very heavy demand on glycolytic energy metabolism. While glycolytic ATP generation is rapid, so also is the production of lactic acid, the accumulation of which can result in significant disruptions of acid-base balance. Activities of this type place a heavy demand on the bicarbonate buffering system and may warrant bicarbonate loading.

Of studies indicating bicarbonate loading to be effective, the majority have addressed predominately anaerobic activities [22, 23, 25-27, 30-35]. Among these studies, four stand out [32-35]. All examined the effectiveness of bicarbonate loading using similar exercise protocols progressing from low-intensity aerobic exercise to high-intensity anaerobic exercise, with time to exhaustion being evaluated in the anaerobic exercise bout. The sodium bicarbonate dosage was 300 mg/kg, administered 3 h before the beginning of the exercise bout. All these studies showed significant increases in time to fatigue with bicarbonate loading, with improvements ranging from 19% to 98%. Figure 17.2 is

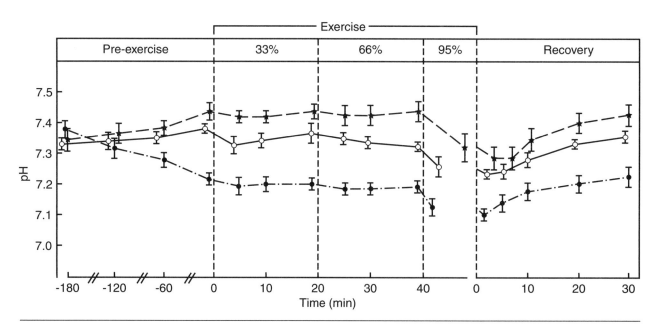

Figure 17.2 Representative time-course changes in plasma pH in response to bicarbonate loading with 300 mg/kg followed 3 h later by steady state submaximal exercise and exercise to exhaustion.

★ = $NaHCO_3$; ○ = placebo; ● = NH_4CL

Reprinted, by permission, from N. L. Jones, J. Sutton, R. Taylor, and C. Toews, 1977, "Effect of pH on cardiorespiratory and metabolic responses to exercise," *Journal of Applied Physiology* 43 (6): 959-64.

representative of the experimental protocol and also the pH changes observed in each of these studies.

Kots et al. [36] and Bouissou et al. [37] evaluated the effect of bicarbonate loading during high-intensity cycling exercise that would lead to exhaustion in approximately 2 to 3 min and reported significant increases in time to exhaustion of 20% and 22%, respectively. Five additional studies have evaluated anaerobic performance on a cycle ergometer during a fixed-time exercise bout of 60 to 240 sec. In each case the amount of work performed was significantly improved with bicarbonate loading [24-27].

Although all these studies indicate that bicarbonate loading will either improve endurance time to exhaustion or improve total work output (signifying a delay in the onset of fatigue), the results do not necessarily equate with improved performance time (the primary interest of most competitive athletes). To determine the effect of bicarbonate loading on performance time, Wilkes et al. [30] evaluated 800-m (875 yd) performance in trained runners. The results indicated a significant, 2.9-sec improvement with bicarbonate loading. These findings were later supported by a similar study demonstrating 400-m (437 yd) run time to be improved by approximately 1.5 sec with bicarbonate loading [31]. To put all of these performance improvements with bicarbonate loading in perspective, consider the recent feats of 200/400-m (219/437 yd) sprinter Michael Johnson. His 1996 200-m world-record performance of 19.32 sec bested the previous record time by 0.40 sec, a record that had stood for 17 years. This was an improvement of only 2.03%, but this difference is considered by many to have "shattered" the existing record. Likewise, Johnson's 1999 400-m (437 yd) world record of 43.18 sec lowered the previous record time by 0.11 sec, a record that had stood for 11 years. Again, even though this improvement is less than 0.3%, it is considered a huge improvement in performance.

While not all bicarbonate-loading studies of anaerobic exercise show significant improvements in performance, the studies that do so all appear to have been well controlled and well designed. Consequently, a strong case can be made for the efficacy of bicarbonate loading during anaerobic exercise.

Aerobic

Exercise categorized as aerobic consists of either submaximal- or maximal-intensity activities with a duration of approximately 10 min or longer. Typically this equates to an exercise intensity of less than about 90% of $\dot{V}O_2$max.

One of the first studies, performed at the Harvard Fatigue Laboratory, showed a run duration of 15 min to be improved by 3 to 5 min with the administration of alkaline salts [21]. Although this study has many shortcomings, it prompted questions regarding the efficacy of bicarbonate loading during aerobic work. The four prominent studies mentioned in the anaerobic category also evaluated the effect of bicarbonate loading during 20 min of steady state low-level (33% $\dot{V}O_2$max) and moderate-level (66% $\dot{V}O_2$max) aerobic exercise and showed no significant physiological changes [32-35]. Runners exercising to exhaustion at an intensity equating with their 4 mM blood lactate concentration reported no significant changes in run performance with bicarbonate loading [58]. Potteiger et al. [45] reported that bicarbonate loading did not have any significant effect on exercise heart rate or perceived exertion during a 30-min treadmill run at an intensity corresponding to the lactate threshold. In addition, two other studies have indicated that sodium bicarbonate does not attenuate the $\dot{V}O_2$ slow component (upward drift in $\dot{V}O_2$) during constant-load cycling [59, 60].

In stark contrast, McNaughton et al. [28] reported that bicarbonate loading increased total work output by approximately 14% during 60 min of cycling. Throughout the entire 60-min ride, plasma pH and HCO_3^- were significantly higher, and $[La^-]$ was significantly lower, than during control and placebo conditions. In fact, throughout the entire exercise bout, plasma pH and HCO_3^- never decreased below resting levels. This elevation and maintenance of acid-base balance appears to be the only plausible explanation for the difference in findings reported among aerobic studies.

Before 1999, essentially all bicarbonate-loading studies on aerobic exercise indicated no performance-enhancing effects, clearly suggesting that bicarbonate loading is not effective during this type of work. However, it is also clear that the recent physiological and exercise performance data warrant further investigation [28]. Consequently, caution is in order before one makes a definitive statement about the effectiveness of bicarbonate loading during aerobic work.

Interval

Interval exercise consists of repeated bouts of activity with each bout separated by a relatively brief rest period. The exercise bouts are typically characterized as high intensity and anaerobic, with a duration ranging from ~10 sec to 3 to 4 min. By far the greatest support for the effectiveness of bicarbonate loading is derived from studies using interval exercise protocols. Each exercise bout performed during this type of exercise places a heavy demand on rapid energy production. This emphasizes glycolytic metabolism, with its resultant production and accumulation of lactic acid, for the generation of ATP. The rest interval following each exercise bout allows the muscle an opportunity to try to accommodate the alteration in acid-base balance imposed by the exercise and at least partially recover its force-generating capability before performing the next exercise bout. In a specified time period, the amount of work that can be performed during this type of work is significantly greater than during a single work bout; however, a potentially severe acid-base challenge is also imposed on the bicarbonate buffering system. This was clearly illustrated in two similar interval exercise protocols that showed a [lactate] of 32.1 mM, the highest ever reported in exercising humans; a blood pH of 6.80; a muscle pH of 6.41; and a base excess value of –34 mEq/L [10, 61].

While several studies have reported bicarbonate loading to be ineffective during a single bout of anaerobic exercise, it was suggested that a single bout of high-intensity exercise might be insufficient to lower intracellular pH [22]. To test this hypothesis, subjects were bicarbonate loaded before performing four 1-min cycling bouts at 125% of $\dot{V}O_2$max with a 1-min rest period between bouts, followed by a fifth bout to exhaustion. The results indicated a 42% improvement in time to exhaustion during the bicarbonate-loading trial as compared with a placebo trial. These results have been substantiated in subsequent studies using similar cycling exercise protocols [48, 54]. In a study of swimmers performing five 100-yd (91.4 m) sprints at near maximal effort with a 2-min rest interval after each sprint, performance time was not influenced in the first three sprints but was significantly faster in the fourth and fifth sprints [62]. Cyclists performing ten 10-sec sprints with a 50-sec rest interval after each sprint demonstrated significantly greater peak power and average power with bicarbonate loading compared to a placebo [43].

The results of these studies presented a strong argument for the effectiveness of bicarbonate loading during repeated-bout exercise. This led to two studies evaluating the effectiveness of bicarbonate loading during high-volume resistance exercise [40, 47]. Investigators in both studies attempted to maximize several of the variables consistently associated with improved cycling and running performance (trained subjects, interval exercise protocol, dosage of 300 mg/kg, 105-min ingestion period). The first study had subjects perform four sets of 12 repetitions of a leg press with a fifth set to volitional fatigue at a resistance equaling ~70% of their 1-RM. Four of six subjects improved performance by an average of 16%; however, the overall mean was not statistically significant [47]. A similar study had subjects perform five maximal sets of leg press exercise with each set to volitional fatigue. Overall, the investigators considered this a higher-intensity exercise protocol than that used by Webster et al. [47] and thought it to be more similar to actual resistance training practices. However, once again, there was no difference in exercise performance [40].

When one compares the physiological demands of repeated bouts of high-volume resistance exercise to those for repeated bouts of cycling exercise, it is apparent that high-volume resistance exercise is not as metabolically challenging at the whole-body level. At the whole-body level, resistance training typically does not elicit metabolic rates greater than approximately 50% $\dot{V}O_2$max [63, 64], whereas repeated cycling bouts can demand upward of 125% $\dot{V}O_2$max. In addition, in each of the resistance exercise studies cited earlier, the acid-base challenge was significantly less (higher plasma pH and lower plasma lactate) than that reported during repeated bouts of cycling [40, 47].

Overall, the data from interval exercise suggest that as long as the whole-body metabolic rate is significantly elevated, bicarbonate loading can be effective in enhancing performance in the later bouts. Despite the interval nature of high-volume resistance training, it does not appear that this type of exercise significantly elevates whole-body metabolic rate, and accordingly, bicarbonate loading does not appear to influence exercise performance of this kind.

In addition to the pre-exercise and exercise measures of acid-base balance reported in the research previously cited, many of these studies presented some postexercise acid-base data [22, 24-28, 32, 36, 40, 47]. These data indicate that the postexercise plasma pH is often higher with bicarbonate loading. The higher pH provides a more optimal environment for the efflux of lactate from the cell, evidenced by a higher postexercise [lactate], thereby speeding the recovery of the intracellular acid-base status. The influence of bicarbonate loading on the recovery of force after exercise has been addressed in only one study [65]. During recovery from a high-intensity exercise bout on a cycle ergometer, functional electrical stimulations were applied to the quadriceps femoris at 10-min intervals for 40 min. Normalized knee torque was significantly greater at each measurement time, indicating that bicarbonate loading reduces postexercise fatigue and enhances recovery. Although postexercise fatigue and recovery have not been evaluated in the first couple of minutes after maximal exercise, the data from this study provide a plausible hypothesis for the enhanced performance often demonstrated with bicarbonate loading during interval exercise.

Although the focus of this review has been on the effect of bicarbonate loading on muscle fatigue, discussion is also warranted on the influence of this practice on a subject's perceived sensations of fatigue during exercise. The first study to report the effect of bicarbonate loading on perceived feelings of fatigue had subjects perform an incremental cycle exercise test until exhaustion [66]. Participants reported no differences in the subjective feelings of fatigue during the test, and the authors suggested that "the change in the acid-base state of the arterial blood is not one of the mechanisms underlying the feelings of fatigue." Two other studies presented the same findings, one after performance of approximately ten 60-sec cycling bouts [67] and one after performance of a single maximal 60-sec cycling bout [27]. In contrast, two later studies [46, 68] specifically addressing the question of the effect of bicarbonate loading on perceived effort indicated that the sensation of fatigue in the arms and legs was inversely related to plasma pH and HCO_3^- and that these sensations were attenuated with bicarbonate loading. While the studies presenting perceived exertion data are equivocal, until further work is reported it is advisable to give strong consideration to the findings of both Robertson et al. [68] and Swank and Robertson [46] for the very reason that these studies were specifically designed to investigate perceived effort. The other studies, with the exception of that of Poulus et al. [66] evaluated perceived effort as one of many variables.

Data on the response of females to bicarbonate loading are quite limited. It has been reported that prior to 1993 only 3% of the subjects in bicarbonate-loading studies were female [56]. Since then, three studies have investigated the effect of bicarbonate loading in just women. While the acid-base responses to bicarbonate loading are similar among studies, the performance data are again equivocal. One study indicated that bicarbonate loading had no effect on performance of a single 600-m (656 yd) run [69] or on the duration of intermittent bouts of 60-sec cycling exercise [67]. Another showed that it enhanced work output during a single maximal 60-sec cycling bout [27].

Ethical Implications

$NaHCO_3$ is not on the United States Olympic Committee (USOC) or the International Olympic Committee (IOC) banned substance list [70]. Consequently, no individual has ever been disqualified from competition for its use. In a nonathletic setting, $NaHCO_3$ may be ingested in relatively small amounts to treat an "upset stomach" or may be administered in the clinical life-threatening condition of metabolic acidosis. However, athletes ingest relatively large amounts of $NaHCO_3$ for the singularly expressed purpose of enhancing exercise performance. Bicarbonate loading, by definition, is in violation of the USOC/IOC doping law, which prohibits "the administration or use by a competing athlete of any foreign substance to the body or of any physiological substance taken in abnormal quantity or taken by an abnormal route of entry into the body with the sole intention of increasing in an artificial and unfair manner his/her performance in competition" [70], thereby "qualifying" $NaHCO_3$ as a banned substance. This

presents a conflict between the "letter of the law" (it isn't tested, so there is no chance of getting punished for its use) and the "principle of the law" (it is illegal, so you shouldn't use it).

Only one study has investigated the effect of bicarbonate loading on urinary pH in an effort to detect individuals who have participated in this practice [41]. In 65 subjects, urine pH 1 hr after an 800-m (875 yd) time trial was significantly elevated in the bicarbonate-loading trial. The data indicated that selecting a urinary pH of 7.0 would detect 92% of individuals taking $NaHCO_3$ with no false-positive tests. It was noted in this study that other potential factors may contribute to an alkaline urinary pH, but their impact with bicarbonate loading was not evaluated.

Summary and Implications for Future Research

After nearly 70 years of systematic evaluation of the physiological and exercise performance responses to bicarbonate loading, it is still somewhat difficult to make many conclusive statements about this practice. However, the bottom-line question most often asked is "Does bicarbonate loading work?"—and the answer is a resounding "maybe." Figure 17.3 outlines some of the "conclusive" statements that one can make about the

---

- The optimal dosage appears to be 300 mg/kg.
- Acute dosages above 300 mg/kg, while effective in enhancing some types of exercise performance, almost always lead to undesirable gastrointestinal symptoms.
- The time necessary for an acute administration dosage of $NaHCO_3$ to elicit the greatest acid-base changes appears to be 90-105 min.
- Bicarbonate loading does not appear to enhance exercise performance during single bouts of maximal activity of less than about 50-s duration.
- Bicarbonate loading appears to enhance performance of single bouts of maximal intensity exercise of approximately 1-7-min duration.
- Bicarbonate loading does not appear to enhance performance of single bouts of submaximal intensity exercise.
- Bicarbonate loading appears to enhance exercise performance of repeated bouts of short-duration, high-intensity exercise, providing the whole-body metabolic rate is great enough to challenge the bicarbonate buffering system.

Figure 17.3 Summary of conclusions that can be drawn about the practice of bicarbonate loading.

practice. Bicarbonate loading based on these conclusions would maximize the likelihood of producing significant performance changes.

Despite these "conclusive" statements, there are still numerous questions surrounding this practice that warrant further study. The following are some suggestions for further research. First, what is the optimal dosage and administration period for ingesting $NaHCO_3$ in several amounts over a longer period of time? Most researchers agree that the optimal acute $NaHCO_3$ dosage is 300 mg/kg over a 90- to 120-min time period; however, there are still undesirable gastrointestinal symptoms in some subjects. The recent work of McNaughton et al. [29] has challenged this optimal dosage/administration conclusion. Their data indicate that a larger total dosage of $NaHCO_3$ can be tolerated without the undesirable symptoms, elicit significant acid-base changes, and enhance exercise performance if the $NaHCO_3$ is administered in several smaller amounts over a longer period of time rather than as a single bolus. It is very possible that the nonsignificant exercise performance findings demonstrated in many bicarbonate-loading studies can be explained, at least in part, by the negative gastrointestinal effects observed in some individuals with the acute 300 mg/kg dosage. Because the experimental design of most bicarbonate-loading studies is limited by a small number of subjects, resulting in a lack of statistical power, a single subject experiencing gastrointestinal symptoms decreases the chances that the study will show statistically significant differences [56].

Second, is bicarbonate loading warranted in competitive "endurance" events? It is generally assumed that exercise such as a 10-km (6.2 miles) run or a road cycling race does not warrant bicarbonate loading because it is predominately aerobic and the disruption of acid-base status is not a primary cause of muscle fatigue. However, tactical competitions are often performed at a steady pace equating with anywhere from 60% to 90% of $\dot{V}O_2$max for most of the race, followed by a supramaximal effort to exhaustion at the end of the race that typically lasts 1 to 4 min. The exercise intensity and duration at the end of the race constitute precisely the type of activity that has been repeatedly demonstrated to be enhanced with bicarbonate loading. The only study to evaluate this question had trained collegiate runners run on a treadmill at their lactate threshold for 30 min and then to exhaustion at 110% of their $\dot{V}O_2$max [45]. A nonsignificant 65-sec increase in time to exhaustion was reported in the bicarbonate-loading trial as compared with the placebo trial. However, once again, a major shortcoming in the experimental design was the small number of subjects (n = 7). A statistical power analysis revealed that with 12 subjects the results would have been significant. Further studies using more subjects and using exercise protocols that mimic the tactical conditions seen in competitive settings are needed.

Third, does bicarbonate loading enhance long-duration exercise performance? As indicated previously, these activities are predominately aerobic, and disruption of acid-base status is typically not thought to be a primary cause of muscle fatigue. However, McNaughton et al. [28] recently reported that bicarbonate loading improved work output by 14% during 60 min of cycling. These findings concur with those of Potteiger et al. [71], who used sodium citrate as a buffering agent and demonstrated a 3% faster ride during a 30-km (18.6 miles) cycling time trial. Considering that only one bicarbonate-loading study has dealt with performance during an exercise bout as long as 60 min, additional studies are needed.

Fourth, is there any difference between men and women in their physiological and performance responses to bicarbonate loading? As is typical with much of the research in exercise science, very few studies of women have been reported. Of the three bicarbonate studies that do include women [27, 67, 69], two [67, 69] indicate that bicarbonate loading is ineffective in enhancing exercise performance, and one [27] indicates that it is effective. Given the few studies and the conflicting findings, further study is clearly warranted.

Finally, what is the effect of bicarbonate loading during high-intensity exercise in the heat? Exercise performance is significantly compromised by hyperthermia, and exercise in this situation is characterized by significantly greater accumulation of lactic acid even during steady state activities. The greater accumulation results from not only a significant elevation in nonoxidative glycogenolytic metabolism, but also from a significant decrease in intracellular buffering capacity. The combination of these two factors presents a physiological environment that significantly stresses the HCO_3^- buffer system and might benefit from bicarbonate loading.

References

1. Metzger, J.M. and R.H. Fitts, Role of intracellular pH in muscle fatigue. J Appl Physiol, 1987. 62(4): p. 1392-1397.

2. Jones, N.L., Hydrogen ion balance during exercise. Clin Sci, 1980. 59(2): p. 85-91.

3. Fitts, R.H., J.B. Courtright, D.H. Kim, and F.A. Witzmann. Muscle fatigue with prolonged exercise: contractile and biochemical alterations. Am J Physiol, 1982. 242(1): p. C65-C73.

4. Bigland-Ritchie, B. and J.J. Woods, Changes in muscle contractile properties and neural control during human muscular fatigue. Muscle Nerve, 1984. 7(9): p. 691-699.

5. Mainwood, G.W. and J.M. Renaud, The effect of acid-base balance on fatigue of skeletal muscle. Can J Physiol Pharmacol, 1985. 63(5): p. 403-416.

6. Mainwood, G.W., J.M. Renaud, and M.J. Mason, The pH dependence of the contractile response of fatigued skeletal muscle. Can J Physiol Pharmacol, 1987. 65(4): p. 648-658.

7. Guyton, A.C. and J.E. Hall, Textbook of Medical Physiology. 9th ed. 1996, Philadelphia: Saunders.

8. Sahlin, K., A. Alvestrand, R. Brandt, E. Hultman, Intracellular pH and bicarbonate concentration in human muscle during recovery from exercise. J Appl Physiol, 1978. 45(3): p. 474-480.

9. Sahlin, K., R.C. Harris, B. Nylind, E. Hultman, Lactate content and pH in muscle obtained after dynamic exercise. Pflugers Arch, 1976. 367(2): p. 143-149.

10. Hermansen, L. and J.-B. Osnes, Blood and muscle pH after maximal exercise in man. J Appl Physiol, 1972. 32(3): p. 304-308.

11. Fabiato, A. and F. Fabiato, Effects of pH on the myofilaments and the sarcoplasmic reticulum of skinned cells from cardiac and skeletal muscles. J Physiol (Lond), 1978. 276: p. 233-255.

12. Inesi, G. and T.L. Hill, Calcium and proton dependence of sarcoplasmic reticulum ATPase. Biophys J, 1983. 44(2): p. 271-280.

13. Fuchs, F., Y. Reddy, and F.N. Briggs, The interaction of cations with the calcium-binding site of troponin. Biochim Biophys Acta, 1970. 221(2): p. 407-409.

14. Donaldson, S.K.B., L. Hermansen, and L. Bolles, Differential direct effects of H^+ on Ca^{2+} activated force of skinned fibres from soleus, cardiac and adductor magnus muscles of rabbits. Pflugers Arch, 1978. 376: p. 55-65.

15. Ui, M., A role of phosphofructokinase in pH-dependent regulation of glycolysis. Biochim Biophys Acta, 1966. 124(2): p. 310-322.

16. Dobson, G.P., E. Yamamoto, and P.W. Hochachka, Phosphofructokinase control in muscle: nature and reversal of pH-dependent ATP inhibition. Am J Physiol, 1986. 250(1 Pt 2): p. R71-R76.

17. Lowry, O.H. and J.V. Passonneau, Kinetic evidence for multiple binding sites on phosphofructokinase. J Biol Chem, 1966. 241(10): p. 2268-2279.

18. Trivedi, B. and W.H. Danforth, Effect of pH on the kinetics of frog muscle phosphofructokinase. J Biol Chem, 1966. 241(17): p. 4110-4112.

19. Newsholme, E.A., A.R. Leech, Biochemistry for the Medical Sciences. 1986, Great Britain: Wiley.

20. Brooks, G.A., T.D. Fahey, T.P. White, K.M. Baldwin, Exercise Physiology: Human Bioenergetics and Its Application. 3rd ed. 2000, Mountain View, CA: Mayfield Publishing Company.

21. Dennig, H., J.H. Talbot, H.T. Edwards, D.B. Dill, Effect of acidosis and alkalosis upon capacity for work. J Clin Invest, 1931. 9: p. 601-613.

22. Costill, D.L., F. Verstappen, H. Kuipers, E. Janssen, W. Fink, Acid-base balance during repeated bouts of exercise: influence of HCO_3^-. Int J Sports Med, 1984. 5(5): p. 228-231.

23. Horswill, C.A., D.L. Costill, W.J. Fink, M.G. Flynn, J.P. Kirwan, J.B. Mitchell, et al., Influence of sodium bicarbonate on sprint performance: relationship to dosage. Med Sci Sports Exerc, 1988. 20(6): p. 566-569.

24. McNaughton, L.R. and R. Cedaro, The effect of sodium bicarbonate on rowing ergometer performance in elite rowers. Aust J Sci Med Sport, 1991. Sept: p. 66-69.

25. McNaughton, L.R., Sodium bicarbonate ingestion and its effects on anaerobic exercise of various durations. J Sports Sci, 1992. 10(5): p. 425-435.

26. McNaughton, L.R., Bicarbonate ingestion: effects of dosage on 60 s cycle ergometry. J Sports Sci, 1992. 10(5): p. 415-423.

27. McNaughton, L.R., S. Ford, and C. Newbold, Effect of sodium bicarbonate ingestion on high intensity exercise in moderately trained women. J Strength Cond Res, 1997. 11(2): p. 98-102.

28. McNaughton, L., B. Dalton, and G. Palmer, Sodium bicarbonate can be used as an ergogenic aid in high-intensity, competitive cycle ergometry of 1 h duration. Eur J Appl Physiol, 1999. 80(1): p. 64-69.

29. McNaughton, L., K. Backx, G. Palmer, N. Strange, Effects of chronic bicarbonate ingestion on the performance of high-intensity work. Eur J Appl Physiol, 1999. 80(4): p. 333-336.

30. Wilkes, D., N. Gledhill, and R. Smyth, Effect of acute induced metabolic alkalosis on 800-m racing time. Med Sci Sports Exerc, 1983. 15(4): p. 277-280.

31. Goldfinch, J., L. McNaughton, and P. Davies, Induced metabolic alkalosis and its effects on 400-m racing time. Eur J Appl Physiol, 1988. 57(1): p. 45-48.

32. Jones, N.L., J.R. Sutton, R. Taylor, C.L. Toews, Effect of pH on cardiorespiratory and metabolic responses to exercise. J Appl Physiol, 1977. 43(6): p. 959-964.

33. Sutton, J.R., N.L. Jones, and C.L. Toews, Effect of acidosis and alkalosis on muscle metabolism. Aust J Sports Med, 1979. 11(4): p. 95-99.

34. Sutton, J.R., N.L. Jones, and C.L. Toews, Effect of pH on muscle glycolysis during exercise. Clin Sci, 1981. 61: p. 331-338.

35. Rupp, J.C., R.L. Bartels, W. Zuelzer, E.L. Fox, R.N. Clark, Effect of sodium bicarbonate ingestion on blood and muscle pH and exercise performance. Med Sci Sports Exerc, 1983. 15(2): p. 115.

36. Kots, Y.M., E.V. Ozolina, and O.L. Vinogradova, Effect of alimentary alkalemia on maximal duration of anaerobic work and lactate concentration in muscles and blood. Human Physiol, 1983. 9: p. 169-174.

37. Bouissou, P., G. Defer, C.Y. Guezennec, P.Y. Estrade, B. Serrurier, Metabolic and blood catecholamine responses to exercise during alkalosis. Med Sci Sports Exerc, 1988. 20(3): p. 228-232.

38. Maughan, R.J., Exercise-induced muscle cramp: a prospective biochemical study in marathon runners. J Sports Sci, 1986. 4(1): p. 31-34.

39. Pfefferle, K.P. and J.G. Wilkinson, Induced alkalosis and supramaximal cycling in trained and untrained men. Med Sci Sports Exerc, 1988. 20(2): p. S25.

40. Portington, K.J., D.D. Pascoe, M.J. Webster, L.H. Anderson, R.R. Rutland, L.B. Gladden, Effect of induced alkalosis on exhaustive leg press performance. Med Sci Sports Exerc, 1998. 30(4): p. 523-528.

41. McKenzie, D.C., Changes in urinary pH following bicarbonate loading. Can J Sport Sci, 1988. 13(4): p. 254-256.

42. Inbar, O., A. Rotstein, I. Jacobs, P. Kaiser, R. Dlin, R. Dotan, The effects of alkaline treatment on short-term maximal exercise. J Sport Sci, 1983. 1: p. 95-104.

43. Lavender, G. and S.R. Bird, Effect of sodium bicarbonate ingestion upon repeated sprints. Br J Sports Med, 1989. 23(1): p. 41-45.

44. McCartney, N., G.J. Heigenhauser, and N.L. Jones, Effects of pH on maximal power output and fatigue during short-term dynamic exercise. J Appl Physiol, 1983. 55(1 Pt 1): p. 225-229.

45. Potteiger, J.A., M.J. Webster, G.L. Nickel, M.D. Haub, R.J. Palmer, The effects of buffer ingestion on metabolic factors related to distance running performance. Eur J Appl Physiol, 1996. 72(4): p. 365-371.

46. Swank, A. and R.J. Robertson, Effect of induced alkalosis on perception of exertion during intermittent exercise. J Appl Physiol, 1989. 67(5): p. 1862-1867.

47. Webster, M.J., M.N. Webster, R.E. Crawford, L.B. Gladden, Effect of sodium bicarbonate ingestion on exhaustive resistance exercise performance. Med Sci Sports Exerc, 1993. 25(8): p. 960-965.

48. Wijnen, S., F. Verstappen, and H. Kuipers, The influence of intravenous $NaHCO_3$ administration on interval exercise: acid-base balance and endurance. Int J Sports Med, 1984. 5: p. 130-132.

49. Parry-Billings, M. and D.P. MacLaren, The effect of sodium bicarbonate and sodium citrate ingestion on anaerobic power during intermittent exercise. Eur J Appl Physiol, 1986. 55(5): p. 524-529.

50. Aschenbach, W., J. Ocel, L. Craft, C. Ward, E. Spangenburg, J. Williams, Effect of oral sodium loading on high-intensity arm ergometry in college wrestlers. Med Sci Sports Exerc, 2000. 32(3): p. 669-675.

51. Brien, D.M. and D.C. McKenzie, The effect of induced alkalosis and acidosis on plasma lactate and work output in elite oarsmen. Eur J Appl Physiol, 1989. 58(8): p. 797-802.

52. Parkhouse, W.S. and D.C. McKenzie, Possible contribution of skeletal muscle buffers to enhanced anaerobic performance: a brief review. Med Sci Sports Exerc, 1984. 16(4): p. 328-338.

53. Sharp, R.L., D.L. Costill, W.J. Fink, D.S. King, Effects of eight weeks of bicycle ergometer sprint training on human muscle buffer capacity. Int J Sports Med, 1986. 7(1): p. 13-17.

54. McKenzie, D.C., K.D. Coutts, D.R. Stirling, H.H. Hoeben, G. Kuzara, Maximal work production following two levels of artificially induced metabolic alkalosis. J Sports Sci, 1986. 4(1): p. 35-38.

55. Downs, N.M. and P.A. Stonebridge, Gastric rupture due to excessive sodium bicarbonate ingestion. Scott Med J, 1989. 34(5): p. 534-535.

56. Matson, L.G. and Z.V. Tran, Effects of sodium bicarbonate ingestion on anaerobic performance: a meta-analytic review. Int J Sport Nutr, 1993. 3(1): p. 2-28.

57. Linderman, J.K. and K.L. Gosselink, The effects of sodium bicarbonate ingestion on exercise performance. Sports Med, 1994. 18(2): p. 75-80.

58. George, K.P. and D.P. MacLaren, The effect of induced alkalosis and acidosis on endurance running at an intensity corresponding to 4 mM blood lactate. Ergonomics, 1988. 31(11): p. 1639-1645.

59. Zoladz, J.A., K. Duda, J. Majerczak, J. Domanski, J. Emmerich, Metabolic alkalosis induced by pre-exercise ingestion of $NaHCO_3$ does not modulate the slow component of VO_2 kinetics in humans. J Physiol Pharmacol, 1997. 48(2): p. 211-223.

60. Heck, K.L., J.A. Potteiger, K.L. Nau, J.M. Schroeder, Sodium bicarbonate ingestion does not attenuate the VO_2 slow component during constant-load exercise. Int J Sport Nutr, 1998. 8(1): p. 60-69.

61. Osnes, J.-B. and L. Hermansen, Acid-base balance after maximal exercise of short duration. J Appl Physiol, 1972. 31(1): p. 59-63.

62. Gao, J.P., D.L. Costill, C.A. Horswill, S.H. Park, Sodium bicarbonate ingestion improves performance in interval swimming. Eur J Appl Physiol, 1988. 58(1-2): p. 171-174.

63. Dudley, G.A., P.A. Tesch, R.T. Harris, C.L. Golden, P. Buchanan, Influence of eccentric actions on the metabolic cost of resistance exercise. Aviat Space Environ Med, 1991. 62(7): p. 678-682.

64. Wilmore, J.H., R.B. Parr, and P. Ward, Energy cost of circuit weight training. Med Sci Sports Exerc, 1978. 10: p. 75-78.

65. Verbitsky, O., J. Mizrahi, M. Levin, E. Isakov, Effect of ingested sodium bicarbonate on muscle force, fatigue, and recovery. J Appl Physiol, 1997. 83(2): 333-337.

66. Poulus, A.J., H.J. Docter, and H.G. Westra, Acid-base balance and subjective feelings of fatigue during physical exercise. Eur J Appl Physiol, 1974. 33: p. 207-213.

67. Kozak-Collins, K., E.R. Burke, and R.B. Schoene, Sodium bicarbonate ingestion does not improve performance in women cyclists. Med Sci Sports Exerc, 1994. 26(12): p. 1510-1515.

68. Robertson, R.J., J.E. Falkel, A.L. Drash, A.M. Swank, K.F. Metz, S.A. Spungen, et al., Effect of induced alkalosis on physical work capacity during arm and leg exercise. Ergonomics, 1987. 30(1): p. 19-31.

69. Tiryaki, G.R. and H.A. Atterbom, The effects of sodium bicarbonate and sodium citrate on 600 m running time of trained females. J Sports Med Phys Fit, 1995. 35(3): p. 194-198.

70. Education, CoSARa, USOC/IOC Banned Drugs. 1986, Colorado Springs, CO: United States Olympic Committee/ International Olympic Committee.

71. Potteiger, J.A., G.L. Nickel, M.J. Webster, M.D. Haub, R.J. Palmer, Sodium citrate ingestion enhances 30 km cycling performance. Int J Sport Med, 1996. 17(1): p. 17-21.

Herbals As Ergogenic Aids

Melvin H. Williams, PhD, FACSM

J. David Branch, PhD, FACSM

All nutrients essential for life may be obtained from animal or plant foods we consume. As discussed in a previous chapter, several nutrients may possess ergogenic potential for athletes under special circumstances, such as carbohydrate loading for marathon runners. Other than essential nutrients, animal and plant foods contain naturally occurring substances that are referred to respectively as zoochemicals and phytochemicals (American Dietetic Association, 1999). One zoochemical, creatine, is derived from muscle tissue; its efficacy and safety as a nutritional ergogenic are evaluated in chapter 16. This chapter focuses on herbals, a class of phytochemicals that may induce physiologic actions in the body conducive to enhanced physical performance.

Herbals As Drugs

Conventional and medical dictionaries variously define an herbal as equivalent to a botanical, specifically as a flowering plant with various parts, including leaves, bark, berries, roots, gums, seeds, stems, and flowers. Herbals contain numerous phytochemicals (variously known as phytonutrients, phytoceuticals, or nutraceuticals) thought to have nutritive or medicinal value. Defined in pharmacological terms, herbals or botanicals are drugs made from part of a plant (Zeisel, 1999).

Herbs have been used as medicine throughout history. Winslow and Kroll (1998) reported that the earliest evidence of human use of plants for healing dates back to the Neanderthal period. Blumenthal and colleagues (2000) indicated that the ancient Greek physicians Hippocrates, Dioscorides, and Galen were medical herbalists. Winslow and Kroll (1998) further note that botanical gardens were created to grow medicinal plants for medical schools in the 16th century, and that homemade herbal remedies were common in the U.S. colonial period. With the advent of modern pharmaceutical techniques in the 20th century, herbal medicine came to be regarded as quackery by practitioners of conventional medicine and its use discouraged. However, several reports (Angell and Kassirer, 1998; Winslow and Kroll, 1998) indicate that the use of herbal medicine is becoming increasingly accepted in Western societies, as documented by the establishment of the

Office of Alternative Medicine by the National Institutes of Health in the United States and publication of *The Complete German Commission E Monographs: Therapeutic Guide to Herbal Medicines* (Bundesanzeiger, 1998). Additionally, the World Health Organization has encouraged developing countries to use traditional plant medicines to fulfill a need unmet by modern systems (Winslow and Kroll, 1998).

Medicinal herbs are precursors to conventional medicines, as specific individual, active compounds have been identified and standardized. About 30% of all modern drugs are derived from plants, including atropine *(Atropa belladonna)*, digoxin *(Digitalis purpurea)*, codeine *(Papaver somniferum)*, quinine *(Cinchona officinalis)*, reserpine *(Rauvolfia serpentina)*, and taxol *(Taxus brevifolia)* (Winslow and Kroll, 1998). In many countries, such as Germany, herbs are classified as prescription drugs. Some examples, from *Herbal Medicine: Expanded Commission E Monographs* (Blumenthal et al., 2000), are presented in table 18.1.

Herbals As Nutrients

In the United States, the Dietary Supplement Health and Education Act (DSHEA) of 1994 defines a dietary supplement as a product intended to supplement the diet to enhance health that bears or contains one or more of the following dietary ingredients: a vitamin, mineral, amino acid, herb or other botanical and not represented as a conventional food or as a sole item of a meal or diet. Given the increasing popularity of dietary supplements in North America, several government agencies have been developed to monitor and regulate their use, including the Office of Dietary Supplements within the National Institutes of Health in the United States and the Office of Natural Health Products in Canada.

Multivitamin/mineral tablets reign as the most popular dietary supplement, particularly supplements containing antioxidants, such as vitamin C, vitamin E, and selenium; but herbal preparations are also very popular. For example, Winslow and Kroll (1998) indicated that over 20,000 herbs and related products are used in the United States, while Angell and Kassirer (1998), citing data from the Presidential Commission on Dietary Supplement Labels, note that some 1500 to 1800 botanical products are sold

Table 18.1 Herbs Used Medicinally for Various Health Problems

System/Organ	Health problem	Medicinal herb
Cardiovascular	High cholesterol	Soy lecithin
	Hypertension	Garlic
Dermatological	Eczema	Walnut leaf
	Skin itching	Butcher's broom
Endocrine	Fatigue	Kola nut
	PMS	Chaste tree fruit
Gastrointestinal	Appetite	Cinnamon bark
	Irritable colon	Psyllium seed husk
Immune	Convalescence	Eleuthero root
	Free radicals	Ginkgo biloba
Liver	Cirrhosis	Milk thistle fruit
	Hepatitis	Soy phospholipid
Neural	Anxiety	St. John's wort
	Memory	Ginkgo biloba
Respiratory	Asthma	Ephedra
	Colds	Echinacea
Musculoskeletal	Joint pain	Arnica flower (external)
	Muscle spasm	Cayenne pepper
Urinary	Kidney stones	Goldenrod
	Urinary infection	Horseradish

in the United States as dietary supplements. Commercial herbal preparations come in many forms, including tablets, capsules, liquids, powders, tinctures, extracts, compresses, creams, lotions, salves, and oils. Many supplements contain multiple herbs.

Most herbal dietary supplements are marketed for their medicinal properties to enhance one's health status. In one sense, herbals that help prevent or remedy an illness may be ergogenic as they may enable the athlete to train more effectively and, hopefully, compete more effectively. Use of medicinal herbs is widespread among some Western societies, suggesting that athletes may also use herbals for medicinal purposes. However, although medicinal applications of herbal dietary supplements may benefit the health status of the physically active individual, they are not designed to be ergogenic.

Herbals As Ergogenic Aids

Phytochemicals and zoochemicals have been used to increase physical performance capacity for centuries, particularly for military combat. Ancient Greeks consumed sesame seeds, the legendary Norse warriors (Berserkers) used bufotenine before combat, and the Andean Indians and Australian aborigines chewed,

respectively, coca leaves and the pituri plant for stimulating and anti-fatiguing effects (Williams, 1974).

Herbals As Pharmacological Ergogenics

From the standpoint of classification as an ergogenic aid, herbs may be considered either a pharmacological or a nutritional aid. Zeisel (1999), discussing the regulation of nutraceuticals, noted that it is often difficult to distinguish among nutrients and drugs, indicating that a dietary supplement can be foodlike at some times and druglike at other times, and that under present conceptualizations the boundary at which a food ingredient becomes a drug is not well defined. Zeisel notes further that some dietary supplements are druglike when ingested in amounts that could never be achieved in the diet, even though they are essential nutrients when ingested in smaller amounts. For example, niacin is an essential vitamin found in small amounts in the diet, but dietary supplements containing megadoses may be used to treat hypercholesteremia. Zeisel indicates that when the dosage of food components, botanicals, or their extracts exceeds levels achievable in normal diets, their bioactivity can be druglike. Indeed, many countries in Europe regulate herbs as drugs (Blumenthal et al., 2000).

Every major drug category discussed in this text has a historical or contemporary herbal counterpart. For example, androstenedione, an anabolic, may be derived from wild yams and is marketed as a dietary supplement. Likewise, there are herbal diuretics, analgesics, depressants, stimulants, and social/recreational herbals. Indeed, even specific drugs to which entire chapters in this text are devoted, such as caffeine (*Coffea arabica*), cocaine (*Erythroxylon coca*), ephedrine (*Ephedra sinica*), and marijuana (*Cannabis sativa*), may technically be classified as herbals.

Herbals As Nutritional Ergogenics

In the United States, most herbs are regulated as dietary supplements under the DSHEA. Thus, for the purposes of this text, herbals have been classified as nutritional ergogenic aids. In this regard, numerous functional foods (sport bars, sport drinks) and dietary supplements containing herbals are marketed to physically active individuals. Such products are marketed to increase energy, induce weight loss, promote muscle growth, or induce other physiological or metabolic responses that may enhance exercise performance. For example, marketed as an all-natural nutritional supplement formulated specifically for runners, R-1 contains several ingredients, including Panax and Siberian ginseng, which the company alleges have been shown to increase energy levels, endurance, and oxygen utilization while shortening the body's recovery time. Another herbal product,

SportPharm, contains multiple herbals, including Thermadrene, Ma Huang, Guarana, caffeine, purple willow bark, cayenne pepper, and ginger root, designed to increase mental alertness, stimulate fat-burning metabolism, and help enhance physical performance.

The DSHEA permits general structure/function claims, such as the claim that a product contains substances essential in production of energy. Unless documented by scientific research, however, specific claims, such as that a product increases $\dot{V}O_2$max, may not be made. As noted later in the discussion of individual herbals, such supporting research is generally not available.

General Efficacy, Quality, Safety, and Permissibility of Herbs

Preceding a discussion of individual herbal products with ergogenic potential, some general comments on herbal efficacy, quality, safety, and legality appear to be relevant. Details regarding specific herbals, particularly quality and safety, may be obtained from the Web sites listed in figure 18.1.

Efficacy and Quality

Craig (1999) recently noted that different herbs may contain a wide variety of active phytochemicals, including flavonoids, terpenoids, lignans, sulfides, polyphenolics, carotenoids, coumarins, saponins, plant sterols, curcumins, and phthalides, and that each may influence major health-related and sport-related physiological functions in the body, such as DNA formation, enzyme activity, and antioxidant processes. Balentine and others (1999) indicated that currently there is great interest in determining the role of phytonutrients in promoting improved health and well-being and in reducing cancer, cardiovascular disease, and the effects of aging.

Chang (2000) notes that sufficient evidence exists to suggest that extracts of medicinal herbs, once they are isolated in their pure state, can produce pharmacological effects that differ significantly from that of the whole herb. Furthermore, research supports beneficial medicinal effects of specific herbs for specific health problems, as documented in *Herbal Medicine: Expanded Commission E Monographs* (Blumenthal et al., 2000) and *WHO Monographs on Selected Medicinal Plants* (World Health Organization, 1999A). Nevertheless, according to Chang (1999), the process of evaluating medicinal herbs is complex, and there is a need to carefully define a research strategy that addresses a solution to safe and efficacious herbal products. One possibility is to distill the pharmacological activity of a herb into a chemical suitable for drug development, while another approach is to develop a standardized herbal extract that yields consistent pharmacological activity.

In Germany, Wagner (1999) notes that most of the herbal drugs, even mixtures of herbal drugs, are registered as conventional drugs; this means that they meet the same stringent criteria of quality, efficacy, and safety as synthetic drugs. However, such is not the case in the United States. Winslow and Kroll (1998) pointed out that currently the DSHEA requires no proof of efficacy and sets no standards for quality control for products labeled as dietary supplements. Indeed, Winslow and Kroll (1998) indicated that dietary supplement labels may be incorrect, accidentally or intentionally, and that the product may contain additives—such as steroids, nonsteroidal anti-inflammatory agents, sedatives, or stimulants—that may be the source of the therapeutic effect.

According to Rotblatt (1999B), standardization of herbal products is difficult; products from different manufacturers vary considerably because it is inherently difficult to control all the factors that affect a plant's chemical composition. Environmental conditions such as sunlight and rainfall, as well as manufacturing processes such as selecting, drying, purifying, extracting, and storing herbs, can create substantial variability in product quality, for example the concentration of plant chemicals within different products. Rotblatt compares herbal products to wines in this regard. Wine (a botanical product) derived from the same species of grape may vary substantially from one winery to another; even wine originating in the same vineyard can vary from year to year.

Currently, the United States Pharmacopoeia (USP) is establishing analytical standards for certain botanical

American Botanical Council
http://www.herbalgram.org

Consumer Lab
www.consumerlab.com

Food and Drug Administration
Safety Information: The Special Nutritionals Adverse Event Monitoring System
www.fda/gov/medwatch

National Center for Complementary and Alternative Medicine
http://nccam.nih.gov

United States Pharmacopeia
www.usp.org

Figure 18.1 Web sites containing information on herbal efficacy, quality, or safety.

products. Manufacturers that meet these standards can place an official "NF" for "National Formulary" on their labels (Rotblatt, 1999B). The National Center for Complementary and Alternative Medicine has indicated that standardized extracts or standardized products are generally considered the highest-quality herbal products that a consumer can buy. Additionally, herbs must comply with Good Manufacturing Practice (GMP) regulations for foods, and the Food and Drug Administration is considering more extensive GMP regulations for dietary supplements (Rotblatt, 1999B).

Safety

Safety of herbal dietary supplements is an important issue. Angell and Kassirer (1998) note that a major portion of the world's population depends almost exclusively on herbal products and other alternative methods as the primary defense against or treatment for disease and various organic disorders. In this regard, Rotblatt (1999B) points out that serious side effects from herbal medicines are still relatively rare, especially compared with those for pharmaceutical drugs; adverse effects of appropriately prescribed pharmaceuticals were recently estimated to cause 106,000 deaths per year in hospitalized patients, whereas herbs may be less toxic because of weaker pharmacological activity, less consistent use, and a poorly established mechanism for recognizing and reporting adverse outcomes.

Many people may believe that if it's natural, it's harmless. Nevertheless, several reviewers (Angell and Kassirer, 1998; Consumers Union, 1998; Cupp, 1999; Fugh-Berman, 2000; Miller, 1998; Nortier et al., 2000; Winslow and Kroll, 1998) have presented some precautions for the use of herbals. Just like conventional drugs, herbal medicinals may have adverse side effects in some conditions; for example, ginseng may exacerbate hypertension. Some botanicals are toxic at high doses; for example, excess intake of herbal Ma Huang, as a source of ephedrine, may cause cardiac arrhythmias and death. Adverse herb/herb or herb/drug interactions may occur; for example, echinacea could cause hepatotoxicity and therefore should not be used with other possible hepatotoxic drugs such as anabolic steroids. Herbals may contain harmful contaminants; for example, a Chinese herbal weight-reducing dietary supplement contained a nephrotoxic and carcinogenic herb (*Aristolochia fangchi*) that caused renal disease or urothelial cancer in nearly half the individuals taking it. Moreover, thinking that herbals are safe and effective, individuals may forgo potentially curative care.

As Winslow and Kroll (1998) note, currently the DSHEA requires no proof of safety for products labeled as supplements. The burden lies with the FDA to prove a product unsafe, rather than with a company to prove that its product is safe; however, other counties, such as Germany, France, and Canada, enforce standards of herb safety assessment on manufacturers.

Permissibility

The International Olympic Committee (2000), in the Olympic Movement Anti-Doping Code, defines doping as the use of an expedient (substance or method) which is potentially harmful to athletes' health and/or capable of enhancing their performance. Several plant-derived drugs that might be construed to be herbals are prohibited or their use is limited, for example cocaine, caffeine, and ephedrine—all stimulants. However the list does not include every member of a prohibited class, such as stimulants, but provides the identifying phrase "and related substances." A related substance is any substance having pharmacological action and/or chemical structure similar to a prohibited substance. Theoretically, use of a herbal stimulant could be construed as doping.

In general, however, use of most herbal dietary supplements is currently permitted by the IOC and related sport governing associations. Nevertheless, many of the over-the-counter dietary supplements may contain prohibited substances. For example, products such as Energy Rise, Excel, Action Caps, or Super Charge may contain Ma Huang, or Chinese ephedra, as do many herbal weight loss supplements. Caffeine may also be found in supplements targeted to athletes. Thus, athletes who may be tested for drug use should read supplement labels carefully. Additionally, case studies have shown that herbal dietary supplements may be spiked with drugs whose use is prohibited by the IOC (Ros et al., 1999).

Purported Herbal Ergogenics

Herbal dietary supplements, like drugs, may be used to induce ergogenic effects in various ways. Some are theorized to enhance energy production, possibly by influencing metabolic pathways or enhancing physiological factors important to exercise; increased mitochondrial oxidation, myocardial activity, capillarization, and hemoglobin concentration are some proposed mechanisms. Other herbals are thought to benefit psychological processes important to some sports; some may stimulate psychological processes, whereas others may reduce excess anxiety that may impair performance in a given sports, particularly in precision-target sports such as archery, riflery, and pistol shooting.

Some of the most popular purported ergogenic herbals are theorized to modify body composition favorably. For example, Grunewald and Bailey (1993), in a survey of 624 commercially available supplements targeted toward bodybuilding athletes, noted that many of the supplements included herbals, such as gamma-oryzanol and yohimbine. The U.S. Olympic Committee (1996) has indicated that many herbal and plant products are alleged to be anabolic alternatives designed to increase weight and strength gains, and such herbals may contain steroidal compounds (Bernardo et al., 1996). Other herbals are marketed to induce weight loss. Excess body mass, particularly excess body fat, may be disadvantageous to athletes in several ways, increasing the energy costs of body movement and diminishing aesthetic appearance in judged sports. Thus, numerous athletes are interested in minimizing body fat to gain a mechanical edge or a more aesthetic appearance.

Unfortunately, with a few exceptions (particularly the voluminous research database on ginseng supplementation), research on the ergogenic effects of herbal supplements is limited. Although most herbal ergogenics have not been shown to be effective or have been inadequately studied, according to Blendon and others (2001) many users would continue to take them even if they were shown in scientifically conducted clinical studies to be ineffective. The following discussion highlights available research regarding the theory, efficacy, safety, and permissibility of selected herbal supplements purported to possess ergogenic potential.

Bee Pollen

Pollen consists of male germ spores mixed with nectar from seed-bearing plants. It is collected in a meshlike pollen trap as honeybees enter the hive and is marketed as the dietary supplement, bee pollen. Tyler (1993) indicated that the chemical constituents of bee pollen have been rather extensively investigated, and although the different components vary greatly in quantity among pollens of different species, some general ranges are available. Carbohydrates may range from 50% to 60%, lipids are extremely variable and range from 1% to 20%, and protein ranges from about 6% to 28%. Pollens may also contain small amounts of vitamins, minerals, and plant phytochemicals, such as flavonoids, terpenes, and sterols. Commercial supplements are available in tablets, capsules, extracts, and the like.

It has been alleged that bee pollen provides relief for various health problems, including anemia, bodily weakness, and weight loss, although none of the identified constituents of pollen has been linked to any related therapeutic activity (Tyler, 1993).

Theory

The mechanism underlying the purported ergogenicity of bee pollen is not known, but several theories have been proposed. On the basis of his observations with sprinters, Remi Korchemny, a former Russian track coach, speculated that bee pollen stimulates rapid recuperation

of adenosine triphosphate and enhances recovery, a phenomenon he referred to as a super second wind (Dunnett and Crossen, 1980). Additionally, children with anemia reportedly increased their red blood cell (RBC) count through bee pollen ingestion, a finding that may have been extrapolated to enhanced aerobic endurance performance (Dunnett and Crossen, 1980; Steben et al., 1976). At its height of popularity, a snack bar containing bee pollen was an "official snack food" of the 1987 Pan American Games in Indianapolis (Tyler, 1993).

Efficacy

Bee pollen as an effective ergogenic aid has been supported by anecdotal evidence. Abebe Bikila, the great two-time Olympic marathon champion, ate scrapings from the bottoms of beehives all his life and claimed it was the secret to his endurance, while Lasse Viren, the famous Finnish distance runner from the early 1970s, was also an advocate of bee pollen (Dunnett and Crossen, 1980). Chandler and Hawkins (1984) cited claims of increased energy production and improved postexercise recovery rates, mostly based on testimonial evidence.

However, there is little scientific support that bee pollen is an effective ergogenic aid, either to enhance recovery from strenuous exercise or to improve aerobic endurance capacity.

Several studies have evaluated the effect of bee pollen supplementation on recovery during intense exercise. In a double-blind, placebo-controlled study, Steben and others (1976) investigated the effect of bee pollen on average performance time (yards/sec) of 27 college swimmers in 12 repeat 200-yd (183 m) swim intervals. Daily for eight weeks of swim training, one group consumed a placebo; one group consumed 10 bee pollen tablets (total dosage not reported); and one group consumed half of both the placebo and bee pollen. Although all groups improved their performance and increased their hemoglobin levels by training, the statistical analysis revealed no significant differences among the groups for either variable. Woodhouse and others (1987) evaluated the effect of bee pollen supplementation on recovery time in five highly trained distance runners. In a three-week, double-blind, placebo-controlled, repeated-measures counterbalanced crossover study, subjects consumed a placebo, 1350 mg, or 2700 mg of bee pollen daily during each one-week period. At the end of each week, subjects performed six repeat treadmill runs to exhaustion at a speed of 7 miles/hr (11.2 km/hr) on a 15% uphill grade with 10-min rest interval between each run. Dependent variables included the run time of each repeat, the total run time for all six treadmill runs, and the rating of perceived exertion (RPE) 30 sec into each run. Although there was a fatiguing effect on both the time to exhaustion and the RPE in subsequent runs within each trial, there were no significant differences between the treatments.

Bee pollen supplementation has also been studied for its effects on hemoglobin and aerobic exercise endurance performance. In a double-blind, placebo-controlled study, Steben and Bourdreaux (1978) compared the effects of placebo, bee pollen in capsules, and a bee pollen extract preparation on performance in male cross country runners during a 12-week period of training. Bee pollen dosages equivalent to four capsules were consumed daily. Although a training effect did occur, there were no significant differences among the groups for changes in hemoglobin, hematocrit, and time on a 3-mile (4.8 km) run. In a double-blind, placebo-controlled study, Maughan and Evans (1982) evaluated the effect of six weeks of supplementation with pollen extract on exercise performance in adolescent swimmers. They reported no significant differences between the groups on $\dot{V}O_2$max, hemoglobin, hematocrit, grip strength, quadriceps strength, or quadriceps endurance. Chandler and Hawkins (1984), using 46 healthy males and females in a double-blind, placebo-control protocol, evaluated the ergogenic effects of 75 days of supplementation with commercial bee pollen (400 mg/day). They reported no significant differences between the groups for pretest and posttest measures of $\dot{V}O_2$max, grip strength, percent body fat, or body weight.

Thus, there are no reputable published studies supporting an ergogenic effect of bee pollen supplementation on recovery from high-intensity, repeat interval-type exercise or on hemoglobin, hematocrit status, or aerobic endurance performance.

Safety

Containing mostly nutrients, bee pollen may be safe for most individuals. However, ingestion of bee pollen may cause serious reactions in some allergic individuals. Numerous case reports in the medical literature have documented adverse reactions following bee pollen ingestion, including headache, nausea, diarrhea, abdominal pain, and anaphylaxis, a life-threatening medical emergency (Geyman, 1994; Tyler, 1993). Athletes with allergies should use extreme caution.

Permissibility

Bee pollen supplementation is permissible.

Capsicum (Capsaicin)

The capsicum species *(C. annuum; C. frutescens)*, native to tropical America, incorporates such peppers as the cayenne, red, and chili. Chili is the Aztec name for the cayenne pepper, and it has been used by Native Americans as food and medicine for over 9000 years (Blumenthal et al., 2000).

Tyler (1993) indicates that the medicinal properties of the capsicum species are attributable to a compound known as capsaicin, although other capsaicinoids are also present (Blumenthal et al., 2000). German pharmacopeial grade contains not less than 0.4% capsaicinoids. In the German Pharmacopoeia, capsaicin is normally used externally as a topical ointment, but Tyler (1993) indicated that it is also taken internally. Although its exact mechanisms are not fully understood, capsaicin is regarded as a neuropathic pain reliever, possibly blocking pain fibers by depleting substance P, the neurotransmitter mediating pain signals to the brain. Capsaicin is found in over-the-counter topical analgesic drug products used as counterirritant preparations for relief of arthritis pain (Blumenthal et al., 2000; Tyler, 1993).

Theory

Although blocking pain may be an underlying ergogenic mechanism for some athletic endeavors, capsaicin has not been studied in this regard. The USP has classified capsaicin as a stimulant; and on the basis of their previous research, Lim and others (1997) have related its physiological action to caffeine—that is, ingestion may induce sympathetic activation of the central nervous system, increasing catecholamine secretion and enhancing lipid oxidation, sparing the use of glycogen and improving aerobic endurance exercise capacity.

Efficacy

Some research supports this hypothesis, as Glickman-Weiss and others (1998) found that males, while at rest and exposed to immersion in cold water (22 °C), had a significant 75% decrease in carbohydrate for energy provision when fed capsaicin (2 mg/kg) as compared to a 47% decrease in the placebo trial. However, other studies presented different findings. Matsuo and others (1996) found that a capsaicin-supplemented diet for seven days did not influence liver or muscle glycogen content in rats that engaged in running training during the study. Lim and others (1997), using a repeated-measures, placebo, crossover design, evaluated the effect of a breakfast meal containing 10 g of dried hot red pepper on energy substrate use in male runners during rest (2.5 hr after meal) and exercise (cycle ergometry for 1 hr at 150 W, about 60% $\dot{V}O_2$max). For the red pepper trial, plasma epinephrine and norepinephrine concentrations were significantly elevated after 30 min, but not at 60 and 150 min of rest. The hot pepper meal significantly elevated the respiratory quotient (RQ) and blood lactate levels at rest and during exercise, but there was no effect on oxygen consumption or energy expenditure during rest or exercise. These results suggest that contrary to the theory of glycogen sparing, hot red pepper ingestion stimulates carbohydrate oxidation at rest and during exercise. The authors suggested that hot red pepper ingestion before exercise could decrease endurance performance in athletes because of associated muscle and/or liver glycogen depletion; however, no performance data were presented. Currently, no scientific evidence is available to support either an ergogenic or ergolytic effect of capsaicin supplementation. Additional research is merited.

Safety

As a dietary ingredient or supplement, capsaicin appears to be relatively safe. Some individuals may be allergic to cayenne preparations. Additionally, cayenne preparations are very irritable to mucous membranes, particularly in the eyes (Blumenthal et al., 2000).

Permissibility

Capsaicin supplementation appears to be legal.

Gamma-Oryzanol

Gamma-oryzanol, a mixture of ferulic acid esters of sterol and triterpene alcohols including campesterol, stigmasterol, and β-sitosterol, occurs in rice *(Oryza stavia)* bran oil at a level of 1% to 2%. Gamma-oryzanol serves as a natural antioxidant, and some research has shown that supplementation can lower serum cholesterol levels (Scavariello and Arellano, 1998).

Theory

As an ergogenic aid, Wheeler and Garleb (1991) indicated that gamma-oryzanol is used in the belief that its ingredients may elicit anabolic effects via increased testosterone production, increased release of human growth hormone, or rapid conversion to androgens. However, they reported that, in animals, injection of gamma-oryzanol has been shown to suppress luteinizing hormone release, reduce growth hormone synthesis and release, and increase the release of catecholamine, dopamine, and norepinephrine in the brain—suggesting that this metabolic milieu may actually reduce testosterone and human growth hormone production. Additionally, Fry and others (1997) indicated that the ferulic acid esters appear to be the active portion of gamma-oryzanol and may be involved in augmentation of norepinephrine levels, which may account for its proposed performance-enhancing effects.

Efficacy

The only available published study does not support an ergogenic effect of gamma-oryzanol supplementation in humans. In a randomized, placebo-controlled study, Fry and others (1997) assigned weight-trained males into placebo control or supplemented groups, the latter receiving 500 mg/day of gamma-oryzanol for nine weeks

of periodized resistance exercise training. Both groups were tested for hormonal and cholesterol status and exercise performance before and after four and nine weeks of supplementation. There were no differences between groups for circulating concentrations of hormones (testosterone, cortisol, estradiol, human growth hormone, insulin), for catecholamine-sensitive resting cardiovascular responses, or for blood lipids including total and high-density lipoprotein cholesterol. Although both groups demonstrated significant increases in vertical jump performance and one-repetition maximum (1-RM) muscular strength for the bench press and squat, there were no significant differences between the two groups.

Safety

Animal research has shown no adverse side effects, even with doses of 1000 mg gamma-oryzanol per day; and no adverse effects, such as gastrointestinal distress, were observed in humans consuming 500 mg/day (Fry et al., 1997).

Permissibility

Currently, gamma-oryzanol supplementation is not prohibited by the IOC.

Ginkgo Biloba

The Chinese ginkgo tree is the world's most ancient extant, having originated 200 million years ago, and is the source for *Ginkgo biloba* leaf extract, specifically proprietary extract EGb 761 (Blumenthal et al., 2000). In Germany, the standardized extract contains 24% flavonoid glycosides and 6% terpene lactones from green leaves. The three major flavonoids are quercetin, kaempferol, and isorhamnetin; the major terpenoids are ginkgolides (A, B, and C) and bilobalide (Blumenthal et al., 2000; Cott, 1995; Curtis-Prior et al., 1999).

Curtis-Prior and others (1999) note that *G. biloba* exerts its mode of action when its active ingredients, the flavonoids and terpenoids, work in concert. One of the tissue-level effects is stimulated release of endothelium-derived relaxing factor, which may enhance microcirculation (Cott, 1995). Most *G. biloba* supplementation research has been conducted in the elderly population, primarily for the vasoregulatory and cognition-enhancing effects (Blumenthal et al., 2000; Curtis-Prior, 1999). The German Commission E indicated that improvement of blood flow, particularly microcirculation, and increased memory performance are pharmacological effects of *G. biloba* that have been established experimentally (Blumenthal et al., 2000).

Theory

Improved microcirculation could be ergogenic for aerobic endurance athletes.

Efficacy

Ginkgo biloba has been shown to improve exercise performance, as evaluated by walking distance, in patients with peripheral arterial disease (PAD). In a meta-analysis of five placebo-control clinical trials, Schneider (1992) reported a highly significant therapeutic effect of *G. biloba* EGb 761 for the treatment of PAD. The global effect size was estimated as 0.75, meaning that the mean increase in walking distance obtained with *G. biloba* extract was 0.75 standard deviation higher than that achieved with placebo. Several major studies subsequent to this meta-analysis also showed beneficial effects. In a double-blind, placebo-controlled study with 60 patients, Blume and others (1996) reported a significant improvement in treadmill walking distance following *G. biloba* supplementation (3×40 mg for 24 weeks). Using the same experimental design and *G. biloba* dosage in a multicenter clinical trial, Peters and others (1998) also reported significantly longer walking distance compared to that in the placebo group. As the Doppler index values did not change in this latter study, the investigators speculated that the improvement in walking distance may have been attributable to improved nutrition to tissues and microcirculation rather than changes in macrocirculation.

Although *G. biloba* supplementation may improve exercise endurance in patients with PAD, there is no evidence that similar effects occur in healthy young or older athletes.

Safety

Ginkgo biloba may cause hypersensitivity reactions in some individuals, including headaches, allergic skin reactions, and gastrointestinal distress (Blumenthal et al., 2000). Additionally, concomitant intake with other blood thinners, such as aspirin, may increase bleeding (Cupp, 1999).

Permissibility

Currently, use of *G. biloba* as an ergogenic aid is not prohibited by the International Olympic Committee.

Ginseng

Ginseng is one of the most popular herbal dietary supplements worldwide. Current sales in the United States are over \$300 million annually (Bahrke and Morgan, 2000). Ginseng consists of several species belonging to the plant family Araliaceae. The two major forms are Chinese, Korean, or Asian ginseng, which belongs to the genus Panax, and Siberian or Russian ginseng, which belongs to the genus Eleutherococcus (Vogler et al., 1999). Other forms include *Panax japonicus* (Japan, India), *P. vietnamenis* (Vietnam), and *P. quinquefolius* (American or North American) (Bahrke and Morgan, 1994; Vogler et al., 1999).

There are many types and grades of ginseng, depending on the origin, root maturity, parts of the root used, and methods of raw material preparation or processing (Blumenthal et al., 2000). Although *Eleutherococcus senticosus* Maxim is marketed as Siberian ginseng in the United States and Blumenthal (1991) has noted that it is a legitimate form of ginseng, Tyler (1993) stated that it does not belong to the same genus as the true ginsengs and that knowledgeable persons prefer the designation eleuthero. Indeed, in *Herbal Medicine,* Blumenthal and others (2000) treat the ginseng root and the eleuthero root separately, but do refer to eleuthero as Siberian ginseng. Nevertheless, the two plants share some common physiological attributes and have been the most widely researched.

The Chinese ginseng root consists of the dried main and lateral root of *P. ginseng* C.A. Meyer *(P. ginseng)* and their preparations in effective dosage. The biologically active constituents in *P. ginseng* are a complex mixture of triterpene saponins known as ginsenosides. The root contains 2% to 3% ginsenosides, among which Rg_1, Rc, Rd, Rb_1, Rb_2, and Rb_0 are quantitatively the most important (Blumenthal et al., 2000)

Siberian, or Russian, ginseng consists of the dried roots and rhizome of *E. senticosus*, and contains phenolics, polysaccharides, and eleutherosides A-G, the total content ranging between 0.6% to 0.9%. Eleutherosides B, B_1, and E are representative of three classes of compounds collectively called eleutherosides (Blumenthal et al., 2000). In China, *E. senticosus* is known as wujiaseng or ciwujia (Tyler, 1993), and the proposed active ingredients are ciwujianosides, a series of triterpenoid glycosides derived from the leaves of *Acanthopanax (Eleutherococcus) senticosus* Harms (Cheuvront et al., 1999).

Ginseng has been used for its purported tonic effects for centuries. In ancient Chinese medicine, documented 2000 years ago, dried ginseng was used to revitalize and replenish vital energy, to build resistance; its effects were on the whole body, not specific organs or systems—an effect somewhat equivalent to that of the multivitamin tablet in Western conventional medicine (Blumenthal et al., 2000). In a related vein, Soviet researchers used the term adaptogen to describe the ability of *E. senticosus* to increase nonspecific resistance in an organism under stressful conditions (Brekhman and Dardymov, 1969). These effects have been attributed to the numerous ginsenosides or eleutherosides, but ginseng also possesses other substances that may have insulinomimetic and antioxidant properties (Blumenthal et al., 2000). Today, ginseng is included in the Pharmacopoeias of numerous countries, not only Asian countries such as China and

Japan, but also Western nations including Germany, the United Kingdom, and Russia.

Theory

Herbal ginseng supplements, using such labels as Ginseng Energy, are marketed to physically active individuals. Indeed, the German Commission E approved ginseng as a tonic for invigoration in times of fatigue and declining capacity for work and concentration (Blumenthal et al., 2000), while the World Health Organization (1999B) indicated that ginseng could be used as a prophylactic agent for enhancement of mental and physical capacities in cases of weakness, exhaustion, tiredness, and loss of concentration. These effects certainly would be important for athletes, but how ginseng elicits them is not known.

Although ginseng extracts from the Araliaceae family may contain numerous substances including sterols, glycans, flavonoids, amino acids, vitamins, and trace elements (Liu and Xiao, 1992; Ng and Yeung, 1986), all of which may elicit various physiological responses in humans, the ergogenic effect of ginseng is attributed to the ginsenosides or eleutherosides (Brekhman and Dardymov, 1969; Carr, 1986; Chong and Oberholzer, 1988).

Ginseng is theorized to influence the hypothalamic-pituitary-adrenal cortex axis, possibly mitigating the catabolic effects of the stress hormone cortisol, which is secreted by the adrenal gland. Given these theorized anti-stress effects, one theory of ginseng supplementation is that it enhances sport performance by allowing athletes to train more intensely, induces an antifatiguing effect, and increases stamina during competition (Williams, 1998).

Other theories have been proposed to explain the potential ergogenic effect on aerobic endurance capacity, including favorable metabolic, hematologic, and cardiovascular functions. Animal studies have shown that ginseng supplementation (4 days of 10 and 20 mg/kg day) resulted in higher liver and skeletal muscle glycogen levels after exhaustive exercise, the authors suggesting that ginsenosides, particularly Rg_1 and Rb_1, enhance exercise endurance by altering fuel homeostasis during prolonged exercise (Wang and Lee, 1998). In another animal study, using a 2×2 factorial design with exercise and ginseng as the independent variables, rats supplemented with the standardized *P. ginseng* extract G115 (50 mg/kg for 12 weeks) increased the capillary density, mitochondrial content, and oxidative capacity of the red gastrocnemius muscle to an extent similar to that seen with physical exercise training. However, when exercise training and ginseng supplementation were combined, the effects obtained with ginseng separately were not potentiated by exercise training. This finding suggests that ginseng may benefit exercise performance

in nonexercisers but not in exercisers (Ferrando et al., 1999). Other researchers have theorized that ginseng may enhance myocardial metabolism (Liu and Xiao, 1992), increase hemoglobin (Baranov, 1982), induce vasodilation (Carr, 1986), and increase oxygen extraction by muscles (Tesch et al., 1987).

Given these postulates, much of the research involving the ergogenicity of ginseng supplementation has focused on cardiovascular or aerobic endurance performance, with some emphasis on psychomotor performance. It should be noted, however, that although numerous theories have been advanced in attempts to explain the alleged ergogenic effects of ginseng supplementation, an underlying mechanism has yet to be determined.

Efficacy

Many of the marketing claims relative to increased energy or exercise performance are based on either testimonial evidence or poorly controlled ginseng research studies conducted several decades ago. Although numerous studies evaluated the ergogenicity of ginseng supplementation, many unfortunately possessed research design flaws, including no control or placebo group, no double-blind protocol, no randomization of order of treatment, no statistical analysis, or the use of nonstandardized commercial ginseng preparations containing other potential ergogenic substances. These experimental design irregularities have been detailed by Bahrke and Morgan (1994), who indicated that there is a lack of controlled research demonstrating the ability of ginseng to improve or prolong performance. Numerous studies have been conducted subsequent to that 1994 review, and the findings continue to support this viewpoint. Several of these studies with *P. ginseng, E. senticosus,* and *P. quinquefolium* are highlighted here.

Four recent randomized, double-blind, placebo-controlled studies have shown no significant effect of *P. ginseng* supplementation on physiologic, metabolic, or performance aspects of exercise. Allen and others (1998) found no significant effect of *P. ginseng* (200 mg day of a 7% ginsenoside solution for 3 weeks) on $\dot{V}O_2$peak, plasma lactate, heart rate, RPE, or time to exhaustion on a symptom-limited, graded cycle ergometer exercise test in young, moderately fit men and women. Engels and his associates (1996) reported no ergogenic effect of *P. ginseng* (200 mg/day; 4% ginsenosides; 8 weeks) on $\dot{V}O_2$, heart rate, minute ventilation, respiratory exchange ratio, blood lactate, or maximal work performance of adult females on a graded maximal bicycle ergometer test to exhaustion. In a similar study with healthy men, Engels and Wirth (1997) reported no beneficial effect of two doses of *P. ginseng* (G115; 200 or 400 mg/day for 8 weeks) on $\dot{V}O_2$, minute ventilation, heart rate, respiratory exchange ratio, blood lactic acid concentration, or RPE during either submaximal or maximal aerobic exercise. Ziemba and others (1999) found no ergogenic effect of *P. ginseng* (350 mg/day for 6 weeks) on $\dot{V}O_2$max or lactate threshold in 15 soccer players during an incremental cycle ergometer test. However, they reported that *P. ginseng* supplementation shortened multiple-choice reaction time both before and during the latter stages of the exercise protocol. Such an effect may be of benefit to athletes who must react quickly in sport. This finding merits additional research.

Three randomized, double-blind, placebo-controlled studies also have shown no significant effect of *E. senticosus* (provided either as *E. senticosus* Maxim or as ciwujia) on physiologic, metabolic, or performance aspects of exercise. Using 20 highly trained distance runners as subjects, Dowling and others (1996) revealed no significant effect of *E. senticosus* Maxim L (3.4 ml daily for 6 weeks) on submaximal or maximal $\dot{V}O_2$, minute ventilation, RPE, respiratory exchange ratio, or serum lactate during either submaximal or maximal exercise; nor was maximal treadmill time to exhaustion affected. Subjects were tested at baseline, every two weeks during the supplementation period, and two weeks after cessation of supplementation. Ciwujia is the main active ingredient in the commercial product Endurox. Endurox is marketed to endurance athletes, and literature published by its manufacturers suggests that it can increase fat oxidation (possibly sparing muscle glycogen), increase oxygen consumption, reduce lactate accumulation, and improve heart rate recovery after exercise. However, most of these claims are based on clinical studies with poor experimental designs. Plowman and others (1999) noted that none of the studies followed a randomized crossover or double-blind protocol, nor was the use of a placebo mentioned. None have been published in peer-reviewed journals. Moreover, published research does not support these marketing claims. Cheuvront and others (1999), using a double-blind, placebo-controlled, repeated-measures crossover design, reported that Endurox supplementation (800 mg for 7 days) had no significant effect on $\dot{V}O_2$, minute ventilation, RER, heart rate, blood pressure, RPE, blood lactate, or serum glycerol during cycle ergometry performance for 30 min at 25% peak $\dot{V}O_2$ followed by 10 min at 65% peak $\dot{V}O_2$. Plowman and others (1999), using the same research protocol, reported no significant effect of Endurox supplementation (800 mg for 10 days) on $\dot{V}O_2$, RER, heart rate, and RPE during a self-selected, submaximal 30-min workout on a StairMaster 4000PT.

Limited research evaluating the ergogenicity of North American ginseng is available, and what is available is not supportive. For example, using a randomized, placebo-controlled crossover design, Morris and others (1996) reported no significant ergogenic effect of standardized

P. quinquefolium (8 or 16 mg/kg/day for 7 days) on $\dot{V}O_2$, RPE, blood glucose and lactate levels, or cycle ergometer exercise time to exhaustion at 75% $\dot{V}O_2$max.

Relative to ergogenicity for exercise, ginseng is the most widely studied herbal dietary supplement. Overall, detailed reviews indicate that ginseng is not an effective ergogenic aid. Vogler and others (1999) conducted a systematic review of double-blind, randomized, placebo-controlled trials, evaluating the efficacy of ginseng root extract for various indications, including physical and psychomotor performance. They concluded that the efficacy of ginseng root extract is not established beyond reasonable doubt for any of these indications. In a recent update of their 1994 review, which includes an additional 35 reports, Bahrke and Morgan (2000) conclude again that although more well-controlled research is needed, there is an absence of compelling research evidence regarding the efficacy of ginseng use to improve physical performance in humans.

Safety and Quality

Commercial ginseng preparations may vary in quality. G115 is the registered trademark of a proprietary extract of *P. ginseng* standardized to 4% ginsenosides (Blumenthal et al., 2000). G115R is marketed as Ginsana, Gericomplex, and Geriatric Pharmaton. However, these preparations may contain some or all of the following substances in addition to G115: vitamins, minerals, trace elements, and dimethylaminoethanol bitartrate (Dowling et al., 1996). Commercial products may also suffer from poor quality control. Recent assays of commercial ginseng preparations revealed ginsenoside or ciwujianoside concentrations ranging from 0% to 9.0%, with over 10% of the products containing no detectible ginsenosides; one product contained large amounts of ephedrine (Cheuvront et al., 1999; Consumers Union, 1995; Cui et al., 1994; Schardt, 1999B).

Blumenthal and others (2000) note that although commercial ginseng preparations appear to have relatively low acute or chronic toxicity when taken in dosages recommended by the manufacturer, a ginseng-abuse syndrome has been reported, with such symptoms as high blood pressure, nervousness, and sleeplessness. These effects may be attributed to the postulated stimulant effect of ginseng, or possibly to additional substances in the commercial preparation such as the stimulants caffeine or ephedrine. Ginseng may also increase blood pressure by interacting with other stimulant drugs (Cupp, 1999). Individuals who desire to experiment with ginseng supplementation should consult with their physicians.

Permissibility

Currently, ginseng supplementation as a sport ergogenic is legal. However, athletes subject to drug testing should be aware that some commercial ginseng products may contain drugs, such as ephedrine, that are prohibited by the International Olympic Committee.

Hydroxycitric Acid

Hydroxycitric acid (HCA), derived from the tropical fruit *Garcinia cambogia,* is available as a herbal supplement and promoted as a weight loss agent (Kriketos et al., 1999). As a competitive inhibitor of citrate lyase, HCA has been hypothesized to modify citric acid cycle metabolism to promote fatty acid oxidation (Heymsfield et al., 1998; Kriketos et al., 1999).

Theory

Supplementation with HCA may be theorized to enhance performance in several ways. Loss of excess body fat could provide a mechanical advantage, while increased fatty acid oxidation could spare muscle glycogen and enhance aerobic endurance performance.

Efficacy

Data from human studies do not support a fat-burning role for HCA supplementation. Kriketos and others (1999), in a double-blind, placebo-controlled, randomized crossover study, reported no significant effect of HCA supplementation (3.0 g/day for 3 days) on serum energy substrates, RQ, or energy expenditure either during rest or during moderately intense exercise (30 min at 40% $\dot{V}O_2$max and 15 min at 60% $\dot{V}O_2$max) in sedentary males. They concluded that these data do not support the hypothesis that HCA supplementation alters the short-term rate of fat oxidation in the fasting state during rest or moderate exercise. Changes in body composition were not reported. Heymsfield and others (1998) reported no significant differences in weight loss between two groups of obese individuals receiving either a placebo or HCA supplementation (1.5 g/day for 3 months). Collectively, these data indicate that HCA is not an effective supplement for weight loss, but no exercise performance effects were studied.

Safety

There appear to be few human data indicating that HCA supplementation conveys significant health risks, although Schardt (1999A) noted that the pharmaceutical firm Hoffman-LaRoche tried to turn HCA into a drug in the 1980s but dropped the idea because of side effects, such as testicular atrophy, in animals.

Permissibility

Currently, HCA is found in herbal weight loss dietary supplements, and its use is not prohibited by the IOC.

Kava Kava

Kava kava, or kava, is the peeled and dried root of *Piper methysticum* G. Forster, a centuries-old South Pacific herb used as a ritual beverage for its relaxing or calming properties. Kava root contains greater than 3.5% kava lactones (kava pyrones) calculated as kavain. The recommended therapeutic dose of kava is about 60 to 120 mg/day of the kava pyrones, but the amount in supplements varies widely among brands in the United States (Blumenthal et al., 2000; Rotblatt, 1999A).

The neuropharmacologic effects of kava include analgesia and sedation. The mechanism is not clear, but the gamma-aminobutyric acid or norepinephrine neuroreceptors may be involved. Kava has the ability to relax skeletal muscles, yet does not act as a central nervous system depressant (Blumenthal et al., 2000).

Theory

Excess anxiety or hand tremor may disrupt performance in many sports, such as archery and pistol shooting. Alcohol and beta blockers, anxiolytic drugs, have been used by athletes to mitigate some of the adverse effects of anxiety, so their use has been prohibited for ergogenic purposes in such sports (Williams, 1991). Moreover, although synthetic anxiolytic drugs are effective for treating anxiety, they are burdened with adverse health effects (Pittler and Ernst, 2000) and their use also may be prohibited. Kava kava has been marketed for its antidepressant or anti-anxiety effects, a possible alternative to the prohibited or potentially risky ergogenic drugs.

Efficacy

In a recent systematic review and meta-analysis, Pittler and Ernst (2000) reported a superiority of kava extract over placebo in seven reviewed trials, and the meta-analysis of these trials suggests a significant difference in the reduction of anxiety in favor of kava extract. The authors concluded that kava extract is a herbal treatment option for anxiety that is worthy of consideration. Blumenthal and others (2000) also reported that numerous clinical studies support the relative efficacy of kava extracts for reduction of symptoms in patients with anxiety disorders, these substances comparing effectively with prescription antidepressants without associated tolerance problems.

Unfortunately, no research evaluating the potential ergogenic effect of kava kava supplementation on exercise or sport performance has been uncovered.

Safety

As with any sedative agent, excess kava intake or concomitant use with other sedatives, such as alcohol, may depress the central nervous system, impairing the ability to drive or operate other equipment. The American Herbal Products Association recommends that individuals who are pregnant, nursing, or taking a prescription drug should consult a health care practitioner before using kava. Continuous intake may lead to yellow discoloration of the skin, but this is reversible with discontinuation (Blumenthal et al., 2000; Rotblatt, 1999A).

Permissibility

Currently, kava use as an ergogenic aid is not specifically prohibited by the IOC.

St. John's Wort

St. John's wort (SJW) consists of the dried, aboveground parts of *Hypericum perforatum,* a perennial herb from the plant family Hypericaceae. In Europe, SJW blooms near the birthday of John the Baptist, hence its name. St. John's wort contains many phytochemicals, including flavonoids, phenolic acids, sterols, tannins, two naphthodianthrones (hypericin and pseudohypericin), and a phloroglucinol derivative (hyperforin) (Blumenthal et al., 2000).

Historically, SJW was used as a herbal tea by Hippocrates and other Greek physicians to treat neurologic conditions, and it eventually evolved as a herbal antidepressant. Today in Germany, SJW is more widely prescribed than Prozac for mild to moderate depression (NCCAM, 2000). As low levels of the neurotransmitter serotonin are associated with depression, SJW is thought to act similarly to conventional synaptic serotonin-reuptake inhibitors, helping to maintain optimal brain serotonin levels (Blumenthal et al., 2000; NCCAM, 2000). Hyperforin is thought to be the primary active ingredient in the antidepressant activity (Blumenthal et al., 2000), but hypericin and pseudohypericin may also be important. The USP requires not less than 3.0% of hyperforin. St. John's wort is available in various forms, including tinctures and dry standardized extract in capsules and tablets. It may also be brewed as tea and may be found in some functional foods, such as Robert's Gourmet St. John's Wort Tortilla Chips, but in lesser amounts.

Theory

Comparable to kava kava, SJW may be theorized to reduce anxiety and hand tremor in some athletes (Anderson, 1998), which could enhance performance in sports such as archery. Additionally, as serotonin is involved in appetite control, SJW is theorized to help induce weight loss, which could confer a mechanical advantage to some athletes.

Efficacy

Considerable evidence suggests that SJW may be an effective antidepressant. A review and meta-analysis of 23 European clinical studies concluded that SJW possesses antidepressant effects in cases of mild to moderate depression, although no long-term studies have been conducted (Linde et al., 1996). In their review, Blumenthal and others (2000) note that although additional research is warranted, the modern therapeutic application of SJW for mild to moderate depression is supported by its history of use in traditional medicine, in vivo experiments in animals, pharmacodynamic studies in humans, human clinical studies, and meta-analyses. Additionally, eight studies of good methodological quality suggest that SJW is more effective than placebo in the treatment of mild to moderate depression, but less effective than tricyclic antidepressants (Gaster and Holroyd, 2000). Currently, a large-scale clinical study is under way in the United States to evaluate the efficacy of SJW to treat depression (NCCAM, 2000).

Although the use of SJW may help treat mild depression and reduce anxiety in some athletes, an effect that could benefit performance in precision-target sports, unfortunately this ergogenic potential has not been investigated.

St. John's wort is also used as part of herbal fen phen, a natural dietary supplement weight loss pill also containing ephedrine marketed to replace the prescription obesity drug combination (fenfluramine and phentermine; fen phen) pulled from the market because of concerns that fenfluramine caused heart valve problems (Ernst, 1999). Although ephedrine, a potent stimulant, may be effective in increasing thermogenesis and body weight loss in obese individuals, no studies are available to indicate that ephedrine will promote leanness in athletes who are relatively lean (Clarkson and Thompson, 1997), nor are any data available to support such an effect for SJW.

Safety

St. John's wort or hypericum extracts may interfere with liver function and resultant drug metabolism (Ernst, 1999). Combining SJW with other antidepressants, such as Prozac, may lead to increased sedation or serotonin excess, with changes in mental stress, tremor, headache, and restlessness (Cupp, 1999; Ernst, 1999). St. John's wort also may interact adversely with numerous other drugs, including oral contraceptives, statins, and beta blockers (Consumers Union, 2000).

Permissibility

Currently, the use of SJW supplements is not prohibited by the IOC.

Tribulus Terrestris

According to Antonio and others (2000B), *Tribulus terrestris,* commonly known as puncture vine, is an herbal preparation that has been used medicinally as a diuretic and as treatment for hypertension, hypercholesterolemia, and colic pains; it has also been used for centuries in Europe as treatment for impotence. The purported active ingredients are saponins and protodioscin.

Theory

Tribulus terrestris supplementation may stimulate luteinizing hormone from the pituitary gland, enhancing plasma testosterone levels and promoting skeletal muscle hypertrophy (Antonio et al., 2000B).

Efficacy

Three research studies presented at the year 2000 meeting of the American College of Sports Medicine presented some preliminary data showing that use of a dietary supplement containing *T. terrestris,* as well as other herbal compounds, had no effect on serum testosterone (Street et al., 2000) and produced only a trend toward increases in lean body mass and muscular strength (Antonio et al., 2000A). Supplement capsules each contained 250 mg *T. terrestris,* 100 mg 7-isopropoxyiso-flavone, 100 mg Avena sativea, and 50 mg saw palmetto; and subjects consumed daily, for up to 10 weeks, one capsule for every 10 kg body mass. In the third study, 10 highly trained competitive cyclists consumed a supplement containing *T. terrestris* and ipriflavone or a placebo for 38 days, including 23 days of normal training and 11 days of intensified training. The investigators reported no significant differences between the treatments for total testosterone, the total testosterone:cortisol ratio, or average power and $\dot{V}O_2$ during a 12.5-km (7.8 miles) cycle performance trial. However, the free testosterone:cortisol ratio was higher following *T. terrestris* supplementation, a finding the authors attributed to lower cortisol and a tendency for free testosterone to be higher. Also, when they adjusted the performance times for differences in absolute $\dot{V}O_2$peak, a significant treatment effect favoring the *T. terrestris* group was observed for time to completion of the performance trial (McGregor et al., 2000).

In the only published study uncovered, *T. terrestris* supplementation had no significant ergogenic effects. Using a double-blind, placebo-controlled design, Antonio and others (2000B) evaluated the ergogenicity of a standardized *T. terrestris* supplement (standardized extract to 45% saponins and protodyosin). Fifteen resistance-trained males were randomly assigned to a placebo or a commercial (Metabolic Response Modifiers) *T. terrestris* product group; the dosage was 3.21 mg/kg body weight daily for eight weeks. Subjects engaged in periodized resistance training during the supplementation period. Body weight, body composition, maximal strength, muscular endurance, and mood states were determined before and after the supplementation period.

No significant differences attributable to *T. terrestris* were noted in any of the dependent variables. Plasma testosterone or luteinizing hormone levels were not measured.

Safety

Antonio and others (2000B) reported no adverse health effects of short-term supplementation with *T. terrestris,* but they did note that some forms of *T. terrestris* have been shown to induce neuromuscular dysfunction in sheep, although the underlying mechanisms are unknown.

Permissibility

Currently, *T. terrestris* supplementation is not proscribed by the IOC.

Yohimbine

Yohimbe bark, derived from the evergreen yohimbe tree common in West Africa, has been used as a sexual aphrodisiac for centuries. Yohimbine, an indole alkaloid obtained from the yohimbe and other related trees, is believed to be the active constituent, and yohimbine hydrochloride has been prescribed for functional impotence. The proposed mechanism of action of yohimbine is to block presynaptic α_2-adrenergic receptors, which may have various physiological effects in the body, including one important to treating impotence (Blumenthal et al., 2000). Yohimbine is also an FDA-approved prescription drug used for pupil dilation.

Theory

On the basis of the purported sexual functions, yohimbe bark and related products have been marketed in the United States as alternatives to anabolic steroids to enhance athletic performance. Yohimbine may be also ergogenic in other ways. Galitzky and others (1988) reported that oral yohimbine supplementation (0.2 mg/kg) elevated plasma glycerol and non-esterified fatty acids in fasting, healthy subjects; and the lipid-mobilizing action of yohimbine was reinforced during physical exercise. Plasma norepinephrine concentrations were increased (40-50%) after oral yohimbine administration. These investigators suggested that the lipid-mobilizing effect of yohimbine could be attributable to the increase in synaptic norepinephrine, a decrease in α2-adrenoceptor stimulation of human fat cell α2-adrenoceptors, or a blockade of presynaptic α2-adrenoceptors. Thus, it may be theorized that yohimbine functions comparably to caffeine, mobilizing fatty acids to spare muscle glycogen or promote weight loss.

Efficacy

No studies have been uncovered on possible anabolic effects of yohimbine supplementation. Additionally, no studies are available to indicate that yohimbine when used alone has ergogenic effects comparable to those of caffeine. Actually, when used in conjunction with caffeine and ephedrine, yohimbine may possibly be ergolytic. Waluga and others (1998) reported that the addition of yohimbine to a diet containing caffeine and ephedrine decreased ejection fraction and increased cardiac load during dynamic cycle ergometer exercise, which might be considered to be unfavorable responses during exercise. However, subjects were obese women, not physically active individuals, and no actual performance data were presented.

Loss of excess body fat may be ergogenic for some athletes. In a randomized, placebo-controlled study with female obese outpatients, Kucio and others (1991) supplemented a three-week low-energy diet (1000 calories/day) with 5 mg yohimbine orally four times a day. The yohimbine significantly increased the mean weight loss in patients compared to placebo (3.55 vs. 2.21 kg). The investigators noted that although yohimbine had no effect on lipolysis, a steady level of effort-induced energy expenditure and sympathetic system activity was maintained. Again, however, subjects were not physically active individuals, and no performance data were obtained.

Safety

Blumenthal and others (2000) indicate that yohimbe bark or yohimbine should be used with caution; side effects include nervous excitation, tremor, sleeplessness, anxiety, tachycardia, and increased blood pressure. They note that yohimbine can significantly increase blood pressure at oral doses of only 15 to 20 mg and may interact with prescribed drugs, such as tricyclic antidepressants, to cause a hypertensive crisis. The German Commission E does not recommend it as therapeutic.

Permissibility

Currently, yohimbine supplementation is not prohibited by the IOC. However, an analysis of commercial yohimbe products sold in the United States revealed that few products contained any appreciable levels of yohimbine, raising concerns of quality control (Blumenthal et al., 2000). Yohimbine supplements marketed as anabolics could contain proscribed substances.

Conclusion

As noted in the preface to this book, much of what we know about the efficacy and adverse effects of PES is anecdotal, and research is often laden with methodological problems, for example poor research design and use of various substances whose purity and content are often suspect. This is particularly relevant to many purported herbal ergogenics.

In *Nutrients as Ergogenic Aids for Sports and Exercise,* Bucci (1993) noted that the use of herbs to affect physical performance remained largely unstudied. Although the situation has improved somewhat in the past decade, there still remains a dearth of well-controlled research evaluating the efficacy of purported herbal ergogenics in relation to human exercise or sport performance. Future research efforts require careful attention to experimental design, particularly use of randomized, double-blind, placebo-controlled, crossover designs. Investigators must analyze the purported herbal ergogenic in order to confirm its contents. Standardized dosages in accordance with established recommendations should be used. Commercial products, many containing a blend of multiple herbals, need to be studied to evaluate marketing claims. Urinalysis or other tests should be employed to document subject compliance. The sample size should be sufficient to provide adequate statistical power. Only through the use of rigorous experimental control can the ergogenicity of purported herbal ergogenic aids be adequately evaluated.

Many contemporary herbal medicines have survived for centuries, and as this review indicates, several may have therapeutic medicinal (although not ergogenic) value applicable to physically active individuals. Moreover, even if they were not to be shown by scientific research to confer health or sport performance benefits, many individuals would continue to use herbal supplements (Blendon et al., 2001). However, individuals who desire to use herbal supplements should consult appropriate health care professionals before doing so because not all herbal supplements are safe, particularly when used in excessive amounts or when combined with other herbs or drugs. Moreover, many commercial herbal products may not contain significant amounts, or any, of the active ingredient and may contain contaminants (Carlson and Thompson, 1998; Consumers Union, 1998).

In the 1996 *The Drug Free Handbook,* the USOC indicates that there is no scientific evidence to support the ergogenic claims of herbal products and that the contents and safety of these products cannot be guaranteed—statements supported by this review. Although several herbal supplements theoretically may be effective, their ergogenicity has not been investigated. When buying herbal supplements as ergogenic aids, the athlete should be aware of the old Latin saying, *caveat emptor*—let the buyer beware.

Additional Readings

Blumenthal, M., Goldberg, A., and Brinckmann, J. *Herbal medicine.* Newton, MA: Integrative Medicine Communications, 2000.

Pierce, A. *The American Pharmaceutical Association practical guide to natural medicine.* New York: Morrow, 1999.

Tyler, V.E. *The honest herbal: A sensible guide to the use of herbs and related remedies.* New York: Pharmaceutical Products Press, 1993.

References

Allen, J.D., McLung, J., Nelson, A.G., and Welsch, M. Ginseng supplementation does not enhance healthy young adults' peak aerobic exercise performance. Journal of the American College of Nutrition 17:462-466, 1998.

American Dietetic Association. Position of the American Dietetic Association: Functional foods. Journal of the American Dietetic Association 99:1278-1285, 1999.

Anderson, O. St. John's wort: A nice mood-lifter for rueful runners? Running Research News 14(3):1, 7-10, 1998.

Angell, M., and Kassirer, J.P. Alterative medicine: The risks of untested and unregulated remedies. New England Journal of Medicine 339:839-841, 1998.

Antonio, J., Uelmen, J., Ehler, L., Raether, J., and Sanders, M. Influence of a Tribulus-containing supplement on body composition and strength in football players and bodybuilders. Medicine and Science in Sports and Exercise 32:S61, 2000A. (Abstract)

Antonio, J., Uelmen, J., Rodriguez, R., and Earnest, C. The effects of Tribulus terrestris on body composition and exercise performance in resistance-trained males. International Journal of Sport Nutrition and Exercise Metabolism 10:208-215, 2000B.

Bahrke, M.S., and Morgan, W.P. Evaluation of the ergogenic properties of ginseng. Sports Medicine 18:229-248, 1994.

Bahrke, M.S., and Morgan, W.P. Evaluation of the ergogenic properties of ginseng: An update. Sports Medicine 29:113-133, 2000.

Balentine, D.A., Albano, M.C., and Nair, M.G. Role of medicinal plants, herbs, and spices in protecting human health. Nutrition Reviews 57:S41-S45, 1999.

Baranov, A.I. Medicinal uses of ginseng and related plants in the Soviet Union: Recent trends in Soviet literature. Journal of Ethnopharmacology 6:339-353, 1982.

Bernardo, R.R., Pinto, A.V., and Parente, J.P. Steroidal saponins from Smilax officinalis. Phytochemistry 43:465-469, 1996.

Blendon, R.J., DesRoches, C.M., Benson, J.M., Brodie, M., and Altman, D.E. Americans' views on the use and regulation of dietary supplements. Archives of Internal Medicine 161:805-810, 2001.

Blume, J., Kieser, M., and Holscher, U. Placebo-controlled double-blind study of the effectiveness of Ginkgo biloba special extract EGb 761 in trained patients with intermittent claudication. Vasa 25:265-274, 1996.

Blumenthal, M. The different uses of different ginsengs. Whole Foods, February, 50-52, 1991.

Blumenthal, M., Goldberg, A., and Brinckmann, J. Herbal Medicine. Newton, MA: Integrative Medicine Communications, 2000.

Brekhman, I.I., and Dardymov, I.V. New substances of plant origin which increase nonspecific resistance. Annual Review of Pharmacology 9:419-428, 1969.

Bucci, L.R. Nutrients as Ergogenic Aids for Sports and Exercise. Boca Raton, FL: CRC Press, 1993.

Bundesanzeiger (BAnz). Monographien der Kommission E (Zulassungs- und Aufbereitungskommission am BGA fur den humanmed. Bereich, phytotherapeutische Therapie-richtung und Stoffgruppe). Cologne: Bundesgesundheitsamt (BGA), 1998.

Carlson, M., and Thompson, R.D. Liquid chromatographic determination of methylxanthines and catechins in herbal preparations containing guarana. Journal of AOAC International 81:691-701, 1998.

Carr, C.J. Natural plant products that enhance performance and endurance. In: Enhancers of Performance and Endurance, ed. C.J. Carr and E. Jokl. Hillsdale, NJ: Erlbaum, 1986, pp. 139-192.

Chandler, J.V., and Hawkins, J.D. The effect of bee pollen on physiological performance. International Journal of Biosocial Research 6:107-114, 1984.

Chang, J. Medicinal herbs: Drugs or dietary supplements? Biochemical Pharmacology 59:211-219, 2000.

Chang, J. Scientific evaluation of traditional Chinese medicine under DSHEA: A conundrum. Journal of Alternative and Complementary Medicine 5:181-189, 1999.

Cheuvront, S.N., Moffatt, R.J., Biggerstaff, K.D., Bearden, S., and McDonough, P. Effect of ENDUROX™ on metabolic responses to submaximal exercise. International Journal of Sport Nutrition 9:434-442, 1999.

Chong, S.K., and Oberholzer, V.G. Ginseng: Is there a clinical use in medicine? Postgraduate Medicine Journal 64:841-846, 1988.

Clarkson, P., and Thompson, H. Drugs and sport. Sports Medicine 24:366-384, 1997.

Consumers Union. Herbal roulette. Consumer Reports 7(11):698-705, 1995.

Consumers Union. Uprooting herbal myths. Consumer Reports on Health 10(10):6-7, 1998.

Consumers Union. St John's wort: Not so benign. Consumer Reports on Health 12(6):6, 2000.

Cott, J. NCDEU update: Natural product formulations available in Europe for psychotropic indications. Psychopharmacology Bulletin 31:745-751, 1995.

Craig, W.J. Health promoting properties of common herbs. American Journal of Clinical Nutrition 70:491S-499S, 1999.

Cui, J., Garle, M., Eneroth, P., and Bjorkhem, I. What do commercial ginseng preparations contain? Lancet 344:134, 1994.

Cupp, M.J. Herbal remedies: Adverse effects and drug interactions. American Family Physician 59:1239-1245, 1999.

Curtis-Prior, P., Vere, D., and Fray, P. Therapeutic value of Ginkgo biloba in reducing symptoms of decline in mental function. Journal of Pharmacy and Pharmacology 51:535-541, 1999.

Dowling, E.A., Redondo, D.R., Branch, J.D., Jones, S., McNabb, G., and Williams, M.H. Effect of Eleutherococcus senticosus on submaximal and maximal exercise performance. Medicine and Science in Sports and Exercise 28:482-489, 1996.

Dunnett, W., and Crossen, D. The bee pollen promise. Runner's World 15:53-54, 1980.

Engels, H-J., Said, J.M., and Wirth, J.C. Failure of chronic ginseng supplementation to affect work performance and energy metabolism in healthy adult females. Nutrition Research 16:1295-1305, 1996.

Engels, H-J., and Wirth, J.C. No ergogenic effects of ginseng (Panax ginseng C. A. Meyer) during graded maximal aerobic exercise. Journal of the American Dietetic Association 97:1110-1115, 1997.

Ernst, E. Second thoughts about safety of St. John's wort. Lancet 254(9195):2014-2016, 1999.

Ferrando, A., Vila, L., Voces, J.A., Cabral, A.C., Alvarez, A.I., and Prieto, J.G. Effects of a standardized Panax ginseng extract on the skeletal muscle of the rat: A comparative study in animals at rest and under exercise. Planta Medica 65:239-244, 1999.

Fry, A.C., Bonner, E., Lewis, D.L., Johnson, R.L., Stone, M.H., and Kraemer, W.J. The effects of gamma-oryzanol supplementation during resistance exercise training. International Journal of Sport Nutrition 7:318-329, 1997.

Fugh-Berman, A. Herb-drug interactions. Lancet 355(9198):134-138, 2000.

Galitzky, J., Taouis, M., Berlan, M., Riviere, D., Garrigues, M., and Lafontan, M. Alpha 2-antagonist compounds and lipid mobilization: Evidence for a lipid mobilizing effect of oral yohimbine in healthy male volunteers. European Journal of Clinical Investigation 18:587-594, 1988.

Gaster, B., and Holroyd, J. St. John's wort for depression: A systematic review. Archives of Internal Medicine 160:152-156, 2000.

Geyman, J.P. Anaphylactic reaction after ingestion of bee pollen. Journal of the American Board of Family Practitioners 7:250-252, 1994.

Glickman-Weiss, E.L., Hearon, C.M., Nelson, A.G., and Day, R. Does capsaicin affect physiologic and thermal responses of males during immersion in 22 degrees C? Aviation Space and Environmental Medicine 69:1095-1099, 1998.

Grunewald, K.K., and Bailey, R.S. Commercially marketed supplements for bodybuilding athletes. Sports Medicine 15:90-103, 1993.

Heymsfield, S.B., Allison, D.B., Vasselli, J.R., Pietrobelli, A., Greenfield, D., and Nunez, C. Garcinia cambogia (hydrocitric acid) as a potential antiobesity agent: A randomized controlled trial. JAMA 280:1596-1600, 1998.

International Olympic Committee. The Olympic Movement Anti-Doping Code. Lausanne: International Olympic Committee, 2000.

Kriketos, A.D., Thompson, H.R., Green, H., and Hill, J.O. (-)-Hydroxycitric acid does not affect energy expenditure and substrate oxidation in adult males in a post-absorptive state. International Journal of Obesity and Related Metabolic Disorders 23:867-873, 1999.

Kucio, C., Jonderko, K., and Piskorska, D. Does yohimbine act as a slimming drug? Israel Journal of Medical Sciences 27:550-556, 1991.

Lim, K., Yoshioka, M., Kikuzato, S., Kiyonaga, A., Tanaka, H., Shindo, M., and Suzuki, M. Dietary red pepper ingestion increases carbohydrate oxidation at rest and during exercise in runners. Medicine and Science in Sports and Exercise 29:355-361, 1997.

Linde, K., Ramirez, G., Mulrow, C.D., Weidenhammer, W., and Melchart, D. St. John's wort for depression: An overview and meta-analysis of randomized clinical trials. British Medical Journal 313:253-258, 1996.

Liu, C.X., and Xiao, P.G. Recent advances on ginseng research in China. Journal of Ethnopharmacology 36:27-38, 1992.

Matsuo, T., Yoshioka, M., and Suzuki, M. Capsaicin in diet does not affect glycogen contents in the liver and skeletal muscle of rats before and after exercise. Journal of Nutritional Science and Vitaminology (Tokyo) 42:249-256, 1996.

Maughan, R., and Evans, S. Effects of pollen extract upon adolescent swimmers. British Journal of Sports Medicine 16:142-145, 1982.

McGregor, S.J., Snyder, A.R., and Pizza, F.X. Herbal supplementation in highly trained cyclists during a period of intensified competition. Medicine and Science in Sports and Exercise 32:S117, 2000. (Abstract)

Miller, L.G. Herbal medicinal: Selected clinical considerations focusing on known or potential drug-herb interactions. Archives of Internal Medicine 158:2200-2211, 1998.

Morris, A.C., Jacobs, I., McLellan, T.M., Klugerman, A., Wang, L.C., and Zamecnik, J. No ergogenic effect of ginseng ingestion. International Journal of Sport Nutrition 6:263-271, 1996.

NCAAM. St. John's Wort. National Center for Complementary and Alternative Medicine fact sheet. NCAAM Clearinghouse, May 24, 2000.

Ng, T.B., and Yeung, H.W. Scientific basis of the therapeutic effects of ginseng. In: Folk Medicine: The Art and the Science. Washington, DC: American Chemical Society, 1986, pp. 138-151.

Nortier, J.L., Martinez, M.M., Schmeiser, H.H., Arlt, V.M., Bieler, C.A., Petein, M., Depierreux, M.F., De Pauw, L., Abramowicz, D., Vereerstraeten, P., and Vanherweghem, J. Urothelial carcinoma associated with the use of a Chinese herb. New England Journal of Medicine 342:1686-1692, 2000.

Peters, H., Kieser, M., and Holscher, U. Demonstration of the efficacy of ginkgo biloba special extract EGb 761 on intermittent claudication: A placebo-controlled, double-blind multicenter trial. Vasa 27:106-110, 1998.

Pittler, M.H., and Ernst, E. Efficacy of kava extract for treating anxiety: Systematic review and meta-analysis. Journal of Clinical Psychopharmacology 20:84-89, 2000.

Plowman, S.A., Dustman, K., Walicek, H., Corless, C., and Ehlers, G. The effects of ENDUROX™ on the physiological responses to stair-stepping exercise. Research Quarterly for Exercise and Sport 70:385-388, 1999.

Ros, J.J., Pelders, M.G., and De Smet, P.A. A case of positive doping associated with a botanical food supplement. Pharmacy World and Science 21:44-46, 1999.

Rotblatt, M.D. Cranberry, feverfew, horse chestnut, and kava. Western Journal of Medicine 171:195-198, 1999A.

Rotblatt, M.D. Herbal medicine: A practical guide to safety and quality assurance. Western Journal of Medicine 171:172-175, 1999B.

Scavariello, E.M., and Arellano, D.B. Gamma-oryzanol: An important component in rice bran oil. Archivos Latinoamericanos de Nutricion 48:7-12, 1998.

Schardt, D. Fat burners. Nutrition Action Health Letter 26(6):9-11, 1999A.

Schardt, D. Ginseng. Nutrition Action Health Letter 26(4):10-11, 1999B.

Schneider, B. Ginkgo biloba extract in peripheral arterial diseases: Meta-analysis of controlled clinical studies. Arzneimittelforschung 42:428-436, 1992.

Steben, R.E., and Bourdreaux, P. The effects of pollen and pollen extracts on selected blood factors and performance of athletes. Journal of Sports Medicine and Physical Fitness 18:221-226, 1978.

Steben, R.E., Wells, J.C., and Harless, I.L. The effect of bee pollen tablets on the improvement of certain blood factors and performance of male collegiate swimmers. Athletic Training 11:124-126, 1976.

Street, C., Antonio, J., and Scally, M.C. The effects of Tribulus terrestris on endocrine status in recreational bodybuilders: A preliminary report. Medicine and Science in Sports and Exercise 32:S61, 2000. (Abstract)

Tesch, P.A., Johansson, H., and Kaiser, P. Effekten av ginseng, vitaminer och mineraler pafysisk arbetsformaga hos medelalders man. Lartidningen 84:4326-4328, 1987.

Tyler, V.E. The Honest Herbal: A Sensible Guide to the Use of Herbs and Related Remedies. New York: Pharmaceutical Products Press, 1993.

United States Olympic Committee. The Drug Free Handbook. Colorado Springs, CO: United States Olympic Committee, 1996.

Vogler, B.K., Pittler, M.H., and Ernst, E. The efficacy of ginseng: A systematic review of randomized clinical trials. European Journal of Clinical Pharmacology 55:567-575, 1999.

Wagner, H. Phytomedicine research in Germany. Environmental Health Perspectives 107:779-781, 1999.

Waluga, M., Janusz, M., Karpel, E., Hartleb, M., and Nowak, A. Cardiovascular effects of ephedrine, caffeine and yohimbine measured by thoracic electrical bioimpedance in obese women. Clinical Physiology 18:69-76, 1998.

Wang, L.C., and Lee, T.F. Effect of ginseng saponins on exercise performance in non-trained rats. Planta Medica 64:130-133, 1998.

Wheeler, K.B., and Garleb, K.A. Gamma oryzanol-plant sterol supplementation: Metabolic, endocrine, and physiologic effects. International Journal of Sport Nutrition 1:170-177, 1991.

Williams, M.H. Drugs and Athletic Performance. Springfield, IL: Charles C Thomas, 1974.

Williams, M.H. Alcohol, marijuana, and beta blockers. In: Ergogenics: Enhancement of Performance in Exercise and Sport, ed. D.R. Lamb and M.H. Williams. Dubuque, IA: AC/Brown & Benchmark, 1991, pp. 331-372.

Williams, M.H. The Ergogenics Edge: Pushing the Limits of Sports Performance. Champaign, IL: Human Kinetics, 1998.

Winslow, L.C., and Kroll, D.J. Herbs as medicines. Archives of Internal Medicine 158:2192-2199, 1998.

Woodhouse, M.L., Williams, M.H., and Jackson, C.W. The effects of varying doses of orally ingested bee pollen extract upon selected performance variables. Athletic Training 22:26-28, 1987.

World Health Organization. WHO Monographs on Selected Medicinal Plants. Geneva: World Health Organization, 1999A.

World Health Organization. Ginseng radix. WHO Monographs on Selected Medicinal Plants. Geneva: World Health Organization, 1999B, pp. 168-182.

Zeisel, S.H. Regulation of "Nutraceuticals." Science 285: 1853-1855, 1999.

Ziemba, A.W., Chmura, J., Kaciuba-Uscilko, H., Nazar, K., Wisnik, P., and Gawronski, W. Ginseng treatment improves psychomotor performance at rest and during graded exercise in young athletes. International Journal of Sport Nutrition 9:371-377, 1999.

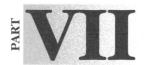
Social and Recreational Drugs

CHAPTER

19

Alcohol Use in Sport and Exercise

Robert D. Stainback, PhD

Rachelle Jansevics Cohen, PhD

Alcohol has been a part of human culture since at least 8000 B.C. (Goodwin and Gabrielli, 1997). Throughout history, it has been a tool for celebration, pleasure, performance enhancement, and medical purposes. Drinking ethanol (the form of alcohol intended for oral consumption) is legal in the United States for those ages 21 and older. Alcohol has a history of use in medical practice as an antiseptic, anesthetic, and sedative, as well as in the detoxification of an individual from alcohol (Lucia, 1963). It is now commonly used for sedation in liquid medications such as cough syrups.

History of Alcohol Use in Sport and Exercise

There has been a strong association between alcohol use and sport in the United States and in other Westernized cultures. Historical accounts suggest that the distant roots of this relationship perhaps lie in the competition of war. For example, in 1777, Frederick the Great, King of Prussia, commenting on the importance of beer to his soldiers, said:

> My people must drink beer. His majesty was brought up on beer and so were his officers and soldiers. Many battles have been fought and won by soldiers nourished on beer, and the King does not believe that coffee-drinking soldiers can be depended on to endure hardships or to beat the enemies. (Johnson, 1988, p. 71)

More contemporarily, beer has claimed a high-profile status in sport. Beer drinking is commonplace in activities

ranging from postgame parties among club rugby teams to afternoons at the baseball park. As Johnson aptly suggested in "Sports and Suds," his 1988 *Sports Illustrated* article, "beer and sport have come to be as inseparable in the American lexicon as mom and apple pie, God and country, ham and eggs, Jack and Jill, and, of course, suds and Spuds" (p. 70).

Literature and film also have supported the alcohol-sport relationship. Ardolino (1991) suggested that bars have been incorporated in stories about sport figures to provide settings for character development. For example, the sports bar Cheers, also the name of the successful television sitcom, is owned by Sam Malone, an alcoholic ex-Boston Red Sox pitcher. As they enjoy sporting events on TV, the Cheers regulars exemplify the communal and festive atmosphere of the bar, which becomes a place where friendships are forged within the context of the common interest of sport.

The alcohol-sport relationship is bolstered further by the fact that the demographics of beer drinkers and sport fans strongly overlap. Johnson (1988) perceptively comments, "beer drinkers and sports fans are one and the same—indivisible, inseparable, identical! No one drinks more beer than a sports fan, and no one likes sports more than a beer drinker" (p. 74). This observation may exaggerate in the interest of making a point, but the beer-drinking habits of sport fans are not unnoticed by corporate America, in particular beer brewers. In 1953, August A. Busch Jr., president of the Anheuser-Busch brewery, recognized the potential profitability of the alcohol-sport relationship when he purchased the baseball St. Louis Cardinals. His investment paid off in a handsome way; from 1953 to 1978, Anheuser-Busch annual sales grew from less than 6 million to more than 35 million barrels. In a 1978 interview with the *Sporting News,* Mr. Busch attributed this sales growth in part to the company's association with baseball (Johnson, 1988).

Fully realizing the potential of sport affiliation, Anheuser-Busch and Miller breweries escalated their investments in sport-related advertising during the 1970s. This increase in investment has forged a symbiotic relationship between breweries and sport such that the beer industry profits from the efficient expenditure of advertising dollars and the sport world depends on advertising revenue from the beer companies. For a more detailed review of this relationship as well as its effects on the general population, in particular on youth, see Stainback (1997, pp. 26-31).

Before further discussion of alcohol and sport, some background on alcoholic beverages and clarification of some important terms will be useful. In order of escalating alcohol concentrations, alcoholic beverages are produced in the forms of beers (approximately 4% by volume alcohol), wines (12-20%), liqueurs (22-50%), and distilled spirits (40-50% or 80 to 100 proof) (Blum, 1984). A "standard" drink typically contains 0.5 oz (16 g) of pure alcohol, which corresponds approximately with 12 oz (373 g) of beer, 2.5 oz (78 g) to 4.2 oz (131 g) of wine, or 1 oz (31 g) to 1.3 oz (40 g) of distilled spirits. Blood alcohol concentration (BAC) is the measurement to determine the concentration of alcohol in the bloodstream. Blood alcohol concentration levels are expressed as the number of grams (g) of alcohol per 100 milliliters (ml) of blood and are usually indicated as a percentage. Since 100 g in 100 ml would equal 100%, 100 milligrams (mg) of alcohol in 100 ml of blood is reported as 0.10% (Ray and Ksir, 1993). A BAC at the .l0 level is considered legal intoxication in most states. For the sake of simplicity this chapter refers to levels of BAC in numeric form only (e.g., .10 represents 100 mg/100 ml).

Since there are individual differences in the response to volume of alcohol consumed, BAC is the best standard by which to relate the effects of alcohol across individuals. An unfortunate weakness in the alcohol literature is that BAC is not reported in many studies, making it difficult to interpret outcomes in a single study and to compare results from multiple studies. Rather than discuss this shortcoming of the literature repeatedly, it is mentioned here so that the reader can be aware of it. Reviews of studies in the following sections refer to BAC when it is appropriate and available. Otherwise, the reviews present what the author reports with respect to alcohol consumption.

Terminology used to describe problems related to alcohol use varies with the literature. For purposes of this chapter, the terms "alcohol abuse" and "alcohol dependence" (also referred to as alcoholism) are used diagnostically as described in the fourth edition (DSM-IV) of the American Psychiatric Association's *Diagnostic and Statistical Manual of Mental Disorders* (1994). Individuals having these diagnoses are referred to as "alcohol abusers" and "alcoholics," respectively. These disorders are described later in the section "Adverse Reactions to Alcohol." It is important to understand at this juncture, however, that the criteria for these diagnoses do not include volume of alcohol consumed, but rather focus on how the alcohol affects the physical and psychosocial functioning of the individual. Therefore, individuals could be diagnosed with alcohol abuse or alcohol dependence who drink differing amounts of alcohol. "Problem drinking" and "problem drinker," terms from the behavioral psychology literature, refer to drinking patterns that create problems for the drinker but do not necessarily meet DSM-IV diagnostic criteria for alcohol abuse or dependence. "Social drinking," unlike the other terms, refers to drinking patterns that are not associated with recurrent medical, psychological, or social problems.

The following sections of this chapter briefly review clinical pharmacology and health effects of alcohol, alcohol use in the general U.S. population and among sport participants, ergolytic and ergogenic effects of alcohol on sport performance, and legislation and policy issues related to alcohol use in sport.

Clinical Pharmacology of Alcohol

This section reviews absorption and metabolism of alcohol, acute effects of alcohol, and adverse reactions to alcohol.

Absorption and Metabolism of Alcohol

When alcohol is ingested, it quickly begins to be absorbed unaltered and directly into the body, starting with small amounts in the mouth. More alcohol is absorbed in the stomach; however, the most absorption of alcohol occurs in the small intestine (Beers and Berkow, 1999). Several factors influence the rate of absorption, including the type of alcoholic beverage and the speed of its consumption, the concentration of alcohol and the presence of other chemicals in the beverage, stomach contents and variables influencing stomach emptying time (e.g., beverage carbonation, condition of the stomach tissues, emotional states such as fear and anger), gastric motility, and body weight (Blum, 1984; Mannaioni, 1984). Alcohol quickly crosses the blood-brain barrier and therefore acts as an almost instantaneous central nervous system (CNS) depressant. Since alcohol readily diffuses across capillary walls and cell membranes, it is distributed rapidly and unmodified throughout the blood, tissues, and organs (Blum, 1984). However, alcohol does not distribute significantly into fatty tissue; therefore, all other important variables being equal, a person who weighs 180 lb (81.6 kg) and is lean will experience a lower blood alcohol level than a person who weighs 180 lb with more body fat after drinking the same amount of alcohol (Ray and Ksir, 1993). Because the average male has a lower proportion of body fat and a higher proportion of body water than the average female (and therefore for a given weight more volume to distribute alcohol), males typically reach lower blood alcohol levels after consuming the same amount of alcohol as females. A recent review by Graham et al. (1998) also has shown that adjusting alcohol dosage for total body water eliminates gender differences in peak blood alcohol levels.

Although a small amount of alcohol (2-10%) is excreted in the urine, sweat, and breath, the liver metabolizes the majority of alcohol (90-98%; Diamond and Jay, 2000). Unlike most other drugs, alcohol is metabolized at a constant rate regardless of its concentration in the blood. The rate for a typical adult is about 0.25 to 0.3 oz (7 to 10 g) of 100% alcohol per hour (Ray and Ksir, 1993). Although the metabolic rate is constant in a given person, there are individual variations in response to alcohol based on differences in the activities of liver enzyme systems responsible for metabolism. Factors that influence these liver enzyme systems include age (Dufour and Fuller, 1995), menstrual cycle (Reichman et al., 1993), heredity (Diamond and Jay, 2000; Schuckit, 1994), race (Chen et al., 1999), liver disease, and experience with alcohol and other drug consumption (Mannaioni, 1984; Ray and Ksir, 1993).

Individual alcohol metabolic rates largely determine the time required to function without behavioral decrements after drinking. Behavioral impairments are associated with specific blood alcohol concentrations (BAC, also known as blood alcohol levels or BAL). Assuming consumption of standard drink quantities of 0.5 oz (16 g) of pure alcohol and no tolerance to alcohol, table 19.1 (from Ray and Ksir, 1993) shows approximate BAC levels expected as a result of gender, body weight, and number and type of alcoholic beverage consumed. Table 19.2 (from Corry and Cimbolic, 1985) shows various behavioral effects of increasing BAC levels. As suggested in table 19.2, the behavioral effects of alcohol range from pleasant and euphoric feelings at low BAC levels to death by respiratory failure at BAC levels approximating .45.

Table 19.1 Relationships Among Gender, Weight, Alcohol Consumption, and Blood Alcohol Level

Absolute alcohol (oz)	Beverage intake per hour	Blood alcohol levels (g/100 ml)					
		Female (100 lb)	Male (100 lb)	Female (150 lb)	Male (150 lb)	Female (200 lb)	Male (200 lb)
1/2	1 oz spirits[‡] 1 glass wine 1 can beer	0.045	0.037	0.03	0.025	0.022	0.019
1	2 oz spirits 2 glasses wine 2 cans beer	0.090	0.075	0.06	0.050	0.045	0.037
2	4 oz spirits 4 glasses wine 4 cans beer	0.180	0.150	0.12	0.100	0.090	0.070
3	6 oz spirits 6 glasses wine 6 cans beer	0.270	0.220	0.18	0.150	0.130	0.110
4	8 oz spirits 8 glasses wine 8 cans beer	0.360	0.300	0.24	0.200	0.180	0.150
5	10 oz spirits 10 glasses wine 10 cans beer	0.450	0.370	0.30	0.250	0.220	0.180

[‡]100-proof spirits.

From O. Ray and C. Ksir, 1993, *Drugs, society and human behavior* (New York NY: McGraw-Hill Companies), 194. Reproduced with permission of the McGraw-Hill Companies.

Table 19.2   Blood Alcohol Level and Behavioral Effects

Present blood alcohol level	Average effects
.02	Reached after approximately one drink; light or moderate drinkers experience some pleasant feelings (e.g., sense of warmth and well-being).
.04	Most people feel relaxed, energetic, and happy. Time seems to pass quickly. Skin may flush, and motor skills may be slightly impaired.
.05	More observable effects begin to occur. Individual may experience lightheadedness, giddiness, lowered inhibitions, and impaired judgment. Coordination may be slightly altered.
.06	Further impairment of judgment; individual's ability to make rational decisions concerning personal capabilities is affected (e.g., driving a car). May become "a lover or a fighter."
.08	Muscle coordination definitely impaired and reaction time increased; driving ability suspect. Heavy pulse and slow breathing. Sensory feelings of numbness in the cheeks, lips, and extremities may occur.
.10	Clear deterioration of coordination and reaction time. Individual may stagger, and speech may become fuzzy. Judgment and memory further affected (legally drunk, in most states).
.15	All individuals experience a definite impairment of balance and movement. Large increases in reaction time.
.20	Marked depression in motor and sensory capability; slurred speech, double vision, difficulty standing and walking may all be present. Decidedly intoxicated.
.30	Individual is confused or stuporous; unable to comprehend what is seen or heard. May lose consciousness (passes out) at this level.
.40	Usually unconscious. Alcohol has become deep anesthetic. Skin may be sweaty and clammy.
.45	Circulatory and respiration functions are depressed and can stop altogether.
.50	Near death.

From *Drugs, Facts, Alternatives, and Decisions, 1st edition*, by J.M. Corry and P. Cimbolic © 1985. Reprinted with permission of Wadsworth, an imprint of the Wadsworth Group, a division of Thomson Learning. Fax 800 730-2215.

Acute Effects of Alcohol

There are several acute effects of alcohol ingestion that may have a direct bearing on athletic performance. One such effect is the dilation of blood vessels close to the surface of the skin, which acts to increase heat loss in cold weather. A related effect is the tendency for alcohol to suppress the body's temperature regulation system, especially when larger amounts of alcohol are ingested. Therefore, contrary to the popularly held belief that alcohol increases body temperature and warmth in cold weather, it in fact may result in loss of body heat and, in severe cases, hypothermia (Diamond and Jay, 2000).

Alcohol also is a diuretic, leading to increased urine production. This effect may result in dehydration and a possible disruption in electrolyte balance (Wiese, Shlipak, and Browner, 2000). Alcohol also stimulates appetite and the production of gastric secretion (Schlaadt and Shannon, 1994). Additionally, it has an anticoagulant effect; therefore, in the event of an injury, blood is likely to be lost at a higher rate than if alcohol had not been ingested (Criqui, 1998). Binge drinking episodes have been associated with an increased susceptibility to

bacterial and viral infection (Szabo, 1999), although this effect is more common among chronic heavy drinkers. Seizure thresholds are elevated while BAC is increasing; however, threshold levels are reduced as BAC decreases, which may prompt seizures in recently abstinent heavy drinkers (Goodwin and Gabrielli, 1997). Yet another acute effect is the suppression of rapid eye movement (REM) sleep, resulting in disturbed sleep patterns (Schuckit, 1994).

Adverse Reactions to Alcohol

As a person consumes alcohol over time, the CNS adapts to this situation and alcohol has a lesser effect, or, to state this differently, it takes more alcohol to achieve the same desired effect (Beers and Berkow, 1999). This phenomenon, known as tolerance, occurs both in acute and in chronic drinking. In a single acute drinking episode, tolerance can be observed in what is known as the Mellanby effect, whereby a person exhibits more intoxication at a given BAC level when the BAC is rising as compared to when it is falling (Martin and Moss, 1993). In chronic drinkers, inebriation may not be observed despite extremely high BAC. Gradual tolerance, therefore, explains why an alcohol-dependent individual can operate a motor vehicle without apparent impairment with a BAC well over the legal limits of intoxication or, as one author observed, why an individual can walk into an emergency room with minimal signs of inebriation despite a BAC of .35, which would produce coma or stupor in a nondependent individual.

As an individual consumes more and more alcohol over time and the CNS continues to adapt, the person is at risk for experiencing withdrawal when alcohol is suddenly discontinued. In this case, neurons are no longer repressed by alcohol and a variety of symptoms, such as anxiety, tremor, irritability, increased heart rate, nausea, vomiting, diarrhea, seizures, perceptual distortions, and delirium tremens may emerge. These symptoms vary in terms of their severity, the most critical being seizures and delirium tremens. These conditions constitute a medical emergency and may be life threatening (O'Brien, 1997). Alcohol-withdrawal seizures are experienced by about one-third of alcohol-dependent individuals and typically develop in 12 to 24 hr after the last drink. It is noteworthy that alcohol-withdrawal convulsions have been observed in nonchronic drinkers after binges lasting five to seven days (Diamond and Jay, 2000). Delirium tremens, on the other hand, is characterized by agitation, cognitive disorientation, hallucinations and/or delusions, and sympathetic nervous system hyperactivity (Erwin, Williams, and Speir, 1998). These symptoms usually are manifested two to four days after the person discontinues alcohol. Patients experiencing delirium tremens are often combative and terrified of the perceptual disturbances they are experiencing. These conditions can be avoided with early medical intervention and are managed with other CNS depressants, such as benzodiazepines, which are gradually decreased until a patient is drug and alcohol free.

In both the nonchronic and chronic drinker, a lesser version of withdrawal, known as a hangover, is quite common. Symptoms include nausea, vomiting, headache, and thirst (Wiese, Shlipak, and Browner, 2000). This is problematic for athletes in that performance can be compromised by these symptoms and by the dehydration that is responsible for excessive thirst.

Should excessive alcohol use continue, an individual is at risk for developing alcohol abuse or dependence. Alcohol dependence, as defined by the fourth edition of the *Diagnostic and Statistical Manual of Mental Disorders* (DSM-IV) (American Psychiatric Association, 1994) refers to serious impairment of a person's life due to alcohol use. Symptoms for this disorder may include tolerance; withdrawal; inability to cut down or control drinking despite desire to do so; devotion of a great deal

of time to obtaining, using, or recovering from the effects of alcohol; reduction or cessation in one's occupational, recreational, and social activities due to alcohol use; and continued drinking despite knowledge of its detrimental effects (e.g., physical or psychological problems). Abuse is a lesser diagnosis requiring occurrences of at least one of the following: recurrent alcohol use causing a failure to meet major role obligations at work, school, or home; recurrent alcohol use in dangerous situations (e.g., drinking and driving); recurrent alcohol-related legal problems; or continued alcohol use despite persistent alcohol-related social or interpersonal problems. In both diagnoses, maladaptive alcohol use must lead to impairment and/or distress.

One complication experienced by many alcohol-dependent individuals is cross tolerance (Evans, O'Brien, and Chafetz, 1991). This effect may occur when a person addicted to alcohol begins substituting another drug with similar, CNS-depressant qualities, such as benzodiazepines, for alcohol. In this case, the alcohol-tolerant individual may require larger doses of benzodiazepines to obtain inebriation than another person not tolerant to the effects of alcohol. Another common problem is that using alcohol in combination with other drugs often has a potentiating effect; each drug augments the activity of the other drug. This is especially a concern with alcohol and other sedatives. Mixing small amounts of these substances can have devastating results, including death (O'Brien, 1997).

When excessive amounts of alcohol are rapidly ingested, overdose may occur. This is rare because loss of consciousness usually occurs prior to overdose. However, alcohol overdoses have been documented, especially in teenagers and young adults who are engaging in drinking "games" or contests. The amount of alcohol required to induce death varies according to tolerance and other factors; however, a quart of whiskey or its equivalent, if rapidly consumed, is sufficient to cause death due to arrested respiration and heartbeat (Evans, O'Brien, and Chafetz, 1991).

Health Effects of Alcohol

This section outlines the effects of alcohol on physical health and discusses common psychosocial consequences of alcohol abuse.

Effects of Alcohol on Physical Health

The focus of many recent studies (e.g., Camargo et al., 1997; Gaziano et al., 2000; San Jose et al., 1999) and reviews (Gronbaek et al., 1997; Svardsudd, 1998) has been on the relationship between alcohol consumption and mortality. These studies have suggested that light-to-moderate levels of alcohol consumption (levels are defined differently across studies, but generally range between less than one drink per day and three drinks per day) may reduce mortality. A J- or U-shaped relationship between alcohol consumption and mortality has been reported (e.g., Camargo et al., 1997; Gaziano et al., 2000), showing higher mortality in abstainers and heavy drinkers than in moderate drinkers. However, a number of inconsistencies and methodological concerns have been reported regarding this literature, making interpretation of results problematic (Andreasson, 1998; Fillmore et al., 1998; Svardsudd, 1998).

While researchers continue to investigate potential positive health effects of moderate alcohol consumption, there are numerous well-documented negative health effects associated with alcohol abuse and dependence that, when combined with the deleterious health effects of addiction to nicotine and other drugs, have exacted a tremendous burden on the well-being of Americans (McGinnis and Foege, 1999). Alcoholics who continue to drink face a life expectancy at least 15 years shorter than nondependent individuals (Diamond and Jay, 2000), and they have mortality rates 2.5 (Schlaadt and Shannon, 1994) to 3.3 (Rossow and Amundsen, 1997) times higher than the population at large, due primarily to accidents, suicide, homicide, and a variety of health problems. Alcohol-related pathologies occur in various body systems, including, but not limited to, the CNS (O'Brien, 1997), cardiovascular (Puddey et al., 1999), gastrointestinal (Lawrence, 2000), reproductive (Wetterling et al., 1999), and immune (Cook, 1998; MacGregor and Louria, 1997) systems; many of these pathologies are related to nutritional deficits associated with excessive use of alcohol. Researchers typically find thiamine, folate, pyridoxine, niacin, vitamin A, potassium, magnesium, calcium, zinc, and phosphorus deficiencies among alcoholics (Schuckit, 1994). With the notable exceptions of CNS damage and liver cirrhosis, many of these health problems are reversible with abstinence, proper medical treatment, and the introduction of thiamine supplements (Diamond and Jay, 2000).

Although these conditions are found primarily among alcoholics, nondependent drinkers may experience significant health problems as well. For example, alcohol-induced blackouts may be experienced by nondependent binge drinkers. During a blackout, a severely intoxicated person maintains consciousness, but, when sober, has no recollection of some or all of the events that occurred while intoxicated. There is no disruption in recall of new information or long-term memory (O'Brien, 1997).

Another condition experienced by some nondependent binge drinkers with no history of heart disease is known as the "holiday heart syndrome." After binge drinking, an individual with this condition experiences depressed cardiac functioning and arrhythmias (Greenspan and Schaal, 1983). Also, since it easily crosses the placenta, alcohol in quantities as low as one to two drinks per day increases the risk of growth retardation (Mills et al., 1984) and information-processing difficulties (Jacobson et al., 1993) in a child born to a woman consuming alcohol. Fetal alcohol syndrome, an irreversible collection of abnormalities, including mental retardation, facial anomalies, growth deficiencies, and microcephaly (Jain, 1998), is a risk for children of mothers who drink more than four to five drinks per day during pregnancy.

Psychosocial Consequences of Alcohol Abuse

A number of negative psychosocial consequences tend to occur secondary to alcohol abuse and dependence. The consequences often associated with athletes include academic difficulties at both the high school and college levels. For example, excessive drinking has been associated with decreased academic performance, especially among students with formerly high academic performance (Wood, Sher, and McGowan, 2000). A frequent scenario is that of athletes who fail classes (due to absenteeism, poor study habits, and the late submission of assignments) and are therefore deemed ineligible for athletic participation. Whereas the causes of these academic problems vary, and may include the time and energy commitment of sport participation itself, alcohol use should not be overlooked as a plausible reason for poor academic performance and missed classes.

Ineligibility for sport participation can have a direct effect on an athlete's job prospects as well. Those desiring a career in professional athletics may not be given opportunities for exposure if their academic performance prohibits participation. If excessive alcohol consumption is the explanation for such difficulties, vocational problems may ensue. Individuals experiencing alcohol abuse or dependence often report spotty job histories, absenteeism, alcohol-related job loss, on-the-job accidents, and poor performance related to drinking. The National Institute of Alcohol Abuse estimates that 50% of referrals to employee assistance programs for job-performance issues are related to alcohol use (Evans, O'Brien, and Chafetz, 1991).

Individuals who drink excessively also are more likely to have contact with law enforcement agencies. In fact, alcohol is the substance most likely to be related to both violent and nonviolent crime in this country as compared to any other drug (Dawkins, 1997). Alcohol impairs judgment, and inebriated individuals often experience difficulties in determining their ability to operate motor vehicles after drinking. In 1996, alcohol was implicated as a contributing factor in 4% of motor vehicle deaths in the United States (Rouse, 1998). Lowered inhibitions related to alcohol use appear to contribute to public intoxication charges and incidences of violence and crime. Approximately one of every three arrests in the United States is associated with alcohol (Carson, Butcher and Mineka, 2000). For instance, alcohol has been identified as a contributing factor in 50% of homicides (Bennett and Lehman, 1996), 40% of assault cases, and 50% of rapes (Seto and Barbaree, 1995). It should be noted that alcohol-dependent individuals are not responsible for the majority of these crimes; in fact most are committed by nondependent individuals (Evans, O'Brien, and Chafetz, 1991).

Alcohol also exacts a toll on families. Excessive alcohol use is associated with higher divorce rates (Fillmore et al., 1994) and higher incidences of both spouse and child abuse (Van Hightower and Gordon, 1998). Frequent, heavy drinkers often gravitate toward others with similar drinking patterns and away from friends and family who express concern about their drinking.

There is a high rate of comorbidity between alcohol abuse and dependence and a variety of psychological disorders. The highest comorbidity rates occur with depression, anxiety disorders, schizophrenia, antisocial personality disorder, bipolar disorder, and other drug dependencies (American Psychiatric Association, 1994). Studies indicate that up to 50% of alcohol-addicted individuals attempt suicide and that about 10% to 15% actually commit suicide (Becker, 2000); these rates are significantly higher than for the population at large. It is often difficult to determine causal direction between addiction and related psychological disorders—for example, whether alcohol dependence and deterioration of one's life contributed to depression, or whether an individual's depression spurred increased alcohol intake as a coping mechanism. Addiction and depression frequently exacerbate one another as a person's life spirals out of control.

Alcohol Use in the General United States Population

A brief description of alcohol use and consequences in the general U.S. population will give the reader a context for considering alcohol use among sport participants. Alcohol is the third leading source of calories in the American diet, behind breads and sweets ("Vital Statistics," 1993). This is the case despite adult abstinence rates across the United States ranging from 30% to 70%. Of those who drink, the vast majority (approximately 80%) of people drink without significant alcohol-related negative consequences (see review in United States Department of Heath and Human Services [USDHHS], 1993).

Recent epidemiological data indicate that per capita alcohol consumption in the United States reached a 35-year low in 1995 (most of the recent decrease in alcohol consumption can be attributed to decreases in use of spirits). From 1990 to 1997, overall per capita alcohol consumption decreased by 11% (Nephew et al., 1999). Despite decreases in apparent alcohol consumption in the United States, Midanik and Greenfield (2000) found that trends in self-reported social consequences (e.g., fights/arguments, accidents/legal problems, health problems) of alcohol use and alcohol dependence symptoms have remained stable.

Recent data from the National Household Survey on Drug Abuse (Substance Abuse and Mental Health Services Administration, 1999) indicated that alcohol remained the clear drug of choice in the United States relative to nicotine and illicit drugs (table 19.3). The 1998 version of this annual survey included a nationally representative sample of the civilian noninstitutionalized population of the United States aged 12 years and older. The survey indicated that 81% of the target population reported lifetime use of alcohol, 64% reported use in the past year, and 52% reported use in the past month. The incidence of other drug use pales in comparison to these figures.

Alcohol Use Among Secondary School and College Students

In their recent survey results of secondary school students, Johnston, O'Malley, and Bachman (2000) reported that alcohol use is typical in this population. They reported lifetime use rates of 52% for 8th graders, 71% for 10th graders, and 80% for 12th graders. Of concern in this population is the rate of heavy or binge drinking (reported incidence of five or more drinks in a row in the prior two weeks). Fifteen percent of 8th graders, 26% of 10th graders, and 31% of 12th graders reported binge drinking. This style of drinking has been associated with significant negative consequences (i.e., adverse effects on social life; physical health; happiness; home life; work, studies, or employment opportunities; finances) in the Canadian general population aged 15 years and older (Room, Bondy, and Ferris, 1995). Binge drinking also has been linked to a reduction in the average number of years of education completed beyond high school (Cook and Moore, 1993). Despite negative consequences associated with binge drinking, other data in the Johnston, O'Malley, and Bachman (2000) survey indicate that many students do not perceive binge drinking as potentially harmful and do not disapprove of it.

Binge drinking also is a troubling issue among college students. Although noncollege age peers and high school students have shown a net decrease in binge drinking since 1980, college students have maintained a high rate

Table 19.3 Percentage and Estimated Number* of Users of Illicit Drugs, Alcohol, and Tobacco in the United States**

| | Time period | | | | | |
| | Lifetime | | Past year | | Past month | |
Drug	%	Number of users (thousands)	%	Number of users (thousands)	%	Number of users (thousands)
Any illicit drug use[1]	35.8	78,123	10.6	23,115	6.2	13,615
Marijuana or hashish	33.0	72,070	8.6	18,710	5.0	11,016
Cocaine	10.6	23,089	1.7	3811	0.8	1750
Crack	2.0	4476	0.4	971	0.2	437
Inhalants	5.8	12,589	0.9	2009	0.3	713
Hallucinogens	9.9	21,607	1.6	3565	0.7	1514
PCP	3.5	7640	0.2	346	0.0	91
LSD	7.9	17,223	0.8	1806	0.3	655
Heroin	1.1	2371	0.1	253	0.1	130
Nonmedical use of any psychotherapeutic[2]	9.2	20,193	2.6	5759	1.1	2477
Stimulants	4.4	9614	0.7	1489	0.3	633
Sedatives	2.1	4640	0.2	522	0.1	210
Tranquilizers	3.5	7726	0.9	1940	0.3	655
Analgesics	5.3	11,595	1.9	4070	0.8	1709
Any illicit drug other than marijuana[1]	18.9	41,337	4.9	10,788	2.5	5388
Alcohol	81.3	177,512	64.0	139,807	51.7	112,850
Binge alcohol use[3]	—	—	—	—	15.6	32,950
Heavy alcohol use[3]	—	—	—	—	5.9	12,427
Cigarettes	69.7	152,313	30.6	66,735	27.7	60,406
Smokeless tobacco	17.2	37,667	4.4	9582	3.1	6730

*In thousands

**Sample is from a noninstitutionalized population age 12 and older reporting use in their lifetime, the past year, and the past month; 1998 (n = 25,500).

[1]"Any illicit drug" indicates use at least once of marijuana/hashish, cocaine (including crack), inhalants, hallucinogens (including PCP and LSD), heroin, or any prescription-type psychotherapeutic used nonmedically. "Any illicit drug other than marijuana" indicates use at least once of any of these listed drugs, regardless of marijuana/hashish use; marijuana/hashish users who also have used any of the other listed drugs are included.

[2]Nonmedical use of any prescription-type stimulant, sedative, tranquilizer, or analgesic. Does not include over-the-counter drugs.

[3]Binge alcohol use is defined as drinking five or more drinks on the same occasion on at least one day in the past 30 days. By "occasion" is meant at the same time or within a couple hours of each other. Heavy alcohol use is defined as drinking five or more drinks on the same occasion on each of five or more days in the past 30 days. All heavy alcohol users are also binge alcohol users.

Data gathered from *Summary of Findings from the 1998 National Household Survey on Drug Abuse* (pp. 62-67) by the Substance Abuse and Mental Health Services Administration, 1999, Rockville, MD.

of this drinking style; 38% of college students reported binge drinking in 1996 (Johnston, O'Malley, and Bachman, 1998). Another survey of college students' alcohol use indicated that while binge drinking showed little change from 1993 to 1997, it remained at a level that was problematic (Wechsler et al., 1998). These survey results indicated that two in five students were binge drinkers, one in five was an abstainer, and one in five was a frequent binge drinker (students reporting binging

three or more times in a two-week period). These researchers defined binge drinking as at least five drinks in a row for men or four drinks in a row for women during the two weeks prior to the survey. Their results also indicated that among students who drank alcohol there were increases in frequency of drinking, drunkenness, drinking to get drunk, and alcohol-related problems (including drinking and driving). Binge drinkers also were at increased risk for various alcohol-related problems including driving after drinking, damaging property, and suffering personal injury. Fraternities and sororities appeared to be the center of binge drinking, with two-thirds of fraternity and sorority members reporting binge drinking.

Alcohol Use in Sport

To gain an appreciation of the significance of alcohol use among sport participants, it is necessary to explore the relationship between physical activity and alcohol use. Specifically, do sport participants differ from nonparticipants with respect to frequency and quantity of alcohol use and frequency of high-risk or binge drinking? Further, what consequences, if any, result from these differences? The following subsections discuss alcohol use among athletes at the secondary, collegiate or amateur, and professional levels, comparing use among these groups to that of their age mates in the general population.

Secondary Level

There is evidence suggesting a relationship between sport participation and alcohol use in secondary school students. In a three-year prospective study of a population-based cohort of adolescents aged 12 to 16 years old, Aaron et al. (1995) found a significant relationship between leisure-time physical activity and initiation of alcohol use. Males who participated in competitive athletics were significantly more likely than nonathletes to begin drinking. No association between physical activity and initiation of alcohol use was noted for females. Another study (Rainey et al., 1996) showed in a sample of 12th-grade students that highly active athletes drank more frequently than their less active and sedentary peers and also were more inclined toward binge drinking (defined as five or more drinks in a row during the last 30 days).

While alcohol use among adolescents is commonplace (Johnston, O'Malley, and Bachman, 2000), the Aaron et al. (1995) and Rainey et al. (1996) studies of alcohol use in the subpopulation of adolescents participating in sport give reason for pause and concern. It appears that athletes are initiating alcohol use at a rate that is at least comparable to that of their nonathletic peers and, in the case of males, perhaps at a greater rate. Athletes also appear to be drinking more frequently and in higher volumes than their peers. This high-consumption drinking is more likely to be done in social settings and situations that pose risk. For example, Mayer et al. (1998), reporting on survey results with 9th and 12th graders, found that those reporting five or more drinks on one occasion in the last two weeks (binge drinking) were more likely to report drinking with peers, in large groups of underage persons, and away from home.

Collegiate and Amateur Level

Given the levels of drinking among secondary school (Johnston, O'Malley, and Bachman, 2000) and college students (Wechsler et al., 1998), it is not surprising that college athletes have been found to be consuming alcohol at a rate at or above that of their peers. For example, Leichliter et al. (1998) found that, relative to nonathletes, both male and female intercollegiate athletes consumed significantly more alcohol per week, binge drank more often, and experienced more adverse consequences related to their alcohol use. Unfortunately, in addition to binge drinking, college athletes appear to engage in other risk-taking behaviors more than their nonathlete peers. For example, Nattiv, Puffer, and Green (1997), in a multicenter, cross-sectional study including seven major collegiate institutions in the United States, found that athletes engaged in a number of high-risk behaviors more frequently than their nonathlete peers. The survey showed, for instance, that athletes were less likely to always wear seat belts, were more likely to ride as a passenger with a driver under the influence of alcohol or drugs, reported greater quantity and frequency of alcoholic beverage use, reported less contraceptive use, and reported more involvement in physical fighting. Male athletes reported more risk-taking behavior than female athletes, and athletes in contact sports showed more risk taking than athletes in noncontact sports. In addition, this study showed that athletes with one high risk-taking behavior tended to report multiple risk-taking behaviors. Kokotailo et al. (1996) also found that male athletes reported more high-risk behaviors than their female athlete peers, and in some areas (e.g., infrequent seat belt use, riding in a car with a driver under the influence of alcohol) were more prone to high-risk behaviors than male nonathletes.

According to Nattiv, Puffer, and Green (1997), female athletes reported a number of high-risk behaviors more frequently than their peers, including greater frequency of alcohol use and greater quantity of alcohol per sitting. Conversely, Kokotailo et al. (1996) found that in contrast to male athletes, female athletes generally reported fewer risk-taking behaviors than their female nonathlete peers. Other researchers focusing on female collegiate athletes (e.g., Bower and Martin, 1999; Martin, 1998) reported alcohol use behavior similar to that for the general college student population. For instance, in a study of alcohol and drug use in African American female basketball players, Bower and Martin found that 72% of women reported alcohol use and 46% reported binge drinking (defined in this study as four or more drinks per drinking episode). In a population of female college athletes representing a variety of sports, Martin found a 60% rate of binge drinking. Interestingly, in both studies, female athletes reported a significant reduction in quantity and frequency of alcohol use during their competitive season; this suggested that they viewed alcohol use as incompatible with high-level athletic performance.

Although data on amateur, postcollegiate athletes' use of alcohol are less available than information on drinking in collegiate athletes, there are reports indicating that alcohol use by serious recreational athletes may exceed use by their nonexercising peers. Gutgesell, Timmerman, and Keller (1996), in a study of long-distance runners, found that running was associated with increased alcohol consumption except among those reporting a history of problem alcohol behavior. These researchers also found that male and female runners reported more occasions of drinking than matched controls. Runners with scores on an alcohol abuse screening instrument that were suggestive of a history of problem drinking reported drinking less than controls with similar scores. This result suggests that running may help those with alcohol problems maintain a sober state; the data did not address this issue directly, however.

Professional Level

Reports of alcohol and drug abuse among professional athletes are common in the media; however, studies documenting alcohol use in this population are infrequent. In a survey of 262 male athletes in a professional sport league (the league was not indicated by the author) regarding their alcohol and drug use, Malone (1991) found that alcohol was the only drug that many players reported using regularly. Virtually all of the athletes reported lifetime use of alcohol, and 93% reported alcohol use in the last 30 days. Roughly one-third of the athletes reported two or more drinking occasions in the last two weeks when they consumed more than five drinks in a row. According to Malone, comparing these athletes' reported use of alcohol to that in a comparable age group in the general population suggested that a greater proportion of these athletes were drinkers. However, reported other-drug use in the last 12 months among these athletes was significantly lower than for their age mates in the general population.

The results of the Malone (1991) study clearly indicate that alcohol was the drug of choice among these male professional athletes. Further, 40 (15%) of the athletes were rated as problem drinkers based on their responses to the Michigan Alcoholism Screening Test, a commonly used self-report screening instrument for problem drinking. A participant-observer study conducted by Gallmeier (1988), with a group of minor league hockey players, adds support to the idea that heavy alcohol use is not an uncommon practice among professional athletes. As a part of the study, the researcher became part of the hockey team during the season, participating in "all the activities that the players were involved in with the exception of actually playing the game" (Gallmeier, 1988, p. 2). The author found that the most common drug activity among the players was team drinking sessions after all home games and many road games. "The players called these events 'juicing sessions' and believed they were necessary for developing team solidarity" (Gallmeier, 1988, p.3). These two studies, one using a survey methodology and the other behavioral observation, suggest that alcohol use is a frequent practice among professional athletes and may cause problems for some athletes.

Ergolytic and Ergogenic Effects of Alcohol on Sport Performance

In the late 1800s, athletes used alcohol as a stimulant to release inhibitions and decrease feelings of fatigue in events requiring extreme exertion or brief maximal effort (Boje, as cited in Williams, 1991). Jokl (1968) reported alcohol use by European athletes at the turn of the century. For example, he reported incidents of marathon runners consuming large quantities of cognac during competition and cyclists drinking rum and champagne during 24-hr races. The athletes' rationale for alcohol consumption apparently was for refreshment and strength restoration. Pistol shooters also have been known to use alcohol to decrease anxiety levels, thus allowing for maximal performance. Prior to 1968, alcohol use was proscribed as a doping agent by the International Olympic Committee (IOC), leading to two pistol shooters' disqualification in the 1968 Olympics because of alleged alcohol use (Shephard, 1972). However, for the 1972 Munich Olympics, alcohol was not included among the proscribed doping agents (Fischbach, as cited in Williams, 1991) despite being referred to as "gold water" by pistol-shooting athletes.

Historical evidence suggests that athletes have used alcohol in hopes of achieving ergogenic effects on sport performance; however, scientific research indicates that alcohol is rarely an ergogenic aid. Indeed, in most cases alcohol use detracts from athletic performance (i.e., has ergolytic effects). Stainback (1997) summarized some of the conclusions of the American College of Sports Medicine (ACSM, 1982) in its position stand on alcohol use in sport as follows:

- Alcohol in small (1.5-2.0 oz [44-59 ml]) to moderate (3-4 oz [89-118 ml]) amounts has negative effects on a variety of psychomotor skills, including reaction time, eye-hand coordination, accuracy, balance, and complex coordination or gross-motor skills.
- Alcohol apparently has little or no beneficial effects on metabolic or physiological functions underlying

physical performance (e.g., energy metabolism and functions that contribute to oxygen consumption and maximal oxygen consumption, heart rate, stroke volume, cardiac output). Furthermore, in those studies demonstrating significant effects, changes appear to decrease performance. Alcohol may adversely affect body temperature regulation during prolonged exercise in cold temperatures.

- Alcohol will not improve and potentially may decrease muscular work capacity (Stainback, 1997, pp. 63-64).

The following sections address each of the three areas referred to in the ACSM position stand regarding the effects of acute alcohol ingestion on sport performance. A final discussion deals with the performance effects of social drinking as an individual lifestyle choice.

Psychomotor Effects

Although it may be tempting to consume alcohol for its potential positive effects on psychological well-being or for its tension-reduction properties, in the majority of sport circumstances alcohol ingestion is likely to impair psychomotor skills that underlie sport performance. It has been suggested that alcohol may increase an athlete's self-confidence (Shephard, 1972). However, more recent evidence indicates that the risks for a decline in psychomotor skills (and therefore decreased performance) that are associated with alcohol consumption outweigh the potential benefits on self-confidence or tension levels for most individuals. Much of the research on alcohol's effects on human psychomotor performance and cognitive function has focused on skills related to automobile driving. A recent review of this literature (Kerr and Hindmarch, 1998) indicates that greater alcohol-related deficits are observed as dose levels increase and tasks become more complex. These authors also noted the large interindividual and interoccasional differences in the effects of alcohol on performance. That is, different people respond differently to the effects of alcohol, and the same person responds differently on separate drinking occasions. Generally, complex skills that require CNS processing capacity are impaired at lower BAC levels (Mitchell, 1985). It has been found that psychomotor tasks involving divided attention, tracking, visual search, and recognition and response are impaired with BAC levels as low as .015 (Moskowitz, Burns, and Williams, 1985). In contrast, Mitchell noted that other psychomotor skills, such as simple reaction time, may show no or relatively small alcohol-related deficits at BAC levels approaching .10.

The effect of alcohol consumption on sport performance is largely dependent on the amount of alcohol consumed, the skill demands placed on the athlete by the sport, and the individual's particular response to alcohol. Since alcohol has significant anti-anxiety and anti-tremor effects (Koller and Biary, 1984), its consumption may affect performance in sports requiring steady hands and aiming. These sports include pistol shooting, archery, billiards, and darts. There also are aiming components in sports such as fencing and the modern pentathlon. In a review of alcohol and anti-anxiety drugs in sport, Reilly (1996) indicated that there are differential effects of alcohol on performance in archery and dart throwing. Reilly and Halliday (1985) found differential effects of alcohol (levels of BAC at .02 and .05) on archery-related tasks. Arm steadiness deteriorated and reaction time increased at both BAC levels (possible impairments), and a clearer loose (valuable in promoting a smoother release) occurred at .02 (possible enhancement). No alcohol-related effects were found for muscular strength and endurance. Reilly concluded that alcohol showed differential effects on archery-related tasks depending on dose levels, components of the task analyzed, and individual susceptibility to the drug's effects. Since no performance data were reported, alcohol's ergogenic properties were not evaluated directly. Also, because subjects had no specific archery training and the tests were performed in a noncompetitive laboratory setting, results cannot be directly extrapolated to competitive archery. Reilly also noted that the negative effects of alcohol on some aspects of archery would not necessarily apply to other aiming sports such as darts and pistol shooting. In these sports, the weight load on the arm is significantly less than in archery, making it more likely that alcohol will produce greater arm steadiness. Decrements in reaction time in the archery study that have potential to reduce performance do not apply because the timing of the release is at the total discretion of the subject.

A study by Golby (1989) provides evidence that alcohol may induce changes in the composition of factors influencing skilled performance. This study examined the effects of two levels of alcohol dose (0.5 g pure alcohol per kg body weight and 1 g pure alcohol per kg body weight) and a placebo condition on a soccer ball-control slalom task. Various performance outcomes (e.g., time to complete the task, number of errors made by touching cones, number of times the ball went out of control) and reference tests were included as measures. The latter were included to identify alterations in performance strategy used to maintain performance while level of alcohol dose changed. Choice of these tests was based on their potential to predict performance on the soccer skill since they were thought to rely on many of the information-processing and ability factors judged to be critical to the successful performance of the skill. The results indicate that the low dose of alcohol produced significant decreases in the time needed to complete the soccer slalom (performance-enhancing effect) when compared with the placebo condition. This effect on performance was reversed in the higher-alcohol-dose condition: there were significant increases in performance time, but the times were still faster than in the placebo condition. The pattern of dependent-measure results indicated that performance strategies were unchanged between the placebo and low-alcohol-dose conditions. However, in the higher-alcohol-dose condition, the pattern of results indicated the emergence of a "response-impairment" factor, which the author suggested may be interpreted as subjects changing performance composition (as indicated by a compensatory increase in foot speed) in response to the effects of alcohol on information-processing capacity. The author indicated major limitations of the study (e.g., lack of data to support selection of reference tests known to be related to abilities required by the soccer task; inclusion of a broad range of skill levels in the subject pool, perhaps masking individual differences in performance strategy changes between performers with high and low skill levels), suggesting that the results should be regarded as preliminary.

Effects on Metabolic and Physiological Functions Underlying Sport Performance

A conclusion of the ACSM (1982) position was that alcohol has few or no beneficial effects on metabolic and physiological responses to exercise. Moreover, in those studies indicating significant effects, the alcohol-induced changes adversely affected performance.

Studies since publication of the ACSM position stand have largely corroborated these conclusions. For example, Heikkonen (1989) found that in young healthy male subjects there were minor detrimental effects on exercise-induced changes in hormonal and metabolic activities in response to alcohol. In this study, subjects performed an exhaustive ergometer exercise during alcohol intoxication, hangover (BAC approached 0), and before alcohol intoxication. Among other findings, Heikkonen reported that physical exercise heightened and prolonged alcohol's depressant effect on testosterone; that alcohol consumption immediately pre- or postexercise attenuated the human growth hormone secretion increase typically found following exercise; and that alcohol taken immediately prior to exercise inhibited the usual increase in blood glucose levels in response to exercise, causing mild hypoglycemia in recovery from exercise after fasting. This hypoglycemic effect also was found, interestingly, after exercise during hangover. Other studies similarly showed that alcohol yielded no beneficial influences on

metabolic or work performance measures (Bond, Franks, and Howley, 1984; Borg, Domserius, and Kaijser, 1990). Borg and colleagues also found that moderate doses of alcohol had no effect on subjects' perceived exertion.

Although studies since publication of the ACSM position stand have largely supported the idea that alcohol has no beneficial effects on metabolic and physiological responses to exercise, there have been results inconsistent with this conclusion. For example, Amusa and Muoboghare (1986) found differential alcohol-related effects on physiological responses to exercise. These investigators studied the effects of three BAC levels (.03, .05, .10) on various physical measures and found no effect of alcohol on resting blood pressure or on blood pressure, heart rate, and oxygen uptake during exercise. Conversely, they found that alcohol at the studied dosages increased the resting heart rate, work duration, and recovery rate. The authors suggested that alcohol's apparent positive effect on work duration was mediated by its effect on resting heart rate, which may have salutary effects on fatigue, or by its depressant or inhibitory effect on the brain, which may reduce perception of fatigue. This is an interesting speculation; however, there is presently limited support for this hypothesis.

The ACSM position stand cited studies that noted a significant loss of body heat and a resulting drop in body temperature in response to alcohol, suggesting that alcohol may impair temperature regulation. Desruelle, Boisvert, and Candas (1996) found that for subjects exercising in a warm environment there was significant variation in response to alcohol ingestion, with no consistent effect on thermoregulatory response. The authors reported no significant changes in skin and body temperature and in sweat rate, suggesting that the body's capacity to accommodate to exogenous and endogenous heat was not fundamentally altered by alcohol. However, similarly to previous research, this study indicated significant interindividual variation in response to alcohol. Some subjects had a highly sensitive regulatory system, showing mean increases in their body temperature and sweating in response to alcohol ingestion, while others were relatively unaffected by alcohol consumption. In a related study focusing on the effects of alcohol on responses to exercise in a warm environment, Saini et al. (1995) found that alcohol ingestion enhanced body fluid losses, apparently because of a suppressive effect on plasma arginine vasopressin, a hormone involved in body fluid and electrolyte regulation that is normally stimulated during warm-weather exercising to preserve physiological homeostasis. This alcohol-related effect, along with the documented diuretic effect of alcohol, enhances the probability of dehydration in athletes exercising or competing in a warm environment.

Effects on Tests of Fitness Components

Similar to research on alcohol's effects on metabolic and physiological functions underlying performance, the ACSM position stand indicated that alcohol either had no beneficial effects on muscular work capacity or had detrimental effects on performance. For example, findings cited in the ACSM position stand indicated that alcohol might have adverse effects on dynamic muscular strength, isometric grip strength, dynamometer strength, power, and ergographic muscular output. Other ACSM-cited studies indicated no effect of alcohol on muscular strength, local muscular endurance, physical performance capacity, exercise time at maximum levels, or exercise time to exhaustion.

More recent studies corroborate the ACSM conclusions. For example, Houmard et al. (1987) found that 18 well-trained male runners consuming either low levels of alcohol (BAC level less than .05) or no alcohol showed no significant differences in performance levels on a 5-mile (8 km) treadmill run. The authors concluded that performance in endurance exercise was unaffected by alcohol ingestion at low levels. McNaughton and Preece (1986) found that alcohol in varying amounts had no positive effects on performances in the 100-, 200-, 400-, 800-, and 1500-m (109, 219, 437, 874, and 1640 yd) track events. In all of these events, alcohol had negative effects on performance except in the 100-m event, where performance remained stable. Finally, Bond, Gresham, Balkissoon, and Clearwater (1984) demonstrated no effect of small (0.34 g/kg) or moderate (0.69 g/kg) doses of alcohol on torque-generating capacities during elbow flexion and extension and knee extension exercises.

Social Drinking and Sport Performance

Although the majority of studies on alcohol's effects on sport performance have focused on acute effects of alcohol consumption, perhaps a more critical issue given the incidence of drinking among athletes is the effects of social drinking on athletic performance. Specifically, it is important to understand the potential cumulative effects of social drinking on fitness levels and other performance-related criteria, as well as its effects on performance given alcohol consumption the night before a competition.

With respect to the first issue, the effect of social drinking on fitness- and performance-related criteria, the epidemiological data, though inconsistent, suggest that moderate alcohol consumption confers neither benefits nor detriments to physical performance (see review by Williams, 1991). In an attempt to distinguish harm-producing from non-harm-producing drinking levels with respect to cognitive functioning in sober social drinkers, Parsons and Nixon (1998) reviewed studies published since 1986 that involved the relationship between cognitive functioning and sober social drinking. Their conclusions support a testable alcohol-causal-threshold hypothesis suggesting that persons consuming five or six standard drinks per occasion (0.42 oz [12 g]) pure alcohol per drink (note that the standard drink in this study contains less alcohol, by 4 g, than the standard drink defined earlier in the chapter), five to seven days a week over a year or more, will manifest some cognitive inefficiencies; that mild cognitive deficits will occur at seven to nine standard drinks per day; and that moderate cognitive deficits similar to those found in diagnosed alcoholics will occur at 10 or more standard drinks per day. The authors indicated that these values are for males. For females, the number of drinks per day would be reduced by one drink, and possibly two drinks at the higher levels. The authors also emphasized that these hypotheses point the way for future research on this important public health issue.

With respect to the second issue, the potential for performance decrements related to alcohol consumption the previous night, it appears that the amount of alcohol consumed is the primary operative factor. This area has received limited research attention; however, it appears that potential performance decrements the morning following a drinking episode are dose dependent. For example, MacDonald and Svoboda (as cited in Williams, 1991) found that one drink consumed nightly for 10 days did not significantly affect measures of strength, power, and physiological response to aerobic exercise performed the next morning. O'Brien (1993) found that the aerobic performance of rugby players was adversely affected following consumption of varying amounts of alcohol the previous night. No alcohol effects on anaerobic performance were observed. O'Brien also found significant individual variability of players in next-day effects of alcohol on aerobic performance. Some players demonstrated extreme sensitivity to small amounts of alcohol consumed the previous night and therefore showed significant decrements in their aerobic performance relative to their peers. Other players consumed substantially more alcohol and showed equal, and in some cases lesser, ill effects on aerobic performance the following morning than their peers. Karvinin, Miettinen, and Ahlman (1962) also found that alcohol consumption of an average of 1.67 g of alcohol per kg body weight (as reported by Williams [1991], about eight drinks in this study) significantly impaired next-day aerobic performance. However, there were no alcohol effects on tests of static strength or power the following morning.

Another important consideration with respect to social drinking among athletes is the well-known diuretic effect of alcohol (Williams, 1991). It is not uncommon for athletes to drink alcohol the night before competition or perhaps following an endurance event such as the marathon. Because of alcohol's diuretic properties, consumption before any event that entails appreciable fluid loss through sweating may cause dehydration and resulting decrements in performance. Furthermore, for the athlete in a state of dehydration and with an empty stomach following such an event, alcohol would be rapidly absorbed and concentrated in the body. Since even small amounts of alcohol can impair psychomotor skills, it is unwise for any athlete in such a dehydrated state to consume alcohol and drive an automobile or perform other potentially dangerous tasks involving psychomotor skills.

Conclusion

The best conclusion based on the sport literature to date is that alcohol lacks ergogenic qualities for practically all sport applications. Although the effects of alcohol might produce some performance enhancement in aiming sports—for instance, archery and shooting sports—that render the athlete susceptible to excessive anxiety, available evidence is ambiguous at best. Use of alcohol in these sport competitions has been banned by some sport organizations (e.g., the National Collegiate Athletic Association [NCAA] has banned alcohol use in rifle competitions; see **http://www.ncaa.org/sports_ sciences/drugtesting/banned_list.html**). Sports requiring complex psychomotor skills appear to be most susceptible to the effects of alcohol. Other sport-related functions, such as metabolic and physiological processes and muscular work capacity, demonstrate few or no beneficial alcohol-related effects or show decreases in performance. Social drinking has not been found to be ergolytic. Excessive consumption the night before a competition, however, may produce decreased performance.

Given the conclusion that alcohol at best yields no consistent ergogenic effects and at worst produces decrements (sometimes substantial), what might be prudent recommendations to give to athletes with respect to drinking? The ACSM position stand, although two decades old, offers advice that is still useful:

> Serious and continuing efforts should be made to educate athletes, coaches, health and physical educators, physicians, trainers, the sports media, and the general public regarding the effects of acute alcohol ingestion upon human physical performance and on the potential acute and chronic problems of excessive alcohol consumption. (ACSM, 1982, p. ix)

Recent articles in the popular sport and coaching literature have contributed to this educational effort (e.g., Clark, 1998; Coleman, 1997; Deakin, 1999; Williams, 1998). These efforts have been apparent in this literature for over two decades (see Stainback, 1997, p. 69); however, the educational task is an unending one as new challenges are faced with each new generation of athletes. With respect to specific recommendations on alcohol consumption, ACSM recommends a guideline originating from Anstie's rule (as cited in ACSM, 1982). This rule defines as moderate, safe drinking for adults no more than 0.5 oz (16 g) of pure alcohol per 51 lb (23 kg) of body weight per day. This amount is equivalent to three bottles of beer (4.2% alcohol), three 4 oz (124 g) glasses of 13% wine, or 3 oz (93 g) of 50% whiskey for a 150-lb (68 kg) person.

Although this is a guideline recommended by ACSM, a "safe" level of alcohol consumption for an individual is a questionable concept (Thakker, 1998). Indeed, Room, Bondy, and Ferris (1995) suggest "with respect to casualty, social and interactional problems, at least, there appears to be no such thing as a drinking pattern with zero risk" (p. 511). Since non-harm-producing levels of alcohol consumption appear to vary with the individual, it seems that each individual must make a decision with respect to the use of alcohol based on that person's appraisal of the applicable risks. There are guidelines available for low-risk consumption (e.g., Bondy et al., 1999), but they must be interpreted within the framework of the individual's risks for alcohol abuse and other negative consequences of alcohol consumption.

Legislation and Policy Issues

Because alcohol use pervades Western society, efforts have been made by public and private institutions to reduce the negative consequences of drinking. Historically, prevention efforts have focused on heavy drinking involved in alcohol abuse and alcoholism. However, more recent efforts have broadened the target to include social, legal, and economic factors influencing alcohol use. This change in focus recognizes that alcohol use is commonplace in American society, as well as the associated problems. Indeed, light or moderate drinkers account for the majority of alcohol-related problems because they represent a greater proportion of the overall population than individuals consuming larger quantities do (Kreitman, 1986). To accommodate the broader focus of prevention efforts, the public health model has been used as a guide to generate ideas for programs and approaches that will reduce the harm associated with alcohol use. In this model, harms are recognized as outcomes of interactions between the drinker (host), the drug itself (alcohol), and the physical and social environment (Fischer et al., 1997). Generally, strategies that focus on host factors pertain to individual characteristics that place a person at risk for alcohol problems (e.g., age, gender, family history). Other strategies are directed toward alcohol itself and environmental factors surrounding its use that contribute to risk (e.g., alcohol availability, alcohol control laws, alcohol warning placed on containers, efforts to prevent alcohol-related problems in the workplace). For an extensive review of these prevention approaches, see the USDHHS report on alcohol and health (1997).

Sport is an important socializing institution in the United States and other parts of the world. Teenagers in particular are avid sport participants; a recent study (Pate et al., 2000) of a nationally representative sample of U.S. high school students indicated that approximately 70% of males and 53% of females participated in one or more sport teams. Further, youth involved in sport demonstrate alcohol- and drug-related attitudes and behaviors that are similar to those of their nonathlete peers (Stuck, 1990). In view of this broad overlap between alcohol use and sport participation, alcohol abuse prevention efforts are important to the general well-being of sport participants.

Although a comprehensive discussion of alcohol-related prevention efforts is beyond the scope of this chapter, it seems appropriate to briefly review legislation and policy issues important to sport. The development of legislation and policies is an example of an environmental prevention strategy intended to influence alcohol consumption levels or to prevent negative consequences of alcohol consumption. Laws and policies are a mechanism for communicating society's attitudes regarding alcohol use and provide a foundation for other prevention approaches, such as education (Funkhouser, Goplerud, and Bass, 1992). These alcohol-related policies may be classified into overlapping categories: public and institutional (Toomey and Wagenaar, 1999). Some examples of legislation intended to prevent alcohol and drug abuse are the Drug-Free Workplace Act (1988) and the Drug-Free Schools and Communities Act (1986). These legislative acts and other policy-directed measures have been successful at mobilizing preventive efforts nationwide in the public and private sectors (Toomey and Wagenaar, 1999). Another prominent example of legislative measures that have shown desirable effects on prevention of alcohol-related problems is the section titled "National Minimum Drinking Age" found in Title 23 of the U.S. Code Annotated at section 158 ("23 U.S.C.A.," 1990) encouraging all states to raise the minimum legal drinking age to 21. Higher minimum legal drinking ages have been associated with lower incidences of alcohol purchase, alcohol use, and impaired driving among 16-20 year olds (Yu and Shacket, 1998) and lower rates of suicide among 18-20 year olds

(Birckmayer and Hemenway, 1999). This act and related legislation appears to have contributed to significant decreases in alcohol-related traffic crashes and fatalities among drivers ages 16 to 24 (Yi et al., 1999).

Alcohol-Related Policies in Sport

Policies at the sport organizational level also may have a significant influence on alcohol and drug use and consequences. The majority of sport leagues or organizations (amateur and professional) have adopted policies that discourage alcohol and drug use and provide mechanisms for assisting athletes who need intervention (see Wadler and Hainline, 1989, for examples). Many of these policies, however, focus primarily on drug abuse, devoting limited attention to alcohol use by athletes. For example, Young and Young (1989) found in a survey of 272 women's sport programs in the NCAA that 68% of Division I and 53% of Division II programs lacked a departmental policy addressing alcohol use by athletes. This is unfortunate, because policies are an excellent way of communicating expectations regarding alcohol use and setting specific guidelines for efforts to prevent alcohol-related problems among athletes.

At the professional level, there is evidence of specific policies that address alcohol and drug use and actions that will be taken both to prevent substance-related problems and to treat individuals experiencing substance abuse or dependence. Substance abuse-related policy statements for major professional sport leagues in the United States can be found on the World Wide Web at **http://sports.findlaw.com/drugs/policy/index.html**.

For sports in which alcohol use may potentially confer an ergogenic effect (e.g., archery, shooting sports), some amateur sport organizations have specifically banned these substances in competitions. For instance, the NCAA has banned alcohol use in rifle competitions (see the NCAA banned drug classes, 2000-01, at **http://www.ncaa.org/sports_sciences/drugtesting/banned_list.html**). The IOC and the United States Anti-Doping Agency (USADA, the independent anti-doping agency for Olympic sports in the United States) also have briefly addressed alcohol in their policy statements. Both organizations have indicated that "where the rules of a responsible authority so provide, tests will be conducted for ethanol" (**http://www.usantidoping.org/files/2000_iocprohibited_sub.pdf**). This statement indicates that these amateur sport-governing bodies have left much discretion to governing bodies of specific sports regarding policies on alcohol. As Reilly points out, however, for sports that discourage alcohol use in competition there is "disharmony in standards for what constitutes legality" (Reilly, 1996, p. 159). He reports that standards range from banning any use of alcohol (e.g., in the modern pentathlon, fencing, and shooting) to setting specific BAC levels that are considered maximum allowable. Variability in standards related to alcohol use in sport reflects apparent ambivalence on ways to handle a drug that is legally used and widely accepted throughout much of the world, but whose use is severely restricted in other parts of the world (e.g., in many countries in the Middle East). Given this disparity of societal views regarding alcohol use, it is likely that alcohol-related policies in sport will remain diverse and in many cases nonspecific.

Conclusion

Alcohol use is commonplace in the United States, and alcohol-related problems occur both in dependent and nondependent drinkers. Sport participants are not immune to these problems; indeed there is evidence that athletes participate in more high-risk behaviors generally, including drinking-related risk behaviors, than their age peers. With reference to alcohol use and sport performance, the literature indicates no consistent alcohol-related ergogenic effects, and in most cases the effects are ergolytic. Although ACSM provides guidelines for safe drinking, alcohol consumption carries with it inherent risks that vary across individuals. Therefore, individuals, taking into account their personal risks for alcohol-related negative consequences, should make appropriate decisions regarding alcohol use.

References

23 U.S.C.A. 158 (West 1990 and Supp. 1996).

Aaron, D.J., Dearwater, S.R., Anderson, R., Olsen, T., Kriska, A.M., and LaPorte, R.E. 1995. Physical activity and the initiation of high-risk health behaviors in adolescents. Medicine and Science in Sports and Exercise 27: 1639-1645.

American College of Sports Medicine. 1982. The use of alcohol in sports. Medicine and Science in Sports and Exercise 14: ix-xi.

American Psychiatric Association. 1994. Diagnostic and statistical manual of mental disorders, 4th ed. Washington, DC: American Psychiatric Association.

Amusa, L.O., and Muoboghare, P.A. 1986. The effect of three dosages of alcohol on physical performance. SNIPES Journal (Patiala, India) 9(2): 46-53.

Andreasson, S. 1998. Alcohol and J-shaped curves. Alcoholism: Clinical and Experimental Research 22: 359S-364S.

Ardolino, F. 1991. Dives, dark clubhouses, deceptive dreamscapes, and clean, well-lighted places in sports literature and film. Aethlon. 8(2): 35-54.

Becker, U. 2000. Alcohol and suicide attempts. Journal of Psychosomatic Research 48: 243.

Beers, M.H., and Berkow, R., eds. 1999. Merck manual of diagnosis and treatment. Whitehouse Station, NJ: Merck Research Laboratories, Merck & Co.

Bennett, J.B., and Lehman, W.E.K. 1996. Alcohol, antagonism, and witnessing violence in the workplace: Drinking climates and social alienation-integration. In Violence in the workplace, ed. G.R. Vandenbos and E.Q. Bulatao, 105-152. Washington, DC: American Psychological Association.

Birckmayer, J., and Hemenway, D. 1999. Minimum-age drinking laws and youth suicide. American Journal of Public Health 89: 1365-1368.

Blum, K. 1984. Handbook of abusable drugs. New York: Gardner.

Bond, V., Franks, B.D., and Howley, E.T. 1984. Alcohol, cardiorespiratory function and work performance. British Journal of Sports Medicine 18(3): 203-206.

Bond, V., Gresham, K.E., Balkissoon, B., and Clearwater, H.E. 1984. Effects of small and moderate doses of alcohol on peak torque and average torque in an isokinetic contraction. Scandinavian Journal of Sports Science 6(1): 1-5.

Bondy, S.J., Rehm, J., Ashley, M.J., Walsh, G., Single, E., and Room, R. 1999. Low-risk drinking guidelines: The scientific evidence. Canadian Journal of Public Health 90: 264-270.

Borg, G., Domserius, M., and Kaijser, L. 1990. Effect of alcohol on perceived exertion in relation to heart rate and blood lactate. European Journal of Applied Physiology and Occupational Physiology 60: 382-384.

Bower, B.L., and Martin, M. 1999. African American female basketball players: An examination of alcohol and drug behaviors. Journal of American College Health 48(3): 129-133.

Camargo, C.A., Hennekens, C.H., Gaziano, J.M., Glynn, R.J., Manson, J.E., and Stampfer, M.J. 1997. Prospective study of moderate alcohol consumption and mortality in U.S. male physicians. Archives of Internal Medicine 157(1): 79-85.

Carson, R.C., Butcher, J.N., and Mineka, S. 2000. Abnormal psychology and modern life, 11th ed. Needham Heights, MA: Allyn & Bacon.

Chen, Y.C., Lu, R.B., Peng, G.S., Wang, M.F., Wang, H.K., Ko, H.C., Chang, Y.C., Lu, J.J., Li, T.K., and Yin, S.J. 1999. Alcohol metabolism and cardiovascular response in an alcohol patient homozygous for the ALDH2*2 variant gene allele. Alcoholism: Clinical and Experimental Research 23: 1853-1860.

Clark, K. 1998. Alcohol to enhance athletic performance? Alcohol in weight management? ACSM'S Health and Fitness Journal 2(1): 38-39.

Coleman, E. 1997. Alcohol and performance. Sports Medicine Digest (Hagerstown, MD) 19(2): 23.

Cook, P.J., and Moore, M.F. 1993. Drinking and schooling. Journal of Health Economics 12: 411-429.

Cook, R.T. 1998. Alcohol abuse, alcoholism, and damage to the immune system—a review. Alcohol: Clinical and Experimental Research 22: 1927-1942.

Corry, J.M., and Cimbolic, P. 1985. Drugs: Facts, alternatives, decisions. Belmont, CA: Wadsworth.

Criqui, M.H. 1998. Do known cardiovascular risk factors mediate the effects of alcohol on cardiovascular disease? Novartis Foundation Symposium 216: 159-167.

Dawkins, M.P. 1997. Drug use and violent crime among adolescents. Adolescence 32: 395-405.

Dawson, D.A. 2000. Alcohol consumption, alcohol dependence, and all-cause mortality. Alcoholism: Clinical and Experimental Research 24(1): 72-81.

Deakin, V. 1999. Alcohol: The legal drug in sport. Sports Coach (Canberra, Australia) 22(2): 22-23.

Desruelle, A., Boisvert, P., and Candas, V. 1996. Alcohol and its variable effect on human thermoregulatory response to exercise in warm environment. European Journal of Applied Physiology and Occupational Physiology 74: 572-574.

Diamond, I., and Jay, C.A. 2000. Alcoholism and alcohol abuse. In Cecil textbook of medicine, 21st ed., ed. L. Goldman and J.C. Bennett, 1: 49-54. Philadelphia: Saunders.

Drug-Free Schools and Communities Act of 1986, 20 U.S.C.A. 3171 et seq. (West 1990 and Supp. 1996).

Drug-Free Workplace Act of 1988, 41 U.S.C.A. 701 et seq. (West Supp. 1996).

Dufour, M., and Fuller, R.K. 1995. Alcohol and the elderly. Annual Review of Medicine 46: 123-132.

Erwin, W.E., Williams, D.B., and Speir, W.A. 1998. Delirium tremens. Southern Medical Journal 91: 425-432.

Evans, G., O'Brien, R., and Chafetz, M., eds. 1991. The encyclopedia of alcoholism, 2nd ed. New York: Facts on File and Greenspring, Inc.

Fillmore, K.M., Golding, J.M., Graves, K.L., Kniep, S., Leino, E.V., Romelsjo, A., Shoemaker, C., Ager, C.R., Allebeck, P., and Ferrer, H.P. 1998. Alcohol consumption and mortality. I. Addiction 93: 183-203.

Fillmore, K.M., Golding, J.M., Leino, E.V., Ager, C.R., and Ferrer, H.P. 1994. Societal-level predictors of group drinking patterns: A research synthesis from the Collaborative Alcohol-Related Longitudinal Project. American Journal of Public Health 84: 247-253.

Fischer, B., Kendall, P., Rehm, J., and Room, R. 1997. Charting WHO—goals for licit and illicit drugs for the year 2000: Are we "on track"? Public Health 111(5): 271-275.

Funkhouser, J.E., Goplerud, E.N., and Bass, R.O. 1992. Current status of prevention programs. In A promising future: Alcohol and other drug problem prevention services improvement (OSAP Monograph No. 10, DHHS Publication No. ADM-92-1807), ed. M.A. Jansen, S. Becker, M. Klitzner, and K. Stewart, 17-82. Rockville, MD: Office for Substance Abuse Prevention.

Gallmeier, C.P. 1988. Juicing, burning, and tooting: Observing drug use among professional hockey players. Arena Review 12(1): 1-12.

Gaziano, J.M., Gaziano, T.A., Glynn, R.J., Sesso, H.D., Ajani, U.A., Stampfer, M.J., Manson, J.E., Hennekens, C.H., and Buring, J.E. 2000. Light-to-moderate alcohol consumption and mortality in the Physician's Health Study enrollment cohort. Journal of the American College of Cardiology 35(1): 96-105.

Golby, J. 1989. Use of factor analysis in the study of alcohol-induced strategy changes in skilled performance on a soccer test. Perceptual and Motor Skills 68(1): 147-156.

Goodwin, D.W., and Gabrielli, W.F. 1997. Alcohol: Clinical aspects. In Substance abuse: A comprehensive textbook, ed. J.H. Lowinson, P. Ruiz, M.A. Mill, and G. Langrod, 142-148. Baltimore: Williams & Wilkins.

Graham, K., Wilsnack, R., Dawson, D., and Vogeltanz, N. 1998. Should alcohol consumption measures be adjusted for gender differences? Addiction 93: 1137-1147.

Greenspan, A.J., and Schaal, S.F. 1983. The "holiday heart": Electrophysiologic studies of alcohol effects in alcoholics. Annals of Internal Medicine 98: 135.

Gronbaek, M.N., Iversen, L., Olsen, J., Becker, P.U., Hardt, F., and Sorensen, T.I. 1997. (Ovid Abstract). Sensible drinking limits. Ugeskrift for Laeger 159: 5939-5945.

Gutgesell, M.E., Timmerman, M., and Keller, A. 1996. Reported alcohol use and behavior in long-distance runners. Medicine and Science in Sports and Exercise 28: 1063-1070.

Heikkonen, E. 1989. Endocrine and metabolic changes induced by alcohol and physical exercise in healthy males. Helsinki, Finland: Turku.

Houmard, J.A., Langenfeld, M.E., Wiley, R.L., and Siefert, J. 1987. Effects of acute ingestion of small amounts of alcohol on 5-mile run times. Journal of Sports Medicine and Physical Fitness (Torino, Italy) 27: 253-257.

Jacobson, S.W., Jacobson, J.L., Sokol, R.J., Martier, S.S., and Ager, J.W. 1993. Prenatal alcohol exposure and infant information processing ability. Child Development 64: 1706-1721.

Jain, L. 1998. Maternal substance abuse. Indian Journal of Pediatrics 65(2): 283-289.

Johnson, W.O. 1988, August 8. Sports and suds: The beer business and the sports world have brewed up a potent partnership. Sports Illustrated 69: 68-82.

Johnston, L.D., O'Malley, P.M., and Bachman, J.G. 1998. National survey results on drug use from the monitoring the future study, 1975-1997. Vol. II: College students and young adults. (NIH Publication No. 98-4346). Rockville, MD: National Institute on Drug Abuse.

Johnston, L.D., O'Malley, P.M., and Bachman, J.G. 2000. The monitoring the future study: National results on adolescent drug use: Overview of key findings, 1999 (NIH Publication No. 00-4690). Bethesda, MD: National Institute on Drug Abuse.

Jokl, E. 1968. Notes on doping. Medicine and sport: Vol. 1: Exercise and altitude, ed. E. Jokl (series ed.) and E. Jokl and P. Jokl (vol. eds.), 55-57. Basel, Switzerland: Karger.

Karvinin, E., Miettinen, A., and Ahlman, K. 1962. Physical performance during hangover. Quarterly Journal of Studies on Alcohol 23: 208-215.

Kerr, J.S., and Hindmarch, I. 1998. The effects of alcohol alone or in combination with other drugs on information processing, task performance, and subjective responses. Human Psychopharmacology 13(1): 1-9.

Kokotailo, P.K., Henry, B.C., Koscik, R.E., Fleming, M.F., and Landry, G.L. 1996. Substance use and other health risk behaviors in collegiate athletes. Clinical Journal of Sport Medicine 6: 183-189.

Koller, W.C., and Biary, N. 1984. Effects of alcohol on tremors. Comparison with propranolol. Neurology 34: 221-222.

Kreitman, N. 1986. Alcohol consumption and the prevention paradox. British Journal of Addiction 81: 353-363.

Lawrence, S.P. 2000. Advances in the treatment of hepatitis C. Advances in Internal Medicine 45: 65-105.

Leichliter, J.S., Meilman, P.W., Presley, C.A., and Cashin, J.R. 1998. Alcohol use and related consequences among students with varying levels of involvement in college athletics. Journal of American College Health 46: 257-262.

Lucia, S.P. 1963. The antiquity of alcohol in diet and medicine. In Alcohol and civilization, ed. S.P. Lucia. New York: McGraw-Hill.

MacGregor, R.R., and Louria, D.B. 1997. Alcohol and infection. Current Clinical Topics in Infectious Diseases 17: 291-315.

Malone, D.L. 1991. The nature and extent of drug and alcohol use within a professional sports league. Ph.D. diss., University of Pittsburgh. Dissertation Abstracts International 52: 2823A.

Mannaioni, P.F. 1984. Clinical pharmacology of drug dependence. Padua, Italy: Piccin.

Martin, C.S., and Moss, H.B. 1993. Measurement of acute tolerance to alcohol in human subjects. Alcoholism: Clinical and Experimental Research 17: 211-216.

Martin, M. 1998. The use of alcohol among NCAA Division I female college basketball, softball, and volleyball athletes. Journal of Athletic Training 33(2): 163-167.

Mayer, R.R., Forster, J.L., Murray, D.M., and Wagenaar, A.C. 1998. Social settings and situations of underage drinking. Journal of Studies on Alcohol 59: 207-215.

McGinnis, J.M., and Foege, W.H. 1999. Mortality and morbidity attributable to use of addictive substances in the United States. Proceedings of the Association of American Physicians 111(2): 109-118.

McNaughton, L., and Preece, D. 1986. Alcohol and its effects on sprint and middle distance running. British Journal of Sports Medicine 20(2): 56-59.

Midanik, L.T., and Greenfield, T.K. 2000. Trends in social consequences and dependence symptoms in the United States: The national alcohol surveys, 1984-1995. American Journal of Public Health 90(1): 53-56.

Mills, J.L., Graubard, B.I., Harley, E.E., Rhoads, G.G., and Berendes, H.W. 1984. Maternal alcohol consumption and birth weight: How much drinking is safe during pregnancy? Journal of the American Medical Association 252: 1875-1879.

Mitchell, M. 1985. Alcohol-induced impairment of central nervous system function: Behavioral skills involved in driving. Journal of Studies on Alcohol Supplement 10: 109-116.

Moskowitz, H., Burns, M.M., and Williams, A.F. 1985. Skills performance at low blood alcohol levels. Journal of Studies on Alcohol 46: 482-485.

Nattiv, A., Puffer, J.C., and Green, G.A. 1997. Lifestyles and health risks of collegiate athletes: A multi-center study. Clinical Journal of Sport Medicine 7: 262-272.

Nephew, T.M., Williams, G.D., Stinson, F.S., Nguyen, K., and Dufour, M.C. 1999. Apparent per capita alcohol consumption: National, state, and regional trends, 1977-1997 (NIAAA Surveillance Report No. 51). Bethesda, MD: National Institute on Alcohol Abuse and Alcoholism.

O'Brien, C.P. 1993. Alcohol and sport: Impact of social drinking on recreational and competitive sports performance [Guest Editorial]. Sports Medicine 15: 71-77.

O'Brien, C.P. 1997. Approach to the problem of alcohol abuse and dependence. In Textbook of internal medicine, ed. W.N. Kelley, 168-171. Philadelphia: Lippincott-Raven.

Parsons, O.A., and Nixon, S.J. 1998. Cognitive functioning in sober social drinkers: A review of the research since 1986. Journal of Studies on Alcohol 59: 180-190.

Pate, R.R., Trost, S.G., Levin, S., and Dowda, M. 2000. Sports participation and health-related behaviors among US youth. Archives of Pediatric and Adolescent Medicine 154: 904-911.

Puddey, I.B., Rakic, V., Dimmitt, S.B., and Beilin, L.J. 1999. Influence of pattern of drinking on cardiovascular disease and cardiovascular risk factors—a review. Addiction 94(5): 649-663.

Rainey, C.J., McKeown, R.E., Sargent, R.G., and Valois, R.F. 1996. Patterns of tobacco and alcohol use among sedentary, exercising, nonathletic, and athletic youth. Journal of School Health 66(1): 27-32.

Ray, O., and Ksir, C. 1993. Drugs, society, and human behavior. St. Louis: Mosby.

Reichman, M.E., Judd, J.T., Longcope, C., Schatzkin, A., Cleridence, B.A., Nair, P.P., Campbell, W.S., and Taylor, R.R. 1993. Effects of alcohol consumption on plasma and urinary hormone concentrations in premenopausal women. Journal of the National Cancer Institute 86: 722-727.

Reilly, T. 1996. Alcohol, anti-anxiety drugs and sport. In Drugs in sport, ed. D.R. Mottram, 144-172. London: Spon.

Reilly, T., and Halliday, F. 1985. Influence of alcohol ingestion on tasks related to archery. Journal of Human Ergology 14(2): 99-104.

Room, R., Bondy, S.J., and Ferris, J. 1995. The risk of harm to oneself from drinking, Canada 1989. Addiction 90: 499-513.

Rossow, I., and Amundsen, A. 1997. Alcohol abuse and mortality: A 40-year prospective study of Norwegian conscripts. Social Science Medicine 44: 261-267.

Rouse, B.A., ed. 1998. Substance abuse and mental health statistics source book. Rockville, MD: Department of Health and Human Services.

Saini, J., Boisvert, P., Speigel, K., Candas, V., and Brandenberger, G. 1995. Influence of alcohol on the hydromineral hormone responses to exercise in a warm environment. European Journal of Applied Physiology and Occupational Physiology 72: 32-36.

San Jose, B., van de Mheen, H., van Oers, J.A., Mackenbach, J.P., and Garretsen, H.F. 1999. The U-shaped curve: Various health measures and alcohol drinking patterns. Journal of Studies on Alcohol 60: 725-731.

Schlaadt, R.G., and Shannon, P.T. 1994. Drugs: Use, misuse and abuse. Englewood Cliffs, NJ: Prentice Hall.

Schuckit, M.A. 1994. Alcohol and alcoholism. In Harrison's principles of internal medicine, ed. R.J. Isselbacker, E. Braunwald, J.D. Wilson, J.D. Martin, J.B. Fauci, and A.S. Kasper, 2420-2425. New York: McGraw-Hill.

Seto, M.C., and Barbaree, H.E. 1995. The role of alcohol in sexual aggression. Clinical Psychology Review 15: 546-566.

Shephard, R.J. 1972. Alive man: The physiology of physical activity. Springfield, IL: Charles C Thomas.

Stainback, R.D. 1997. Alcohol and sport. Champaign, IL: Human Kinetics.

Stuck, M.F. 1990. Adolescent worlds: Drug use and athletic activity. New York: Praeger.

Substance Abuse and Mental Health Services Administration. 1999. Summary of findings from the 1998 national household survey on drug abuse (DHHS Publication No. SMA 99-3328). Rockville, MD: Substance Abuse and Mental Health Services Administration.

Svardsudd, K. 1998. Moderate alcohol consumption and cardiovascular disease: Is this their evidence for a preventive effect? Alcoholism: Clinical and Experimental Research 22(7 Suppl): 307S-314S.

Szabo, G. 1999. Consequences of alcohol consumption on host defense. Alcohol and Alcoholism 34: 830-841.

Thakker, K. 1998. An overview of health risks and benefits of alcohol consumption. Alcoholism: Clinical and Experimental Research 22(7 Suppl): 285S-298S.

Toomey, T.L., and Wagenaar, A.C. 1999. Policy options for prevention: The case of alcohol. Journal of Public Health Policy 20(2): 192-213.

U.S. Department of Health and Human Services. 1993. Eighth special report to the U.S. Congress on alcohol and health (Contract No. ADM-281-91-0003). Rockville, MD: National Institute on Alcohol Abuse and Alcoholism.

U.S. Department of Health and Human Services. 1997. Ninth special report to the U.S. Congress on alcohol and health (NIH Publication No. 97-4017). Rockville, MD: National Institute on Alcohol Abuse and Alcoholism.

Van Hightower, N.R., and Gorton, J. 1998. Domestic violence among patients at two rural health care clinics: Prevalence and social correlates. Public Health Nursing 15(5): 355-362.

Vital statistics. 1993. The Edell Health Letter 12 (March): 5.

Wadler, G.I., and Hainline, B. 1989. Drugs and the athlete. Philadelphia: Davis.

Wechsler, H., Dowdall, G.W., Maenner, G., Gledhill-Hoyt, J., and Lee, H. 1998. Changes in binge drinking and related problems among American college students between 1993 and 1997: Results of the Harvard School of Public Health College Alcohol Study. Journal of American College Health 47(2): 57-68.

Wetterling, T., Veltrup, C., Driessen, M., and John, U. 1999. Drinking pattern and alcohol related medical disorders. Alcohol and Alcoholism 34(3): 330-336.

Wiese, J.G., Shlipak, M.G., and Browner, W.S. 2000. The alcohol hangover. Annals of Internal Medicine 132: 897-902.

Williams, M.H. 1991. Alcohol, marijuana, and beta blockers. In Perspectives in exercise science and sports medicine: Vol. 4: Ergogenics—enhancement of performance in exercise and sport, ed. D.R. Lamb and M.H. Williams, 331-372. Dubuque, IA: Brown & Benchmark.

Williams, M.H. 1998. Alcohol intake and sport performance. Strength and Conditioning 20(2): 16-17.

Wood, P.K., Sher, K.J., and McGowan, A.K. 2000. Collegiate alcohol involvement and role attainment: Findings from a prospective high-risk study. Journal of Studies in Alcohol 61: 278-289.

Yi, H., Stinson, F.S., Williams, G.D., and Bertolucci, D. 1999. Trends in alcohol-related fatal traffic crashes, United States, 1975-97 (NIAAA Surveillance Report No. 49). Bethesda, MD: National Institute on Alcohol Abuse and Alcoholism.

Young, D.S., and Young, D.B. 1989. Drug testing and student-athlete assistance programs in National Collegiate Athletic Association women's sports. Journal of Applied Research in Coaching and Athletics 4(2): 94-108.

Yu, J., and Shacket, R.W. 1998. Long-term changes in underage drinking and impaired driving after the establishment of drinking age laws in New York State. Alcoholism: Clinical and Experimental Research 22: 1443-1449.

CHAPTER 20

Cannabis: Clinical Pharmacology and Performance Effects in Humans

Stephen J. Heishman, PhD

Humans have used the plant *Cannabis sativa* to make rope and clothing and for medicinal purposes for thousands of years. The ancient Greeks and Romans knew about the strength of cannabis or hemp rope, and the Chinese emperor Shen-Nung wrote about the medicinal properties of cannabis in 2700 B.C.—making it one of the oldest drugs in recorded history (Adams and Martin 1996). The intoxicating and euphoric effects of cannabis had been identified by 1400 B.C. in India. Today, in countries that conduct surveys regarding drug use, cannabis is the most widely used illicit drug. Recreational users of cannabis typically seek the euphoric and relaxing effects of the drug. However, the addictive effects of cannabis are evident in individuals seeking treatment for cannabis dependence who report significant psychiatric and psychosocial distress, including withdrawal symptoms (Stephens, Roffman, and Simpson 1993; Budney et al. 1998; Budney, Novy, and Hughes 1999). Recently, in the United States, a growing movement has focused attention on the medicinal properties of smoked cannabis, which brings us full circle with the ancient Chinese and Indians. The purpose of this chapter is to review briefly the clinical pharmacology of cannabis with an emphasis on its performance and health effects, which are most salient to athletes who may use cannabis.

Source of Cannabis

The plant *C. sativa* contains more than 400 chemicals, of which about 60 are referred to as cannabinoids. The primary psychoactive cannabinoid, delta-9-tetrahydrocannabinol (THC), was isolated in 1964. Cannabinoids are found in the resin that is secreted by the flowering tops and leaves of the plant. The concentration of THC varies greatly between the three main preparations of the cannabis plant: marijuana (comparable to the preparation referred to by the Indian names *bhang* and *ganja*), hashish *(charas)*, and hash oil.

Marijuana consists of the dried and crushed leaves and flowering tops of the plant. Sinsemilla refers to a preparation of only the flowering tops of the unfertilized female plant and typically has a higher THC concentration than marijuana. In 1999, the average THC concentration of seized commercial-grade marijuana in the United

States was 5.2%; the average for sinsemilla was 13.4% THC (personal communication, Robert Brown, Drug Enforcement Agency). Marijuana is typically smoked as small hand-rolled cigarettes (joints) or through a water pipe. Of recent popularity is the smoking of blunts, which are hollowed cigar wrappers filled with marijuana. Hashish consists of the resin of the plant and usually takes the form of dried cakes. The THC concentration of hashish is 5 to 10 times that of marijuana. Hash oil is a dark, viscous liquid that can contain THC concentrations up to 80%.

Prevalence of Cannabis Use

Cannabis is by far the most widely used illicit drug in the United States, accounting for 75% of all reported illicit drug use in 1999. Recent surveys indicate that 34.6% of the U.S. population over age 12 (76.4 million people) report having used marijuana at least once in their lifetime; and 5.1% (11.1 million) are current users, reporting use in the past month (Substance Abuse and Mental Health Services Administration 2000). Cannabis use is most frequent among young adults, aged 18 to 25; use is rare in adults older than 35 years. This suggests that the majority of individuals use cannabis on a recreational basis and stop using as they mature. However, of those reporting current use of cannabis, 25% report having used it on 20 to 30 days during the past month. Daily, chronic cannabis users are at high risk for experiencing the adverse health and cognitive effects of long-term cannabis use (see later).

Clinical Pharmacology

Numerous studies have documented the complex pharmacology of cannabis in humans, including its unique psychological "high" and the adverse cognitive and performance effects caused by acute doses. During the past decade, advances in cannabinoid neurochemistry have given us a glimpse at the brain mechanisms underlying many of the effects of cannabis.

Endogenous Cannabinoid System

Like many other therapeutic and nontherapeutic drugs, THC binds to receptors, proteins embedded in cell membranes that initiate a cascade of physiological events culminating in some measurable response, such as euphoria or increased pulse. Studies have shown that the behavioral, physiological, mood, and cognitive effects produced by THC are mediated through a specific cannabinoid receptor (CB1), which is located in the central and peripheral nervous systems (Matsuda et al. 1990; Gerard et al. 1991; Ledent et al. 1999). A second cannabinoid receptor subtype (CB2) appears to be concentrated in the peripheral immune system (Munro, Thomas, and Abu-Shaar 1993). The identification of specific cannabinoid receptors has led to the discovery of a group of endogenous cannabinoids, such as anandamide, that also bind to the CB1 receptor and mimic the effects of THC (Devane et al. 1992).

Recently, a selective CB1 receptor antagonist, SR141716, has been developed. Antagonist drugs bind to the receptor site; but they do not initiate any effect, and prevent the drug from binding to the receptor. In the first human study, Huestis et al. (2001) found that SR141716 dose-dependently blocked the psychoactive effects and the increased pulse produced by smoked marijuana. These findings suggest that CB1 receptors play an important role in mediating the effects of THC in humans.

Pharmacodynamics

Cannabis produces distinct changes in mood, physiology, psychomotor performance, and cognitive functioning. A subsequent section reviews the acute effects of cannabis on performance and cognition. The most commonly reported mood change after smoking cannabis is the psychological "high," which is characterized by feelings of euphoria and relaxation. The "high" serves as the primary reinforcing (motivating) factor among recreational users of the drug. Clinical laboratory studies with experienced cannabis users have shown that the subjective "high" begins within the first few puffs, lasts for several hours, and is dose related, such that larger doses produce greater responses (Huestis, Henningfield, and Cone 1992; Heishman, Arasteh, and Stitzer 1997). Other psychological effects of cannabis include increased intensity of sensory experiences, talkativeness, laughter, and perceptual distortions, such as an altered sense of time (Hall, Solowij, and Lemon 1994; Heishman and Stitzer 1989).

The most reliable physiological effects of cannabis are increased pulse and conjunctival injection (red eyes). Smoking one marijuana cigarette produced peak increases in heart rate of 25 to 35 beats per minute over baseline; the peak was at 10 min after smoking, and the heart rate declined gradually over the next 75 min (Heishman, Stitzer, and Yingling 1989). As with the psychological effects, the cardiovascular effects are dose dependent.

Pharmacokinetics

The pharmacokinetics (absorption, distribution, metabolism, and excretion) of THC are complex. When cannabis is smoked, THC is rapidly absorbed into the bloodstream from the lungs and reaches the brain within 8 to 10 sec. This rate of absorption accounts for the rapid onset of effects from smoked cannabis. Plasma concentration of THC peaks immediately at the end of smoking (Huestis, Sampson et al. 1992) in the range of 80 to 160 ng/ml (Heishman et al. 1990; Azorlosa et al. 1992; Huestis, Henningfield, and Cone 1992). Because THC is a highly lipophilic molecule, it leaves the blood rapidly and is deposited in the fatty tissues of the body. As a result, plasma THC concentration falls below 20 ng/ml within 30 to 45 min after smoking.

Delta-9-tetrahydrocannabinol is extensively metabolized in the liver. The principal inactive metabolite is 11-nor-9-carboxy-delta-9-tetrahydrocannabinol (THC-COOH), which is the compound tested for in urine drug tests. Because THC is stored in fat tissue and slowly released back into the bloodstream, urinary levels of THC-COOH can remain elevated for some time, resulting in a positive drug test. In occasional cannabis users, THC-COOH can be detected in urine for two to three days after the smoking of one marijuana cigarette; however, in daily users, who have larger stores of THC, urinary cannabinoids might be detected for up to several weeks. For these reasons and because the dose of THC ingested is rarely known, it is very difficult to determine the time of cannabis smoking from a single cannabinoid-positive urine test. Because cannabis can impair psychomotor and cognitive abilities critical for driving, there has been interest in determining the relationship between plasma THC or THC-COOH concentration and performance. However, this knowledge has proved elusive because while THC concentration is decreasing during the first 30 to 45 min after smoking, performance impairment is increasing. The issue of impairment of performance by cannabis the day after smoking is discussed in a subsequent section.

Use in Clinical Medicine

Cannabis has been used for thousands of years to treat various maladies, such as gout, rheumatism, malaria, headache, and constipation. In the United States, the late 19th and early 20th centuries saw the development and marketing of nearly 30 legal cannabis preparations, which found some popularity as analgesic, anticonvulsant, and muscle-relaxant medications. However, as more effective drugs were developed for most illnesses, the therapeutic use of cannabis declined; and in 1941, cannabis was removed from the U.S. Pharmacopoeia.

In 1987, an oral formulation of synthetic THC, dronabinol (Marinol), was approved by the Food and

Drug Administration. Although THC remains in Schedule I, Marinol is a Schedule III drug because its formulation in sesame oil, slow onset of action, and relatively weak reinforcing effects result in a lower abuse potential than for smoked cannabis (Calhoun, Galloway, and Smith 1998). Marinol is indicated for the treatment of anorexia associated with weight loss in autoimmune deficiency syndrome patients and for nausea and vomiting associated with cancer chemotherapy.

In its recent report, *Marijuana and Medicine,* the Institute on Medicine (IOM) concluded that the scientific data indicated a potential therapeutic benefit for cannabinoid drugs, especially THC, for pain relief, control of nausea and vomiting, and appetite stimulation (Joy, Watson, and Benson 1999). The report also acknowledged that more effective medications exist for such symptoms and that the therapeutic efficacy of cannabinoids is modest. However, the IOM recommended that clinical trials be conducted with the purpose of developing rapid-onset and safe delivery systems (e.g., inhaler) of cannabinoids.

Acute and Chronic Health Effects

As previously mentioned, one of the most reliable acute effects of cannabis is an increased heart rate (tachycardia) observed shortly after smoking, which can last for 1 to 2 hr. In healthy, young cannabis users, this tachycardia probably has no clinical significance, primarily because tolerance develops to the cardiovascular effects of cannabis (Hall et al. 1994). However, in nontolerant users with cardiovascular disease (e.g., hypertension or atherosclerosis), a rapid increase in heart rate may have adverse medical consequences. The acute toxicity of cannabis is low. Thus, it is extremely unlikely that someone could achieve a lethal dose by smoking or eating cannabis preparations.

Because many individuals use cannabis repeatedly over a number of years, there has been considerable research on the chronic health effects of cannabis. Studies have shown that THC can alter cellular metabolism and DNA synthesis. Animal studies have consistently indicated that cannabis smoke is mutagenic, and thus potentially carcinogenic, and that THC and other cannabinoids impair the immune system (Hall et al. 1994). However, in humans, the evidence for immune system damage is not consistent, with some studies indicating adverse effects and others suggesting no effect. Similarly, the limited research in humans is inconsistent regarding cannabis-induced reproductive system dysfunction.

In contrast to these questionable adverse effects of cannabis, there is clear evidence that cannabis smoking produces respiratory pathology. Tashkin and colleagues (Tashkin et al. 1987; Wu et al. 1988; Fligiel et al. 1997; Roth et al. 1998) have demonstrated that cannabis smokers exhibit significant airway inflammation, increased tar inhalation and retention and blood carboxyhemoglobin levels, and bronchial histopathology. Such pulmonary insult results in increased risk of chronic bronchitis and pathology leading to lung cancer. In general, the effects of cannabis and tobacco are additive with respect to these respiratory diseases.

Use of Cannabis in Sport

There is no evidence in the literature that athletes use cannabis to enhance their performance in competitive events (Wagner 1991; Catlin and Murray 1996). As detailed in the following section, cannabis typically impairs psychomotor abilities and cognitive processing. Physical work capacity as measured with a bicycle ergometer is also significantly diminished after smoking marijuana (Steadward and Singh 1975). Anecdotal reports suggest that athletes may use cannabis to relax and be loose before competition or to relax after an intense workout, but there is no empirical support for this (Wagner 1991). Epidemiological studies indicate that individuals who use anabolic-androgenic steroids are more likely to use other drugs of abuse, including cannabis, than those who don't use steroids. For example, 19% of college students using steroids reported using cannabis daily during the previous year compared to 4% of those not using steroids (Meilman et al. 1995). Kindlundh et al. (1999) found that drug use was more common among adolescents who were using steroids for fun or because of peer pressure compared with those using steroids to improve appearance or enhance athletic performance.

Marijuana is listed as a banned substance by the International Olympic Committee (IOC). During Olympic competition, if an athlete's urine tests positive for cannabinoids, sanctions can follow. Outside of Olympic competition, cases are referred to the various international sport federations, each of which has its own rules on sanctions for marijuana use. Federations that ban marijuana in competition, such as the International Ski Federation, could impose sanctions on member athletes. If, however, a federation does not ban marijuana, sanctions might be imposed by a national team. Although there is no scientific evidence that cannabis enhances performance, there are other reasons for its classification as a banned substance. In sports that entail speed and agility (e.g., skiing, bobsledding), safety is a great concern; and cannabis can impair psychomotor skills, coordination, and cognitive functions. Other arguments for banning cannabis are that in most countries it is an illegal drug and that Olympic athletes are role models for younger athletes (Catlin and Murray 1996).

The 1998 Winter Olympics in Nagano, Japan, provided a highly publicized instance of the supposed use of cannabis in sport. After Ross Rebagliati won the gold medal in snowboarding, his urine tested positive for THC-COOH, the primary cannabinoid metabolite. The IOC board voted 3 to 2 to disqualify Rebagliati and asked him to return the medal. Rebagliati claimed that the positive test was due to environmental exposure to cannabis smoke. However, laboratory studies have shown that in order to test positive from passive marijuana smoke inhalation, one must endure noxious smoke conditions in an enclosed space for an extended period of time (Perez-Reyes et al. 1983; Cone and Johnson 1986). The Canadian Olympic Association appealed the IOC's decision to the Committee for the Arbitration of Sport. On a legal technicality, the committee ruled that because the IOC did not have an agreement with the International Ski Federation on cannabis use, the IOC could not disqualify Rebagliati. In restoring the medal, the committee avoided the controversial issue of recreational cannabis use.

Performance Effects of Cannabis

The performance effects of acute cannabis administration have been investigated in numerous laboratory studies over the past several decades (Chait and Pierri 1992; Beardsley and Kelly 1999). This literature derives primarily from the fields of behavioral and clinical pharmacology and not from sports medicine. Cannabis has not been a focus of the sports medicine field, probably because athletes do not use cannabis to enhance their performance. Thus, data from some studies (e.g., motor skills) may relate more directly to sport than data from other studies (e.g., cognitive processing).

This overview of the literature deals with the effects of cannabis on sensory, motor, attentional, and cognitive abilities. The chronic effect of cannabis on cognitive functioning is summarized next. The section concludes with a brief discussion of two behavioral effects of marijuana that have received much research attention, next-day or hangover effects and an amotivational syndrome. Unless otherwise noted, the studies reviewed in this section were conducted with experienced cannabis users who smoked research cigarettes containing marijuana, which were provided by the National Institute on Drug Abuse. These marijuana cigarettes resemble an unfiltered tobacco cigarette in size, weigh 700 to 900 mg, and are assayed to determine the percentage of THC by weight. Doses are typically manipulated through the use of cigarettes that differ in THC content or through variation in the number of puffs administered to subjects. Placebo marijuana cigarettes, which have had the THC removed chemically from the plant material, are also available. When burned, placebo cigarettes smell exactly the same as active-marijuana cigarettes.

Sensory Abilities

A frequently used measure of central nervous system (CNS) functioning is the critical flicker frequency (CFF) threshold. The task requires subjects to view a light stimulus and to note the point (CFF threshold) at which the steady light begins to flicker (and vice versa), as the frequency of the light is manipulated. An increase in CFF threshold indicates increased cortical and behavioral arousal, whereas a decrease suggests lowered CNS arousal (Smith and Misiak 1976). Surprisingly, few studies have investigated the effect of cannabis on CFF threshold. Block, Farinpour, and Braverman (1992) reported that one marijuana cigarette (2.6% THC) decreased CFF threshold compared with placebo. However, Liguori, Gatto, and Robinson (1998) reported that one marijuana cigarette (1.8% and 4.0% THC) did not affect CFF threshold. Methodological differences between the studies may account for the conflicting results. More studies are needed to clarify the effect of cannabis on CFF threshold.

An increase in the subjective passage of time relative to clock time—more a perceptual process than a sensory ability—is a commonly reported effect of cannabis. This typically results in subjects either overestimating an experimenter-generated time interval (Chait, Fischman, and Schuster 1985) or underproducing a subject-generated interval (Chait and Perry 1994). However, Heishman et al. (1997) found that 3.6% THC marijuana cigarettes (4, 8, or 16 puffs) had no effect on either time estimation or production.

Motor Abilities

In their review, Chait and Pierri (1992) indicated that cannabis moderately impaired balance (increased body sway) and hand steadiness. Consistent with this motor impairment, one marijuana cigarette (1.5% or 4.0% THC) was found to decrease postural balance as subjects attempted to maintain balance while standing on a moving platform (Greenberg et al. 1994; Liguori et al. 1998). The circular lights test is another measure of gross-motor coordination in which subjects extinguish lights by pressing buttons that are arranged in a circle on a wall-mounted panel. Cone et al. (1986) found that two marijuana cigarettes (2.8% THC) impaired performance on the circular lights task, whereas Heishman, Stitzer, and Bigelow (1988) reported no effect of marijuana (1.3% and 2.7% THC, two cigarettes) on circular lights performance.

The effect of cannabis on fine-motor control has also been examined. The time taken to sort a deck of playing cards was increased after the smoking of one 2.9% THC marijuana cigarette (Chait et al. 1985). In contrast, several studies have shown that cannabis did not influence finger tapping rate (Chait and Pierri 1992), which is considered to be a measure of pure motor activity.

Attentional Abilities

Attention is a broad psychological construct encompassing behaviors such as searching, scanning, and detecting visual and auditory stimuli for brief or long periods of time (Kinchla 1992). In nearly all tests assessing attention, responding is measured in some temporal form, such as reaction or response time, time off target, or response rate. Response accuracy may also be reported. Because of differential drug effects, a distinction between focused, selective, divided, and sustained attention can be instructive.

Focused attention can be defined as attending to one task for a brief period of time, usually 5 min or less. A relatively large number of studies have investigated the effects of cannabis on focused attention, including reaction time tests. One study showed that marijuana (1.8% and 3.6% THC) slowed responding on a simple, visual reaction time task (Wilson et al. 1994), whereas others have not found marijuana to impair simple reaction time performance (Chait and Pierri 1992; Foltin et al. 1993; Heishman et al. 1997). In contrast, marijuana has been consistently shown to impair complex or choice reaction time tasks (Block et al. 1992; Chait and Pierri 1992).

Another commonly used test of psychomotor skills and focused attention is the digit symbol substitution test (DSST), which requires subjects to type a pattern associated with each numeral from 1 to 9 (McLeod et al. 1982). In general, cannabis impairs performance on the DSST. In concentrations ranging from 1.8% to 3.6% THC, marijuana has been shown to decrease number of attempted responses (speed) and/or decrease number of correct responses (accuracy) on the DSST (Heishman et al. 1988, 1989, 1997; Azorlosa et al. 1992; Kelly, Foltin, and Fischman 1993; Chait and Perry 1994). Oral THC (10 and 20 mg) also impaired DSST performance (Kamien et al. 1994). However, other studies have shown no effect of marijuana (1.3-3.6% THC) on the DSST (Chait et al. 1985; Foltin et al. 1993; Azorlosa, Greenwald, and Stitzer 1995). The reasons for a lack of effect in these latter studies is unclear because doses of marijuana were comparable across studies; and in one study (Azorlosa et al. 1995), task presentation was identical to that in the studies reporting impairment. Marijuana (1.2% THC) also impaired selective attention as evidenced by slower responding and greater interference scores in the Stroop color naming test (Hooker and Jones 1987).

Divided attention has generally been shown to be impaired by cannabis. Most divided-attention tests consist of a central or primary task and a secondary or peripheral task. Several studies have shown that marijuana impaired detection accuracy and/or stimulus reaction time in one or both test components (Chait, Corwin, and Johanson 1988; Perez-Reyes et al. 1988; Marks and MacAvoy

1989; Azorlosa et al. 1992; Chait and Perry 1994). Kelly, Foltin, Emurian, and Fischman (1993) used a complex, 5-min divided-attention test in which an arithmetic task was presented in the center of the video monitor and three other stimulus-detection tasks were presented in the corners of the monitor. Performance was impaired in a dose-related manner after the smoking of one marijuana cigarette (2.0% or 3.5% THC). This finding illustrates that cannabis disrupts performance in complex tasks requiring the ability to shift attention between various stimuli. These same abilities are required when one is operating a motor vehicle. In a study of drivers who reported smoking marijuana within 2 hr of driving, 56% indicated that marijuana did not adversely affect their driving ability. However, laboratory tests that model various components of driving (Moskowitz 1985; Liguori et al. 1998; Kurzthaler et al. 1999) and tests of on-road driving (Robbe 1994) were impaired by cannabis. Thus, driving under the influence of cannabis may play a causative role in traffic accidents and injuries (Bates and Blakely 1999).

Cannabis also impairs sustained attention. In a 30-min vigilance task, hashish users exhibited more false alarms than nonusing control subjects (Bahri and Amir 1994). This finding is consistent with the observation that the impairing effects of cannabis on sustained attention are most evident in tests that last 30 to 60 min; tests with durations of 10 min are typically not adversely affected by cannabis (Chait and Pierri 1992).

Cognitive Abilities

Cannabis has been shown to impair learning in the repeated-acquisition and performance of response sequence tasks, which comprise separate acquisition (learning) and performance components (Bickel, Hughes, and Higgins 1990). This task allows independent assessment of drug effects on acquisition of new information and on performance of previously learned information. Increased errors in the acquisition phase were reported after subjects smoked marijuana (Kelly, Foltin, and Fischman 1993) and oral THC (Kamien et al. 1994). However, other studies have shown no effect of marijuana on this test (Foltin and Fischman 1990; Foltin et al. 1993). Block et al. (1992) reported that one 2.6% THC marijuana cigarette impaired paired-associative learning.

One of the most reliable behavioral effects of cannabis is the impairment of memory processes. Numerous studies have shown that smoked marijuana decreased the number of words or digits recalled and/or increased the number of intrusion errors in immediate or delayed tests of free recall after presentation of information to be remembered (Chait et al. 1985; Hooker and Jones 1987; Heishman et al. 1989, 1990, 1997; Azorlosa et al. 1992; Block et al.

1992; Kelly, Foltin, Emurian, and Fischman 1993). Using an extensive battery of cognitive tests, Block et al. (1992) reported that marijuana (2.6% THC) slowed response time for producing word associations; slowed the reading of prose; and impaired tests of reading comprehension, verbal expression, and mathematics. Heishman et al. (1990) also found that simple addition and subtraction skills were impaired by the smoking of one, two, or four marijuana cigarettes (2.6% THC). Finally, Kelly, Foltin, Emurian, and Fischman (1993) reported that marijuana (2.0% and 3.5% THC) slowed response time in a spatial orientation test requiring subjects to determine whether number and letters were displayed normally or as a mirror image when they were rotated between 90° and 270°.

Chronic Effects of Cannabis on Cognition

Numerous studies, including those from cultures in which cannabis use is very common, indicate that the cognitive consequences from chronic cannabis use are subtle. Functions most readily affected include memory, attention, and the processing of complex information (Block and Ghoneim 1993; Fletcher et al. 1996; Hall et al. 1994). Whether such subtle impairment affects daily functioning is not known. Research indicates that impairment increases with duration of cannabis use; typically, cognitive deficits are observed only after 5 to 10 years of use. Recent evidence indicates that cognitive impairment may persist for some time after cannabis use has ceased (Pope, Gruber, and Yurgelun-Todd 1995; Pope and Yurgelun-Todd 1996). Gruber and Pope (2000) recently reported that long-term, frequent cannabis users were impaired on tests of memory and mental flexibility compared with occasional users 28 days after being abstinent from cannabis. Whether such residual cognitive deficits resolve after longer periods of abstinence or persist permanently will have to be resolved by future research.

Next-Day or Hangover Effects

Over the years, an intriguing research question with important practical implications has been whether cannabis impairs performance beyond the period of acute intoxication, which typically lasts 2 to 6 hr after a person has smoked one or two cigarettes. Recently, studies have documented performance decrements 12 to 24 hr after the smoking of marijuana (Pope et al. 1995). One series of studies showed that 24 hr after smoking one marijuana cigarette (2.2% THC), experienced aircraft pilots were impaired in attempting to land a plane in a flight simulator (Yesavage et al. 1985; Leirer, Yesavage, and Morrow 1991); however, a third study failed to replicate this next-day effect (Leirer, Yesavage, and

Morrow 1989). In another series of studies, a comprehensive battery of tests revealed that only time estimation (Chait et al. 1985) and memory (Chait 1990) were impaired 9 to 17 hr after subjects smoked two marijuana cigarettes (2.1-2.9% THC), leading the authors to conclude that evidence for next-day performance effects of marijuana was weak. Yet another series of studies showed next-day impairment on tests of memory and mental arithmetic after the smoking of two or four marijuana cigarettes (2.6% THC) over a 4-hr period (Heishman et al. 1990), but not after one marijuana cigarette (Heishman et al. 1990; Fant et al. 1998). Thus, residual impairment appears to be a dose-related phenomenon, with effects more likely to be observed at higher cannabis doses.

Amotivational Syndrome

A long-standing, controversial issue has been the amotivational syndrome allegedly caused by heavy, chronic cannabis use. This syndrome has been characterized by feelings of lethargy and apathy and an absence of goal-directed behavior (McGlothin and West 1968; Kupfer et al. 1973). However, studies conducted in countries where segments of the population use cannabis heavily (Comitas 1976; Stefanis, Dornbush, and Fink 1977; Page 1983), as well as laboratory studies in North America (Mendelson et al. 1976; Kagel, Battalio, and Miles 1980; Kelly et al. 1990), have not found empirical support for an amotivational syndrome. Foltin and colleagues (Foltin et al. 1989; Foltin, Fischman, Brady, Bernstein, Capriotti, Nellis, and Kelly 1990; Foltin, Fischman, Brady, Bernstein, Nellis, and Kelly 1990) have conducted several inpatient studies lasting 15 to 18 days with subjects reporting weekly marijuana use. Subjects were required to perform low-probability tasks such as the DSST, word sorting, and vigilance to gain access to more highly desired (high probability) work and recreational activities. On days when subjects smoked active marijuana, the amount of time they spent on low-probability tasks increased, which is inconsistent with an amotivational syndrome. Additionally, the effect of marijuana on time spent on low- versus high-probability activities differed for work and recreational activities, indicating that the behavioral effects of marijuana are context dependent and not readily predicted by a simplistic amotivational hypothesis (Beardsley and Kelly 1999).

Summary of Performance Effects

Laboratory studies in which subjects smoked marijuana have documented that marijuana impaired sensory-perceptual abilities by increasing the subjective passage of time relative to clock time. Marijuana impaired gross-motor coordination as measured by body sway and postural balance. However, inconsistent findings have been reported for fine-motor control; hand steadiness was impaired, whereas several studies showed no effect of marijuana on finger tapping. Marijuana has been shown to impair complex, but not simple, reaction time tests. A majority of studies have shown that marijuana disrupted performance on the DSST. Complex divided-attention tests, including driving a vehicle, were readily impaired by marijuana, as were tests requiring sustained attention for more than 30 min. Numerous studies have documented that smoked marijuana and oral THC impaired learning, memory, and other cognitive processes. The chronic use of cannabis results in subtle cognitive impairment in memory, attention, and information processing. Residual or next-day impairment is not a robust phenomenon, but some studies suggest that it is dose related. Empirical evidence does not support a cannabis-induced amotivational syndrome.

Legal Status of Cannabis

In the United States, cannabis (marijuana) and THC were classified as Schedule I drugs under the Comprehensive Drug Abuse Prevention and Control Act of 1970. Schedule I drugs are considered to have the highest abuse potential and no recognized medical use and carry the stiffest penalties (fines and jail terms) for illegal possession, manufacturing, and distribution. Over the years, several petitions have been sent to the Drug Enforcement Administration requesting that marijuana be rescheduled so that it could be prescribed for medical purposes. All of these petitions have failed to change the federal status of marijuana. However, as of the November 2000 election, nine states (Alaska, Arizona, California, Colorado, Hawaii, Maine, Nevada, Oregon, and Washington) have some form of medical marijuana law through either ballot initiatives or legislative action.

Conclusion

Millions of people throughout the world smoke or consume cannabis preparations in search of an altered state of consciousness, characterized by euphoria and relaxation. However, cannabis adversely affects psychomotor performance and cognitive functioning, and for this reason, athletes typically do not use cannabis before competitions. Although there is no evidence that cannabis enhances performance, there are anecdotal reports that athletes smoke cannabis to relax before competition or after intense workouts. Cannabis has been banned by the IOC and various international sport federations during competition because of safety concerns. Considerable progress has been made over the past decade on the neurophysiology and neuropharmacology of the cannabinoid system. The goal of future research will be to explore the functional significance of

this neuroscientific knowledge with respect to human behavior. The end result may be the development of novel therapeutic agents for the treatment of conditions known to have cannabinoid involvement, such as memory loss, movement disorders, and mood disturbances.

References

Adams, I.B., and B.R. Martin. 1996. Cannabis: pharmacology and toxicology in animals and humans. *Addiction* 91: 1585-1614.

Azorlosa, J.L., M.K. Greenwald, and M.L. Stitzer. 1995. Marijuana smoking: effects of varying puff volume and breathhold duration. *Journal of Pharmacology and Experimental Therapeutics* 272: 560-569.

Azorlosa, J.L., S.J. Heishman, M.L. Stitzer, and J.M. Mahaffey. 1992. Marijuana smoking: effect of varying Δ^9-tetrahydrocannabinol content and number of puffs. *Journal of Pharmacology and Experimental Therapeutics* 261: 114-122.

Bahri, T., and T. Amir. 1994. Effect of hashish on vigilance performance. *Perceptual and Motor Skills* 78: 11-16.

Bates, M.N., and T.A. Blakely. 1999. Role of cannabis in motor vehicle crashes. *Epidemiologic Reviews* 21: 222-232.

Beardsley, P.M., and T.H. Kelly. 1999. Acute effects of cannabis on human behavior and central nervous system function. In *The Health Effects of Cannabis,* ed. H. Kalant, W. Corrigall, W. Hall, and R. Smart, 127-169. Toronto: Addiction Research Foundation.

Bickel, W.K., J.R. Hughes, and S.T. Higgins. 1990. Human behavioral pharmacology of benzodiazepines: effects on repeated acquisition and performance of response chains. *Drug Development Research* 20: 53-65.

Block, R.I., R. Farinpour, and K. Braverman. 1992. Acute effects of marijuana on cognition: relationships to chronic effects and smoking techniques. *Pharmacology Biochemistry and Behavior* 43: 907-917.

Block, R.I., and M.M. Ghoneim. 1993. Effects of chronic marijuana use on human cognition. *Psychopharmacology* 110: 219-228.

Budney, A.J., P.L. Novy, and J.R. Hughes. 1999. Marijuana withdrawal among adults seeking treatment for marijuana dependence. *Addiction* 94: 1311-1321.

Budney, A.J., K.J. Radonovich, S.T. Higgins, and C.J. Wong. 1998. Adults seeking treatment for marijuana dependence: a comparison with cocaine-dependent treatment seekers. *Experimental and Clinical Psychopharmacology* 6: 419-426.

Calhoun, S.R., G.P. Galloway, and D.E. Smith. 1998. Abuse potential of dronabinol (Marinol). *Journal of Psychoactive Drugs* 30: 187-196.

Catlin, D.H., and T.H. Murray. 1996. Performance-enhancing drugs, fair competition, and Olympic sport. *Journal of the American Medical Association* 276: 231-237.

Chait, L.D. 1990. Subjective and behavioral effects of marijuana the morning after smoking. *Psychopharmacology* 100: 328-333.

Chait, L.D., R.L. Corwin, and C.E. Johanson. 1988. A cumulative dosing procedure for administering marijuana smoke to humans. *Pharmacology Biochemistry and Behavior* 29: 553-557.

Chait, L.D., M.W. Fischman, and C.R. Schuster. 1985. "Hangover" effects the morning after marijuana smoking. *Drug and Alcohol Dependence* 15: 229-238.

Chait, L.D., and J.L. Perry. 1994. Acute and residual effects of alcohol and marijuana, alone and in combination, on mood and performance. *Psychopharmacology* 115: 340-349.

Chait, L.D., and J. Pierri. 1992. Effects of smoked marijuana on human performance: a critical review. In *Marijuana/Cannabinoids: Neurobiology and Neurophysiology,* ed. L. Murphy and A. Bartke, 387-423. Boca Raton, FL: CRC Press.

Comitas, L. 1976. Cannabis and work in Jamaica: a refutation of the amotivational syndrome. *Annals of the New York Academy of Science* 282: 24-32.

Cone, E.J., and R.E. Johnson. 1986. Contact highs and urinary cannabinoid excretion after passive exposure to marijuana smoke. *Clinical Pharmacology and Therapeutics* 40: 247-256.

Cone, E.J., R.E. Johnson, J.D. Moore, and J.D. Roache. 1986. Acute effects of smoking marijuana on hormones, subjective effects and performance in male human subjects. *Pharmacology Biochemistry and Behavior* 24: 1749-1754.

Devane, W.A., L. Hanus, A. Breuer, R.G. Pertwee, L.A. Stevenson, G. Griffin, D. Gibson, A. Mandelbaum, A. Etinger, and R. Mechoulam. 1992. Isolation and structure of a brain constituent that binds to the cannabinoid receptor. *Science* 258: 1946-1949.

Fant, R.V., S.J. Heishman, E.B. Bunker, and W.B. Pickworth. 1998. Acute and residual effects of marijuana in humans. *Pharmacology Biochemistry and Behavior* 60: 777-784.

Fletcher, J.M., J.B. Page, D.J. Francis, K. Copeland, M.J. Naus, C.M. Davis, R. Morris, D. Krauskopf, and P. Satz. 1996. Cognitive correlates of long-term cannabis use in Costa Rican men. *Archives of General Psychiatry* 53: 1051-1057.

Fligiel, S.E., M.D. Roth, E.C. Kleerup, S.H. Barsky, M.S. Simmons, and D.P. Tashkin. 1997. Tracheobronchial histopathology in habitual smokers of cocaine, marijuana, and/or tobacco. *Chest* 112: 319-326.

Foltin, R.W., and M.W. Fischman. 1990. The effects of combinations of intranasal cocaine, smoked marijuana, and task performance on heart rate and blood pressure. *Pharmacology Biochemistry and Behavior* 36: 311-315.

Foltin, R.W., M.W. Fischman, J.V. Brady, D.J. Bernstein, R.M. Capriotti, M.J. Nellis, and T.H. Kelly. 1990. Motivational effects of smoked marijuana: behavioral contingencies and low-probability activities. *Journal of the Experimental Analysis of Behavior* 53: 5-19.

Foltin, R.W., M.W. Fischman, J.V. Brady, D.J. Bernstein, M.J. Nellis, and T.H. Kelly. 1990. Marijuana and behavioral contingencies. *Drug Development Research* 20: 67-80.

Foltin, R.W., M.W. Fischman, J.V. Brady, T.H. Kelly, D.J. Bernstein, and M.J. Nellis. 1989. Motivational effects of smoked marijuana: behavioral contingencies and high-probability recreational activities. *Pharmacology Biochemistry and Behavior* 34: 871-877.

Foltin, R.W., M.W. Fischman, P.A. Pippen, and T.H. Kelly. 1993. Behavioral effects of cocaine alone and in combination with ethanol or marijuana in humans. *Drug and Alcohol Dependence* 32: 93-106.

Gerard, C.M., C. Mollereau, G. Vassart, and M. Parmentier. 1991. Molecular cloning of a human cannabinoid receptor which is also expressed in testis. *Biochemical Journal* 279: 129-134.

Greenberg, H.S., S.A.S. Werness, J.E. Pugh, R.O. Andrus, D.J. Anderson, and E.F. Domino. 1994. Short-term effects of smoking marijuana on balance in patients with multiple sclerosis and normal volunteers. *Clinical Pharmacology and Therapeutics* 55: 324-328.

Gruber, A.J., and H.G. Pope Jr. 2000. Residual neuropsychological effects of cannabis. Paper presented at the World Psychiatric Association International Jubilee Congress, Paris.

Hall, W., N. Solowij, and J. Lemon. 1994. *The Health and Psychological Consequences of Cannabis Use.* Canberra: Australian Government Publishing Service.

Heishman, S.J., K. Arasteh, and M.L. Stitzer. 1997. Comparative effects of alcohol and marijuana on mood, memory, and performance. *Pharmacology Biochemistry and Behavior* 58: 93-101.

Heishman, S.J., M.A. Huestis, J.E. Henningfield, and E.J. Cone. 1990. Acute and residual effects of marijuana: profiles of plasma THC levels, physiological, subjective, and performance measures. *Pharmacology Biochemistry and Behavior* 37: 561-565.

Heishman, S.J., and M.L. Stitzer. 1989. Effects of *d*-amphetamine, secobarbital, and marijuana on choice behavior: social versus nonsocial options. *Psychopharmacology* 99: 156-162.

Heishman, S.J., M.L. Stitzer, and G.E. Bigelow. 1988. Alcohol and marijuana: comparative dose effect profiles in humans. *Pharmacology Biochemistry and Behavior* 31: 649-655.

Heishman, S.J., M.L. Stitzer, and J.E. Yingling. 1989. Effects of tetrahydrocannabinol content on marijuana smoking behavior, subjective reports, and performance. *Pharmacology Biochemistry and Behavior* 34: 173-179.

Hooker, W.D., and R.T. Jones. 1987. Increased susceptibility to memory intrusions and the Stroop interference effect during acute marijuana intoxication. *Psychopharmacology* 91: 20-24.

Huestis, M.A., D.A. Gorelick, S.J. Heishman, K.L. Preston, R.A. Nelson, E.T. Moolchan, and R.A. Frank. 2001. Blockade of smoked marijuana effects in humans by the CB1-selective cannabinoid receptor antagonist SR141716. *Archives of General Psychiatry* 58: 322-328.

Huestis, M.A., J.E. Henningfield, and E.J. Cone. 1992. Blood cannabinoids. I. Absorption of THC and formation of 11-OH-THC and THCCOOH during and after smoking marijuana. *Journal of Analytical Toxicology* 16: 276-282.

Huestis, M.A., A.H. Sampson, B.J. Holicky, J.E. Henningfield, and E.J. Cone. 1992. Characterization of the absorption phase of marijuana smoking. *Clinical Pharmacology and Therapeutics* 52: 31-41.

Joy, J.E., S.J. Watson Jr., and J.A. Benson, eds. 1999. *Marijuana and Medicine: Assessing the Data Base.* Washington, DC: National Academy Press.

Kagel, J.H., R.C. Battalio, and C.G. Miles. 1980. Marihuana and work performance: results from an experiment. *Journal of Human Resources* 15: 373-395.

Kamien, J.B., W.K. Bickel, S.T. Higgins, and J.R. Hughes. 1994. The effects of Δ^9-tetrahydrocannabinol on repeated acquisition and performance of response sequences and on self-reports in humans. *Behavioural Pharmacology* 5: 71-78.

Kelly, T.H., R.W. Foltin, C.S. Emurian, and M.W. Fischman. 1990. Multidimensional behavioral effects of marijuana. *Progress in Neuro-Psychopharmacology and Biological Psychiatry* 14: 885-902.

Kelly, T.H., R.W. Foltin, C.S. Emurian, and M.W. Fischman. 1993. Performance-based testing for drugs of abuse: dose and time profiles of marijuana, amphetamine, alcohol, and diazepam. *Journal of Analytical Toxicology* 17: 264-272.

Kelly, T.H., R.W. Foltin, and M.W. Fischman. 1993. Effects of smoked marijuana on heart rate, drug ratings and task performance by humans. *Behavioural Pharmacology* 4: 167-178.

Kinchla, R.A. 1992. Attention. *Annual Review of Psychology* 43: 711-742.

Kindlundh, A.M.S., D.G.L. Isacson, L. Berglund, and F. Nyberg. 1999. Factors associated with adolescent use of doping agents: anabolic-androgenic steroids. *Addiction* 94: 543-553.

Kupfer, D.J., T. Detre, J. Koral, and P. Fajans. 1973. A comment on the "amotivational syndrome" in marijuana smokers. *American Journal of Psychiatry* 130: 1319-1322.

Kurzthaler, I., M. Hummer, C. Miller, B. Sperner-Unterweger, V. Günther, H. Wechdorn, H-J. Battista, and W.W. Fleischhacker. 1999. Effect of cannabis use on cognitive functions and driving ability. *Journal of Clinical Psychiatry* 60: 395-399.

Ledent, C., O. Valverde, G. Cossu, F. Petitet, J.F. Aubert, F. Beslot, G.A. Bohme, A. Imperato, T. Pedrazzini, B.P. Roques, G. Vassart, W. Fratta, and M. Parmentier. 1999. Unresponsiveness to cannabinoids and reduced addictive effects of opiates in CB1 receptor knockout mice. *Science* 283: 401-404.

Leirer, V.O., J.A. Yesavage, and D.G. Morrow. 1989. Marijuana, aging, and task difficulty effects on pilot performance. *Aviation Space and Environmental Medicine* 60: 1145-1152.

Leirer, V.O., J.A. Yesavage, and D.G. Morrow. 1991. Marijuana carry-over effects on aircraft pilot performance. *Aviation Space and Environmental Medicine* 62: 221-227.

Liguori, A., C.P. Gatto, and J.H. Robinson. 1998. Effects of marijuana on equilibrium, psychomotor performance, and simulated driving. *Behavioural Pharmacology* 9: 599-609.

Marks, D.F., and M.G. MacAvoy. 1989. Divided attention performance in cannabis users and non-users following alcohol and cannabis separately and in combination. *Psychopharmacology* 99: 397-401.

Matsuda, L.A., S.J. Lolait, M.J. Brownstein, A.C. Young, and T.I. Bonner. 1990. Structure of a cannabinoid receptor and functional expression of the cloned cDNA. *Nature* 346: 561-564.

McGlothin, W.H., and L.J. West. 1968. The marihuana problem: an overview. *American Journal of Psychiatry* 125: 370-378.

McLeod, D.R., R.R. Griffiths, G.E. Bigelow, and J. Yingling. 1982. An automated version of the digit symbol substitution task (DSST). *Behavioral Research Methods and Instrumentation* 14: 463-466.

Meilman, P.W., R.K. Crace, C.A. Presley, and R. Lyerla. 1995. Beyond performance enhancement: polypharmacy among collegiate users of steroids. *Journal of American College Health* 44: 98-104.

Mendelson, J.H., J.C. Kuehnle, I. Greenberg, and N.K. Mello. 1976. Operant acquisition of marihuana in man. *Journal of Pharmacology and Experimental Therapeutics* 198: 42-53.

Moskowitz, H. 1985. Marihuana and driving. *Accident Analysis and Prevention* 17: 323-345.

Munro, S., K.L. Thomas, and M. Abu-Shaar. 1993. Molecular characterization of a peripheral receptor for cannabinoids. *Nature* 365: 61-65.

Page, J.B. 1983. The amotivational syndrome hypothesis and the Costa Rica study: relationship between methods and results. *Journal of Psychoactive Drugs* 15: 261-267.

Perez-Reyes, M., S. Di Guiseppi, A.P. Mason, and K.H. Davis. 1983. Passive inhalation of marijuana smoke and urinary excretion of cannabinoids. *Clinical Pharmacology and Therapeutics* 34: 36-41.

Perez-Reyes, M., R.E. Hicks, J. Bumberry, A.R. Jeffcoat, and C.E. Cook. 1988. Interaction between marihuana and ethanol: effects on psychomotor performance. *Alcoholism: Clinical and Experimental Research* 12: 268-276.

Pope, H.G. Jr., A.J. Gruber, and D. Yurgelun-Todd. 1995. The residual neuropsychological effects of cannabis: the current status of research. *Drug and Alcohol Dependence* 38: 25-34.

Pope, H.G. Jr., and D. Yurgelun-Todd. 1996. The residual cognitive effects of heavy marijuana use in college students. *Journal of the American Medical Association* 275: 521-527.

Robbe, H.W.J. 1994. *Influence of Marijuana on Driving.* Maastricht: University of Limburg.

Roth, M.D., A. Arora, S.H. Barsky, E.C. Kleerup, M. Simmons, and D.P. Tashkin. 1998. Airway inflammation in young marijuana and tobacco smokers. *American Journal of Respiratory and Critical Care Medicine* 157: 928-937.

Smith, J.M., and H. Misiak. 1976. Critical Flicker Frequency (CFF) and psychotropic drugs in normal human subjects—a review. *Psychopharmacology* 47: 175-182.

Steadward, R.D., and M. Singh. 1975. The effects of smoking marihuana on physical performance. *Medicine and Science in Sports* 7: 309-311.

Stefanis, C., R. Dornbush, and M. Fink. 1977. *Hashish: Studies of Long-term Use.* New York: Raven Press.

Stephens, R.S., R.A. Roffman, and E.E. Simpson. 1993. Adult marijuana users seeking treatment. *Journal of Consulting and Clinical Psychology* 61: 1100-1104.

Substance Abuse and Mental Health Services Administration. 2000. *Summary of Findings from the 1999 National Household Survey on Drug Abuse.* Washington, DC: U.S. Government Printing Office.

Tashkin, D.P., A.H. Coulson, V.A. Clark, M. Simmons, L.B. Bourque, S. Duann, G.H. Spivey, and H. Gong. 1987. Respiratory symptoms and lung function in habitual heavy smokers of marijuana alone, smokers of marijuana and tobacco, smokers of tobacco alone, and nonsmokers. *American Review of Respiratory Disease* 135: 209-216.

Wagner, J.C. 1991. Enhancement of athletic performance with drugs: an overview. *Sports Medicine* 12: 250-265.

Wilson, W.H., E.H. Ellinwood, R.J. Mathew, and K. Johnson. 1994. Effects of marijuana on performance of a computerized cognitive-neuromotor test battery. *Psychiatry Research* 51: 115-125.

Wu, T-C., D.P. Tashkin, B. Djahed, and J.E. Rose. 1988. Pulmonary hazards of smoking marijuana as compared with tobacco. *New England Journal of Medicine* 318: 347-351.

Yesavage, J.A., V.O. Leirer, M. Denari, and L.E. Hollister. 1985. Carry-over effects of marijuana intoxication on aircraft pilot performance: a preliminary report. *American Journal of Psychiatry* 142: 1325-1329.

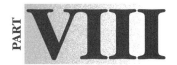

PART VIII

Stimulants

CHAPTER 21

Amphetamines

Steven B. Karch, MD

Before amphetamines were ever invented, athletes chewed coca leaves in the hope of gaining a competitive edge. Before that they used caffeine (Karch 1998). In fact, stimulants of one sort or another have been used as performance-enhancing drugs for nearly two centuries. Cocaine and amphetamine have certain common mechanisms of action, and their use by athletes is hardly surprising. What is surprising is that actual performance improvement has been so difficult to demonstrate. The preponderance of evidence suggests that amphetamine improves physical performance by masking pain and fatigue, but even then, not by very much (Borg, Edstrom et al. 1972; Dekhuijzen, Machiels et al. 1999). However, in today's fiercely competitive environment, performance improvements amounting to less than 1% may make the difference between a gold medal and a bronze. There is also evidence that the performance of some mental tasks may be improved by amphetamine (Mattay, Callicott et al. 2000). Whether improved mental performance translates into enhanced athletic performance has never been proven, but it is certainly possible. This chapter reviews the pharmacology and toxicology of amphetamine and amphetamine-like substances that have been and continue to be abused by athletes.

History

In the late 19th century, race walking was a popular sport in England and the United States. In 1876 the reigning champion, an American named Edward P. Weston, accepted a challenge by the leading British race walker and sailed to England to compete in a 24-hr, 115-mile (185 km) ultramarathon. The race began on the evening of February 8, 1876, at the Royal Agricultural Hall, located in a London suburb (Karch 1998). Weston was 37

years old. His English opponent was a few years younger, and a faster walker, but he lacked Weston's endurance. The race venue was poorly ventilated and quickly became overheated. Foot pain and dehydration caused the Englishman to quit at 14 hr, after completing only 65.5 miles (105 km). Physicians in attendance at the race reported that he did not look well; his pulse and temperature were elevated, his blood pressure was decreased, and his feet badly were blistered. Weston was in much better shape and kept walking in spite of the heat. Foot blisters caused him to pause briefly after 17 hr, but he continued walking for the full 24 hr, managing to complete 109.5 miles (176 km). Both competitors maintained their fluid intake during the race, drinking tea and coffee, along with egg yolks and Liebig extract, the latter being an 1870s equivalent of Gatorade (Finaly 1992). After the race it was revealed that Weston had also been chewing coca leaves. When reporters found out, a furor ensued. In a letter to *The Lancet,* Weston later admitted he had been chewing coca leaf but claimed that he did not believe it had helped him. In fact, he claimed, it made him sleepy (Weston 1876).

Amphetamine did not become commercially available until nearly one-half century after the London race. It was invented, quite by accident, by a UCLA graduate student named Gordon Alles, who was trying to synthesize ephedrine. In the 1930s ephedrine, obtained from the ephedra plant, was the only effective drug available for treating asthma. Concerned that the supply of naturally occurring ephedrine might not be sufficient, chemists worldwide tried to produce synthetic ephedrine. Alles failed in his attempt to synthesize ephedrine, but he did manage to produce a molecule called phenylisopropylamine, later named dextroamphetamine. A Japanese chemist named Ogata was equally unsuccessful in his attempts at synthesizing ephedrine, but he accidentally produced a related stimulant: d-phenyl-isopropylmethylamine hydrochloride, later known as methamphetamine.

Ogata sold the rights for methamphetamine to the British pharmaceutical giant Burroughs Wellcome Company, which sold methamphetamine in the United States under the brand name Methedrine until 1968. In 1932, the Smith, Kline and French Company began promoting the use of a nasal decongestant inhaler containing a racemic mixture of dl-amphetamine called Benzedrine. It took the general public very little time to notice that Benzedrine was something more than a nasal decongestant.

Taken in moderate doses, dl-amphetamine increases the ability to sustain attention over prolonged periods of time and also improves the ability to perform monotonous tasks (Heishman and Karch 2000). Those effects alone probably explain why, during World War II, troops of both the Allied and Axis forces were supplied with amphetamines. It is not clear when athletes first began to experiment with amphetamine, but in June of 1957 the board of trustees of the American Medical Association (AMA) appointed the ad hoc Committee on Amphetamines and Athletes to investigate, in conjunction with the National Collegiate Athletic Association (NCAA) and other sport federations, "alleged widespread use of amphetamine substance by coaches, trainers and athletes to improve athletic performance" (Karpovich 1959).

The AMA sponsored the studies of two early sports medicine researchers, Henry Beecher and Gene Smith, at Harvard. Separate papers were published by *JAMA* in 1959, one by Karpovich and one by Smith and Beecher. The findings of both papers suggested that amphetamine had an effect on performance, but not very much, and only at higher doses. In an accompanying editorial, a *JAMA* editor affirmed the research findings and went on to point out that, in spite of alleged widespread abuse of these drugs by athletes, the NCAA and the other sporting federations had been unable to uncover any convincing evidence that a problem really existed. One reason for the failure may have been the federation's inability to detect amphetamine. The technology used to test urine for drugs (the enzyme-multiplied immunoassay technique) did not become available until the end of the Vietnam War.

The sporting federation might not have been able to detect any problems, but that did not mean that athletes were not using amphetamine. Just one year later, a Danish cyclist named Knut Jensen died at the Rome Summer Olympics. His death was attributed to the combined use of amphetamines and nicotinyl tartrate (not strychnine, as has been widely reported in the press). Jensen's death was followed almost immediately by the amphetamine-related death of a British cyclist named Tommy Simpson during a televised stage of the Tour de France. The occurrence of such highly publicized deaths finally forced the International Olympic Committee (IOC) to draw up a list of banned substances. Stimulants, including caffeine and ephedrine, as well as amphetamine, were the first class of drugs to be banned by the IOC. Random drug testing, including tests for amphetamines, began in 1968 at the Winter Olympics in Grenoble, France, and continued in the Mexico City Summer Games.

Amphetamine abuse declined during the 1980s and 1990s, whether as result of the highly publicized deaths of Jensen and Simpson or as a consequence of the ready availability of cocaine, as well as other adrenergic agonists such as clenbuterol, is not clear. The magnitude of the problem has always been difficult to assess, because the IOC and the IOC's newly formed World Anti-Doping Agency do not publish information on testing results but divulge only the number of tests performed.

More recently, attention has focused on athletes disqualified for having used common over-the-counter cold remedies containing ephedrine, pseudoephedrine (a naturally occurring isomer of ephedrine), or phenylpropanolamine (now withdrawn from the market in the United States). These compounds bear strong structural similarities to amphetamine and, while not nearly so potent, share some of the actions as well. Convincing controlled, double-blinded experiments with volunteer athletes show that if these related compounds are taken in sufficiently large doses (greater than those recommended on package inserts), they can improve performance and endurance (Bell, Jacobs et al. 1998; Bell and Jacobs 1999).

The serious complications associated with amphetamine abuse are essentially the same as for cocaine: arrhythmic sudden cardiac death, stroke, psychosis, and rhabdomyolysis (Karch 1996). Most case reports of amphetamine toxicity are to be found in the older literature. Mentions were uncommon during the 1980s; but episodes of toxicity are now more frequent, though still uncommon when compared to mentions of cocaine toxicity. Reports of serious adverse events related to use of dl-amphetamine are rarer still. According to the most recent Drug Abuse Warning Network report, there are still 10 cocaine-related deaths for every death attributed to methamphetamine (Kissin, Garfield et al. 2000). The far less potent dl-amphetamine does not even rate a mention in the government's top-100 list of drug-related deaths.

There is very little evidence to suggest that significant numbers of athletes take amphetamines. Still, the suggestion that an athlete might be taking amphetamine to improve performance is, at least, biologically plausible. And even if the older amphetamines do not seem to be very popular with today's competitive athletes, there is interest in other amphetamine-like drugs that clearly do enhance performance.

At the Atlanta Olympic Games, several Russian athletes were caught using a new drug called bromantan. Bromantan is a derivative of amantadine, originally synthesized by chemists working for the Russian army. It exhibits the same psychostimulant effects on brain dopamine, norepinephrine, and serotonin metabolism as would be expected with any phenylethylamine (Grekhova, Gainetdinov et al. 1995). Studies published in the Russian literature indicate that the use of bromantan substantially improves both athletic and mental performance. Even before bromantan was detected in Atlanta, athletes had been abusing a related psychostimulant called Sydnocarb (3-(beta-phenylisopropyl)-N-phenylcarbamoylsyd-nonimine). Sydnocarb is used in Russia to treat a variety of psychiatric disorders. Animal studies suggest that Sydnocarb is a stimulant and that its effects are very much like those of methamphetamine, though less potent (Biniaurishvili, Vein et al. 1984; Shashkov, Lakota et al. 1991).

Metabolism

Amphetamines are commonly referred to as sympathomimetic amines because they stimulate the sympathetic nervous system. All sympathomimetic amines share basic structural features with a molecule called phenylethylamine: a benzene ring and an ethylamine side chain. Substitution at either of the carbon atoms in the ethylamine side chain or on the benzene ring determines receptor binding and physiologic activity. In addition to an ethylamine side chain, epinephrine and norepinephrine also have hydroxyl groups substituted at positions 3 and 4 of the benzene ring. Before the structure of epinephrine was known, benzene rings with hydroxyl substitutions at positions 3 and 4 were referred to as "catechols." Hence the term "catecholamine" is often used interchangeably, but incorrectly, with the term "sympathomimetic."

Methamphetamine, "designer" amphetamines like MDMA (N-methyl-3,4-methylenedioxy-amphetamine), and naturally occurring sympathomimetics like ephedrine and cathinone (khat), do not have hydroxyl substitutions and are not catecholamines, though they are sympathomimetic agents and do produce many of the same effects as catecholamines, albeit indirectly. They cause nerve endings to release norepinephrine, and they also act directly on some of the same receptors as true catecholamines, but with different degrees of affinity (Hoffman and Lefkowitz 1996).

Indirectly acting sympathomimetics, which do not have hydroxyl substitutions on the benzene ring, differ from true catecholamines in two very important ways: (1) true catecholamines are destroyed in the gastrointestinal tract, but indirectly acting agents are not; and (2) unsubstituted indirect agents readily cross the blood-brain barrier, but true catecholamines cannot. Amphetamines are therefore central nervous system stimulants, but exogenously administered epinephrine and norepinephrine are not (Hoffman and Lefkowitz 1996). Drugs such as Sydnocarb and bromantan are not catecholamines, or even phenylethylamines, but they do

exert amphetamine-like actions within the central nervous system, altering the metabolism of neurotransmitters in much the same fashion as amphetamines (Musshoff 2000).

Clinical measurements, and the results of one large autopsy series, have shown that 10% to 20% of a given dose of methamphetamine is N-demethylated to form amphetamine and ephedrine. Both of these metabolites are also psychoactive (Caldwell, Dring et al. 1972a; Cho and Wright 1978; Karch, Stephens et al. 1999). Accordingly, the detection of amphetamine or ephedrine in a urine sample, along with methamphetamine, is not proof that either of those drugs were also ingested but only that they are present. Conversely, the integrity of a urine sample might well be questioned if it were found to contain only methamphetamine and none of the metabolites. Indeed, in federally regulated workplace testing programs, a urine specimen, even one containing very high methamphetamine concentrations, cannot be reported as positive unless certain minimum concentrations of amphetamine are also present.

Naturally occurring compounds, such as ephedrine and pseudoephedrine, as well as synthetic compounds like amphetamine and methamphetamine, affect the body in two ways: by interfering with the body's normal metabolism of neurotransmitters and also by acting directly on some of the same receptors as norepinephrine. Thus the principal effects exerted by all amphetamine-like drugs (figure 21.1) are similar to the effects that

amineptine	mesocarb
amfepramone	methamphetamine
amiphenazole	methoxyphen-amine
ampheta-mine	methylephedrine
bambuterol	methylphenidate
bromantan	niketha-mide
caffeine	norfenfluramine
carphedon	parahydroxyamphetamine
cathine	pemoline
cocaine	pentylentetrazol
cropropamide	phendimetrazine
crotethamide	phentermine
ephedrine	phenylpropanolamine
etamivan	pholedrine
etilamphetamine	pipradol
etilefrine	prolintane
fencamfamine	propylhexedrine
fenetylline	pseudo-ephedrine
fenfluramine	reproterol
formoterol	salbutamol
heptaminol	salmeterol
methylendioxyamphetamine	selegiline
mefenorex	strychnine
mephen-termine	terbutaline

Figure 21.1 Prohibited amphetamines and other stimulant drugs. This is not an exhaustive list of prohibited substances. Many substances that do not appear on this list are prohibited under the term "and related substances."

would be produced by the direct administration of norepinephrine. The principal difference is that hydroxyl groups at position 3 and 4 on the benzene ring prevent the absorption of norepinephrine from the gastrointestinal tract. Agents such as amphetamine and methamphetamine are readily abused and abusable.

Pharmacokinetics

Ten milligrams of oral methamphetamine results in peak plasma concentrations of 30 ng/ml 1 hr after ingestion (Lebish, Finkle et al. 1970). Peak methamphetamine blood concentrations after smoking and injecting are comparable, with both routes producing higher blood concentrations than the oral route (Cook, Jeffcoat et al. 1992, 1993; Perez, Arsura et al. 1999). In seven patients presenting at an emergency room with evidence of amphetamine toxicity, plasma concentrations ranged from 105 ng/ml to 560 ng/ml (Lebish, Finkle et al. 1970). Over the course of several days, between one-third and one-half of a given dose of methamphetamine will be excreted unchanged in the urine (Cook, Jeffcoat et al. 1992, 1993). If the urine is acidic, the amount of methamphetamine excreted unchanged may increase to over 75%. If the urine is extremely alkaline, the amount excreted unchanged may drop to 2% (Beckett and Rowland 1965a,b). Other metabolites also appear in substantial quantities, including 4-hydroxymethamphetamine, norephedrine, and 4-hydroxynorephedrine (Caldwell, Dring et al. 1972b). The (+) isomer of amphetamine is metabolized more rapidly than the (−) isomer and appears in the urine sooner. Articles in the underground press continue to recommend drinking vinegar as a way to foil urine drug testing. In fact, quite the opposite will occur; acidifying the urine increases the amount of amphetamine excreted and thus increases the probability of a positive urine test.

Methamphetamine concentrations in saliva are much higher than concentrations measured in plasma, and methamphetamine remains detectable in saliva for at least 48 hr (Wan, Matin et al. 1978). There is, unfortunately, great intra-individual variation in the amount of methamphetamine that appears in saliva. In a study of 25 methamphetamine abusers, methamphetamine was found in the hair of 73%, in the nails of 65%, in the sweat of 50%, but in the saliva of only 16% (Suzuki, Inoue et al. 1989). This high degree of unpredictability and the difficulties associated with specimen collection make saliva an unsuitable matrix for methamphetamine testing, especially for athletic competitions.

Possible Ergogenic Effects

All amphetamines, to greater or lesser degree, cause catecholamines to be released from nerve terminals and at the same time prevent catecholamine reuptake. As a consequence, these drugs act as both α- and β-agonists, increasing respiratory rate, heart rate, blood pressure, and metabolic rate. Centrally, increased concentrations of catecholamines lead to increased arousal and alertness. Over and above its effects on the vital signs, amphetamine causes concentrations of plasma free fatty acids to increase (Dekhuijzen, Machiels et al. 1999). It has been suggested that methamphetamine-induced increases in plasma free fatty acid could result in the sparing of glycogen stores within skeletal muscle and thereby improve performance (Pinter and Pattee 1968). Another possible explanation for improved performance might be improved respiratory function; both rate and depth of respiration are increased. Arguing against this possibility is the complete lack of evidence that respiratory function is a limiting factor in elite athletes (Chandler and Blair 1980). In more recent studies, large doses of pseudoephedrine (180 mg) increased both forced vital capacity (FVC) and FVC1, but the ratio between the two was unchanged (Gill, Shield et al. 2000).

The results of studies performed nearly half a century ago suggest that endurance (as evidenced by maximal treadmill time) and maximal heart rate are both increased by amphetamine. But when these studies were performed, the science of exercise physiology was in its early stages, $\dot{V}O_2$max could not be measured, and even the design of the studies would not be considered acceptable by today's standards. For example, in the study by Smith and Beecher (1959), runners were used as their own controls, and times for various distances were compared. During the course of these studies, the ambient temperature varied from 25 °F to 69 °F, and the wind velocity varied from 8 to 23 miles per hour. In spite of the wide variation in experimental conditions, the experimenters were still able to document improved performance, on the order of 1%. In the study by Karpovich (1959), published in *JAMA* at the same time as Smith and Beecher's study, treadmill testing was performed but the protocol used was not specified.

When the effects of amphetamine on aerobic power and anaerobic capacity were finally measured in volunteers, using defined ramping protocols, $\dot{V}O_2$max was found to be unchanged even though lactic acid concentration and endurance time were increased. These findings strongly suggest that amphetamines do nothing to prevent fatigue but simply mask its effects. Indeed, that was the conclusion reached by Borg et al. more than 30 years ago, when he attributed performance improvement to "increased resistance against fatigue" (Borg, Edströstrom et al. 1972; Chandler and Blair 1980; Dekhuijzen, Machiels et al. 1999).

The link between amphetamines and lactate production is disputed. In recent studies in which pseudoephedrine was given to volunteer cyclists, minor increases in maximal performance were documented; but they occurred without any change in lactate production (Gill, Shield et al. 2000). In a randomized, double-blind, crossover study of 22 healthy male athletes who had been given a 180-mg dose of pseudoephedrine, maximum torque produced in an isometric knee extension exercise was much greater than in the controls. Peak power as estimated by an "all-out" 30-sec cycle test was also increased, but the increase was modest and just barely reached statistical significance (p < 0.03). Bench press tasks and total work during the cycle test were not affected by the ingestion of pseudoephedrine, and lactate concentration was unchanged. Of course, it may well be that even though pseudoephedrine has no effect on lactate concentration, amphetamine does; but until the experiments are finally done, conclusions about amphetamine's mode of action remain speculative.

Central Nervous System Effects

There have been so few controlled studies that the behavioral effects of amphetamines are difficult to assess. Identification of any specific amphetamine-related effect is also complicated by polydrug abuse and by the heterogeneous neuropsychological response to amphetamine administration. Positron emission tomography scans of non-drug-using volunteers have shown that memory and the ability to concentrate are increased by amphetamines and that the improvement is most evident in those who have the highest performance at baseline. Those with poor memory capacity at baseline also improve, but not by nearly so much as those with a higher capacity to begin with (Mattay, Callicott et al. 2000). Individuals who are not regular amphetamine abusers do demonstrate some increase in alertness but no measurable improvement in either cognition or memory (Drachman 1977).

Neuropsychological testing of chronic users may also disclose memory impairment and an inability to concentrate, but only in long-term, regular users (Kish, Kalasinsky et al. 1999). While there is considerable overlap in the behavioral abnormalities observed in cocaine and amphetamine abusers, the results of the most recent experimental studies suggest that in contrast to the reinforcing effects of cocaine, which are a consequence of altered dopamine release and reuptake, the reinforcing effects of amphetamine have more to do with alterations in norepinephrine metabolism than dopamine metabolism (Rothman, Baumann et al. 2001).

Drug Testing

Amphetamines can be detected in hair. There is a time lag before drugs appear in hair, but once there, they remain indefinitely. Thus the detection of amphetamine in hair (or of any other drug for that matter) merely proves prior use. Of course, in a zero-tolerance setting, proof of prior use may be all that is required, but other difficulties associated with hair testing limit its usefulness. Results appear to be partly a function of hair color, with darker hair retaining more drug than lighter. This should be a considerable cause for concern if many different racial groups are being tested (Huestis and Cone 1998). Primarily because of this problem, urine testing remains the standard means of drug detection, at least for amphetamines and the other stimulant drugs.

Several different urine screening tests can be used to detect amphetamine. The enzyme-multiplied immuno-assay test (EMIT), the first product designed specifically for detecting abused drugs in urine samples, is still the most widely used. Introduction of this technology was followed a few years later by a slightly different method known as the fluorescence polarization immunoassay. Both of these methods employ specially produced antibodies that are designed to react with both amphetamine and methamphetamine. The tests are calibrated so that positive readings are produced when urine concentrations of amphetamine exceed 300 ng/ml (the original cutoff concentrations used in workplace drug-testing programs).

Depending on the brand of immunoassay used (and there are many), other related compounds, such as ephedrine, pseudoephedrine, and even MDMA, may also be detected. Ephedrine-containing products are popular among weight lifters and bodybuilders. In Europe, ephedrine is still widely used as a cold remedy. The use of ephedrine is not prohibited by the IOC, but urine concentration limits have been set (500 ng/ml cutoff). Some food supplements may contain ephedrine even though no mention of this is made on the label (Ros, Pelders et al. 1999). Provided that confirmatory analysis with gas chromatography-mass spectrometry is performed, ephedrine should not be confused with amphetamine, regardless of the immunoassay results.

Amphetamine Toxicity

There are important differences between cocaine and amphetamine, but essentially the same medical complications are seen with both drugs: sudden cardiac death, myocardial infarction, stroke, and psychosis. All are recognized risks of stimulant abuse, although the incidence of some complications varies. For example, dissecting aneurysm is much more common among amphetamine abusers, while myocardial infarction is more likely to be associated with cocaine use.

Heart Disease

All phenylethylamines can cause catecholamine-mediated cardiotoxicity. The connection was first recognized nearly 50 years ago (Szakacs and Cannon 1958; Szakacs, Dimmette et al. 1959). Experimental animals given doses of dl-amphetamine in quantities not much smaller than those used by addicts exhibit subendocardial hemorrhages, sometimes extensive enough to disrupt the conduction system. When the hemorrhages heal, they are replaced by a scar tissue (myocardial microfibrosis), a very common finding in the hearts of both methamphetamine and cocaine users (figure 21.2). The presence of microfocal myocardial fibrosis is strongly associated with the occurrence of sudden cardiac death (Karch, Stephens et al. 1999).

Increased heart size is also a predictor for sudden death (Zipes and Wellens 1998; Spirito, Bellone et al. 2000), and longtime users of either amphetamine or cocaine have enlarged hearts (Karch, Stephens et al. 1999). The increase in size may not be striking, but comparison of observed weights to standard reference tables usually discloses a 10% to 15% increase above the expected weight. Hypertrophy in stimulant abusers is thought to be catecholamine related, either via some direct effect or via catecholamine-stimulated increases in blood pressure. As ventricular mass increases, coronary artery reserve declines, and myocardial contractility becomes impaired (Strauer 1979). These myocardial

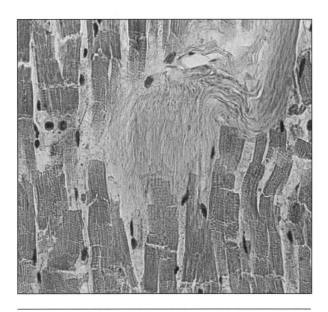

Figure 21.2 Microfocal fibrosis. Note that the scarring process is confined to one or two cells and that the damaged cells are surrounded by normal cells. This pattern of injury is classically seen in cases of catecholamine toxicity, a result of either catecholamine-secreting tumors, such as pheochromocytoma, or stimulant abuse. Scarring of the myocardium is associated with reentry arrhythmias and sudden cardiac death.

abnormalities persist for some time after drug use is discontinued. Studies of asymptomatic users in rehabilitation have shown significant increases in left ventricular mass and posterior wall thickness (Brickner, Willard et al. 1991).

Aortic dissection is a well-recognized complication of methamphetamine abuse (Davis and Swalwell 1996; Swalwell and Davis 1999), but the mechanism is not known; nor is it understood why dissection is seen much more often in amphetamine abusers than in cocaine abusers. Similarly, chest pain and myocardial infarction are common occurrences in cocaine users but are rarely experienced by amphetamine users (Furst, Fallon et al. 1990; Carson, Oldroyd et al. 1987; Huang, Wu et al. 1993; Lam and Goldschlager 1988; Packe, Garton et al. 1990; Marsden and Sheldon 1972), dextrofenfluramine (1990; Evrard and Allaz 1990; Wiener, Tilkian et al. 1990; Derreza, Fine et al. 1997). The disparity is particularly puzzling given the results of postmortem studies showing that methamphetamine abusers are prone to accelerated, multivessel, coronary artery disease (Karch, Stephens et al. 1999). Recent advances in molecular biology may explain why; the rise in body temperature associated with amphetamine use leads to the increased production of myocardial heat shock proteins (Maulik, Wei et al. 1994). Cells produce these proteins in response to stressors such as ischemia and cellular injury (Lindquist 1986), and animals pretreated with amphetamine are resistant to ischemia (Maulik, Engelman et al. 1995). If the same set of responses occurs in humans, that would explain the apparent difference in cardiotoxicity between methamphetamine and cocaine.

Stroke

Methamphetamine use is associated with both hemorrhagic and ischemic stroke, but the mechanism is not always clear (Bostwick 1981). Amphetamine-related hemorrhage is more often intracerebral, or simultaneously intracerebral and subarachnoid, than pure subarachnoid (Perez, Arsura et al. 1999). The incidence of stroke seems to be similar in cocaine and methamphetamine abusers, suggesting drug-related hypertension as the most likely explanation. Rare cases of stroke secondary to vasculitis have been reported in methamphetamine abusers. This syndrome was first described by Citron in 1970 (Citron, Halpern et al. 1970). The histological appearance of Citron's cases is identical to that seen in polyarteritis nodosa. Other reports have described involvement of smaller (Stafford, Bogdanoff et al. 1975) and larger (Bostwick 1981; Shibata, Mori et al. 1991) vessels. A possible explanation for the apparent decline in the number of cases being reported is that vasculitis may have been the result of some contaminant or adulterant introduced during the manufacture of methamphetamine. Vasculitis has also been reported in association with the oral use of methylphenidate (Trugman 1988; Schteinschnaider, Plaghos et al. 2000), fenfluramine (Derby, Myers et al. 1999), phenylpropanolamine (Ryu and Lin 1995), and ephedrine (Mourand, Ducrocq et al. 1999).

Psychosis

Even without developing psychosis, amphetamine users are often restless, tense, and fearful. Delusions of persecution, and ideas of reference are also common, as are auditory, tactile, and visual hallucinations. Reports of amphetamine-related psychotic reactions began to appear shortly after the drug was introduced. The first paper on the subject was published in 1938 (Young and Scoville 1938). As more cases were described, it became apparent that there were striking similarities between the symptoms of amphetamine-induced psychosis and schizophrenia (Connell 1958). Amphetamine-related psychosis seems to be more common than psychosis in cocaine abusers. The difference may be due to methamphetamine's affinity for sigma receptors. The ability to bind sigma receptors and the ability to produce psychosis are related. In animal studies, chronic methamphetamine administration leads to up-regulation of sigma receptors in the substantia nigra, frontal cortex, and cerebellum (Itzhak 1993). Patients with methamphetamine-related psychosis may remain in that state for months after the drug has been discontinued (Iwanami, Sugiyama et al. 1994). Cultural determinants may also have some bearing on the psychiatric manifestations of amphetamine abuse. Methamphetamine psychosis is common in Japan (Iwanami, Sugiyama et al. 1994) but not in the United States.

Magnetic resonance imaging studies of abstinent methamphetamine abusers have shown that, compared to non-drug-using controls, concentrations of N-acetylaspartate (a neuronal marker for cell viability) are significantly reduced in the basal ganglia and frontal white matter. The reduction of activity in the frontal white matter correlates inversely with the logarithm of the lifetime methamphetamine use, a finding indicative of long-term neuronal damage (Ernst, Chang et al. 2000). In spite of the magnetic resonance imaging findings, gross neuroanatomic lesions in chronic methamphetamine abusers have never been identified.

Conclusion

The number of amphetamine-abusing athletes is not known with any certainty, but results of in-competition testing suggest that the number is quite small. One reason for the relative unpopularity of this drug, at least in terms of ergogenic as opposed to "recreational" use, is that benefits appear to be small. Newer chemical agents such as bromantan, which are structurally distinct from amphetamines but which have some common mechanisms of action, are more likely to improve performance and are therefore more likely to be abused.

References

Beckett, A.H. and M. Rowland (1965a). Urinary excretion kinetics of amphetamine in man. *J Pharm Pharmacol* 17(10): 628-639.

Beckett, A.H. and M. Rowland (1965b). Urinary excretion of methylamphetamine in man. *Nature* 206(990): 1260-1261.

Bell, D.G. and I. Jacobs (1999). Combined caffeine and ephedrine ingestion improves run times of Canadian Forces Warrior Test. *Aviat Space Environ Med* 70(4): 325-329.

Bell, D.G., I. Jacobs, et al. (1998). Effects of caffeine, ephedrine and their combination on time to exhaustion during high-intensity exercise. *Eur J Appl Physiol Occup Physiol* 77(5): 427-433.

Biniaurishvili, R.G., A.M. Vein, et al. (1984). [Clinical and electroencephalographic features of the action of the psychic stimulant sydnocarb in various forms of epilepsy]. *Zh Nevropatol Psikhiatr Im S S Korsakova* 84(6): 886-891.

Borg, G., C.G. Edstrom, et al. (1972). Changes in physical performance induced by amphetamine and amobarbital. *Psychopharmacologia (Berl)* 26: 10-18.

Bostwick, D.G. (1981). Amphetamine induced cerebral vasculitis. *Hum Pathol* 12(11): 1031-1033.

Brickner, M.E., J.E. Willard, et al. (1991). Left ventricular hypertrophy associated with chronic cocaine abuse. *Circulation* 84(3): 1130-1135.

Caldwell, J., L. Dring, et al. (1972a). Metabolism of (C-14) methamphetamine in man, the guinea pig, and the rat. *Biochem J* 120: 11-22.

Caldwell, J., L.G. Dring, et al. (1972b). Norephedrines as metabolites of (14C)amphetamine in urine in man. *Biochem J* 129(1): 23-24.

Carson, P., K. Oldroyd, et al. (1987). Myocardial infarction due to amphetamine. *Br Med J (Clin Res Ed)* 294(6586): 1525-1526.

Chandler, I. and S. Blair (1980). The effect of amphetamines on selected physiologic components related to athletic success. *Med Sci Sports Exerc* 12: 65-69.

Cho, A. and J. Wright (1978). Minireview: pathways of metabolism of amphetamine. *Life Sci* 22: 363-372.

Citron, B.P., M. Halpern, et al. (1970). Necrotizing angiitis associated with drug abuse. *N Engl J Med* 283(19): 1003-1011.

Connell, P. (1958). *Amphetamine psychosis.* London: Chapman and Hall.

Cook, C.E., A.R. Jeffcoat, et al. (1992). Pharmacokinetics of oral methamphetamine and effects of repeated daily dosing in humans. *Drug Metab Dispos* 20(6): 856-862.

Cook, C.E., A.R. Jeffcoat, et al. (1993). Pharmacokinetics of methamphetamine self-administered to human subjects by smoking S-(+)-methamphetamine hydrochloride. *Drug Metab Dispos* 21(4): 717-723.

Davis, G.G. and C.I. Swalwell (1996). The incidence of acute cocaine or methamphetamine intoxication in deaths due to ruptured cerebral (berry) aneurysms. *J Forensic Sci* 41(4): 626-628.

Dekhuijzen, P., H. Machiels, et al. (1999). Athletes and doping: effects of drugs on the respiratory system. *Thorax* 54: 1041-1046.

Derby, L.E., M.W. Myers, et al. (1999). Use of dexfenfluramine, fenfluramine and phentermine and the risk of stroke. *Br J Clin Pharmacol* 47(5): 565-569.

Derreza, H., M.D. Fine, et al. (1997). Acute myocardial infarction after use of pseudoephedrine for sinus congestion. *J Am Board Fam Pract* 10(6): 436-438.

Drachman, D.A. (1977). Memory and cognitive function in man: does the cholinergic system have a specific role? *Neurology* 27(8): 783-790.

Ernst, T., L. Chang, et al. (2000). Evidence for long-term neurotoxicity associated with methamphetamine abuse: a 1H MRS study. *Neurology* 54(6): 1344-1349.

Evrard, P. and A.F. Allaz (1990). Myocardial infarction associated with the use of dextrofenfluramine. *Br Med J* 301(6747): 345.

Finaly, M. (1992). Quackery and cookery: Justus von Liebig's extract of meat and the theory of nutrition in the Victorian age. *Bull Hist Med* 66: 404-418.

Furst, S.R., S.P. Fallon, et al. (1990). Myocardial infarction after inhalation of methamphetamine [letter]. *N Engl J Med* 323(16): 1147-1148.

Gill, N.D., A. Shield, et al. (2000). Muscular and cardiorespiratory effects of pseudoephedrine in human athletes. *Br J Clin Pharmacol* 50(3): 205-213.

Grekhova, T.V., R.R. Gainetdinov, et al. (1995). [The effect of bromantane, a new immunostimulant with psychostimulating action, on release and metabolism of dopamine in the dorsal striatum of freely moving rats: a microdialysis study]. *Biull Eksp Biol Med* 119(3): 302-304.

Heishman, S. and S.B. Karch (2000). Drugs and Driving. *Encyclopedia of forensic science.* J. Siegel. London: Academic Press.

Hoffman, B. and R. Lefkowitz (1996). Catecholamines, sympathetic drugs, and adrenergic receptor antagonists. Goodman and Gilman's *The pharmacological basis of therapeutics,* 9th ed. J. Hardman, A. Goodman, L. Gilman, and E. Limbird. New York: McGraw-Hill Health Professions Division.

Huang, C.N., D.J. Wu, et al. (1993). Acute myocardial infarction caused by transnasal inhalation of amphetamine. *Jpn Heart J* 34(6): 815-818.

Huestis, M. and E. Cone (1998). Alternative testing matrices. *Drug abuse handbook.* S. Karch. Boca Raton, FL: CRC Press.

Itzhak, Y. (1993). Repeated methamphetamine-treatment alters brain sigma receptors. *Eur J Pharmacol* 230(2): 243-244.

Iwanami, A., A. Sugiyama, et al. (1994). Patients with methamphetamine psychosis admitted to a psychiatric hospital in Japan. A preliminary report. *Acta Psychiatr Scand* 89(6): 428-432.

Karch, S.B. (1996). *The pathology of drug abuse.* Boca Raton, FL: CRC Press.

Karch, S. (1998). *A brief history of cocaine.* Boca Raton, FL: CRC Press, LLC.

Karch, S.B., B.G. Stephens, et al. (1999). Methamphetamine-related deaths in San Francisco: demographic, pathologic, and toxicologic profiles. *J Forensic Sci* 44(2): 359-368.

Karpovich, P. (1959). Effect of amphetamine sulphate on athletic performance. *JAMA* 170: 558-561.

Kish, S.J., K.S. Kalasinsky, et al. (1999). Brain choline acetyltransferase activity in chronic, human users of cocaine, methamphetamine, and heroin. *Mol Psychiatry* 4(1): 26-32.

Kissin, W., T. Garfield, et al. (2000). Drug abuse warning network. Annual medical examiner data 1998. Bethesda, MD: Department of Health and Human Services, Substance Abuse and Mental Health Administration, Office of Applied Statistics.

Lam, D. and N. Goldschlager (1988). Myocardial injury associated with polysubstance abuse. *Am Heart J* 115(3): 675-680.

Lebish, P., B.S. Finkle, et al. (1970). Determination of amphetamine, methamphetamine, and related amines in blood and urine by gas chromatography with hydrogen-flame ionization detector. *Clin Chem* 16(3): 195-200.

Lindquist, S. (1986). The heat-shock response. *Ann Rev Biochem* 55: 1151-1191.

Marsden, P. and J. Sheldon (1972). Acute poisoning by propylhexedrine. *Br Med J* 1(5802): 730.

Mattay, V.S., J.H. Callicott, et al. (2000). Effects of dextroamphetamine on cognitive performance and cortical activation. *Neuroimage* 12(3): 268-275.

Maulik, N., Z. Wei, et al. (1994). Improved postischemic ventricular functional recovery by amphetamine is linked with its ability to induce heat shock. *Mol Cell Biochem* 137(1): 17-24.

Maulik, N., R.M. Engelman, et al. (1995). Drug-induced heat-shock preconditioning improves postischemic ventricular recovery after cardiopulmonary bypass. *Circulation* 92(9 Suppl): II381-II388.

Mourand, I., X. Ducrocq, et al. (1999). Acute reversible cerebral arteritis associated with parenteral ephedrine use. *Cerebrovasc Dis* 9(6): 355-357.

Musshoff, F. (2000). Illegal or legitimate use? Precursor compounds to amphetamine and methamphetamine. *Drug Metab Rev* 32(1): 15-44.

Packe, G.E., M.J. Garton, et al. (1990). Acute myocardial infarction caused by intravenous amphetamine abuse. *Br Heart J* 64(1): 23-24.

Perez, J.A. Jr., E.L. Arsura, et al. (1999). Methamphetamine-related stroke: four cases. *J Emerg Med* 17(3): 469-471.

Pinter, E. and C. Pattee (1968). Fat-mobilizing action of amphetamine. *J Clin Invest* 47: 394-402.

Ros, J.J., M.G. Pelders, et al. (1999). A case of positive doping associated with a botanical food supplement. *Pharm World Sci* 21(1): 44-46.

Rothman, R.B., M.H. Baumann, et al. (2001). Amphetamine-type central nervous system stimulants release norepinephrine more potently than they release dopamine and serotonin. *Synapse* 39(1): 32-41.

Ryu, S.J. and S.K. Lin (1995). Cerebral arteritis associated with oral use of phenylpropanolamine: report of a case. *J Formos Med Assoc* 94(1-2): 53-55.

Schteinschnaider, A., L.L. Plaghos, et al. (2000). Cerebral arteritis following methylphenidate use. *J Child Neurol* 15(4): 265-267.

Shashkov, V.S., N.G. Lakota, et al. (1991). [Functional changes of the cardiovascular system and their pharmacological correction during suited immersion]. *Kosm Biol Aviakosm Med* 25(6): 33-36.

Shibata, S., K. Mori, et al. (1991). Subarachnoid and intracerebral hemorrhage associated with necrotizing angiitis due to methamphetamine abuse—an autopsy case. *Neurol Med Chir (Tokyo)* 31(1): 49-52.

Smith, G.M. and H.K. Beecher (1959). Amphetamine sulfate and athletic performance. 1. Objective effects. *JAMA* 170(5) 102-118.

Spirito, P., P. Bellone, et al. (2000). Magnitude of left ventricular hypertrophy and risk of sudden death in hypertrophic cardiomyopathy. *N Engl J Med* 342(24): 1778-1785.

Stafford, C.R., B.M. Bogdanoff, et al. (1975). Mononeuropathy multiplex as a complication of amphetamine angiitis. *Neurology* 25(6): 570-572.

Strauer, B.E. (1979). Ventricular function and coronary hemodynamics in hypertensive heart disease. *Am J Cardiol* 44(5): 999-1006.

Suzuki, S., T. Inoue, et al. (1989). Analysis of methamphetamine in hair, nail, sweat, and saliva by mass fragmentography. *J Anal Toxicol* 13(3): 176-178.

Swalwell, C.I. and G.G. Davis (1999). Methamphetamine as a risk factor for acute aortic dissection. *J Forensic Sci* 44(1): 23-26.

Szakacs, J. and Cannon A. (1958). 1-Norepinephrine myocarditis. *Am J Clin Pathol* 30: 425-434.

Szakacs, J., R. Dimmette, et al. (1959). Pathologic implications of the catecholamines epinephrine and norepinephrine. *US Armed Forces Med J* 10: 908-925.

Trugman, J.M. (1988). Cerebral arteritis and oral methylphenidate [letter]. *Lancet* 1(8585): 584-585.

Wan, S.H., S.B. Matin, et al. (1978). Kinetics, salivary excretion of amphetamine isomers, and effect of urinary pH. *Clin Pharmacol Ther* 23(5): 585-590.

Weston, E. (1876). Mr. Weston on the use of coca leaves. *Lancet* 1(March 18): 447-447.

Wiener, I., A.G. Tilkian, et al. (1990). Coronary artery spasm and myocardial infarction in a patient with normal coronary arteries: temporal relationship to pseudoephedrine ingestion. *Cathet Cardiovasc Diagn* 20(1): 51-53.

Young, D. and W. Scoville (1938). Paranoid psychosis in narcolepsy and the possible danger of Benzedrine treatment. *Med Clin N Amer* 22: 637.

Zipes, D.P. and H.J. Wellens (1998). Sudden cardiac death. *Circulation* 98(21): 2334-2351.

Caffeine

Lawrence L. Spriet, PhD

Caffeine is a socially acceptable drug that is consumed worldwide and may be the most widely "abused" drug in the world (37, 48, 75). It is also widely used by athletes in their daily lives and in preparation for and during training and competitions (7, 19, 54). In the athletic world, caffeine is a "controlled or restricted drug," and urinary levels greater than 12 μg/ml after competitions are considered illegal by the International Olympic Committee (IOC) (70). However, most athletes who ingest caffeine before or during exercise would not approach the legal limit after a competition. Therefore, if "legal" levels of caffeine in the body enhance sport performance, caffeine occupies a unique position in the sport world as an acceptable and legal drug and performance-enhancing substance (PES).

For researchers, athletes, and sport personnel over the past 30 years, the most compelling question about caffeine has been whether caffeine ingestion improves performance during athletic activity and competitions. Secondly, if caffeine does improve performance, what are the mechanism(s) responsible for these improvements? Much progress has been made in answering the first question, but answers to the second question have been more difficult to establish. Research in this area has been complicated by the fact that caffeine crosses the membranes of all tissues in the body, including the blood-brain barrier (58). This makes it difficult to independently assess caffeine's effects on the central nervous system (CNS) and the peripheral tissues (e.g., skeletal muscle, adipose tissue, liver) of resting and exercising humans. It also seems likely that different mechanisms are responsible for improving performance during different exercise modalities and in different sports.

The potential mechanisms that contribute to the performance-enhancing effects of caffeine may be categorized as targeting three general areas: peripheral tissues that impact on and include skeletal muscle metabolism, the handling of ions in muscle, and the CNS (62, 63). The first category includes the classic or "metabolic" explanation that has been proposed to explain the endurance exercise improvements. It involves a caffeine- or epinephrine-induced increase in fat availability and muscle fat oxidation with a consequent reduction in muscle carbohydrate use, or "glycogen sparing." The reduced glycogen use early in exercise

increases carbohydrate availability later in exercise, thereby providing the fuel to extend the exercise duration. Other potential metabolic effects include caffeine-induced inhibition of the key glycogenolytic enzyme, glycogen phosphorylase (PHOS), and antagonism of adenosine receptors, which are involved in glucose uptake into the muscle. The second category of mechanisms involves a proposed direct effect of caffeine on skeletal muscle performance via ion handling, including stimulation of Na^+-K^+ adenosinetriphosphatase (ATPase) activity and Ca^{2+} kinetics. The third category involves direct caffeine effects on aspects of the CNS that alter the perception of effort, or motor unit recruitment, or both.

This chapter provides a brief review and update regarding caffeine's ability to increase athletic performance and the mechanisms that may be responsible for these improvements. The reader is encouraged to consult the many review articles that assess the earlier work in this area (32, 54, 62, 63, 67).

Caffeine and Endurance Exercise Performance

This section will briefly touch on key studies of caffeine and exercise, while outlining their relevance. Running and cycling have been studied most extensively in the area of endurance training and caffeine.

Early Studies

The interest in caffeine as a PES during endurance exercise is due in large part to the research from David Costill's laboratory in the late 1970s. Trained cyclists improved their cycle time to exhaustion at 80% of maximal oxygen consumption ($\dot{V}O_2$max) from 75 min in the placebo condition to 96 min after the ingestion of 330 mg of caffeine (16). A second study showed a 20% increase in the work completed during 2 hr of cycling after the ingestion of 250 mg of caffeine (39). These studies reported increased venous free fatty acid concentrations ([FFA]) and decreased respiratory exchange ratios (RER) that translated into calculated increases in fat oxidation of ~30% in the caffeine trials. A third study showed that ingestion of 5 mg of caffeine/ kg body mass (bm) spared muscle glycogen and increased the use of muscle triacylglycerol (TG) (22). In the ensuing decade, most investigators examined the effects of caffeine on selected aspects of whole-body metabolism. Consequently, the reported conclusions regarding the metabolic effects of caffeine and extrapolations to performance were based on changes in venous plasma FFA concentrations and RER. Another common theme during the 1980s was the variability in findings and conclusions. Conlee (15) surveyed the literature in 1991 and concluded that much of the variability in the reported caffeine findings was the result of poor experimental designs and a lack of adequate experimental controls. The factors relating to the experimental design included the exercise modality, the exercise power output, and the caffeine dose. Four additional factors were related to the status of the subjects before the experiment: aerobic training status, nutritional status, previous caffeine use, and individual variation. The training status of the subjects deserves mention as it seems clear that aerobic performance reliability improves with increased training frequency and intensity and the talent level of the subjects. Therefore, performance studies require the use of trained subjects in order to minimize day-to-day variability. The final factor, individual variability, may be the greatest contributor to the variable caffeine results, as large individual differences persist even when most other factors are controlled for. The work published in the 1980s has been extensively reviewed (15, 32, 62, 67).

Recent Endurance Performance and Metabolic Studies

Several well-controlled studies in the 1990s reexamined the performance and metabolic effects of caffeine in well-trained recreational and elite athletes. The athletes were accustomed to intense aerobic training, exercise tests to exhaustion, and race conditions. These experiments examined (1) the effects of 6 to 9 mg caffeine/kg bm (in capsule form) on running and cycling time to exhaustion at 80% to 85% $\dot{V}O_2$max (30, 64, 72); (2) the effects of varying doses of caffeine (2.1-13 mg/kg bm) on cycling performance time to exhaustion at 80% to 85% $\dot{V}O_2$max (31, 55) and 1-hr time trial performance (44); and (3) the effects of 5 mg caffeine/kg bm on performance of repeated 30-min bouts of cycling (5-min rest between bouts) at 85% to 90% $\dot{V}O_2$max (69).

This work produced or confirmed several important findings. Endurance performance was improved by ~20% to 50% compared to that in the placebo trial (32-77 min) after ingestion of varying caffeine doses (3-13 mg/kg bm) in elite and recreationally trained athletes during running or cycling at ~80% to 90% $\dot{V}O_2$max. Without exception, the 3, 5, and 6 mg/kg bm doses produced a performance-enhancing effect with urinary caffeine levels below the IOC acceptable limit. Three of four experiments using a 9 mg/kg dose showed performance increases, whereas 6 of 22 athletes tested in these studies had

urinary caffeine at or above 12 μg/ml. Performance was enhanced with a 13 mg/kg bm dose, but 6 of 9 athletes had urinary caffeine well above 12 μg/ml. The side effects of caffeine ingestion (dizziness, headache, insomnia, and gastrointestinal distress) were rare with doses at or below 6 mg/kg bm, but prevalent at higher doses (9-13 mg/kg bm), and were associated with decreased performance in some athletes at 9 mg/kg bm (31). Withdrawal of caffeine for two or four days in habitual caffeine users (~750 mg/day) did not impair the performance improvements associated with the acute ingestion of 6 mg caffeine/kg bm (72).

Caffeine generally produced no change in venous plasma [norepinephrine] at rest or exercise, a twofold increase in plasma epinephrine (EPI) concentration at rest and exercise, and increased plasma [FFA] at rest, although the increases in [FFA] were often not statistically significant. When elevated [FFA] were present with caffeine at the onset of exercise, they were no longer present after 15 to 20 min of exercise. At the lowest caffeine dose (3 mg/kg bm), performance was increased without a significant increase in plasma venous EPI and FFA. Muscle glycogen utilization was reduced with caffeine ingestion, but the "sparing" was limited to the first 15 min of exercise at ~80% $\dot{V}O_2$max.

Caffeine and Short-Term Exercise Performance

The studies just discussed dealt with the ability of caffeine ingestion to (1) improve performance during running and cycling to exhaustion at a given power output, (2) improve the time taken to complete a fixed amount of work, or (3) increase the amount of work performed in a given amount of time. Generally, the placebo trials in these studies lasted between 40 and 80 min. It has been repeatedly suggested that a shift toward greater fat oxidation and reduced carbohydrate use (glycogen sparing) may contribute to the ability to exercise longer after caffeine ingestion. More recently, there has been interest in the effects of caffeine ingestion on performance of short-term exercise as long as 35 min in duration and as short as 30 sec. If caffeine is a PES during short-term exercise, then the shorter the exercise, the less likely the mechanism will be related to increased fat oxidation and decreased carbohydrate oxidation, as carbohydrate availability does not limit performance in short-term exercise.

Intense Aerobic Exercise, ~20-35 Minutes

Competitive races lasting ~20 to 30 min require athletes to exercise at power outputs of ~85% to 95% $\dot{V}O_2$max. In one study, caffeine (6 mg/kg bm) significantly reduced 1500-m (1640 yd) swim trial time from 21:22 (±38 sec) to 20:59 (±36 sec) (min:sec) in trained distance swimmers (49). The authors reported lower pre-exercise venous plasma [K^+] and higher postexercise venous blood [glucose] with caffeine and suggested that electrolyte balance and exogenous glucose availability may be related to caffeine's performance-enhancing effect. A second study indicated no performance-enhancing effect of caffeine in mildly trained military recruits during cycling to exhaustion (26-27 min) at ~80% $\dot{V}O_2$max at sea level (28). However, cycle time was improved on acute (35 vs. 23 min) and chronic (39 vs. 31 min) exposure to altitude. In a third study, the ingestion of 4.45 mg caffeine/kg bm in capsule form increased run time to exhaustion at 85% $\dot{V}O_2$max from ~32 to ~40 min in trained runners (33). However, the consumption of caffeinated coffee did not increase running performance, even though subjects ingested the same amount of caffeine and reached the same blood caffeine levels during exercise as in the caffeine capsule trial. Even when caffeine was added to decaffeinated coffee there was no improvement in running performance, prompting the authors to conclude that other compounds in coffee must antagonize the performance-enhancing effects of caffeine ingestion in capsules (33). A fourth study also demonstrated that both caffeine (6 mg caffeine/kg bm) and theophylline (4.5 mg/kg bm) increased run time to exhaustion at ~80% $\dot{V}O_2$max from 32.6 ± 3.4 min to 41.2 ± 4.8 min and 37.4 ± 5.0 min, respectively (36).

It is not clear why caffeine is a PES during intense aerobic exercise of 20- to 35-min duration. A strong candidate must be caffeine's effect on the CNS, although studies examining the potential effects on skeletal muscle are lacking.

Graded Exercise Tests, 8 to 20 Minutes

Several investigations showed no effect of moderate doses of caffeine on time to exhaustion and $\dot{V}O_2$max during graded exercise protocols lasting 8 to 20 min (see Dodd et al. [20] for review). However, two studies reported prolonged exercise times when 10 to 15 mg caffeine/kg bm was ingested (26, 50). The first of these studies used 10 and 15 mg caffeine/kg bm doses and reported a small but significant increase in performance. However, the control trial preceded the caffeine trials, leading to the possibility of an order effect. The second study used a 10 mg caffeine/kg bm dose, given 3 hr before cycling, and indicated an increased time to exhaustion. The subjects completed control, placebo, and caffeine trials with the control trials always first and the remaining two trials randomized. Although factors such as habitual caffeine use and time between caffeine ingestion and testing were used to explain the positive findings, it seems that the high caffeine dose and the

order effect are the most likely factors explaining these positive findings.

Unfortunately, no mechanistic information presently exists to explain how these high caffeine doses prolong exercise time during a graded test lasting up to 20 min. One proposal was that the mechanism was related to slowing of muscle glycogenolysis at all power outputs, either through enhanced fat metabolism or through a direct inhibition on glycogen PHOS activity at the higher power outputs (26). If the use of muscle glycogen was delayed as the subject exercised at power outputs above 50% $\dot{V}O_2$max, the production and accumulation of glycolytic by-products associated with fatigue may have been slowed. If local muscle fatigue could be delayed at high power outputs, the completion of an additional power output may be possible. However, this scenario is hard to imagine at the highest power outputs, where energy derived from anaerobic glycolysis is essential for the maintenance of performance. No studies have included the muscle measurements necessary to investigate this problem during short-term graded exercise.

Intense Aerobic Exercise, ~4 to 8 Minutes

Exercise events at high power outputs (~95-110% $\dot{V}O_2$max) that last for ~4 to 8 min require near-maximal or maximal rates of energy provision from both aerobic and anaerobic sources.

In some cases, intense aerobic exercise was preceded by prolonged submaximal exercise. Sasaki et al. (57) ran subjects for 2 hr at ~60% $\dot{V}O_2$max, for 10 min at 80%, and finally to exhaustion at 90% $\dot{V}O_2$max. Ingesting a total of 800 mg of caffeine during the 2 hr of submaximal running did not improve performance during the intense running. Falk et al. (23) had subjects complete a 40-km (25 miles) march at ~40% $\dot{V}O_2$max in the field followed by cycling to exhaustion at 90% $\dot{V}O_2$max in the laboratory. Ingesting 5 mg caffeine/kg bm before the march and again during the march did not improve intense exercise performance (~4-6 min).

Collomp et al. (13) reported that moderate caffeine doses increased cycle time to exhaustion at 100% $\dot{V}O_2$max from 5:20 with placebo to 5:49 in one group and 5:40 in a second group, although the increases were not statistically significant. Wiles et al. (79) reported that coffee ingestion (~150-200 mg caffeine) improved 1500-m (1640 yd) race time on a treadmill by 4.2 sec over that with placebo (4:46.0 vs. 4:50.2). The runners in this study were well trained, but clearly not elite. In a second experiment, subjects consumed coffee or placebo and then ran for 1100 m (1203 yd) at a predetermined pace, then ran a final 400 m (437 yd) as fast as possible. The time to complete the final 400 m was 61.25 sec with coffee and 62.88 sec without. After ingestion of coffee, all subjects ran faster, and the mean $\dot{V}O_2$ during the final 400 m was higher. To document such small changes, the average response to three trials in the caffeine and placebo conditions was determined in both experiments. These findings suggesting that coffee is a PES are completely opposite to the results of Graham et al. (33), who reported no performance-enhancing effect during longer-term exercise.

Jackman et al. (40) examined the effects of caffeine ingestion (6 mg/kg) on the performance in and metabolic responses to three bouts of cycling at 100% $\dot{V}O_2$max. The initial two bouts lasted 2 min whereas bout 3 was to exhaustion, with rest periods of 6 min between bouts. Time to exhaustion in bout 3 was prolonged with caffeine (4.93 ± 0.60 vs. 4.12 ± 0.36 min, n = 14). Muscle and blood lactate measurements suggested a higher production of lactate in the caffeine trial, even in the initial two bouts when the power output was fixed. The glycogenolytic rate was not different during bouts 1 and 2, and less than 50% of the muscle glycogen store was used in either trial during the entire protocol. The authors concluded that the performance-enhancing effect of caffeine during intense aerobic exercise was not associated with glycogen sparing and may be due to increased anaerobic energy provision. It is possible that the elevated EPI levels contributed to the stimulation of muscle glycogenolysis at this exercise intensity. Although Chesley et al. (8) demonstrated that caffeine-induced increases in EPI were not associated with enhanced glycogen breakdown at 80% to 85% $\dot{V}O_2$max, this may not be the case at 100% $\dot{V}O_2$max, where the [EPI] are higher.

Two recent studies from the same laboratory showed significant improvements in time to complete a 2000-m (2187 yd) rowing task on a Concept II rowing ergometer. The studies appear to be identical, one examining the effects of placebo and caffeine on rowing performance in oarswomen (1) and the other in oarsmen (6). In each study subjects completed three familiarization trials before the experimental trials. The ingestion of 6 mg and 9 mg caffeine/kg bm by the women improved rowing time by 0.7% and 1.3%, respectively, compared to the placebo trial performance time of ~8 min (1). Similar doses in the men improved rowing time by 1.2% at both doses compared to the placebo trial performance time of ~7 min (6).

Caffeine appears to be a PES during intense aerobic exercise (~95-110% $\dot{V}O_2$max) lasting ~4 to 8 min, although the improvement is not always statistically significant. When intense aerobic exercise is preceded by long-term submaximal exercise, no performance improvement is reported. The mechanism for the performance enhancement during this type of exercise is not known, but may include enhanced anaerobic energy provision, direct effects of caffeine on muscle ion handling, and a CNS component related to the sensation of effort.

Sprint Exercise, 30 to 90 Seconds

Sprinting is defined as exercise or sporting events at power outputs corresponding to 150% to 300% $\dot{V}O_2$max and lasting less than 90 sec. The amount of energy derived from anaerobic processes would be ~75% to 80% of the total energy in the first 30 sec, ~65% to 70% over 60 sec, and ~55% to 60% over the entire 90-sec period.

Williams et al. (80) reported that caffeine ingestion had no effect on maximal power output or muscular endurance during short, maximal bouts of cycling. Collomp et al. (14) reported that 5 mg caffeine/kg bm did not increase peak power or total work completed during a 30-sec Wingate test, but the same group later reported that 250 mg caffeine produced a 7% improvement in the maximal power output generated during a series of 6-sec sprints at varying force-velocity relationships (2). Greer et al. (35) also examined the effect of 6 mg caffeine/kg bm on performance during a series of four Wingate tests, separated by 6 min of rest between bouts. There was no improvement in peak or average power output in the caffeine trial during the initial two bouts, and the average power output was actually lower in the final two bouts with caffeine.

Collomp et al. (12) examined the effects of 4.3 mg caffeine/kg bm on two 100-m (109 yd) freestyle swims separated by 20 min. In well-trained swimmers, caffeine increased swim velocity by 2% and 4% in the two sprints, respectively, but actual performance times were not reported. In untrained swimmers, caffeine had no effect on sprint times.

Therefore, given the present information, it appears that caffeine is not a PES for sprint performance.

Field Studies

Exercise performance in most laboratory studies is measured as the time taken to reach exhaustion at a given power output, the time taken to complete a given amount of work, or the amount of work that can be performed in a given amount of time (2, 13, 16, 30, 39, 55, 64, 69). However, in the field, performance is usually measured as the time taken to complete a given distance. Consequently, extrapolations from the laboratory to field settings may not be valid. Occasionally, laboratory studies simulate race conditions (1, 6), and other studies measure performance in the field (track, swimming pool) in time trial settings without actual race conditions. However, these studies still do not simulate real competitions. In field studies that do simulate race conditions, it is often impossible to employ the controls required to generate conclusive results. For example, Berglund and Hemmingsson (4) reported that caffeine ingestion increased cross-country ski performance by 1 to 2.5 min compared to that in a control race lasting 1 to 1.5 hr. This improvement occurred at altitude, but not at sea level.

Unfortunately, the weather and snow conditions were variable in both locations, requiring normalization of the performance times in order to compare results. Another field study indicated that ingesting 0, 5, or 9 mg caffeine/kg bm had no effect on 21-km (13 miles) road race performance in hot and humid environments (10). Although subjects acted as their own controls, no subjects received the placebo treatment in all three races to enable assessment of whether differing environmental conditions affected race performance, independent of caffeine.

The problems associated with field trials raise questions about the validity of the results and indicate how difficult it is to perform well-controlled and meaningful field trials. Nevertheless, there is clearly a need for more studies of this type.

Theories of Ergogenicity

As mentioned previously, the mechanisms that may contribute to the performance-enhancing effects of caffeine can be categorized as targeting three general areas. The first area is metabolism, and the most popular explanation is the classic or "metabolic" theory for the ergogenic effects of caffeine during endurance exercise, involving an increase in fat oxidation and reduction in carbohydrate oxidation. The metabolic category also includes factors that may affect muscle metabolism and performance in a direct manner, such as caffeine-induced inhibition of the key glycogenolytic enzyme, glycogen PHOS, and antagonism of adenosine receptors, which are involved in glucose uptake into the muscle. The second category entails a proposed direct effect of caffeine on skeletal muscle performance via ion handling, including Na^+-K^+ ATPase activity and Ca^{2+} kinetics. The third category involves a direct effect of caffeine on portions of the CNS that alter the perception of effort and/or motor unit recruitment.

Metabolic Mechanisms for Improved Exercise Performance

There is evidence that metabolic mechanisms are part of the explanation for the improvement in endurance performance after caffeine ingestion (5-13 mg/kg bm), except at low doses (2-4 mg/kg bm); in the latter case this has not been fully examined. The increased plasma [FFA] at the onset of exercise reported in numerous studies, the glycogen sparing in the initial 15 to 30 min of exercise (22, 64), and increased intramuscular TG use during the first 30 min of exercise (22) suggest a greater role for fat metabolism early in exercise after doses of ≥5 mg caffeine/kg bm. However, recent work has been less supportive of a metabolic explanation.

Chesley et al. (9) reported a variable effect of 9 mg caffeine/kg bm on muscle glycogen sparing during the initial minutes of exercise at 80% to 85% $\dot{V}O_2$max in untrained males. Only 6 of 12 subjects used less glycogen (10% reduction or greater) after caffeine ingestion. In the subjects who did spare muscle glycogen, caffeine improved the energy status of muscle in the early stages of intense exercise, resulting in less phosphocreatine use and lower accumulations of free adenosine monophosphate (AMP). Since AMP is an allosteric activator of the active form of glycogen PHOS, lower accumulations would decrease the flux through PHOS and explain the reduction in muscle glycogen use. It is not presently clear how caffeine defends the energy state of the cell at the onset of intense exercise. However, one hypothesis is that this effect may be due to increased fat availability and a greater provision of the reduced form of nicotinamide adenine dinucleotide (NADH) in the mitochondria at the onset of exercise after caffeine ingestion 1 hr before exercise (9). This would enable greater aerobic energy production from fat-derived NADH and reduce the need for glycogenolysis. In the subjects who did not reduce glycogen use, there were no reductions in phosphocreatine use and free AMP accumulation. It is not clear why some subjects respond to caffeine by glycogen sparing and others do not.

However, in two recent studies, caffeine had no effect on substrate metabolism during exercise. Graham et al. (34) reported that 6 mg caffeine/kg bm did not alter fat and carbohydrate metabolism during 1 hr of cycling at 70% $\dot{V}O_2$max in healthy male subjects. Direct measurements of leg glucose and FFA uptake, as well as lactate and glycerol release, were unaffected by caffeine. Caffeine ingestion did increase pre-exercise [FFA] and appeared to increase fat use early in exercise, but the initial measurements were not made until 10 min into the exercise. However, if fat use was increased in the caffeine trial, it did not result in less glycogen use by the group of subjects in the initial 10 min of exercise (34). Laurent et al. (45) also reported no effect of 6 mg caffeine/kg bm on muscle glycogen use during 2 hr of cycling at 65% $\dot{V}O_2$max in well-trained military personnel who were glycogen- "supercompensated." Glycogen use was monitored with ^{13}C nuclear magnetic resonance spectroscopy, a technique that has not been validated for use in the thigh muscle. Also, in the two most recent studies, only mean glycogen data were reported and the effects of caffeine on individual muscle glycogenolysis were not examined. It is not clear why the more recent studies have reported either a variable sparing effect or no effect of caffeine on muscle glycogenolysis. These results may be related to the exercise power output, the training and dietary status of the subjects, the duration of the exercise period examined, or simply biological variation between subjects. However, it is clear that the recent metabolic data argue against an important metabolic contribution to the performance-enhancement effects of caffeine during aerobic exercise.

It also appears that EPI does not contribute to the metabolic changes that lead to enhanced endurance performance after caffeine ingestion. First, performance was enhanced with 3 mg caffeine/kg without significant increases in plasma EPI and FFA, although FFA were increased twofold at rest (31). Second, an infusion of EPI, designed to produce resting and exercise [EPI] similar to those induced by caffeine, had no effect on plasma [FFA] or muscle glycogenolysis during exercise (8). Third, Van Soeren et al. (73) and Mohr et al. (51) gave caffeine to spinal cord-injured subjects and reported increased plasma [FFA] without changes in [EPI]. These findings suggest that caffeine ingestion affects the mobilization of fat by antagonizing the adenosine receptors in adipose tissue.

A contribution of additional metabolic mechanisms to the performance-enhancing effects of caffeine has been suggested. There is some evidence that caffeine has direct and indirect effects on the transformation of PHOS to its active a (PHOSa) form and on the post-transformational control of PHOSa. Caffeine and the associated increase in circulating [EPI] can increase the activation of PHOS during exercise (8, 9), but the actual flux through PHOS (glycogenolysis) is either unaffected or reduced in some individuals. This reduction in glycogen breakdown may be related to a direct inhibitory effect of caffeine on PHOSa activity (43, 56). This could explain the glycogen sparing that occurs in some individuals at the onset of intense aerobic exercise at 80% to 85% $\dot{V}O_2$max but is not consistent with the suggestion that glycogen use is unaffected during exercise at 100% $\dot{V}O_2$max and sprint exercise at ~200% to 300% $\dot{V}O_2$max. It may be that post-transformational regulation of PHOSa by caffeine is present at the lower aerobic intensities but is overwhelmed by activating factors (inorganic phosphate and free AMP) at the higher power outputs.

Vergauwen et al. (74) reported that adenosine receptors are involved in the stimulation of glucose uptake and transport by insulin and by contractions in rat skeletal muscle. Caffeine, as an adenosine receptor antagonist and at a physiological level (77 μM), decreased glucose uptake during contractions. This suggested that caffeine may also spare the use of extramuscular carbohydrate and force the muscle to rely more heavily on fat oxidation. However, a recent study showed no effect of caffeine on directly measured leg glucose uptake during cycle exercise at 70% $\dot{V}O_2$max, suggesting that other regulatory factors overwhelm the adenosine-related effects (34).

Ion Handling in Skeletal Muscle

Caffeine may alter the handling of ions in skeletal muscle and contribute to a performance-enhancing effect during exercise. Most of the supporting evidence has come from in vitro experiments using pharmacological doses of methylxanthines. The most likely candidates as contributors to performance enhancement in a physiological environment are increased Ca^{2+} release during the later stages of exercise and increased Na^+-K^+ ATPase activity, which may help maintain the membrane potential during exercise. The lowest [methylxanthine] used to demonstrate these effects in vitro approach the actual [methylxanthine] that have been shown to be performance enhancing in exercising humans (46, 67).

It has been demonstrated that pharmacological levels of methylxanthine in vitro affect several steps in the excitation-contraction coupling process in skeletal muscle, (1) increasing the release of Ca^{2+} from the sarcoplasmic reticulum, (2) enhancing troponin/myosin Ca^{2+} sensitivity, and (3) decreasing the reuptake of Ca^{2+} by the sarcoplasmic reticulum (67). In support of this, Tarnopolsky and Cupido (68) recently reported that 6 mg caffeine/kg bm increased the force of contraction during the second minute of a 2-min tetanic (20 Hz) stimulation of the common peroneal nerve in healthy males. Habitual caffeine use did not affect the results, and no potentiation of force was reported at 40-Hz stimulation. Maximal voluntary contraction and peak twitch torque were also not affected by caffeine at either stimulation frequency.

Methylxanthines also stimulate Na^+-K^+ ATPase activity in inactive skeletal muscle, leading to increased rates of K^+ uptake and Na^+ efflux. This attenuates the rise in plasma $[K^+]$ with exercise, which may help maintain the membrane potential in contracting muscle (46, 47). Any of these changes could produce increases in skeletal muscle force production. However, it is presently unclear whether or not these ion-handling effects of caffeine contribute to performance enhancement, given the relatively low [methylxanthine] normally found in humans after caffeine ingestion.

Central Effects of Caffeine

Although it is accepted that caffeine affects the CNS, it is difficult to quantify how much of caffeine's ability to enhance performance is due to central effects. Caffeine is certainly a CNS stimulant, causing increased wakefulness and vigilance (17, 53); and it has been suggested that the increased performance is simply due to increased alertness or improved mood (54). However, the ability of caffeine to delay fatigue points to more complex mechanisms than simply heightened arousal. The following topics are of special interest in a discussion of caffeine's central effects because they also relate to peripheral metabolic effects.

Adenosine Receptor Antagonism

Because caffeine can freely pass through the blood-brain barrier (53), its concentration in the brain and CNS increases rapidly after ingestion, in concert with changes in other body tissues (17). Caffeine increases the concentrations of several brain neurotransmitters, including seratonin, dopamine, acetylcholine, norepinephrine, and glutamate, causing increases in spontaneous locomotor activity and neuronal firing in animals (53). It is generally accepted that the mechanism for neurotransmitter increases is adenosine receptor antagonism, and high adenosine receptor levels in the brain support this hypothesis (17, 25, 27, 60).

Adenosine is a neurotransmitter and a neuromodulator, capable of affecting the release of other neurotransmitters (25). Adenosine and adenosine analogs generally cause lowered motor activity, decreased wakefulness and vigilance, and decreases in other concentrations. Caffeine and adenosine receptor antagonists have the opposite effect by blocking the adenosine receptors. It is generally believed that the inhibition (adenosine) or stimulation (caffeine) of neurotransmitter release is presynaptic (27, 60). It has been demonstrated that caffeine increases the concentration, synthesis, and/or turnover of all major neurotransmitters, including serotonin, dopamine, acetylcholine, NE, and glutamate. These neurotransmitters are all inhibited by adenosine. The consequences of these neurotransmitter changes for performance are currently unknown. Dopamine and serotonin levels have been implicated in the central effects of caffeine on fatigue and behavior (17, 25) and in the development of central fatigue independent of caffeine ingestion (18). It has been suggested that an increase in excitatory neurotransmitters could lead to decreases in motorneuron threshold, resulting in greater motor unit recruitment (76) and subsequently lower perceived exertion for a given power output (11, 54). However, although this continues to be cited as a potential mechanism, it has not been examined during exercise (11, 54).

Ratings of Perceived Exertion

One quantifiable aspect of caffeine's central effects is a lower rating of perceived exertion (RPE) during exercise. Studies have demonstrated that RPE at a given power output was lower after caffeine ingestion compared to control (16) and subjects accomplished a greater amount of work after caffeine ingestion compared to control when RPE was held constant (11, 39). It has been speculated that the lowered RPE with caffeine is due to a decrease in the firing threshold of motorneurons (11, 54) or changes in muscle contraction force (67). Both mechanisms would result in lowered afferent feedback from the working muscle and a lowered RPE: the first mechanism because more motor units would be recruited

for a given task and the second because the force for a given stimulus would be greater. The work of Kalmar and Cafarelli (42) lends support to the second possibility, because their study showed that maximal voluntary contraction force was increased by 3.5% after the ingestion of 6 mg caffeine/kg bm. Another hypothesis is that caffeine directly affects the release of β-endorphins and other hormones that modulate the feelings of discomfort and pain associated with exhaustive exercise (53). A final explanation for the reduced RPE may involve the central fatigue hypothesis (18, 67).

Central Fatigue Hypothesis

Given that caffeine affects the CNS, it is appealing to link it to one proposed mechanism of fatigue currently being investigated, the central fatigue hypothesis. This hypothesis argues that the central component of fatigue caused by exhaustive exercise is due to elevated levels of serotonin or 5-hydroxytryptophan (5-HT) in the brain, caused by an increase in its precursor, tryptophan (TRP) (5, 18). Tryptophan is the only amino acid that is transported in plasma bound to albumin, and it competes for transport into the brain with branch chain amino acids (BCAA). Evidence for the central fatigue theory includes increased levels of brain 5-HT at fatigue, increased plasma free TRP at fatigue caused by high [FFA], and decreased fatigue with BCAA supplementation (5). If caffeine delayed the onset of CNS fatigue via serotonin levels, then it must lower 5-HT levels or inhibit the rise in 5-HT. However, the effects of caffeine on the CNS and peripheral metabolism appear to be contradictory, for two reasons. First, acute caffeine ingestion significantly increased brain 5-HT levels, likely due to increases in brain free TRP levels (25, 53). Second, caffeine ingestion before exercise elevates plasma [FFA] at the onset of exercise, which should increase free TRP, due to competition for albumin binding, and hasten fatigue. It is possible that the rise in 5-HT at the onset of exercise is overridden by other factors such as increased sympathetic drive or favorable metabolic factors. Similarly, since it has been postulated that the ratio of 5-HT to dopamine is a larger determinant in fatigue than the [5-HT] alone (18), the caffeine-induced rises in the two neurotransmitters could offset one another.

In summary, the caffeine-induced mechanism(s) that may delay central fatigue remain to be discovered, but the association between caffeine and the central fatigue hypothesis remains a possibility.

Complications of Studying Caffeine, Exercise Performance, and Metabolism

It is important to mention in a discussion of the performance, metabolic, and central effects of caffeine ingestion that the mechanism(s) of action may not be entirely due to the direct effects of caffeine. Caffeine is a trimethylxanthine compound that is rapidly metabolized in the liver to three dimethylxanthines—paraxanthine, theophylline, and theobromine. These are released into the plasma as the [caffeine] declines and remain in the circulation longer. Although the plasma [dimethylxanthines] levels are not high, paraxanthine and theophylline are potential adenosine antagonists and metabolic stimuli. Therefore, as caffeine and its metabolites are often present at the same time, it is difficult to resolve which tissues are directly or indirectly affected by which compound. Another complication of studying caffeine ingestion is the variability of individual responses, affecting central, metabolic, and exercise performance responses. This affects all categories of subjects, but may be a larger problem with less aerobically fit individuals. Chesley et al. (8) reported a variable glycogen-sparing response to a high caffeine dose (9 mg/kg bm) in untrained men. Only 6 of 12 subjects demonstrated glycogen sparing during 15 min of cycling at ~85% $\dot{V}O_2$max, whereas the sparing response was more uniform in a group of trained men (64). This issue has been further complicated by two recent studies reporting no glycogen sparing on a mean basis in a group of untrained subjects and a group of trained subjects (34, 45). Variability is also present in the performance studies and among all groups of caffeine users, including mild and heavy users, users withdrawn from caffeine, and nonusers. Therefore, although mean results from groups of subjects and athletes predict improved athletic performance, predictions that a given person will improve are less certain.

There is now evidence that ingestion of caffeine in capsules and consumption of coffee containing the same amount of caffeine are not equivalent (33). It appears that additional chemicals in coffee negate the usual performance-enhancing effect. On the other hand, there have been several studies in which caffeine administration in coffee produced improvements in performance (16, 69, 79). The explanation for these discrepant results is unclear at the present time.

The study of caffeine ingestion and exercise performance has been generally limited to male subjects. There have been few attempts to study the response of females to caffeine ingestion at rest and during exercise. It will be important to control for menstrual status in future studies, as estrogen may affect the half-life of caffeine.

Practical Aspects of Ingesting Caffeine

This section will examine and explain the ways in which caffeine is used, as well as the effects of this use by athletes. As always, careful attention to the information that exists regarding the physiological effects of caffeine consumption will prevent the athlete from experiencing side effects and doping issues.

Caffeine Dose

Caffeine is a "controlled or restricted substance" with respect to the IOC. Athletes are permitted up to 12 µg caffeine/ml urine before the level is considered illegal (70). This allows athletes who normally consume caffeine in their diet to continue this practice before competition. An athlete can consume a large amount of caffeine before reaching the "illegal limit." A 154-lb (70 kg) person could drink about three to four mugs or six regular-size cups of drip-percolated coffee (~9 mg caffeine/kg bm) ~1 hr before exercise and then exercise for 1 to 1.5 hr, and a subsequent urine sample would only approach the urinary caffeine limit. Consuming a smaller dose of 3 to 6 mg caffeine/kg bm allows an athlete to legally improve performance if the individual responds to caffeine and participates in an event in which it has been shown to be a PES. A caffeine level above 12 µg/ml suggests that a person has deliberately taken caffeine in capsule, tablet, or suppository form in an attempt to improve performance. Not surprisingly, only a few athletes have been caught with illegal levels during competitions, although formal reports of the frequency of caffeine abuse are rare. One study indicated that 26 of 775 cyclists had illegal urinary caffeine levels when tested after competition (19).

Ingestion of higher doses of caffeine (10-15 mg/kg bm) increases the likelihood of urinary caffeine levels that are "illegal" and worsens the side effects. The optimal dose for improving performance is ~3 to 6 mg/kg bm; at this dose the side effects are minimized and urine levels are well within the legal range.

Urinary Caffeine and Doping

The use of urinary caffeine levels to determine caffeine abuse in sport has been criticized (21). Only 0.5% to 3% of orally ingested caffeine actually reaches the urine, as the majority is metabolized in the liver and the excreted by-products are not measured in doping tests. Other factors that affect the urinary [caffeine] include body weight, gender, and hydration status of the athlete. The time elapsed between caffeine ingestion and urine collection is also important and is affected by exercise duration and environmental conditions. Sport governing bodies may not regard these factors as a problem, since most people caught with illegal levels of caffeine will have used the drug in a doping manner, and the adverse and health effects of even high levels of caffeine abuse seem moderate compared to those of many other PES.

Adverse Effects and Variability in Responses

The adverse effects of caffeine ingestion are well known: anxiety, jitters, inability to focus, gastrointestinal unrest, insomnia, irritability, and, with higher doses, the risk of heart arrhythmias and mild hallucinations. In addition, caffeine-induced adverse effects vary considerably between individuals, as do the metabolic and performance effects. The side effects associated with consuming acute doses of up to 9 mg caffeine/kg bm are not dangerous but can be disconcerting before training or competition. These are reduced with administration of 3 to 6 versus 9 mg caffeine/kg bm. Therefore, it is recommended that athletes use only moderate doses of caffeine before competitions to prevent their experiencing any adverse effects.

There are also concerns for athletes who are habitual consumers of caffeine. Caffeine is a psychoactive substance and, if consumed on a daily basis, can lead to a number of caffeine use disorders, including caffeine intoxication, withdrawal and dependence, and caffeine-induced anxiety and sleep disorders (59, 74, 75). For example, people who consume moderate amounts of caffeine may experience a withdrawal syndrome if they alter their daily intake of caffeine (59).

Another concern is that daily caffeine consumption may predispose people (including athletes) to increased risk for a number of diseases. Although the issue is beyond the scope of this review, many researchers have examined the effect of caffeine on cardiovascular health. Most have concluded that the experimental findings do not support the hypothesis that caffeine or coffee consumption increases the risk of coronary heart disease and stroke (38, 52). There are many other areas of concern regarding caffeine consumption, including pregnancy, cancer, fibrocystic breast disease, calcium and bone health, and reproduction (61).

Habitual Caffeine Consumption

An athlete's normal caffeine intake habits may affect whether acute caffeine ingestion improves performance. Many investigators ask users to refrain from caffeine consumption for 48 to 72 hr prior to experiments. Caffeine metabolism is not increased by use, but the effects of caffeine may be altered by habitual use via alterations in adenosine receptor populations. As reviewed by Graham et al. (32), several studies suggest that chronic caffeine use dampens the EPI response to exercise and caffeine but does not affect plasma [FFA] or exercise RER (3, 72). However, these changes do not dampen the performance enhancement associated with doses of 6 to 9 mg caffeine/kg bm. Endurance performance increased in all subjects when both users and nonusers were examined and users

had abstained from caffeine for 48 to 72 hr before experiments (30, 64). However, the performance results were more variable in a subsequent study with more nonusers (31). Lastly, time to exhaustion at 80% to 85% $\dot{V}O_2$max improved with caffeine and was unaffected by withdrawal (0 to 4 days) in chronic caffeine consumers (72).

Caffeine and High-Carbohydrate Diets

An early investigation suggested that a high-carbohydrate diet and a prerace meal negated the expected increase in plasma [FFA] after caffeine ingestion during 2 hr of exercise at ~75% $\dot{V}O_2$max (77). These results suggested that high-carbohydrate diets negated the performance-enhancing effects of caffeine, although performance was not measured. However, a high-carbohydrate diet and pretrial meal did not prevent caffeine-induced increases in performance in a number of studies using well-trained/recreational runners and cyclists (as reviewed in 62).

Diuretic Effect of Caffeine

It has been suggested that caffeine ingestion may lead to poor hydration status before and during exercise because of the potential diuretic properties of the drug. However, no changes in core temperature, sweat loss, or plasma volume were reported during exercise after caffeine ingestion (24, 29). It has also been demonstrated that urine flow rate, decreases in plasma volume, sweat rate, and heart rate were unaffected by caffeine (~600 mg) ingested in a carbohydrate-electrolyte drink (~2.5 l) during 1 hr at rest and 3 hr of cycling at 60% $\dot{V}O_2$max (78). A recent study also showed no effect of ingesting 4.45 mg caffeine/kg bm (either with water or in coffee) on urine output or hemoconcentration in the blood during 1 hr at rest and 1 hr of exercise at 70% $\dot{V}O_2$max (33). Another recent investigation indicated no effect of adding 150 mg caffeine to a carbohydrate-electrolyte drink on gastrointestinal function in well-trained men when compared to a carbohydrate-electrolyte solution alone or plain water (71). There were no differences between the three drinks for gastric pH, gastroesophageal reflux, or gastrointestinal transit during the pre-exercise, cycling (90 min at ~75% $\dot{V}O_2$max), and postexercise periods. Interestingly, intestinal glucose uptake was increased in the carbohydrate-electrolyte plus caffeine trial (71).

Conclusion

Caffeine ingestion (3-13 mg/kg bm) before exercise increases performance during prolonged endurance cycling and running in the laboratory. Caffeine doses below 9 mg/kg bm generally produce urinary caffeine levels below the IOC allowable limit of 12 μg/ml. Moderate caffeine doses (5-6 mg/kg) appear also to increase short-term intense cycling and rowing performance (~4-8 min) in the laboratory and to decrease 1500-m (1640 yd) swim time (~20 min). Sprint exercise lasting less than 90 sec appears to be unaffected by caffeine. These results are generally reported in well-trained or recreational athletes, but field studies are lacking to confirm whether or not caffeine is a PES in the athletic world. The mechanisms for the improved endurance have not been clearly established. There has been evidence suggesting that caffeine ingestion increases the use of fat and decreases muscle glycogen use during the early stages of endurance exercise, thereby prolonging the availability of muscle carbohydrate and performance. However, recent studies have demonstrated that the caffeine-induced metabolic effects at the onset of exercise are variable and that caffeine has no effect on muscle fuel utilization after 10 min of exercise. These findings imply that caffeine must affect additional processes associated with skeletal muscle and/or the CNS in order to have a performance-enhancing effect during many types of exercise. It has been difficult to separate the central and peripheral effects of caffeine in human performance studies.

References

1. Anderson, M.E., Bruce, C.R., Fraser, S.F., Stepto, N.K., Klein, R., Hopkins, W.G., and Hawley, J.A. Improved 2000-meter rowing performance in competitive oarswomen after caffeine ingestion. *International Journal of Sport Nutrition and Exercise Metabolism* 10: 464-475; 2000.

2. Anselme, F., Collomp, K., Mercier, B., Ahmaidi, S., and Prefaut, C. Caffeine increases maximal anaerobic power and blood lactate concentration. *European Journal of Applied Physiology* 65: 188-191; 1992.

3. Bangsbo, J., Jacobsen, K., Nordberg, N., Christensen, N.J., and Graham, T. Acute and habitual caffeine ingestion and metabolic responses to steady-state exercise. *Journal of Applied Physiology* 72: 1297-1303; 1992.

4. Berglund, B., and Hemmingsson, P. Effects of caffeine ingestion on exercise performance at low and high altitudes in cross country skiers. *International Journal of Sports Medicine* 3: 234-236; 1982.

5. Blomstrand, E.E., and Newsholme, E.A. Glucose-fatty acid cycle and fatigue involving 5-hydroxytryptamine. In *Biochemistry of Exercise IX,* ed. R.J. Maughan and S.M. Shirreffs, 185-195. Champaign, IL: Human Kinetics, 1996.

6. Bruce, C.R., Anderson, M.E., Fraser, S.F., Stepto, N.K., Klein, R., Hopkins, W.G., and Hawley, J.A. Enhancement of 2000-m rowing performance after caffeine ingestion. *Medicine and Science in Sports and Exercise* 32: 1958-1963; 2000.

7. Canadian Centre for Drug Free Sport. *The National School Survey on Drugs and Sport,* 1-12. Ottawa, Ontario, 1993.

8. Chesley, A., Hultman, E., and Spriet, L.L. Effects of epinephrine infusion on muscle glycogenolysis during intense aerobic exercise. *American Journal of Physiology* 268: E127-E134; 1995.

9. Chesley, A., Howlett, R.A., Heigenhauser, G.J.F., Hultman, E., and Spriet, L.L. Regulation of muscle glycogenolytic flux during intense aerobic exercise following caffeine ingestion. *American Journal of Physiology* 275: R596-R603; 1998.

10. Cohen, B.S., Nelson, A.G., Prevost, M.C., Thompson, G.D., Marx, B.D., and Morris, G.S. Effects of caffeine ingestion on endurance racing in heat and humidity. *European Journal of Applied Physiology* 73: 358-363; 1996.

11. Cole, K.J., Costill, D.L., Starling, R.D., Goodpaster, B.H., Trappe, S.W., and Fink, W.J. Effect of caffeine ingestion on perception of effort and subsequent work production. *International Journal of Sport Nutrition* 6: 14-23; 1996.

12. Collomp, K., Caillaud, C., Audran, M., Chanal, J.-L., and Prefaut, C. Influence of acute and chronic bouts of caffeine on performance and catecholamines in the course of maximal exercise. *Comptes Renders de la Societe de Biologie* 184: 87-92; 1990.

13. Collomp, K., Ahmaidi, S., Audran, M., Chanal, J.-L., and Prefaut, C. Effects of caffeine ingestion on performance and anaerobic metabolism during the Wingate test. *International Journal of Sports Medicine* 12: 439-443; 1991.

14. Collomp, K., Ahmaidi, S., Chatard, J.C., Audran, M., and Prefaut, C. Benefits of caffeine ingestion on sprint performance in trained and untrained swimmers. *European Journal of Applied Physiology* 64: 377-380; 1992.

15. Conlee, R.K. Amphetamine, caffeine and cocaine. In *Ergogenics: Enhancement of Performance in Exercise and Sport,* ed. D.R. Lamb and M.H. Williams, 285-330. Indianapolis: Brown and Benchmark, 1991.

16. Costill, D.L., Dalsky, G.P., and Fink, W.J. Effects of caffeine on metabolism and exercise performance. *Medicine and Science in Sports* 10: 155-158; 1978.

17. Daly, J.W. Mechanism of action of caffeine. In *Caffeine, Coffee, and Health,* ed. S. Garattini, 97-150. New York: Raven Press, 1993.

18. Davis, J.M., and Bailey, S.P. Possible mechanisms of central nervous system fatigue during exercise. *Medicine and Science in Sports and Exercise* 29: 45-57; 1997.

19. Delbecke, F.T., and Debachere, M. Caffeine: use and abuse in sport. *International Journal of Sports Medicine* 5: 179-182; 1984.

20. Dodd, S.L., Herb, R.A., and Powers, S.K. Caffeine and exercise performance: an update. *Sports Medicine* 15: 14-23; 1993.

21. Duthel, J.M., Vallon, J.J., Martin, G., Ferret, J.M., Mathieu, R., and Videman, R. Caffeine and sport: role of physical exercise upon elimination. *Medicine and Science in Sports and Exercise* 23: 980-985; 1991.

22. Essig, D., Costill, D.L., and VanHandel, P.J. Effects of

caffeine ingestion on utilization of muscle glycogen and lipid during leg ergometer cycling. *International Journal of Sports Medicine* 1: 86-90; 1980.

23. Falk, B., Burstein, R., Ashkenazi, I., Spilberg, O., Alter, J., Zybler-Katz, J., Rubenstein, A., Bashan, N., and Shapiro, Y. The effect of caffeine ingestion on physical performance after prolonged exercise. *European Journal of Applied Physiology* 59: 168-173; 1989.

24. Falk, B., Burstein, R., Rosenblum, J., Shapiro, Y., Zylber-Katz, E., and Bashan, N. Effects of caffeine ingestion on body fluid balance and thermoregulation during exercise. *Canadian Journal of Physiology and Pharmacology* 68: 889-892; 1990.

25. Fernstrom, J.D., and Fernstrom, M.H. Effects of caffeine on monamine neurotransmitters in the central and peripheral nervous system. In *Caffeine,* ed. P.B. Dews, 107-118. Berlin: Springer-Verlag, 1984.

26. Flinn, S., Gregory, J., McNaughton, L.R., Tristram, S., and Davies, P. Caffeine ingestion prior to incremental cycling to exhaustion in recreational cyclists. *International Journal of Sports Medicine* 11: 188-193; 1990.

27. Fredholm, B.B. Adenosine, adenosine receptors and the actions of caffeine. *Pharmacology and Toxicology* 76: 93-101; 1995.

28. Fulco, C.S., Rock, P.B., Trad, L.A., Rose, M.S., Forte, V.A., Young, P.M., and Cymerman, A. Effect of caffeine on submaximal exercise performance at altitude. *Aviation Space and Environmental Medicine* 65: 539-545; 1994.

29. Gordon, N.F., Myburgh, J.L., Kruger, P.E., Kempff, P.J., Cilliers, J.F., Moolman, J., and Grobler, H.C. Effects of caffeine on thermoregulatory and myocardial function during endurance performance. *South African Medical Journal* 62: 644-647; 1982.

30. Graham, T.E., and Spriet, L.L. Performance and metabolic responses to a high caffeine dose during prolonged exercise. *Journal of Applied Physiology* 71: 2292-2298; 1991.

31. Graham, T.E., and Spriet, L.L. Metabolic, catecholamine and exercise performance responses to varying doses of caffeine. *Journal of Applied Physiology* 78: 867-874; 1995.

32. Graham, T.E., Rush, J.W.E., and Van Soeren, M.H. Caffeine and exercise: metabolism and performance. *Canadian Journal of Applied Physiology* 19: 111-138; 1994.

33. Graham, T.E., Hibbert, E., and Sathasivam, P. Metabolic and exercise endurance effects of coffee and caffeine ingestion. *Journal of Applied Physiology* 85: 883-889; 1998.

34. Graham, T.E., Helge, J.W., MacLean, D.A., Kiens, B., and Richter, E.A. Caffeine ingestion does not alter carbohydrate or fat metabolism in skeletal muscle during exercise. *Journal of Physiology* 529.3: 837-847; 2000.

35. Greer, F., McLean, C., and Graham, T.E. Caffeine, performance, and metabolism during repeated Wingate exercise tests. *Journal of Applied Physiology* 85: 1502-1508; 1998.

36. Greer, F., Friars, D., and Graham, T.E. Comparison of caffeine and theophylline ingestion: exercise metabolism

and endurance. *Journal of Applied Physiology* 89: 1837-1844; 2000.

37. Griffiths, R.R., and Mumford, G.K. Caffeine—a drug of abuse? In *Psychopharmacology: The Fourth Generation of Progress,* ed. F.E. Bloom and D.J. Kupfer, 1699-1713. New York: Raven Press, 1995.

38. Grobbee, D.E., Rimm, E.B., Giovannucci, E., Colditz, G., Stampfer, M., and Willett, W. Coffee, caffeine, and cardiovascular disease in men. *New England Journal of Medicine* 323: 1026-1032; 1990.

39. Ivy, J.L., Costill, D.L., Fink, W.J., and Lower, R.W. Influence of caffeine and carbohydrate feedings on endurance performance. *Medicine and Science in Sports* 11: 6-11; 1979.

40. Jackman, M., Wendling, P., Friars, D., and Graham, T.E. Metabolic, catecholamine and endurance responses to caffeine during intense exercise. *Journal of Applied Physiology* 81: 1658-1663; 1996.

41. Jacobson, T.L., Febbraio, M.A., Arkinstall, M.J., and Hawley, J.A.. Effect of caffeine co-ingested with carbohydrate or fat on metabolism and performance in endurance-trained men. *Experimental Physiology* 86.1; 2001 (in press).

42. Kalmar, J.M., and Cafarelli, E. Effects of caffeine on neuromuscular function. *Journal of Applied Physiology* 87: 801-808; 1999.

43. Kavinsky, P.J., Shechosky, S., and Fletterick, R.J. Synergistic regulation of phosphorylase a by glucose and caffeine. *Journal of Biological Chemistry* 253: 9102-9106; 1978.

44. Kovacs, E.M.R., Stegen, J.H.S., and Brouns, F. Effect of caffeinated drinks on substrate metabolism, caffeine excretion, and performance. *Journal of Applied Physiology* 85: 709-715; 1998.

45. Laurent, D., Schneider, K.E., Prusaczyk, W.P., Franklin, C., Vogel, S.M., Krssak, M., Petersen, K.F., Goforth, H.G., and Shulman, G.I. Effects of caffeine on muscle glycogen utilization and the neuroendocrine axis during exercise. *Journal of Clinical Endocrinology and Metabolism* 85: 2170-2175; 2000.

46. Lindinger, M.I., Graham, T.E., and Spriet, L.L. Caffeine attenuates the exercise-induced increase in plasma [K^+] in humans. *Journal of Applied Physiology* 74: 1149-1155; 1993.

47. Lindinger, M.I., Willmets, R.G., and Hawke, T.J. Stimulation of Na^+, K^+-pump activity in skeletal muscle by methylxanthines: evidence and proposed mechanisms. *Acta Physiologica Scandinavica* 156: 347-353; 1996.

48. Lundsberg, L.S. Caffeine consumption. In *Caffeine,* ed. G.A. Spiller, 199-224. New York: CRC Press, 1998.

49. MacIntosh, B.R., and Wright, B.M. Caffeine ingestion and performance of a 1500-metre swim. *Canadian Journal of Applied Physiology* 20: 168-177; 1995.

50. McNaughton, L. Two levels of caffeine ingestion on blood lactate and free fatty acid responses during incremental exercise. *Research Quarterly of Exercise and Sport* 58: 255-259; 1987.

51. Mohr, T., Van Soeren, M., Graham, T.E., and Kjaer, M. Caffeine ingestion and metabolic responses of tetraplegic humans during electrical cycling. *Journal of Applied Physiology* 85: 979-985; 1998.

52. Myers, M.G., and Basinski, A. Coffee and coronary heart disease. *Archives of Internal Medicine* 152: 1767-1772; 1992.

53. Nehlig, A., Daval, J.-L., and Debry, G. Caffeine and the central nervous system: mechanisms of action, biochemical, metabolic, and psychostimulant effects. *Brain Research Reviews* 17: 139-170; 1992.

54. Nehlig, A., and Debry, G. Caffeine and sports activity: a review. *International Journal of Sports Medicine* 15: 215-223; 1994.

55. Pasman, W.J., VanBaak, M.A., Jeukendrup, A.E., and DeHaan, A. The effect of different dosages of caffeine on endurance performance time. *International Journal of Sports Medicine* 16: 225-230; 1995.

56. Rush, J.W.E., and Spriet, L.L. Skeletal muscle glycogen phosphorylase a kinetics: effects of adenine nucleotides and caffeine. *Journal of Applied Physiology*, 91:2071-2078; 2001.

57. Sasaki, H., Maeda, J., Usui, S., and Ishiko, T. Effect of caffeine ingestion on performance of prolonged strenuous running. *International Journal of Sports Medicine* 8: 261-265; 1987.

58. Sawynok, J., and Yaksh, T.L. Caffeine as an analgesic adjuvant: a review of pharmacology and mechanisms of action. *Pharmacological Reviews* 45: 43-85; 1993.

59. Silverman, K., Evans, S.M., Strain, E.C., and Griffiths, R.R. Withdrawal syndrome after the double-blind cessation of caffeine consumption. *New England Journal of Medicine* 327: 1109-1114; 1992.

60. Snyder, S.H. Adenosine as a mediator of the behavioral effects of xanthines. In *Caffeine,* ed. P.B. Dews, 129-141. Berlin: Springer-Verlag, 1984.

61. Spiller, G.A., ed. *Caffeine,* 1-364. New York: CRC Press, 1998.

62. Spriet, L.L. Caffeine and performance. *International Journal of Sports Nutrition* 5: S84-S99; 1995.

63. Spriet, L.L., and Howlett, R.A. Caffeine. In *Nutrition in Sport—Encyclopaedia of Sports Medicine,* Vol. VII, ed. R.J. Maughan, 379-392. Oxford: Blackwell Science, 2000.

64. Spriet, L.L., MacLean, D.A., Dyck, D.J., Hultman, E., Cederblad, G., and Graham, T.E. Caffeine ingestion and muscle metabolism during prolonged exercise in humans. *American Journal of Physiology* 262: E891-E898; 1992.

65. Strain, E.C., and Griffiths, R.R. Caffeine use disorders. In *Psychiatry,* Vol. I, ed. A. Tasman, J. Kay, and J.A. Lieberman, 779-794. Philadelphia: Saunders, 1997.

66. Strain, E.C., Mumford, G.K., Silverman, K., and Griffiths, R.R. Caffeine dependence syndrome: evidence from case histories and experimental evaluations. *Journal of the American Medical Association* 272: 1043-1048; 1994.

67. Tarnopolsky, M.A. Caffeine and endurance performance. *Sports Medicine* 18: 109-125; 1984.

68. Tarnopolsky, M., and Cupido, C. Caffeine potentiates low frequency skeletal muscle force in habitual and nonhabitual caffeine consumers. *Journal of Applied Physiology* 89: 1719-1724; 2000.

69. Trice, I., and Haymes, E.M. Effects of caffeine ingestion on exercise-induced changes during high-intensity, intermittent exercise. *International Journal of Sports Nutrition* 5: 37-44; 1995.

70. United States Olympic Committee guide to banned medications. *Sports Mediscope* 7: 1-15; 1988.

71. Van Nieuwenhoven, M.A., Brummer, R.-J.M., and Brouns, F. Gastrointestinal function during exercise: comparison of water, sports drink, and sports drink with caffeine. *Journal of Applied Physiology* 89: 1079-1085; 2000.

72. Van Soeren, M.H., and Graham, T.E. Effect of caffeine on metabolism, exercise endurance, and catecholamine responses after withdrawal. *Journal of Applied Physiology* 85: 1493-1501; 1998.

73. Van Soeren, M.H., Mohr, T., Kjaer, M., and Graham, T.E. Acute effects of caffeine ingestion at rest in humans with impaired epinephrine responses. *Journal of Applied Physiology* 80: 999-1005; 1996.

74. Vergauwen, L., Hespel, P., and Richter, E.A. Adenosine receptors mediate synergistic stimulation of glucose uptake and transport by insulin and by contractions in rat skeletal muscle. *Journal of Clinical Investigation* 93: 974-981; 1994.

75. Vianni, R. The consumption of coffee. In *Caffeine, Coffee, and Health,* ed. S. Garratini, 17-42. New York: Raven Press, 1993.

76. Waldeck, B. Sensitization by caffeine of central catecholamine receptors. *Journal of Neural Transmission* 34: 61-72; 1973.

77. Weir, J., Noakes, T.D., Myburgh, K., and Adams, B. A high carbohydrate diet negates the metabolic effect of caffeine during exercise. *Medicine and Science in Sports and Exercise* 19: 100-105; 1987.

78. Wemple, R.D., Lamb, D.R., and McKeever, K.H. Caffeine vs. caffeine-free sports drinks: effects on urine production at rest and during prolonged exercise. *International Journal of Sports Medicine* 18: 40-46; 1997.

79. Wiles, J.D., Bird, S.R., Hopkins, J., and Riley, M. Effect of caffeinated coffee on running speed, respiratory factors, blood lactate and perceived exertion during 1500-m treadmill running. *British Journal of Sports Medicine* 26: 166-120; 1992.

80. Williams, J.H., Signoille, J.F., Barnes, W.S., and Henrich, T.W. Caffeine, maximal power output and fatigue. *British Journal of Sports Medicine,* 229:132-134; 1998.

Cocaine

Robert K. Conlee, PhD

Cocaine is a highly addictive drug derived from the leaves of the plant *Erythroxylon coca,* which grows primarily in the Andean mountains of Peru and Bolivia but is also found in Mexico, Indonesia, and the West Indies. It is a powerful central nervous system stimulant with strong euphoric effects. For centuries, the natives of the Andes have used the drug in its impure form to stave off hunger and fatigue. They do this by chewing coca leaves and extracting the drug into the saliva. It is then absorbed through the mucous lining of the mouth or through the gut after the saliva has been swallowed.

In the late 19th century, scientists began to extract the drug in its purified form and test it for its medicinal benefits. It was determined to have anesthetic value and was used as a topical anesthesia for nasal and ophthalmic surgery. It was during this time that Sigmund Freud (Byck, 1974) published several papers touting the beneficial effects of cocaine for everything from asthma to cancer. Freud also conducted the first published experiment on the ergogenic effects of the drug. Using himself as the experimental subject, he reported that after ingesting cocaine while under fatigued conditions his strength and endurance were improved.

Near the turn of the 20th century, availability of cocaine was relatively uncontrolled. It was being used as an ingredient in various tonics and supplements and was the principal component in the initial formulation of the modern-day soft drink Coca-Cola (Gay et al., 1975). As a result of its widespread use and abuse, the federal government in 1914 classified the drug as a controlled substance under the Harrison Tax Act, a classification it still carries today. Declaring it a controlled substance reduced its availability and use, but over the years cocaine has remained a favorite drug of abuse. In 1985 it was estimated that 5.7 million people or 3% of the population of the United States were chronic users of cocaine (National Institute on Drug Abuse [NIDA], 1999). In 1997 that number had fallen to 3.6 million, but the use among school-age children had increased steadily over that same period (NIDA, 1999).

More germane to the subject of this chapter are the reports that athletes were using cocaine to enhance performance (Wadler and Hainline, 1989). This issue gained notoriety when the press reported in the late 1980s that some prominent athletes had died after using

the drug. The extent of use was only anecdotal, and there are no data today regarding the prevalence of use among athletes to enhance performance. These deaths heightened the interest of the federal government, which in turn called for increased research into the physiological and pharmacological effects of the drug, including an emphasis on the combined effects of cocaine and exercise (Thadani, 1991). Until that time very little was known about the ergogenic effects of cocaine or the combined physiological effects of cocaine and exercise. In fact, the report most frequently cited at the time that ascribed ergogenicity to cocaine was the report by Freud (Byck, 1974), mentioned earlier—and as also mentioned, Freud's results were based on one subject, himself! Today, we have more information regarding the physiological effects of cocaine and a greater understanding of its effects when combined with exercise.

The primary purpose of this chapter is to review the research that has focused on the role of cocaine as an ergogenic substance. At the same time we will review the combined physiological effects of cocaine and exercise. The reader is referred to earlier reviews on these subjects (Conlee, 1991; Wadler and Hainline, 1989). Before treating the specific topics, however, the chapter focuses on the general pharmacology of the drug as a means of understanding the basis for its potential ergogenicity. The chapter also provides information regarding the side effects associated with acute and chronic use of cocaine.

Pharmacology of Cocaine and Method of Consumption

Cocaine is benzoylmethylecgonine ($C_{17}H_{21}NO_4$) and belongs to the tropane family of alkaloids, which also include atropine and scopolamine (Burnett and Adler, 2000; Turner et al., 1988). It is extracted from the leaves of the coca plant and purified into a variety of forms depending on the method of consumption. The most common form of the drug is a white crystalline powderlike compound (cocaine-hydrochloride), which can be insufflated through the nose or dissolved in water and injected intravenously. When inhaled as a powder, the drug is absorbed through the mucosal membranes of the nose into the bloodstream. Because of its vasoconstrictive effects on the vasculature, which significantly reduces blood flow at the local point of contact, the drug limits its own absorption when it is inhaled. Therefore the rate of absorption and thus the rate at which effects begin to appear (1-5 min) are considerably less than if the drug were injected directly into the bloodstream. When the drug is taken intravenously, its central effects are realized almost immediately (approximately 15 sec), but the duration of the effect is shorter (20-30 min) than after inhalation (45-90 min).

The other common form of the drug is the alkaline version, which is derived by treating the hydrochloride salt with ether, thus creating a freebase substance that is sensitive to heat. Because ether is extremely volatile and can explode when heated, this form can be extremely dangerous if heated before all of the ether has evaporated. When the freebase form is heated it makes a crackling sound, so the terms "crack cocaine" and "crack" were coined to describe this alkaline derivative. This form of the drug is inhaled into the lung as a vapor created when the crack cocaine is heated in a special pipe designed for this purpose. The drug is absorbed through the mucosal lining of the lung, and, because of the wide surface area of the alveoli and the broad exposure of the blood to it, absorption and subsequent realization of central effects are rapid (5-10 sec). But, similar to the situation with intravenous injection, the duration of the central effects is short (20 min).

In contrast to the uptake and speed of effects when cocaine is taken in one of its purified forms, the rate of absorption and central stimulation are much slower when the drug is obtained by chewing the raw coca leaves. The amount of the drug obtained by this method varies dramatically depending on the amount of leaves chewed, the time they are chewed, the concentration of the drug in the leaves themselves, and whether the drug is absorbed by the lining of the mouth during chewing or by the gut after it has been swallowed. The onset of effect may not occur for 10 min after chewing begins, and the duration may be an hour. The magnitude of the effect is also considerably less than that with the other methods.

Metabolism and Elimination

Regardless of the method of consumption, once in the blood the cocaine is metabolized and degraded by hepatic esterases and plasma pseudocholinesterase. The half-life for the disappearance of cocaine ranges from 30 to 40 min in humans (Johanson and Fishman, 1989) to 11 to 14 min in rats (Han et al., 1996). The metabolites of cocaine breakdown are eliminated in the urine, and some can be detected for up to six days after cocaine use (Das, 1993; Woolf and Shannon, 1995). Some of the metabolites of cocaine degradation are themselves pharmacologically active; and norcocaine, produced in the liver, has been shown to be hepatotoxic (Turner et al., 1988).

Physiological Effects

The physiological effects of cocaine are generally divided into three categories: anesthesia, central nervous system, and peripheral effects.

Anesthesia

Cocaine has long been recognized for its local anesthetic effects. It was often used for surgery of the eyes and nose, but because of local side effects and its highly addictive nature it is used only rarely for these purposes today. It accomplishes its anesthetic effect by directly blocking the sodium channels of sensory nerves, thus reducing nerve conduction (Ritchie and Greene, 1990).

Central Nervous System

By far the most dramatic effect of cocaine is on the central nervous system. The drug produces a sense of euphoria, which is so exhilarating that users may binge on the drug until exhausted or until they run out of money to purchase it. In studies using monkeys, investigators showed that when given a choice between cocaine and food, social interactions with other monkeys, or even sex, the animal chose cocaine (Aigner and Balster, 1978). This euphoric effect may also explain the increased capacity for work by the native Indians of the Andes who chew coca leaves for the purpose of staving off fatigue (Hanna, 1971). Besides producing the euphoric effect, the drug also reduces the sensation of hunger and increases body temperature.

The mechanism by which cocaine exerts these central effects has been given considerable scientific attention over the last two decades (Hammer, 1995; Lakowski, Galloway, and White, 1992). The events are still not completely elucidated, but the prevailing view is that cocaine blocks the reuptake of several neurotransmitters of the brain such as norepinephrine, serotonin, and dopamine. Of the three, dopamine has received the most attention and seems to be most important to the explanation of the euphoric and addictive effects of the drug (Hammer, 1995; Romach et al., 1999). Deep within the cerebrum is an area called the ventral tegmental area (VTA). Neurons from this area stimulate the nucleus accumbens, which is known to be the center for pleasure and reward in the brain. Researchers have discovered that when a pleasurable event is occurring, it is accompanied by a large increase in the amounts of dopamine released in the nucleus accumbens by neurons originating in the VTA (NIDA, 1999). Normally when a pleasurable event is over, dopamine is taken back into the presynaptic neuron by dopamine transporters, and the sense of pleasure recedes. Cocaine, on the other hand, blocks the reuptake pathway for dopamine, causing a residual overflow of dopamine in the synapse that results in a constant stimulation to the pleasure centers of the nucleus accumbens (Romach et al., 1999). It has also been suggested that cocaine may stimulate the release of dopamine into the synaptic space (Gawin, 1991; Romach et al., 1999), thus initiating the pleasure response, which is then heightened by the inhibition of its reuptake. This mechanism is similar to that ascribed to amphetamines, which produce pharmacological responses similar to those of cocaine but lesser in intensity (Carboni et al., 1989).

Peripheral

Besides its central effects, cocaine initiates a dramatic sympathetic response in the periphery. Levels of epinephrine and norepinephrine rise in the blood (Chiueh and Kopin, 1978; Conlee et al., 1991a,b; Han et al., 1996; Kiritsy-Roy et al., 1990). As a consequence, heart rate and blood pressure increase (Fischman et al., 1976; Fischman, Schuster, and Hatano, 1983). In addition to the hormonal surge, a number of metabolic changes occur, such as an increase in plasma free fatty acids (Conlee et al., 1989) and glucose (Han et al., 1996) and a concomitant decrease in muscle glycogen (Bracken et al., 1988, 1989). It has also been shown that cocaine stimulates an increase in the concentration of corticosterone in the blood, indicative of a stress response (Conlee et al., 1991a; Moldow and Fischman, 1987).

Two mechanisms have been proposed to explain the peripheral sympathetic response to cocaine. The most widely accepted theory is that cocaine blocks the reuptake of norepinephrine at the sympathetic nerve endings (Ritchie and Greene, 1990; Trendelenburg, 1959), similar to the way it blocks dopamine reuptake in the central nervous system. This could explain the elevation in norepinephrine, but not that of epinephrine. The second mechanism is that cocaine stimulates the centers controlling the sympathetic nervous system (Chiueh and Kopin, 1978). Through this mechanism, the adrenal gland is stimulated via the preganglionic neuron from the central nervous system to release both epinephrine and norepinephrine A third possibility is that cocaine stimulates the adrenal gland directly (Conlee et al., 1991b). The physiological and metabolic responses that accompany the sympathetic surge could all occur as a consequence of the hormones released or could result from a direct effect of cocaine on the various organs and tissues being affected, that is, the heart, blood vessels, liver, muscle, and adipose tissue.

Adverse Side Effects

Cocaine is extremely dangerous when consumed in one of its purified forms and on rare occasions can cause death after only a single exposure (NIDA, 1999). The side effects of cocaine are summarized in table 23.1.

Deaths are generally attributed to myocardial infarction secondary to coronary vasospasm, increased myocardial oxygen demand, or coronary thrombosis (Das, 1993). Coronary vasospasm and increased myocardial oxygen demand are both linked to the sympathetic surge that accompanies acute cocaine consumption (Lange et al., 1989). More commonly, an acute dose of cocaine can prompt bizarre, erratic behavior. Users may experience tremors, muscle twitches, vertigo, and paranoia or feelings of restlessness, irritability, and anxiety (NIDA, 1999). Cocaine is also very addictive through its effects on the mesolimbic reward centers of the brain. Addiction leads the user to engage in irrational behavior designed to satisfy the craving for the drug at the expense of other important responsibilities such as family and work and other societal expectations. Use of cocaine in a binge, during which the drug is taken repeatedly and at increasingly higher doses, leads to a state of increasing irritability, restlessness, and paranoia. This may result in a full-blown paranoid psychosis, in which the individual loses touch with reality and experiences auditory hallucinations (NIDA, 1999).

Potential for Ergogenicity

The pharmacological effects of cocaine that may be ergogenic are similar to those of amphetamines and caffeine (Conlee, 1991). The powerful euphoric effect and increased mental alertness may override central perceptions of fatigue and prolong endurance during

Table 23.1 Side Effects of Cocaine

Short-term use	Long-term use
Increased energy	Addiction
Decreased appetite	Irritability and mood disturbances
Mental alertness	
Increased heart rate/ blood pressure	Restlessness
	Paranoia
Constricted blood vessels	Hallucinations
Dilated pupils	Irrational behavior
Euphoria	Violent behavior
Muscle twitches/tremors	Heart failure
Vertigo	Strokes
Paranoia	Seizures
Restlessness	Abdominal pain
Irritability	Nausea
Anxiety	Weight loss
	Malnourishment
	Rhabdomyolosis

Modified from National Institute on Drug Abuse (1999).

high-, moderate-, or low-intensity exercise. The peripheral sympathetic effect may mobilize fuel substrates (i.e., blood glucose and free fatty acids) for the maintenance of adenosine triphosphate (ATP) production and prolong exercise.

Ergogenicity of Cocaine

The ergogenicity of cocaine has been studied in both human and animal research models. The following paragraphs discuss these two types of studies.

Human Studies

For centuries, it has been the practice of indigenous workers in the mountains of Peru and Bolivia to chew coca leaves in order to promote physical stamina (Fischman, 1984; Hanna, 1970; Wadler and Hainline, 1989). Several investigators have evaluated this practice to ascertain its effectiveness. In 1970 Hanna selected six experienced coca chewers and six nonchewers from among the Quechua natives of the Peruvian highlands and had them perform a series of four box-stepping exercises. Sixty minutes before the start of exercise the chewers chewed an undisclosed amount of coca leaves. Both groups then exercised by stepping up and down on boxes at a cadence that became increasingly faster with each bout of stepping. Hanna reported that the chewers had a lower heart rate during the last work bout accompanied by a higher diastolic blood pressure. There was no measurable difference in oxygen consumption between the groups during the exercise; but, when the investigator extrapolated his measurements to maximum exercise, the results suggested that the chewers had a lower predicted maximum oxygen consumption. The author concluded that coca chewing (and by inference, cocaine consumption) altered the cardiovascular response to heavy exercise but did not improve work capacity. The study was hampered by the fact that only the experienced chewers received coca leaves before the exercise tests. Furthermore, the author never discussed the implications of the predicted lower maximum oxygen consumption in the chewing group.

In a follow-up study, Hanna (1971) imposed stricter controls on his research design in an attempt to expand his previous findings. He again used chewers and nonchewers indigenous to Peru, but this time he used a crossover design in which both groups exercised with and without coca chewing. The subjects performed two exercise bouts to exhaustion on a bicycle ergometer, one at a high power output and the other incorporating increasing intensities of work in a ramp protocol. Using this design Hanna confirmed that coca chewing caused a higher heart rate during all intensities of exercise, but no other differences in metabolic responses were evident.

More importantly, the results showed that coca chewing did not improve work time to exhaustion on either test. As a result of this second study, Hanna rejected the claim that the chewing of coca leaves makes work easier.

In a more recent series of experiments, a team of French and Bolivian investigators evaluated the effects of coca chewing on a variety of metabolic and performance indexes during exercise of increasing intensity (Spielvogel et al., 1996) and steady state submaximal exercise (Favier et al., 1996). In the first study (Spielvogel et al.), natives from the Altiplano of Bolivia (3800-m altitude), consisting of experienced coca chewers and nonchewers, were recruited as subjects. The chewers were allowed to chew coca leaves while resting for 60 min. Nonchewers only rested. During this period, in response to the coca challenge, the concentrations of plasma free fatty acids (FFA) were elevated but not those of the adrenergic hormones, epinephrine, or norepinephrine. After 60 min of rest, the subjects then performed an incremental exercise protocol to exhaustion on a bicycle ergometer. During the exercise trial, both peak $\dot{V}O_2$ and work efficiency were unaffected by coca chewing. There was, however, a persistent elevation in FFA in the coca group and a tendency for an elevation of the adrenergic hormones at the highest workload. The authors concluded that coca does not improve maximum exercise capacity or work efficiency, but they speculated that the elevation in FFA resulting from coca chewing may potentially spare muscle glycogen, and that might delay fatigue during more prolonged, submaximal work conditions.

In their second study (Favier et al., 1996), the investigators used the same subjects, but this time subjects performed steady state exercise for 60 min at 65% to 70% $\dot{V}O_2$peak preceded by either 60 min of chewing or nonchewing. Unlike the results of the first study, chewing increased the plasma concentration of norepinephrine and glucose at rest; but, similar to what occurred in the first study, the researchers again observed an elevation in plasma FFA. During exercise the elevated adrenergic response continued in the chewing group, accompanied by an increased use of FFA for energy production. After evaluating the findings, the authors repeated their assertion that the metabolic and hormonal profile at rest and exercise induced by coca chewing had the potential to enhance prolonged exercise by postponing glycogen depletion and may be the explanation for coca chewers' claim that they have increased stamina in the field. Unfortunately, the investigators did not measure exercise endurance in either study, so the question whether chewing coca leaves enhances endurance remained unanswered. Another weakness of this series of studies is that the authors did not incorporate a crossover design. The experienced chewers were the only subjects who chewed the coca leaves; therefore, there was no control for either sensitization or tolerance to the drug that may have existed in this group. One valuable outcome from this study, however, was the measurement of the concentration of cocaine in the blood of the coca leaf chewers (Rerat et al., 1997). The authors confirmed that chewing coca leaves results in a significant increase in the levels of cocaine and its metabolite, benzoylecgonine, in the blood, and that those levels are directly related to the amount of leaves chewed.

The inherent problem with studies of coca chewing is the inability to control the amount of cocaine the subjects are actually absorbing (Rerat et al., 1997). To ascertain the ergogenic effect of cocaine the investigator must quantify the amount of drug being used. Some investigators, therefore, have used purified cocaine in known quantities in an attempt to deduce its ergogenic potential. There are, however, very few of these studies, in contrast to the number of studies done on amphetamines or caffeine (Conlee, 1991), probably because of the highly addictive and potentially dangerous nature of the drug. The first study was that by Sigmund Freud (Byck, 1974) using himself as the subject. In one experiment he tested his grip strength on a hand dynamometer several times over a 2-hr period. Then he inhaled 0.1 g of cocaine, tested himself several times over the ensuing 5 hr, and found that his strength had increased by 15% to 20%. On another occasion he measured his reaction time before and after cocaine use and reported that cocaine decreased reaction time by nearly 30% within 45 min of consuming the drug. Whereas Freud's reports have been given credibility merely for the reason that reviews continue to refer to them (Conlee, 1991; Wadler and Hainline, 1989), it is clear that they do not represent good science. In addition, the fact that Freud became addicted to the drug as a result of his experiments (Gay et al., 1975) supports the concern about doing human research with the drug.

Only a few other human studies have been performed in which the purified drug was administered to test its effects on performance. Theil and Essig (1930) gave 0.1 g cocaine by mouth to untrained subjects prior to exhaustive exercise on a bicycle ergometer. The drug raised resting metabolic rates, and the authors reported that by 30 min after using the drug the subjects generally experienced restlessness and tremors. During exercise the cocainized subjects worked slightly more efficiently as measured by oxygen consumed per unit of work. Work time to exhaustion was also improved. The authors concluded that the improved work output was due to the central euphoric effects of the drug. It was not clear how the drug improved efficiency of work. The following year Herbst and Schellenberg (1931) performed a follow-up study using three physically trained subjects. These investigators reported that 0.1 g of cocaine consumed by mouth raised resting oxygen consumption and minute ventilation. On some occasions the drug caused the subjects to lose equilibrium while sitting upright on the bicycle just before the work began. During exercise, the drug did not appreciably improve the amount of work the subjects could do in 2.5 min on a cycle ergometer set at a resistance of 2100 mkg. It had a slight beneficial effect on oxygen efficiency similar to that reported by Theil and Essig (1930). In contradiction to Theil and Essig, these authors were unable to declare any ergogenic benefit to cocaine under the conditions of their study.

In the only other study reported in the literature involving the effects of cocaine on human performance, Asmussen and Bøje (1948) had four male subjects swallow capsules containing 120 mg of cocaine 15 min before each of two exercise protocols. The two trials involved completing 35 or 450 pedal revolutions on a braked bicycle ergometer in the shortest time possible. Cocaine had no effect on performance time for either test. The flaw in this study was that there was not enough time between the consumption of the drug and the beginning of the exercise tests to allow for the drug to be absorbed out of the gut and have an effect. Van Dyke et al. (1978) showed that the peak in plasma cocaine levels occurred 65 min after consumption in capsule form.

In summary, the human studies, which involved the administration of pure cocaine, have provided little quality evidence for an ergogenic effect of the drug. Freud's work (Byck, 1974) has to be dismissed based on the fact that Freud was the only subject. The two German studies (Herbst and Schellenberg, 1931; Theil and Essig, 1930) produced somewhat conflicting results, but both studies revealed side effects of the drug that raise concern about the ethics of its use even in the laboratory; and the study by Asmussen and Bøje (1948) was prone to failure because of a serious design flaw. Even the four studies of the effects of coca chewing (Hanna, 1970, 1971; Favier et al., 1996; Spielvogel et al., 1996) provided no clear evidence of its efficacy as a work enhancer, testimonials by Peruvian natives to the contrary (Fischman, 1984; Hanna, 1970).

Animal Studies

The first published study of the potential ergogenicity of cocaine using animals was that of Jacob and Michaud in 1961. They injected mice subcutaneously with cocaine in doses ranging from 3 to 100 mg/kg body weight and then forced the animals to swim in water maintained at 20 °C until exhausted. Cocaine at the lower doses had no effect on swim times. The higher doses impaired swimming ability and reduced swim times. The design of this study was hampered by the fact that the water was so cold that the control animals could swim only 5 to 6 min before having to be removed; therefore, the validity of the study has to be questioned.

Little interest in cocaine and exercise was evident in the literature after 1961 until two abstracts appeared in the 1980s. The first (Kershner, Edwards, and Tipton, 1983) indicated that an intraperitoneal (ip) injection of cocaine to rats increased $\dot{V}O_2$max and endurance time on a treadmill running test. The authors concluded that cocaine is ergogenic. The author of the other abstract (Avakian, 1986) stated that chronic administration of cocaine to rats for 26 days significantly reduced endurance time to exhaustion, and concluded that cocaine was ergolytic. Unfortunately, neither of these studies was ever published, and it is therefore difficult to critically evaluate them. Nevertheless, it was these brief reports and the encouragement of NIDA that stimulated renewed interest in the topic and resulted in numerous publications of animal studies on the physiological effects of cocaine and exercise.

In the first of these, Bracken et al. (1988) injected rats with cocaine (20 mg/kg, ip) or saline 20 min before they ran to exhaustion on a motorized treadmill. At rest, cocaine reduced the glycogen concentration in soleus muscle but had no effect on other parameters. During the exhaustive run the saline animals ran for 75 min, whereas the cocaine rats ran for only 29 min. The cocainized animals at exhaustion had blood lactate levels two to three times higher than those of the saline group. Muscle glycogen had been depleted to the same extent in the two groups despite the fact that the cocaine group had run only half as long.

In a follow-up study, the same research group (Bracken et al., 1989) investigated the effects of various doses of the drug on exercise endurance and obtained additional physiological measurements. The doses ranged from 0.1 to 20 mg/kg and were injected ip. As in the authors' earlier study, the highest dose of cocaine caused a reduction of glycogen in soleus muscle at rest. In addition the authors observed an elevation in the concentration of glucose, lactate, norepinephrine, epinephrine, and corticosterone in the blood. At exercise, they found that the two highest doses (12.5 and 20.0 mg/kg) impaired running time to exhaustion and that the lower doses had no effect on performance. They concluded that cocaine was not ergogenic at any dose and was ergolytic at high doses. In this study the authors also reported that cocaine rapidly reduced muscle glycogen stores during exercise and concomitantly elevated blood lactate and norepinephrine levels. The drug had no effect on epinephrine levels. Unfortunately, these latter measurements were made after vastly different running times and only at the end point of exhaustion.

In retrospect (Conlee et al., 1991b), it was felt that studying the animals at exhaustion did not give a clear picture of the physiological responses to exercise and cocaine, because running animals to fatigue imposes abnormal stress on the animal as it is prodded to keep up with the treadmill (Marker et al., 1986). A third study from this group was designed to address these concerns. In that study (Conlee et al., 1991b), animals were pretreated with cocaine or saline and either rested for 30 min or exercised for 30 min on a treadmill. The investigators tried to avoid excessive prodding of the animals in order to limit the stress on the animal to that associated with the exercise itself. The intensity of the exercise was moderate and was similar to that used in the previous two studies. At the end of the exercise period, cocaine treatment, compared to saline treatment, had resulted in a greater depletion of glycogen in fast-twitch muscle tissue, a greater elevation in blood lactate concentrations, and higher blood levels of norepinephrine, epinephrine and dopamine, even though the exercise time was similar for the two groups.

These results confirmed the conclusions of the two previous reports that cocaine causes rapid glycogen depletion and lactacidosis during exercise and that these two conditions could lead to the premature fatigue that occurs when animals run under the influence of cocaine. It was also the first report to clearly show the exaggerated catecholamine response to the combined stress of cocaine and exercise. This group reaffirmed the latter observation in many of their subsequent reports. In particular, Han et al. (1996) reported that the epinephrine response to cocaine exercise was 35 times greater than resting values, 4.4 times higher than with cocaine alone, and 3.9 times higher than with exercise alone. The response for norepinephrine was similar in magnitude.

In the fourth study of the ergogenicity of cocaine from this lab (Braiden, Fellingham, and Conlee, 1994), the group evaluated the effects of cocaine using a treadmill protocol that required the rats to run at high intensity. In the earlier studies the exercise test was of moderate intensity at which the control animals could run for 60 to 120 min. It was reasoned that perhaps the euphoric effects of the drug could enhance the animal's endurance at high intensity before the detrimental physiological effects produced fatigue. Rats were injected with either saline or cocaine (12.5 or 20.0 mg/kg) and then allowed to run on a treadmill at a speed and grade that caused the saline control animals to fatigue after only 14 min. The cocaine-treated animals (20 mg/kg) ran for only 9 min before becoming exhausted. Biochemical measures showed once again that muscle glycogen had been depleted more rapidly and that there was significantly more lactate in muscle and blood at exhaustion in the cocaine group compared to the saline animals. These authors concluded that cocaine was not ergogenic even under high-intensity exercise conditions. Close inspection of the data, however, showed that the low dose tended to improve performance at the beginning of the run, which was the phase of the test during which euphoric effects would have been evident. Since these differences did not achieve statistical significance, the authors concluded no effect.

The aim in further studies from this lab was to ascertain the mechanism by which cocaine elicited its ergolytic effects. It was postulated that the exaggerated rise in catecholamines might have induced the rapid glycogenolytic effect and concomitant lactacidosis. Ojuka et al. (1996), however, concluded that these conditions were not mediated by epinephrine, as they observed glycogen wasting and lactate accumulation in exercising adrenodemedullated rats in the absence of any rise in the hormone. More recently, Conlee et al. (2000) used an α1-receptor-blocking agent to eliminate the effects of elevated norepinephrine. This treatment, which abolished the normal hypertension induced by a sympathetic analog, did not eliminate the glycogenolytic effects of cocaine during exercise. Further work is necessary to elucidate the mechanism by which cocaine exerts its detrimental effects during exercise. It may be that the drug affects the cardiovascular system in such a way that cardiac output is insufficient to meet the demands of the working musculature. Branch and Knuepfer (1994) showed that cocaine in resting, conscious rats reduced cardiac output by 18% to 30% within 1 min of administration.

Finally, this research group studied whether the response to cocaine and exercise was different between animals accustomed or not accustomed to cocaine (Kelly et al., 1995). This experiment was designed to test whether animals experienced either tolerance or sensitization in response to chronic cocaine treatment and whether these adaptations would manifest themselves under the stress of exercise. Animals were conditioned to cocaine through administration of two injections of the drug per day for 14 to 15 days. Nonaccustomed animals received daily saline injections. After this preliminary period, animals from both groups were given injections of saline or cocaine and exercised for 30 min on the treadmill. Generally, the accustomed and nonaccustomed animals responded similarly to a cocaine-exercise challenge, and their responses were like those reported previously; that is, they showed rapid glycogenolysis and lactacidosis. The major difference noted in this study was that the accustomed animals had a higher catecholamine surge during exercise than the unaccustomed rats, indicating that they experienced a sensitizing effect to chronic drug exposure that manifested itself under the stress of exercise. In extrapolating their findings to the human experience, the authors warned that chronic cocaine users might be at substantial risk of a cardiac event if they exercise while under the influence of cocaine, because one of the causative factors is elevated catecholamines (Lange et al., 1989; Das, 1993).

One other animal study published during this era was that of McKeever et al. (1993). These investigators evaluated the effects of intravenously administered cocaine on the hemodynamic and physiological responses of horses to treadmill exercise. In this well-designed study, horses engaged in an incremental treadmill run to exhaustion under four treatment conditions: two saline control runs, one run after 50 mg of cocaine, and one run after 200 mg of cocaine. The treadmill test was of such intensity that the saline control animals were exhausted in approximately 10 min. Contrary to the results of Braiden et al. (1994), who reported that cocaine reduced endurance time to exhaustion in rats at high-intensity exercise, McKeever and colleagues observed that the horses that received the highest dose of cocaine ran 90 sec longer before exhaustion in spite of higher blood lactate levels.

McKeever and colleagues (1993) hypothesized that the central effects of the drug may have masked the symptoms of fatigue, thus allowing the animals to endure longer. On a cautionary note, the investigators also found that cocaine caused higher maximum heart rates and higher blood pressures during exercise in their animals. At the highest dose, one of the animals experienced abnormal cardiac disturbances during the exercise test. These results emphasize the potential risk to individuals who use cocaine and exercise and who have a known or unknown predisposition to cardiovascular failure. Indeed, most premature deaths resulting from cocaine use have been attributed to cardiovascular failure consequent to coronary vasospasm, increased myocardial oxygen demand, or thrombosis (Das, 1993).

The results of McKeever et al. (1993) showing abnormal hemodynamic responses under conditions of cocaine and exercise, coupled with the results of the animal studies from Conlee's lab showing an exaggerated catecholamine response under the same conditions (Conlee et al., 1991b; Han et al., 1996), emphasize the real danger in performing strenuous exercise under the influence of cocaine. Indeed, clinical reports of cardiac events in humans after cocaine use with or without exercise emphasize the need for extreme caution (Cigarroa et al., 1992; Lange et al., 1989; Sloan and Mattioni, 1992).

Ethical Considerations

Cocaine is an illegal drug and is banned as a doping substance by all sport governing bodies. In spite of testimonials and limited research findings that some forms of the drug may enhance performance, there is no competitive instance when the use of cocaine for ergogenic benefits should ever be considered. Use of the drug poses significant health risks and can be lethal even after a single acute exposure. Its addictive nature relegates the chronic user to a life of irrational choices, disappointing social outcomes, and significant debilitating health conditions.

Conclusion

Cocaine is a powerful central stimulant that promotes strong euphoric effects to the pleasure centers of the brain. It is also a strong peripheral sympathetic stimulant that promotes an elevation in the adrenergic hormones. As a result of its central and peripheral effects it has been touted as a potential ergogenic aid. However, research on the effects of cocaine and exercise provides little evidence of its ergogenic potential. The human research studies are hampered by poor designs and provide little reproducible evidence that cocaine in any of its tested forms improves performance. Most animal studies indicate that the drug is not ergogenic but rather ergolytic and that it promotes an exaggerated catecholamine response during exercise that could be deleterious to the cardiovascular system. The one animal study with horses that did demonstrate an ergogenic effect of the drug also showed that it caused abnormal hemodynamic responses during exercise that could pose significant health risks to the user. In view of these findings, cocaine should not be used in conjunction with exercise.

Acknowledgments

The author expresses appreciation to his colleague, Allen Parcell, for his helpful suggestions for improvement of the manuscript. The author's research was supported in part by National Institute on Drug Abuse Grant DA-04382.

References

Aigner, T.G., and R.L. Balster. 1978. Choice behavior in rhesus monkeys: cocaine versus food. *Science* 201: 534-535.

Asmussen, E., and O. Bøje. 1948. The effect of alcohol and some drugs on the capacity for work. *Acta Physiologica Scandinavica* 15: 109-118.

Avakian, E.V. 1986. Effect of chronic cocaine administration on adrenergic and metabolic responses to exercise. *Federation Proceedings* 45: 1060.

Bracken, M.E., D.R. Bracken, A.G. Nelson, and R.K. Conlee. 1988. Effect of cocaine on exercise endurance and glycogen use in rats. *Journal of Applied Physiology* 64: 884-887.

Bracken, M.E., D.R. Bracken, W.W. Winder, and R.K. Conlee. 1989. Effect of various doses of cocaine on endurance capacity in rats. *Journal of Applied Physiology* 66: 377-383.

Braiden, R.W., G.W. Fellingham, and R.K. Conlee. 1994. Effects of cocaine on glycogen metabolism and endurance during high intensity exercise. *Medicine and Science in Sports and Exercise* 26: 695-700.

Branch, C.A., and M.M. Knuepfer. 1994. Causes of differential cardiovascular sensitivity to cocaine I: studies in conscious rats. *Journal of Pharmacology and Experimental Therapeutics* 269: 674-683.

Burnett, L.B., and J. Adler. 2000. Toxicity, Cocaine. *Emergency medicine/toxicology.* eMedicine.com, Inc.

Byck, R., ed. 1974. *Cocaine papers by Sigmund Freud.* New York: Stonehill.

Carboni, E., A. Imperato, L. Perezzani, and G.D. Chiara. 1989. Amphetamine, cocaine, phencyclidine and nomifensine increase extracellular dopamine concentrations preferentially in the nucleus accumbens of freely moving rats. *Neuroscience* 28: 653-661.

Chiueh, C.C., and E.J. Kopin. 1978. Centrally mediated release by cocaine of endogenous epinephrine and norepinephrine from the sympathoadrenal medullary system of anaesthetized rats. *Journal of Pharmacology and Experimental Therapeutics* 205: 148-154.

Cigarroa, C.G., J.D. Boehrer, M.E. Brickner, E.J. Eichhorn, and P.A. Grayburn. 1992. Exaggerated pressor response to treadmill exercise in chronic cocaine abusers with left ventricular hypertrophy. *Circulation* 86: 226-231.

Conlee, R.K. 1991. Amphetamine, caffeine, and cocaine. In *Perspectives in exercise science and sports medicine,* vol. 4, ed. D.R. Lamb and M.H. Williams, 285-330. Dubuque, IA: Brown.

Conlee, R.K., D.W. Barnett, K.P. Kelly, and D.H. Han. 1991a. Effects of cocaine, exercise, and resting conditions on plasma corticosterone and catecholamine concentrations in the rat. *Metabolism* 40 (10): 1043-1047.

Conlee, R.K., D.W. Barnett, K.P. Kelly, and D.H. Han. 1991b. Effects of cocaine on plasma catecholamine and muscle glycogen concentrations during exercise in the rat. *Journal of Applied Physiology* 70: 1323-1327.

Conlee, R.K., T.L. Berg, D.H. Han, K.P. Kelly, and D.W. Barnett. 1989. Cocaine does not alter cardiac glycogen content at rest or during exercise. *Metabolism* 38: 1039-1041.

Conlee, R.K., K.P. Kelly, E.O. Ojuka, and R.L. Hammer. 2000. Cocaine and exercise: α-1 receptor blockade does not alter muscle glycogenolysis or blood lactacidosis. *Journal of Applied Physiology* 88: 77-81.

Das, G. 1993. Cardiovascular effects of cocaine abuse. *Journal of Clinical Pharmacology, Therapy and Toxicology* 31(11): 521-528.

Favier, R., E. Caceres, H. Koubi, B. Sempore, M. Sauvain, and H. Spielvogel. 1996. Effects of coca chewing on hormonal and metabolic responses during prolonged submaximal exercise. *Journal of Applied Physiology* 80: 650-655.

Fischman, M.W. 1984. The behavioral pharmacology of cocaine in humans. In *Cocaine: pharmacology, effects, and treatment of abuse,* ed. J. Grabowski, 72-91. National Institute on Drug Abuse Research Monograph No. 50. Washington, DC: U.S. Government Printing Office.

Fischman, M.W., C.R. Schuster, and Y. Hatano. 1983. A comparison of the subjective and cardiovascular effects of cocaine and lidocaine in humans. *Pharmacology and Biochemistry of Behavior* 18: 123-127.

Fischman, M.W., C.R. Schuster, L. Resnekov, J.F.E. Schick, N.A. Krasnegor, W. Fennell, and D.X. Freedman. 1976. Cardiovascular and subjective effects of intravenous cocaine administration in humans. *Archives of General Psychiatry* 33: 983-989.

Gawin, F.H. 1991. Cocaine addiction: psychology and neurophysiology. *Science* 251: 1580-1586.

Gay, G.R., D.S. Inaba, C.W. Shepherd, and J.A. Newmeyer. 1975. Cocaine: history, epidemiology, human pharmacology and treatment. *Clinical Toxicology* 8(2): 149-178.

Hammer, R.P. Jr., ed. 1995. *The neurobiology of cocaine. Cellular and molecular mechanisms.* New York: CRC Press.

Han, D.H., K.P. Kelly, G.W. Fellingham, and R.K. Conlee. 1996. Cocaine and exercise: temporal changes in plasma levels of catecholamines, lactate, glucose, and cocaine. *American Journal of Physiology* 270: E438-E444.

Hanna, J.M. 1970. The effects of coca chewing on exercise in the Quechua of Peru. *Human Biology* 42: 1-11.

Hanna, J.M. 1971. Further studies on the effects of coca chewing on exercise. *Human Biology* 43: 200-209.

Herbst, R., and P. Schellenberg. 1931. Cocain und muskelarbeit. II. Mitteilung: Weitere Untersuchungen über die Beeinflussung des Gasstoffwechsels. *Arbeitsphysiologie* 4: 203-216.

Jacob, J., and G. Michaud. 1961. Actions de divers agents pharmacologiques sur les temps d'épuisement et le comportement de souris nageant a 20° C. *Archives Internationales de Pharmacodynamie et de Therapie* 133: 101-115.

Johanson, C-E., and M.W. Fischman. 1989. The pharmacology of cocaine related to its abuse. *Pharmacology Reviews* 41: 3-52.

Kelly, K.P., D.H. Han, G.W. Fellingham, W.W. Winder, and R.K. Conlee. 1995. Cocaine and exercise: physiological responses of cocaine-conditioned rats. *Medicine and Science in Sports and Exercise* 27: 65-72.

Kershner, P.L., J.G. Edwards, and C.M. Tipton. 1983. Effect of cocaine on the running performance of rats. *Medicine and Science in Sports and Exercise* 15: 12.

Kiritsy-Roy, J.A., J.B. Halter, S.M. Gordon, M.J. Smith, and L.C. Terry. 1990. Role of the central nervous system in hemodynamic and sympathoadrenal responses to cocaine in rats. *Journal of Pharmacology and Experimental Therapeutics* 225: 154-160.

Lakowski, J.M., M.P. Galloway, and F.J. White, eds. 1992. *Cocaine: pharmacology, physiology, and clinical strategies.* Boca Raton, FL: CRC Press.

Lange, R.A., R.G. Cigarroa, C.W. Yancy, J.E. Willard, J.J. Popma, M.N. Sills, W. McBride, A.S. Kim, and L.D. Hillis. 1989. Cocaine-induced coronary-artery vasoconstriction. *New England Journal of Medicine* 321: 1557-1562.

Marker, J.C., D.A. Arnall, R.K. Conlee, and W.W. Winder. 1986. Effect of adrenodemedullation on metabolic responses to high-intensity exercise. *American Journal of Physiology* 251: R552-R559.

McKeever, K.H., K.W. Hinchcliff, D.F. Gerken, and R.A. Sams. 1993. Effects of cocaine on incremental treadmill exercise in horses. *Journal of Applied Physiology* 75: 2727-2733.

Moldow, R.L., and A.J. Fischman. 1987. Cocaine induced secretion of ACTH, beta-endorphin, and corticosterone. *Peptides* 8: 819-822.

National Institute on Drug Abuse (NIDA). 1999. *Cocaine abuse and addiction.* Research report. NIH Publication No. 99-4342.

Ojuka, E.O., J.D. Bell, G.W. Fellingham, and R.K. Conlee. 1996. Cocaine and exercise: alteration in carbohydrate metabolism in adrenodemedullated rats. *Journal of Applied Physiology* 80: 124-132.

Rerat, C., M. Sauvain, P.P. Rop, E. Ruiz, M. Bresson, and A. Viala. 1997. Liquid chromatographic analysis of cocaine and benzoylecgonine in plasma of traditional coca chewers from Bolivia during exercise. *Journal of Ethnopharmacology* 56: 173-178.

Ritchie, J.M., and N.M. Greene. 1990. Local anesthetics. In *The pharmacological basis of therapeutics* (8th ed.), ed. A.G. Gilman, T.W. Rall, A.S. Nies, and P. Taylor, 311-331. New York: Pergamon Press.

Romach, M.K., P. Glue, K. Kampman, H.L. Kaplan, G.R. Somer, S. Poole, L. Clarke, V. Coffin, J. Cornish, C.P. O'Brien, and E.M. Sellers. 1999. Attenuation of the euphoric effects of cocaine by the dopamine D1/D5 antagonist ecopipam (SCH 39166). *Archives of General Psychiatry* 56: 1101-1106.

Sloan, M.A., and T.A. Mattioni. 1992. Concurrent myocardial and cerebral infarctions after intranasal cocaine use. *Stroke* 23: 427-430.

Spielvogel, H., E. Caceres, H. Koubi, B. Sempore, M. Sauvain, and R. Favier. 1996. Effects of coca chewing on metabolic and hormonal changes during graded incremental exercise to maximum. *Journal of Applied Physiology* 80: 643-649.

Thadani, P., ed. 1991. *Cardiovascular toxicity of cocaine: underlying mechanisms.* DHHS Publication No. (ADM)91-1767. National Institute on Drug Abuse Research Monograph No. 108. Washington, DC: U.S. Government Printing Office.

Theil, D., and B. Essig. 1930. Cocain und muskelarbeit. I. Mitteilung: Der Einfluss auf Leistung und Gasstoffwechsel. *Arbeitsphysiologie* 3: 287-297.

Trendelenburg, V. 1959. The supersensitivity caused by cocaine. *Journal of Pharmacology and Experimental Therapeutics* 125: 55-65.

Turner, C.E., B.S. Urbanek, G.M. Wall, and C.W. Waller, eds. 1988. *Cocaine. An annotated bibliography*, vol. I. Jackson, MS: University Press of Mississippi.

Van Dyke, C., P. Jatlow, J. Ungerer, P.G. Barash, and R. Byck. 1978. Oral cocaine: plasma concentrations and central effects. *Science* 200: 211-213.

Wadler, G.I., and B. Hainline. 1989. *Drugs and the athlete.* Philadelphia: Davis.

Woolf, A.D., and M.W. Shannon. 1995. Clinical toxicology for the pediatrician. *Pediatric Clinics of North America* 42: 317-333.

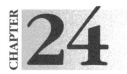

Ephedrine As an Ergogenic Aid

Eric S. Rawson, PhD

Priscilla M. Clarkson, PhD

Ephedrine is classified as a sympathomimetic drug and central nervous system stimulant (Hoffman and Lefkowitz, 1996). The action of ephedrine is similar to that of amphetamines, to which it is structurally related. Its ability to act as a sympathetic agonist and increase thermogenesis has led to its use in weight loss (Clarkson, 1998). As a central nervous system stimulant, it is used to reduce fatigue and increase alertness. Another form of ephedrine is pseudoephedrine, which is found in over-the-counter nasal decongestants (Hoffman and Lefkowitz, 1996). Ephedrine consists of an aromatic ring, an alpha carbon (with attached methyl group), a beta carbon (with attached hydroxyl group), and a terminal amino group (with an attached methyl group). Pseudoephedrine is a stereoisomer of ephedrine.

Ephedrine is available over the counter in 25-mg tablets. In 1997, in part because of the numerous reports of adverse events associated with ephedrine ingestion, the Food and Drug Administration proposed that the maximal daily dose should be not greater than 24 mg and that a single dose not exceed 8 mg. However, the proposal was withdrawn, and at present there are no regulations in this regard. The typical over-the-counter dose of pseudoephedrine in a nasal decongestant is 60 mg every 4 to 6 hr (McKenry and Salerno, 1995). Species of the plant genus Ephedra are the botanical source of ephedrine. Ephedrine and pseudoephedrine are available as a plant extract in products such a Ma Huang and *Ephedra sinica*. It is difficult to provide dosages of ephedrine and pseudoephedrine in these products because of the vast differences in product content and preparation. Various products can supply doses of 1 to 110 mg of ephedrine, and the ephedrine content of many products is often not stated (Turk, 1997). Regardless of the source, ephedrine is banned by the International Olympic Committee (IOC) and the National Collegiate Athletic Association (NCAA). However, pseudoephedrine is not banned by the NCAA (Fuentes and Rosenberg, 1999).

There are few data on the extent of ephedrine use in athletes. Gruber and Pope (1998) noted that of 64 women weight lifters interviewed, 36 (56%) reported taking some form of ephedrine. The 1997 NCAA survey of substance use and abuse habits of college athletes indicated that only 3.4% of the sample reported using

ephedrine, and there were no reports of ephedrine use in the previous surveys. The reason for these discrepant findings is unknown, but it is plausible that an NCAA athlete might be less likely to divulge use of a banned substance than a weight lifter. The prevalence of ephedrine use in professional sport, where there may be no drug testing at all, is almost completely unknown. It is noteworthy that the entrance of professional athletes from the National Basketball Association (NBA) and the National Hockey League (NHL) into the drug-tested arena of the Olympic games has caused concern among NBA and NHL officials. Professional athletes from the NBA and the NHL named to the Olympic team may be subjected to random drug testing for compounds such as ephedrine. There is concern that sanctions from the USOC and IOC could carry over to the NBA and NHL.

Throughout the past 30 years, athletes in a variety of sports have tested positive for ephedrine or pseudoephedrine. Some claimed that they were simply taking over-the-counter cold medicine or that they were ingesting a supplement that they were unaware contained ephedrine. The consequences of these positive drug tests have ranged from rather mild to quite severe. When Linford Christie tested positive for pseudoephedrine at the Seoul Olympics in 1988, the IOC did not punish him. Ultimately, Christie was awarded a silver medal in the 100-m (109 yd) sprint (after Ben Johnson was disqualified from first place for a positive steroid test). In 1988 the USOC allowed eight athletes to compete in Seoul after they tested positive for ephedrine prior to the games; their names were not released. Maria Kisseleva, a synchronized swimmer from Russia, tested positive for ephedrine but claimed that her team physician gave her the product for weight control. She was stripped of her European Duet title, received only a one-month suspension from the European swimming federation, and ultimately won a gold medal at the 2000 Sydney Olympics.

Other athletes have been more severely penalized for ephedrine use. United States swimmer Rick Demont won the 400-m (437 yd) freestyle at the Munich Olympic Games, but prior to the 1500-m (1640 yd) freestyle he tested positive for ephedrine. Demont was unaware that his asthma medication Marax contained ephedrine;

nonetheless, he was banned from competing in the 1500, and his gold medal was revoked. British sprinter Solomon Warisio tested positive for ephedrine at the 1994 European Championships, explaining that he had consumed the supplement Up Your Gas and had been unaware that it contained ephedrine. Warisio received a three-month ban, which caused him to miss the 1994 Commonwealth Games. Argentinean soccer captain Diego Maradona tested positive for "ephedrine and ephedrine-like substances" in the 1994 World Cup. He was banished from the World Cup and banned for two years. The highest-profile pseudoephedrine positive drug test was of 2000 Olympic gold medal gymnast Andreea Raducan. Raducan tested positive for pseudoephedrine at the Olympic Games in Sydney and was stripped of her gold medal, despite the fact that her team physician admitted giving her the medication for cold symptoms.

It is possible that athletes are ingesting ephedrine as part of a cold medication, inadvertently in a nutritional supplement, or purposefully for a performance or weight loss effect. If an athlete tests positive for ephedrine it is difficult to truly know the source. Because products such as Ripped Fuel, Diet Fuel, Ultimate Orange, and Metabolife are not specifically marketed as ephedrine products, athletes who do not pay attention to label ingredients may be unaware that they are ingesting ephedrine. However, "inadvertently" taking a medication or supplement that contains ephedrine has become a convenient excuse for athletes who fail drug tests. Ephedrine is an over-the-counter drug that is widely available, inexpensive, and not tested for in many professional and amateur sports. In this light, it appears that the prevalence of ephedrine use in sport is nearly impossible to determine.

This chapter first details the ephedrine content of supplements and describes the action of ephedrine. Next it presents a review of research studies regarding the efficacy of ephedrine in weight loss and its possible role as a performance booster. Because ephedrine is used by athletes primarily as an ergogenic aid, we give particular attention to review of studies on its role as a performance enhancer. Also to be discussed are the potential adverse effects and safety issues to consider in assessing the various products that contain ephedrine. Because ephedrine can still be purchased over the counter, most people believe it is a safe and harmless product. Therefore, we present detailed discussion of adverse events associated with its use.

Ephedrine Content of Supplements

The ephedrine content of ephedra plants can vary widely and is dependent on where the plant is grown, the type of growing conditions, and the time of harvest (Sagara et al., 1983). This can give rise to large interproduct variability. Sagara et al. (1983) reported the ephedrine content of ephedra plants from China, Pakistan, Russia, as well as of an ephedra plant grown in the laboratory. Plants grown in different regions had 8-, 13-, 3-, 4-, and 3-fold differences in norephedrine, pseudoephedrine, ephedrine, methylephedrine, and total ephedrine alkaloid content, respectively. Gurley et al. (1997) examined the ephedrine alkaloid content of five herbal Ma Huang products (Escalation, Excel, Up Your Gas, Ephedra, and Herbal Ecstasy). The ratio of ephedrine alkaloid content (ephedrine, methylephedrine, and pseudoephedrine) varied markedly among the five products, suggesting that the label claims were indicative of total alkaloid content, not ephedrine content. Further, the variability for ephedrine and methylephedrine content in Herbal Ecstasy exceeded 100% between lots.

Finally, White et al. (1997) determined the variability of ephedrine and pseudoephedrine among capsules from the same lot of Ma Huang. Although the label claimed that each capsule contained 375 mg of Ma Huang per capsule, the amount varied from 368 to 411 mg. Based on per capsule variability, ephedrine content per each four-capsule serving ranged from 15.2 to 23.6 mg.

Herbal preparations are not the only supplements plagued by such variability; even over-the-counter ephedrine supplements may contain variable amounts of the drug. In a study examining the pharmacokinetics of acute and chronic ephedrine ingestion, Pickup et al. (1976) reported lower plasma and urine ephedrine levels than expected. It was subsequently determined that the tablets used in the study contained only 90.9% of the ephedrine claimed on the label.

In addition to potentially ingesting ephedrine and Ma Huang supplements that contain a different amount of the drug than claimed on the label, supplement users should be aware that several factors can influence ephedrine absorption as well. White et al. (1997) evaluated the pharmacokinetic properties of 375 mg of Ma Huang/ ephedra for comparison to previously reported data on ephedrine. Although the half-life, volume of distribution, plasma clearance, and maximum concentration of plasma ephedrine after Ma Huang ingestion were similar to values previously reported following 20 mg of ephedrine ingestion, the values for the absorption rate were considerably lower and the time to reach maximum concentration was longer. This indicates that ephedrine is absorbed much more slowly when ingested as Ma Huang. Gurley et al. (1998) reported that ephedra ingested alone has absorption similar to that of ephedrine, but that ephedra ingested with other herbs has a significantly greater absorption rate from the gut to the blood. The authors were unable to determine which herbs may have increased absorption rates, but all of the formulas that demonstrated increased absorption included a caffeine-containing herb such as Guarana or kola nut. Also, the herbal formula that had the slowest absorption rate (Up Your Gas) was the only tablet formulation, indicating that ephedra from capsules is absorbed faster.

Ephedrine Action

There are two types of adrenergic receptors, α and β. The α-receptors function in vasoconstriction and bladder control, while β-receptors are involved in vasodilation, cardioacceleration, increased myocardial strength, bronchodilation, and stimulation of energy metabolism. Ephedrine is both an α- and β-agonist, and it also functions to enhance release of norepinephrine from sympathetic neurons (Hoffman and Lefkowitz, 1996). In its role as a β-receptor agonist, it has been used to induce bronchodilation in the treatment of asthma symptoms; however, newer drugs that are more selective β2-agonists (less stimulation of β1-receptors in the heart) are now prescribed. Ephedrine is thought to improve exercise performance because it triggers the β1-receptors to increase heart rate and myocardial contraction force and also serves as a central nervous system stimulant.

Ephedrine is also used to promote weight loss. It increases thermogenesis and hence resting energy expenditure by stimulating tissue (muscle) β-receptors to increase substrate metabolism. Adipose tissue contains α- and β-receptors that appear to be involved in the breakdown and mobilization of lipids (Kempen et al., 1994). Ephedrine also functions as an anorectic (appetite suppressor) by activation of adrenergic pathways in the hypothalamus, thereby increasing norepinephrine release (Wellman, 1992). Another way ephedrine could act to suppress appetite is by slowing down the rate at which food exits the stomach, which could affect satiety (Jonderko and Kucio, 1991).

Ephedrine As a Weight Loss Agent

Most studies that dealt with effects of ephedrine on weight loss used predominantly obese individuals as research subjects, so there are few data on its effectiveness as a weight loss agent in normal to slightly above normal-weight individuals. Pasquali et al. (1992) reported that 150 mg of ephedrine per day for two weeks in the course of a six-week, very low calorie diet intervention did not result in a difference in weight loss compared with a placebo. In another study (Pasquali et al., 1987), a longer period of intervention (2 months) did result in greater weight loss, but the difference in weight loss was only 1.8 kg (~4 lb) between the ephedrine group and the placebo group. The increase in weight loss with ephedrine could result from protein sparing caused by stimulation of β2-

receptors, affecting protein synthesis and counteracting lean tissue loss (Dulloo, 1993). Also, ephedrine may prevent the drop in resting metabolic rate associated with low-calorie diets (Pasquali et al., 1992).

Caffeine appears to enhance the effectiveness of ephedrine as a weight loss agent. Although the mechanism of action is not clear (Dulloo et al., 1994), caffeine may boost the effects of ephedrine. Ephedrine stimulates the release of norepinephrine, which in turn stimulates the release of adenosine. Adenosine serves as a prejunctional inhibitor of norepinephrine. Caffeine exerts an antagonistic effect to adenosine and thus potentiates the release of norepinephrine. Several studies showed that a combination of ephedrine and caffeine increased energy expenditure and/or enhanced weight loss in obese subjects (Astrup et al., 1992a, 1992b, 1991; Breum et al., 1994; Toubro et al., 1993). Doses shown to be most effective were 20 mg ephedrine and 200 mg caffeine, three times per day. Toubro et al. (1993) studied the effects of diet restriction (4.2 MJ·day^{-1}) with either ephedrine (20 mg), ephedrine/caffeine (20 mg/200 mg), caffeine (200 mg), or a placebo three times per day for 24 weeks. All groups demonstrated a decrease in body weight, with the greatest decrease for the ephedrine/caffeine combination (16.6 kg [36.6 lb]) and the least for the placebo (13.3 kg [29.3 lb]). It should be noted that the difference between these groups was only 3.3 kg (7.3 lb) over 24 weeks. Astrup and Toubro (1993) estimated that about 80% of weight loss from ephedrine/caffeine was due to an anorectic effect and 20% was due to a thermogenic effect.

Ephedrine has also been coupled with both caffeine and aspirin to further enhance its effectiveness as a weight loss agent. Ephedrine stimulates release of norepinephrine, which stimulates the synthesis of prostaglandins by the activated tissue. Prostaglandins act as prejunctional inhibitors. Aspirin inhibits the synthesis of prostaglandins and serves as a prostaglandin blocker, and thereby may prevent inhibition of norepinephrine release. This effect would enhance the action of ephedrine on sympathetically mediated thermogenesis (Geissler, 1993). Daly et al. (1993) had obese individuals either ingest a combination of ephedrine (75 mg), caffeine (150 mg), and aspirin (330 mg) (ECA) or ingest a placebo for four weeks, with no energy restriction; then the dose of ephedrine was increased to 150 mg·day^{-1} for another four weeks. The mean weight loss over the eight weeks of the study was 2.2 kg (4.9 lb) for the ECA group and 0.7 (1.5 lb) for the placebo.

Ephedrine alone is only mildly effective as a weight loss agent in obesity; when coupled with aspirin and/or caffeine, its effectiveness is improved, but the weight loss is still relatively small compared to prescription drugs for weight loss or with just restricting calories. However, there may be a role for ephedrine or ephedrine combinations as weight loss drugs over the long term (Astrup and Lundsgaard, 1998; Carek and Dickerson, 1999). Although the adverse effects are often generally less than those reported with prescription drugs for weight loss, for some individuals and in high dosages or with prolonged use, adverse effects can be severe (see later section on health concerns). Because withdrawal of these drugs commonly results in weight gain and because use of the drugs is often associated with some adverse effects, drugs may not be the best tool for weight loss in those who are also concerned about athletic performance.

Ephedrine As a Performance Enhancer

Despite the fact that ephedrine and pseudoephedrine are banned by the IOC, few data are available regarding their effects on exercise performance. In fact, these substances were likely placed on the IOC banned substance list based on their structural similarity to amphetamines and assumed performance-enhancing effect (Swain et al., 1997). Only eight studies have examined their ergogenic properties, and there are no documented ergogenic effects of ephedrine or pseudoephedrine when ingested alone. This section reviews the available literature on the effects of ephedrine and pseudoephedrine on physiological and psychological responses to exercise.

Ephedrine

The first available study to examine the effects of ephedrine on exercise performance was published in 1977. Sidney and Lefcoe (1977) examined the effects of 24 mg of ephedrine on a battery of physical performance and fitness tests in 21 healthy males (19-30 years) using a double-blind, placebo-controlled, crossover design. The test battery addressed the effects of ephedrine at rest on physical performance, psychomotor performance, and lung function. When questioned, subjects could not identify whether they received the drug or placebo. Ingestion of ephedrine compared to a placebo resulted in a small (4 mm Hg) yet significant increase in resting diastolic blood pressure. There were no differences in resting heart rate or systolic blood pressure. During a 12-min progressive submaximal treadmill test (40%, 65%, and 85% of $\dot{V}O_2$max) and 5-min recovery, ephedrine caused small increases (3-8 beats·min^{-1}) in heart rate compared to the placebo. Ephedrine had no effect on oxygen uptake, minute ventilation, respiratory gas exchange, and ratings of perceived exertion during submaximal exercise. $\dot{V}O_2$max determined on a treadmill, and all measures taken during this test (maximal ventilation rate, maximal heart rate, maximal respiratory gas exchange, and postexercise lactic acid concentration), were unaffected by ephedrine. Maximal grip strength,

grip endurance, power (vertical jump), anaerobic endurance (timed stair run), time to exhaustion (treadmill test at 85% of maximal heart rate), and postexercise lactic acid concentration were not affected by ephedrine ingestion. Ephedrine ingestion had no effect on reaction time to visual and auditory stimuli, but hand-eye coordination assessed with a pursuit rotor tracking test was statistically improved. Lung function was not changed by drug administration. The authors concluded that 24 mg of ephedrine resulted in small increases in resting blood pressure, exercise, and recovery heart rates, but had no effect on any measures of physical work capacity or lung function in healthy young men. Although ephedrine ingestion increased performance on the hand-eye coordination test in this study, the authors noted that ephedrine may only benefit unskilled subjects tested on a simple psychomotor task and that the effect of ephedrine may disappear in more proficient subjects.

Subsequently, Sidney and Lefcoe (1978) examined the effects of Tedral (24 mg of ephedrine and 130 mg of theophylline) on physical performance, work capacity, and psychomotor performance in 11 male and female track athletes (18-21 years) using a double-blind, placebo-controlled, crossover design. Tedral had no effect on maximal grip strength, grip endurance, vertical jump, time to exhaustion on an anaerobic or aerobic treadmill run, and $\dot{V}O_2$max compared to the placebo. Tedral administration did result in a 4% increase in the number of sit-ups performed in 1 min. Psychomotor performance assessed with a reaction time test (visual stimulus) and hand-eye coordination test (pursuit rotor tracking) was not improved by Tedral ingestion.

No other studies of the effects of ephedrine on exercise performance appeared in the literature until the late 1990s (Bell and Jacobs, 1999; Bell et al., 1998). Bell et al. (1998) investigated the effects of ingestion of caffeine, ephedrine, and their combination on time to exhaustion in eight healthy, male subjects (31 ± 5 years) using a randomized, double-blind, crossover design. The authors chose to combine ephedrine and caffeine based on studies indicating that caffeine induces a "permissive" effect on ephedrine (Astrup et al., 1991; Dulloo et al., 1992). This refers to the concept that caffeine both lowers the threshold concentration required for physiological effects and potentiates the physiological effects of a given ephedrine concentration. Over the testing days, subjects ingested caffeine (5 mg·kg^{-1} body mass), ephedrine (1 mg·kg^{-1} body mass), a combination of the drugs (5 mg·kg^{-1} body mass of caffeine and 1 mg·kg^{-1} body mass of ephedrine), or a placebo. Subjects exercised on a cycle ergometer while exercise intensity was increased (37.5 W·min^{-1}) until they could no longer maintain 50 rpm. Time to exhaustion was increased in the caffeine plus ephedrine condition (approximately 38%) compared to the placebo or caffeine conditions. No differences were found between conditions in oxygen consumption, carbon dioxide production, minute ventilation, and respiratory exchange ratio. Heart rate during exercise was significantly increased for the caffeine plus ephedrine condition compared to the placebo, while ratings of perceived exertion during exercise were significantly lower after caffeine plus ephedrine ingestion compared to placebo. The authors concluded that ingestion of either caffeine or ephedrine alone could not improve exercise performance, but that the combination of caffeine and ephedrine significantly prolonged time to exhaustion compared to a placebo.

In a subsequent study, Bell and Jacobs (1999) examined the effects of ingestion of a combination of caffeine and ephedrine on performance of the Canadian Forces Warrior Test, a 3.2-km (~2 miles) run during which subjects wear 11 kg (24.2 lb) of military gear. One purpose of the study was to examine whether the performance-enhancing effects of combined caffeine and ephedrine ingestion shown under laboratory conditions would occur in a field setting. A second purpose, based on anecdotal reports of fatigue and lethargy from subjects in the prior study, was to determine whether caffeine and ephedrine ingestion could adversely affect exercise performance one day after treatment. Nine healthy male recreational runners completed six balanced and double-blind trials of the run test 2 hr after ingestion of a combination of 375 mg of caffeine and 75 mg ephedrine, or a placebo. Subjects performed three sets (separated by 7 days) of two runs (separated by 24 hr) and were administered treatment in the following manner: Set 1—caffeine and ephedrine trial on day 1 and placebo trial on day 2; Set 2—placebo trial on day 1 and caffeine and ephedrine on day 2; Set 3—placebo on both days. Run times during the caffeine and ephedrine trials were similar and were significantly faster than for control and placebo trials. Exercise performance 24 hr following caffeine and ephedrine ingestion was not affected. The authors concluded that exercise performance on the Canadian Forces Warrior Test was improved by caffeine and ephedrine ingestion, and that this treatment does not cause impaired exercise performance 24 hr later.

Pseudoephedrine

Bright et al. (1981) examined the effects of pseudo-ephedrine in six healthy males (23-28 years) at rest and during submaximal exercise. Subjects ingested a placebo, 60 mg pseudoephedrine, or 120 mg pseudoephedrine in a randomized, double-blind, placebo-controlled, crossover study. Pseudoephedrine consumed 60 min prior to treadmill exercise had no effect on time to reach 85% of maximal predicted heart rate or time to return to baseline heart rate following exercise. Similarly, there

was no effect of the drug on resting, exercise, or recovery blood pressure. Clemons and Crosby (1993) reported the effects of 60 mg of pseudoephedrine ingestion on exercise at greater than 85% of maximal heart rate. Ten healthy female athletes (20.4 ± 1.7 years) participated in a randomized, double-blind, placebo-controlled, crossover study during which they underwent a graded exercise test (Bruce protocol) to exhaustion. Heart rate following pseudoephedrine ingestion was significantly higher at the ends of stages 1, 2, 3, and 4 and also following 8 min of recovery compared to the value with placebo. No significant differences in respiratory exchange ratio, ventilation, oxygen consumption, respiration rate, tidal volume, systolic or diastolic blood pressure, total exercise time, core temperature, or ratings of perceived exertion were found between the drug and placebo conditions. With the exception of increased exercise heart rate (3-6 beats·min^{-1}), these data suggest that 60 mg of pseudoephedrine neither enhances nor impairs physiological or psychological responses to maximal exercise.

Gillies and colleagues (1996) examined the effects of 120 mg of pseudoephedrine ingested 120 min prior to exercise in 10 healthy male cyclists using a randomized, double-blind, placebo-controlled, crossover design. Cycling performance was tested with a 40-km (24.9 miles) time to exhaustion test (approximately 1 hr), and skeletal muscle function was assessed with an isometric fatigue test of the knee extensors (fatigue was defined as the point at which the subjects were unable to maintain a torque $\geq 70\%$ of maximal voluntary contraction). Pseudoephedrine did not influence either time trial performance or isometric muscle fatigue compared to the placebo. None of the subjects were able to identify whether they had ingested the drug or the placebo. Finally, Swain et al. (1997) studied the effects of two dosages of pseudoephedrine (1 mg·kg^{-1} and 2 mg·kg^{-1} of body mass) on exercise performance in 10 male cyclists (18-35 years) using a randomized, double-blind, placebo-controlled, multiple-dose design. Body mass ranged from 57.5 to 90.7 kg (from 127 to 200 lb), so subjects ingested approximately 57 to 90 mg of ephedrine in one trial and 115 to 181 in the other trial. Subjects exercised on a cycle ergometer with increasing resistance (4.905 N every 2 min) until pedal speed could no longer be maintained at 80 rpm. Peak systolic blood pressure during exercise was significantly increased (10.6 mm Hg) in the 1 mg·kg^{-1} group. No significant changes were found in peak diastolic blood pressure, maximal heart rate, ratings of perceived exertion, time to exhaustion, or $\dot{V}O_2$max. In the 2 mg·kg^{-1} group there were no differences in peak systolic or diastolic blood pressure, maximal heart rate, ratings of perceived exertion, time to exhaustion, or $\dot{V}O_2$max. Taken together, data from these four studies indicate that pseudoephedrine supplementation in healthy young subjects does not enhance exercise performance during cycling or treadmill running at submaximal or maximal exercise intensities and has only small effects on selected physiological parameters. Further, there is no indication that pseudoephedrine supplementation reduces perceived exertion during exercise.

Although limited information on the performance-enhancing effects of ephedrine and pseudoephedrine is available at this time, some conclusions can be drawn. Ephedrine supplementation has been shown to have ergogenic effects only when it is ingested with other drugs such as theophylline or caffeine. In fact, there are currently no data to support an ergogenic effect for ephedrine ingestion prior to exercise. It is clear that pseudoephedrine ingestion does not improve exercise performance on submaximal or maximal exercise and does not reduce ratings of perceived exertion during exercise. Furthermore, the increase in heart rate, blood pressure, tremor, and anxiety caused by ephedrine use may actually result in an impairment in athletic performance, especially in doses larger than those used in the research studies.

Health Concerns

Because of its role as a sympathomimetic drug, ephedrine can affect heart rate and blood pressure and result in cardiovascular disturbances. Ephedrine can cause minor adverse effects such as tremor and nervousness or more severe adverse reactions, including myocardial infarction, stroke, seizure, psychosis, and death. Between 1993 and 1997, over 800 adverse events and 34 deaths attributed to ephedrine ingestion were reported to the Food and Drug Administration (1997). Also, few data are available on physiological perturbations, such as heat stress or dehydration, that may exacerbate these negative effects. This section reviews the available literature on the adverse physical and psychological consequences associated with use of ephedrine and related compounds. Most of the studies cited in this section are case reports. While these studies provide some insight into the dangers of ephedrine use, readers must recognize that the incidents they deal with are isolated. Although the adverse events described appear to be linked to ephedrine, there could be other intervening factors as well. At present there are no large-scale epidemiological studies of acute and chronic effects of ephedrine use at any dose.

Ephedrine and Stroke

Bruno et al. (1993) reported ephedrine-related stroke in three patients. Patient 1, a 37-year-old male without stroke risk factors, ingested 153 mg of ephedrine·day^{-1}

for three weeks for weight loss before having a left thalamic infarct. Patient 2 was a 42-year-old-male with a history of hypertension and of drug abuse, which included the ingestion of 100 to 200 mg of ephedrine·day^{-1} for 23 years. He was found dead at home with ephedrine tablets near his body. Finally, patient 3 was an 84-year-old woman who had no history of hypertension or ephedrine use. She died 24 hr after a ruptured aneurysm; the only drug found in her blood was ephedrine.

In 1996, a 23-year-old Tufts University graduate student died of myocardial necrosis, and several empty bottles of a sport product containing ephedrine, designed to enhance muscle mass and burn fat, were found in his room (Theoharides, 1997). Myers et al. (1999) reported a case study of a 20-year-old collegiate wrestler who experienced severe chest pains and syncope after an exercise bout. In an attempt to make weight by losing 4.5 to 6.8 kg (~10 to 15 lb), the athlete had taken a herbal stimulant that contained ephedrine and caffeine for two months. On the day he was hospitalized, the athlete had not ingested food or water, but had ingested the herbal supplement. Urinalysis revealed the presence of ephedrine and documented dehydration. Recently, a case of a stroke in a 33-year-old athlete, with no known vascular risk, was reported (Vahedi et al., 2000). The patient was described as a sportsman who trained intensively 2 hr per day and was perfectly fit before his stroke. He had ingested two multinutrient supplements containing approximately 40 to 60 mg of ephedrine, 400 to 600 mg of caffeine, 6000 mg of creatine monohydrate, and various minerals and amino acids for six weeks prior to his stroke.

Ephedrine Psychosis

In addition to the potential physiological consequences of ephedrine use, there are several reports of psychiatric complications (Capwell, 1995; Doyle and Kargin, 1996; Herridge and O'Brook, 1968; Jacobs and Hirsch, 2000; Roxanas and Spalding, 1977; Whitehouse and Duncan, 1987). The first report of "ephedrine psychosis" appeared in the literature in 1968 (Herridge and O'Brook). Herridge and O'Brook (1968) reported this phenomenon in a 65-year-old man who been hostile and paranoid for two months and a 54-year-old woman who had experienced episodes of psychosis for 10 years. The man was convinced that his wife was being unfaithful with another man, and he claimed to have seen this man and heard the man speaking to his wife on several occasions. In one instance, he believed there was an intruder in his garden at night and began searching outside with an iron bar. After four days of hospitalization, the psychosis disappeared without any pharmacological intervention. At this point, the patient admitted having taken two hundred 60-mg ephedrine tablets a week for years (for asthma and to stay awake while driving), and he had recently increased this amount. Also, this dose of ephedrine had made him impotent.

The woman reported on by Herridge and O'Brook (1968) had pulmonary tuberculosis, asthma, and bouts of bronchitis and reported taking increasing amounts of ephedrine for 20 years (up to seventy-five 15-mg tablets·day^{-1}). In retrospect, the authors noted that her recurrent episodes of psychosis over the 10 years, which included vivid auditory and visual hallucinations, had coincided with exacerbation of her breathing disorders, tremors, and difficulty sleeping. After four days of hospitalization and no ephedrine, the psychosis disappeared. Within one month of discharge her hallucinations returned; and although she denied taking any ephedrine, her urine was positive for ephedrine.

In 1977, Roxanas and Spalding reported three cases of ephedrine psychosis. Case 1 was a 26-year-old man who suddenly felt as if the world was coming to an end, that people had discovered a formula to escape from earth and go to another planet, and that there was a plot to "attack him and amputate his ankles." In addition, he experienced both auditory and visual hallucinations. He had begun taking ephedrine to stay awake at his job, beginning with five 30-mg tablets twice a night and increasing his dosage on the third night to five tablets three times a night. The following day he presented himself to police and asked for protection. Five days after admission to a hospital, all symptoms disappeared.

Case 2 was a 26-year-old man who had behaved oddly and aggressively for several months. He said "I have visions and apparitions of gods and goddesses; I see Isis with white hair, wearing a velvet gown. In one of my past lives I was in Egypt and she used to be a cat." On the day before his admission to the hospital he had taken 300 mg of ephedrine. After his admission, a mental examination showed that he had auditory hallucinations and delusions of persecution and grandeur. Although he had a prior history of drug abuse, he denied taking any drugs except ephedrine in recent weeks. While in the psychiatric hospital he became violent, broke furniture, and attacked a nurse. He admitted to having taken 300 mg of ephedrine on the previous day.

Case 3 was a 30-year-old woman brought to a clinic by her mother, who had noticed a change in her daughter's behavior over two years. The patient became irritable and erratic, began speaking much faster than usual, exhibited paranoia, isolated herself in her bedroom, and refused to care for her children or pay outstanding debts. Her mother reported that her daughter had been ingesting Tedral for her asthma (130 mg theophylline and 24 mg ephedrine) more than appeared necessary. Although the patient denied auditory hallucinations during her interview at the clinic, she frequently talked to herself

and at times burst out laughing. She admitted taking 6 to 10 Tedral tablets daily (780-1300 mg theophylline and 144-240 mg ephedrine). Over three months her condition improved, but not consistently, probably because she refused to discontinue Tedral ingestion. A two-year follow-up revealed that the patient had finally returned to normal after her family had convinced her to change medications. In marked contrast to the cases presented in 1968, in which people had ingested as much as 1700 to 2250 mg of ephedrine·day^{-1}, these three patients had ingested only 144 to 300 mg ephedrine·day^{-1}, for much shorter lengths of time, and still required hospitalization.

In 1987 another instance of ephedrine psychosis was reported in a 59-year-old male who had used ephedrine for asthma for 25 years (Whitehouse and Duncan, 1987). After increasing his dosage to 360 mg·day^{-1}, the man began to experience auditory hallucinations of a woman's cries. Believing a woman was being tortured, and unable to get the police to respond, the man entered the woman's apartment to determine the source of the screams. He was apprehended by police for entering the woman's apartment uninvited and was admitted to a psychiatric ward. The man had no family history or personal history of psychiatric illness. After his ephedrine dose was reduced to 60 mg·day^{-1}, all symptoms disappeared in 13 days.

Whitehouse and Duncan (1987) reviewed 20 cases of ephedrine psychosis. Patients were 19 to 65 years of age, and only two had a previous history of psychiatric illness or family history of psychiatric illness. Ephedrine ingestion ranged from 125 to 2500 mg·day^{-1}, and length of ephedrine ingestion ranged from three days to 25 years. It was noted that 100% of patients experienced delusions, 90% experienced auditory hallucinations, 45% experienced visual hallucinations, and 85% had clear consciousness during these episodes. The authors noted that the main clinical features of ephedrine-induced psychosis were similar to those for amphetamine-induced psychosis.

Capwell (1995) reported the first instance of a psychosis from Ma Huang ingestion. A 45-year-old man, with no history of psychiatric disease or drug abuse, was taken to the emergency room by his wife. After ingesting a herbal supplement for two months to lose weight, he had begun to have personality and behavior changes. He was irritable, had insomnia, and became so disorganized that he was asked to take a leave of absence from work. He became preoccupied with religion and argued with his minister about biblical meanings and the coming "rapture." Eventually he became so aggressive and verbally abusive that his wife insisted he seek medical help. The emergency room physician suggested that he discontinue his Ma Huang ingestion and prescribed a sedative. After three days the man returned to normal.

Doyle and Kargin (1996) reported a case study of a 34-year-old man who had jumped out of an upstairs window trying to flee supposed attackers. Upon examination, the man was agitated and paranoid and had visual hallucinations. He had no prior history of mental illness, but had been ingesting unknown quantities of Ma Huang for 10 days to lose weight. The patient's symptoms resolved rapidly, and he was discharged after two weeks. Recently, Jacobs and Hirsch (2000) reported cases of psychiatric disturbances in two healthy young men. Patient 1 was a 27-year-old male marine sergeant who, after making an error while working as an avionics technician, became agitated and suicidal. The patient had a history of depression, but no history of suicidal tendencies. When questioned, the patient admitted to regular Ma Huang use, but would not disclose the amount or frequency of use. Facing dismissal from the military, he agreed to stop using the herbal supplement. Patient 2 was a 20-year-old male marine private who was evacuated from his ship for evaluation of psychosis and agitation. Prior to this incident, the patient had ingested supplements containing Ma Huang, ginseng, dehydroepiandrosterone (DHEA), and creatine, as well as large amounts of coffee. The patient was treated on an inpatient psychiatric ward for seven days and received antipsychotic medications for three months until he returned to duty.

Other Potential Risks

Few data on the effects of physiological perturbations, such as heat stress, on the pharmacokinetics of sympathomimetic drugs are available. Vanakoski et al. (1993) examined the effects of a sauna on the pharmacokinetics of a 50-mg ephedrine dose in six healthy young women (21 years) using a double-blind, placebo-controlled, crossover design. The sauna (three 10-min sessions at 80 to 100 °C, relative humidity 30-50%) caused a higher absorption rate constant and higher maximum plasma ephedrine concentration compared to control conditions. Although the results were not statistically significant, ephedrine ingestion in the sauna produced greater increases in systolic blood pressure (25.7 vs. 13.0 mm Hg) and heart rate (10.0 vs. 6.5 beats·min^{-1}) than ephedrine ingestion under control conditions. These data suggest that ephedrine is absorbed more rapidly and has more marked effects on cardiovascular function under hot and humid conditions. Athletes often compete in hot and humid environments and should be aware that these conditions could increase the rate of absorption of ephedrine and possibly exacerbate adverse effects.

Recently, Bell et al. (1999) examined the effects of ingestion of ephedrine and caffeine on exercise tolerance under hot and dry conditions. Ten males (39 ± 8 years) exercised on a treadmill at 50% $\dot{V}O_2$peak in a heat chamber (40 °C and 30% relative humidity) until rectal temperature reached 39.3 °C, 95% of peak heart rate was maintained for 3 min, dizziness or nausea required the exercise to be discontinued, or when 3 hr had elapsed. Exercise tolerance time, skin temperature, rectal temperature, and the sensation of thermal comfort were similar under the placebo and the caffeine plus ephedrine conditions. $\dot{V}O_2$, ventilation rate, and heart rate (first 20 min only) were all significantly elevated following caffeine and ephedrine ingestion compared to a placebo. The authors concluded that despite the increase in metabolic rate, heat loss mechanisms were sufficient to offset the increase, so body temperature remained normal. It should be noted again that athletes often compete under hot and humid conditions (in which evaporative cooling is compromised), and it is unknown whether or not heat loss mechanisms would be sufficient to offset the increase in metabolic rate under these conditions.

Conclusion

The ephedrines have been proven effective in producing small losses in body weight due to their anorectic and thermogenic properties. Although adverse effects are associated with their use in recommended doses, the adverse effects are generally milder than for prescription drugs for weight loss. However, these effects, including increased anxiety and headaches, can adversely impact exercise performance, and ephedrines are therefore contraindicated for athletes. Combinations of ephedrine and caffeine, or ephedrine and caffeine and aspirin, have been found to be more effective as weight loss agents than ephedrine alone, but the adverse effects are also increased. Although there are few studies of the efficacy of ephedrine in improving exercise performance, these studies are consistent in their findings of no ergogenic effects. High doses of ephedrine, prolonged use, and even recommended doses in some individuals have been associated with side effects that are sometimes very serious. Several case studies are available to document stroke and psychiatric complications, especially psychosis. Because of the lack of federal regulation of over-the-counter products, there is no assurance of the content of any supplement, and this is true of ephedrine as well. In conclusion, the risks of ephedrine use appear to outweigh any potential ergogenic benefits.

References

Astrup, A, L Breum, S Toubro, P Hein, and F Quaade. 1992a. The effect and safety of an ephedrine/caffeine compound compared to ephedrine, caffeine and placebo in obese subjects on an energy restricted diet. A double blind trial. *International Journal of Obesity and Related Metabolic Disorders* 16 (4):269-277.

Astrup, A, B Buemann, NJ Christensen, S Toubro, G Thorbek, OJ Victor, and F Quaade. 1992b. The effect of ephedrine/caffeine mixture on energy expenditure and body composition in obese women. *Metabolism* 41 (7):686-688.

Astrup, A, and C Lundsgaard. 1998. What do pharmacological approaches to obesity management offer? Linking pharmacological mechanisms of obesity management agents to clinical practice. *Experimental and Clinical Endocrinology and Diabetes* 106 (Suppl 2):29-34.

Astrup, A, and S Toubro. 1993. Thermogenic, metabolic, and cardiovascular responses to ephedrine and caffeine in man. *International Journal of Obesity and Related Metabolic Disorders* 17 (Suppl 1):S41-S43.

Astrup, A, S Toubro, S Cannon, P Hein, and J Madsen. 1991. Thermogenic synergism between ephedrine and caffeine in healthy volunteers: a double-blind, placebo-controlled study. *Metabolism* 40 (3):323-329.

Bell, DG, and I Jacobs. 1999. Combined caffeine and ephedrine ingestion improves run times of Canadian Forces Warrior Test. *Aviation Space and Environmental Medicine* 70 (4):325-329.

Bell, DG, I Jacobs, TM McLellan, M Miyazaki, and CM Sabiston. 1999. Thermal regulation in the heat during exercise after caffeine and ephedrine ingestion. *Aviation Space and Environmental Medicine* 70 (6):583-588.

Bell, DG, I Jacobs, and J Zamecnik. 1998. Effects of caffeine, ephedrine and their combination on time to exhaustion during high-intensity exercise. *European Journal of Applied Physiology* 77 (5):427-433.

Breum, L, JK Pedersen, F Ahlstrom, and J Frimodt-Moller. 1994. Comparison of an ephedrine/caffeine combination and dexfenfluramine in the treatment of obesity. A double-blind multi-centre trial in general practice. *International Journal of Obesity and Related Metabolic Disorders* 18 (2):99-103.

Bright, TP, BW Sandage Jr., and HP Fletcher. 1981. Selected cardiac and metabolic responses to pseudoephedrine with exercise. *Journal of Clinical Pharmacology* 21 (11-12 Pt 1):488-492.

Bruno, A, KB Nolte, and J Chapin. 1993. Stroke associated with ephedrine use. *Neurology* 43 (7):1313-1316.

Capwell, RR. 1995. Ephedrine-induced mania from an herbal diet supplement. *American Journal of Psychiatry* 152 (4):647.

Carek, PJ, and LM Dickerson. 1999. Current concepts in the pharmacological management of obesity. *Drugs* 57 (6):883-904.

Clarkson, PM. 1998. Dietary supplements and pharmaceutical agents for weight loss and gain. In: *Exercise, nutrition and weight control, perspectives in exercise science and sports medicine,* vol. 11, edited by DR Lamb and R Murray. Carmel, IN: Cooper Publishing Group, pp. 349-405.

Clemons, JM, and SL Crosby. 1993. Cardiopulmonary and subjective effects of a 60 mg dose of pseudoephedrine on graded treadmill exercise. *Journal of Sports Medicine and Physical Fitness* 33 (4):405-412.

Daly, PA, DR Krieger, AG Dulloo, JB Young, and L Landsberg. 1993. Ephedrine, caffeine and aspirin: safety and efficacy for treatment of human obesity. *International Journal of Obesity and Related Metabolic Disorders* 17 (Suppl 1):S73-S78.

Doyle, H, and M Kargin. 1996. Herbal stimulant containing ephedrine has also caused psychosis. *British Medical Journal* 313 (7059):756.

Dulloo, AG. 1993. Ephedrine, xanthines and prostaglandin-inhibitors: actions and interactions in the stimulation of thermogenesis. *International Journal of Obesity and Related Metabolic Disorders* 17 (Suppl 1):S35-S40.

Dulloo, AG, J Seydoux, and L Girardier. 1992. Potentiation of the thermogenic antiobesity effects of ephedrine by dietary methylxanthines: adenosine antagonism or phosphodiesterase inhibition? *Metabolism* 41 (11):1233-1241.

Dulloo, AG, J Seydoux, and L Girardier. 1994. Paraxanthine (metabolite of caffeine) mimics caffeine's interaction with sympathetic control of thermogenesis. *American Journal of Physiology* 267 (5 Pt 1):E801-E804.

Food and Drug Administration. 1997. Dietary supplements containing ephedrine alkaloids. Accessed May 5, 2000. Available at **http://vm.cfsan.fda.gov/~lrd/fr97064a.html**.

Fuentes, RJ, and JM Rosenberg, eds. 1999. *Athletic drug reference.* Durham, NC: Glaxo Wellcome Inc., Clean Data, Inc.

Geissler, CA. 1993. Effects of weight loss, ephedrine and aspirin on energy expenditure in obese women. *International Journal of Obesity and Related Metabolic Disorders* 17 (Suppl 1):S45-S48.

Gillies, H, WE Derman, TD Noakes, P Smith, A Evans, and G Gabriels. 1996. Pseudoephedrine is without ergogenic effects during prolonged exercise. *Journal of Applied Physiology* 81 (6):2611-2617.

Gruber, AJ, and HG Pope Jr. 1998. Ephedrine abuse among 36 female weightlifters. *American Journal on Addictions* 7 (4):256-261.

Gurley, BJ, SF Gardner, LM White, and PL Wang. 1998. Ephedrine pharmacokinetics after the ingestion of nutritional supplements containing Ephedra sinica (ma huang). *Therapeutic Drug Monitoring* 20 (4):439-445.

Gurley, BJ, P Wang, and SF Gardner. 1997. Ephedrine alkaloid content of five commercially available herbal products containing Ephedra sinica (ma-huang). *Pharmaceutical Research* 14:5582-5583.

Herridge, CF, and MF O'Brook. 1968. Ephedrine psychosis. *British Medical Journal* 2 (598):160.

Hoffman, BB, and RJ Lefkowitz. 1996. Catecholamines, sympathomimetic drugs, and adrenergic receptor antagonists. In: Goodman and Gilman's *The pharmacological basis of therapeutics,* edited by JG Hardman, LE Limbird, PB Molinoff, RW Ruddon, and AG Gilman. New York: McGraw-Hill, pp. 199-248.

Jacobs, KM, and KA Hirsch. 2000. Psychiatric complications of Ma-huang. *Psychosomatics* 41 (1):58-62.

Jonderko, K, and C Kucio. 1991. Effect of anti-obesity drugs promoting energy expenditure, yohimbine and ephedrine, on gastric emptying in obese patients. *Alimentary Pharmacology and Therapeutics* 5 (4):413-418.

Kempen, KP, WH Saris, JM Senden, PP Menheere, EE Blaak, and MA van Baak. 1994. Effects of energy restriction on acute adrenoceptor and metabolic responses to exercise in obese subjects. *American Journal of Physiology* 267 (5 Pt 1):E694-E701.

McKenry, LM, and E Salerno. 1995. *Mosby's pharmacology in nursing.* St Louis: Mosby, p. 782.

Myers, JB, KM Guskiewicz, and BL Riemann. 1999. Syncope and atypical chest pain in an intercollegiate wrestler: A case report. *Journal of Athletic Training* 34:263-266.

National Collegiate Athletic Association (NCAA). 1997. National Collegiate Athletic Association Study of Research and Abuse Habits of College Student-Athletes. In NCAA research staff document.

Pasquali, R, F Casimirri, N Melchionda, G Grossi, L Bortoluzzi, AM Morselli Labate, C Stefanini, and A Raitano. 1992. Effects of chronic administration of ephedrine during very-low-calorie diets on energy expenditure, protein metabolism and hormone levels in obese subjects. *Clinical Science* 82 (1):85-92.

Pasquali, R, MP Cesari, N Melchionda, C Stefanini, A Raitano, and G Labo. 1987. Does ephedrine promote weight loss in low-energy-adapted obese women? *International Journal of Obesity and Related Metabolic Disorders* 11 (2):163-168.

Pickup, ME, CS May, R Ssendagire, and JW Paterson. 1976. The pharmacokinetics of ephedrine after oral dosage in asthmatics receiving acute and chronic treatment. *British Journal of Clinical Pharmacology* 3 (1):123-134.

Roxanas, MG, and J Spalding. 1977. Ephedrine abuse psychosis. *Medical Journal of Australia* 2 (19):639-640.

Sagara, K, T Oshima, and T Misaki. 1983. A simultaneous determination of norephedrine, pseudoephedrine, ephedrine and methylephedrine in Ephedrae Herba and oriental pharmaceutical preparations by ion-pair high-performance liquid chromatography. *Chemical and Pharmaceutical Bulletin* 31 (7):2359-2365.

Sidney, KH, and NM Lefcoe. 1977. The effects of ephedrine on the physiological and psychological responses to submaximal and maximal exercise in man. *Medicine and Science in Sports and Exercise* 9 (2):95-99.

Sidney, KH, and NM Lefcoe. 1978. Effects of tedral upon exercise performance: a double blind crossover study. In: *Sports medicine,* edited by F Landry and WAR Organ. Miami: Symposium Specialists.

Swain, RA, DM Harsha, J Baenziger, and RM Saywell Jr. 1997. Do pseudoephedrine or phenylpropanolamine improve maximum oxygen uptake and time to exhaustion? *Clinical Journal of Sports Medicine* 7 (3):168-173.

Theoharides, TC. 1997. Sudden death of a healthy college student related to ephedrine toxicity from a ma huang-containing drink. *Journal of Clinical Psychopharmacology* 17 (5):437-439.

Toubro, S, AV Astrup, L Breum, and F Quaade. 1993. Safety and efficacy of long-term treatment with ephedrine, caffeine and an ephedrine/caffeine mixture. *International Journal of Obesity and Related Metabolic Disorders* 17 (Suppl 1):S69-S72.

Turk, MP. 1997. Ephedrine's deadly edge. *U.S. News On Line.* Available at **http://www.usnews.com/usnews/issue/970707/7diet.htm**.

Vahedi, K, V Domigo, P Amarenco, and MG Bousser. 2000. Ischaemic stroke in a sportsman who consumed MaHuang extract and creatine monohydrate for bodybuilding. *Journal of Neurology, Neurosurgery, and Psychiatry* 68:112-113.

Vanakoski, J, C Stromberg, and T Seppälä. 1993. Effects of a sauna on the pharmacokinetics and pharmacodynamics of midazolam and ephedrine in healthy young women. *European Journal of Clinical Pharmacology* 45 (4):377-381.

Wellman, PJ. 1992. Overview of adrenergic anorectic agents. *American Journal of Clinical Nutrition* 55 (1 Suppl):193S-198S.

White, LM, SF Gardner, BJ Gurley, MA Marx, PL Wang, and M Estes. 1997. Pharmacokinetics and cardiovascular effects of ma-huang (Ephedra sinica) in normotensive adults. *Journal of Clinical Pharmacology* 37 (2):116-122.

Whitehouse, AM, and JM Duncan. 1987. Ephedrine psychosis rediscovered. *British Journal of Psychiatry* 150:258-261.

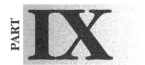
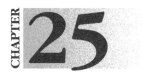

Gamma-Hydroxybutyric Acid

Vincenzo R. Sanguineti, MD

Marion Rudin Frank, EdD

Gamma-hydroxybutyric acid (GHB) is an allegedly benign and presently illicit substance that gained increasing recognition and attention among athletes because of its putative capacity to stimulate the release of growth hormone (GH) and in this way promote muscle buildup and enhance physical performance. It has been promoted in the illegal drug market in different ways that, with time, have changed the description of the major advantages and "natural" functions attributed to the drug.

In this chapter we briefly discuss the chemical GHB and review some of its most common and significant effects—both enhancing and adverse—on the human organism. We then explore in some detail the predominant types of information that have been propagated on this compound and some of its most visible sources. We rely on the material presented on the Internet by "experts" Dan Duchaine, John Morgenthaler, Dan Joy, Ward Dean, and Steven Fowkes. Concurrently we describe the saga of GHB information on the Internet and the typical content of the advertising sites. This discussion illustrates the reality of the ways in which the Internet is used as a source of information—reliable or not—for those interested in such drugs as GHB, whether for performance enhancement or for other purposes.

The Chemical

Gamma-hydroxybutyrate is a natural constituent of the mammalian brain, where hippocampal receptors can be isolated [1], and is also found in non-neuronal tissues, particularly skeletal muscle, heart, and kidney [2], in much higher concentrations than in the brain.

In the brain, according to current medical knowledge, GHB represents a catabolite of gamma-aminobutyric acid (GABA), and it is present at about one-thousandth of the concentration of its parent compound [3]. High-affinity, specific uptake, and energy-dependent transport systems for GHB have been described in the brain, in addition to a class of high-affinity binding sites [3]. Administration of large doses of GHB to animals and humans leads to sedation, and at the highest doses, anesthesia [3]. These effects are prominent when GHB brain levels are over 100-fold the endogenous level [3].

In some animals, GHB administration also induces electroencephalographic and behavioral changes resembling those of human petit mal epilepsy [3]. Gamma-hydroxybutyric acid has been used in humans as an anesthetic adjuvant [3]. It has been reported to lower cerebral energy requirements by slowing cell metabolism and oxygen consumption. Because of this effect it may play a neuroprotective role [3]. However, this effect has not been replicated in animal studies [4]. Administered GHB profoundly affects the cerebral dopaminergic system by a mechanism that remains to be unraveled. It interferes with dopamine transmission by significantly increasing dopamine output [5]. An increase in dopamine output probably plays a significant role in the rewarding response from morphine and alcohol; and, indeed, GHB can suppress opiate and alcohol withdrawal syndromes [6, 7] that are characterized by severe inhibition of dopamine output.

Gamma-hydroxybutyric acid was first synthetically produced by the French surgeon Henry Laborit in 1961 by substitution of a hydroxy group for the amino group present in GABA [8]. Such substitution allows the product to cross the blood-brain barrier, which is largely impermeable to GABA. Laborit had long been interested in anesthetic agents; a decade earlier, in 1951, he had conducted the first human experiments with chlorpromazine as a sedative agent on surgical patients. His observations eventually engendered the systematic use of chlorpromazine (Largactil, Thorazine) in psychiatric patients.

GHB had therefore been tried through the years as an anesthetic induction agent; it is no longer used in this way, however, partly because autonomic responses, such as cardiovascular activation, reflex muscle action, and vocalization [9], continue to be present during anesthetic coma and partly because of the high incidence of myoclonic seizures and vomiting [10].

As mentioned earlier, GHB may also facilitate the release of GH by promoting the slow-wave sleep pattern during which GH release is normally at its peak [11, 12]. This function represented its main original attraction for athletes and bodybuilders.

In Europe GHB is still used occasionally for the treatment of alcohol and opiate dependence as well as narcolepsy. Its sleep-inducing and euphoric effects have also been investigated in the management of fibromyalgia patients [13].

Past and Present Availability

In the past, synthetic forms of GHB were available in health stores as a dietary adjunct and as a sleep inducer and were heavily marketed among athletes as a GH releaser. After a series of acute poisonings, the Food and Drug Administration banned its nonprescription use in November 1990 [14]. Foreign-made GHB could still be found in the underground market, although legislation abroad is also increasingly outlawing it.

The most common type of GHB presently available to users is not even an illegal commercial import but largely homemade. This has been particularly true since February 2000, when GHB became a Schedule I controlled substance [15]. An old recipe for producing GHB at home can be found in "Underground Steroid Handbook for Men and Women, Update 1992" (on p. 15), under the heading "GHB: a home brew" [16]. The author, Dan Duchaine (who advertised himself as the "steroids guru"), gives complete instructions on "how to make GHB in your own kitchen."

The "do-it-yourself" approach has recently been discouraged by some GHB promoters, as the dangers of the substance became more apparent and better documented. John Morgenthaler [14] raised caution about buying bootleg GHB because "there is a lot of bad stuff out there." But he added, "The research for this book, however, has produced no clear cases of adverse effects

attributable to impurities in 'street' GHB." Duchaine, however, continued to advertise how safe it is to home-brew GHB. He also states that "overall, GHB has virtually no toxicity" (Dan Duchaine Q & A on steroids, September 16, 2000, **www.geocities.com/Colosseum/Arena/3322/ZDUCHAINE.HTM**). This is an interesting statement, in view of the impressive data sets to the contrary and in view of his own caveats in the earlier booklet. Finally, five descriptions of how to synthesize GHB, including a "Kitchen Optimized GHB Synthesis" and the link to a kit manufacturer, can be found on the Lycaeum Web site [17].

The Risks and Effects Associated With Gamma-Hydroxybutyric Acid Consumption

Gamma-hydroxybutyric acid was heavily marketed among athletes and bodybuilders because in large doses it produces a significant increase in the release of GH, possibly by activation of a muscarinic cholinergic pathway [18]. However, its effect on the GH is negligible, by admission of its most long-standing supporters [19]. There is no study confirming an anabolic or bodybuilding effect from the drug [20]. Complications from the use of illicit types of GHB emerged initially in California [21]. Use of the drug then expanded to the eastern United States, probably supported by its capacity to give a "high" effect that may represent the major factor in its high potential for abuse. Indeed, GHB is also known as "natural Quaalude" [16] or "Fantasy" or "Grievous Bodily Harm" because of its profound effects on mood and behavior, and it has recently been described as a "prosexual" agent [19] and as a "natural mood enhancer" [22].

Most typically, after ingestion (and depending on the dosing), subjects move from euphoria to experiencing the potent sedative effects of the drug: the same effects that had initially supported its investigation as an anesthetic agent. The reported effects include the following:

Euphoria	Confusion
Seizures	Dizziness
Drowsiness	Unconsciousness/coma
Stiffening of muscles	Agitation
Nausea	Respiratory depression
Disorientation	Hallucinations
Increased confidence	Respiratory arrest/death

It also appears that there is a fine line between the amount required to enhance mood and that which leads to coma [23]. The fact that dosing is at best approximate significantly increases the risk for overdosing. Furthermore, the concomitant use of other central nervous system (CNS) depressants, such as alcohol, augments the intensity of the individual's response to GHB. This combination makes its use particularly dangerous among the dance club crowds, who currently represent the largest group of users. (The FDA has reported over 65 deaths correlated with the use of GHB alone or in combination with other CNS depressants.)

The capacity for the drug to cause disorientation, heightened sensory receptivity, sexual disinhibition, and rapid profound sleep have also made it a drug of choice for sexual predators. This use has reportedly been associated with the death of several young women and eventuated in the Date-Rape Drug Prohibition Act of 2000 signed by President Clinton in February 2000 [15]. This law (HR 2130) makes GHB a Schedule I controlled substance in the same class as heroin, LSD, and cannabis.

A withdrawal syndrome has also been described, implying the development of physical dependence. The syndrome consists of insomnia, anxiety, and tremors that may last for several days [24]. In a case that we reported in the literature concerning a 46-year-old bodybuilder [25], we also observed—in a drug-free, controlled hospital setting—a progressive increase in paranoia with active hallucinations and significant amnesia that lasted for five days after admission.

Clearly, the range of possible adverse reactions to the use of GHB is quite significant. These may include sudden loss of consciousness as in the cases reported by Morgenthaler [14], in which the subjects collapsed and were rushed to an emergency room. (Morgenthaler does not see the reason in these cases for an emergency room visit because of the allegedly benign course of the state of unconsciousness. Other experts have a different opinion on the issue: Li and colleagues recommend a complex management for acute GHB intoxication, addressing the substance's potential for severe morbidity [23].) Some subjects may need to spend a few days in a psychiatric ward, experiencing memory gaps and scary hallucinations [25]. Others may wake up in the process of being raped, as reported by the women who testified against a San Francisco businessman [26]. At times, however, the amnesia that accompanies the quasi-anesthetic level of sleep is such that the subject may not be able to recall the abuse, as was the case with several victims of a disc jockey who was sentenced eventually to 77 years in prison [26] for using GHB as a date-rape drug. Or the subjects may end up in coma and on a respirator, as evidenced by the media-reported cases of a 16-year-old and his friends [26]. Lastly, the victim may die, as in the cases of H. Farias and 15-year-old Samantha Reid, two of the more than 65 deaths attributed to GHB, whose names we include here because they appear in law HR 2130 [15]. Many of these cases may have been athletes convinced to try the drug because of its alleged muscle-enhancing effects [25].

The Public Information Problem

The pattern of misinformation about GHB is a very instructive one, because its path intersected with the growth of the Internet as a media tool and as a marketplace. A close look at the issue raises important questions and may contribute to increased awareness about the use and misuse of the electronic information system.

The oldest documented source of information about GHB that the authors were able to examine is the booklet "Underground Steroid Handbook for Men and Women, Update 1992" by Dan Duchaine, mentioned earlier [16]. This booklet surfaced after the FDA removed GHB from the shelves in 1990. Before then, GHB had been "available over the counter in health food stores, purchased largely by body builders for its ability to aid with fat reduction and muscle-building" [19]. Then, in November of 1990, the FDA banned over-the-counter use of GHB. And in 1992, cases of acute poisoning from GHB were reported in California [21].

Duchaine admitted that one could "get in trouble with GHB." He adds, "Taking too much GHB will result in vomiting, and sometimes in an extremely long sleep (over 12 hours) that you may not be easily wakened from. Oh, and by the way, during this long sleep you may lose control of your bowels and bladder" [16]. However, on his Web page he stated, "And overall, GHB has virtually no toxicity. . . . GHB is a (mostly benign) recreational drug. Those who claim otherwise are just in denial." This type of misinformation is repeated and amplified in other advertisements posted on several Web pages. Even *after* law HR 2130 of February 2000, large Web sites pro-claimed the innocuous characteristics of the product and vested its dangerousness with a series of reframed statements that would lull the nonexpert into a false sense of security about the relative safety of the chemical.

We explored three sites. Of these, we last opened the following site on April 24, 2000 (**http://freehosting2. at.webjump.com/234ba769f/gh/ghb-webjump/ whatis.htm**). It guided us to the Lycaeum drug archive mentioned previously and to the writings of Morgenthaler and Joy. In addition, we explored the site by Dan Duchaine mentioned earlier and the CERI (Cognitive Enhancement Research Institute) site.

It is important to recall that this information was still offered on the Internet at least two months after the signing of law HR 2130. By then a significant amount of clinical data had surfaced pointing to the considerable risks associated with the recreational use of this agent.

Returning to the above Web site, the text mentions "medical reasons" in a statement antithetic to the definition of a Schedule I controlled substance. The statement "GHB is non-toxic" completely disregards information from the clinical reports that have accumulated since the drug received closer attention, including information about acute hospitalizations, rapes, and deaths.

In the first "Recommended Reading" (**Lycaeum.org**), Morgenthaler and Joy discuss in detail the safety of the product [14]. To a casual reader the quantity of scientific references quoted to support the safety and efficacy of GHB may appear quite robust. However, none of the articles cited is more recent than 1980. The two most frequently cited references, in this document as well as in similar ones, are the papers by Laborit (who, being the discoverer of the compound, probably had some investment in it) published in 1964 [8] and 1972 [27]. The often quoted paper by Vickers on the anesthetic safety is from 1969 [9]. Many products were described as benign when initially introduced in the medical pharmacopoeia but proved later to be fraught with risks. Cocaine, LSD, and thalidomide are some egregious examples, but the list is quite long.

The most alarming aspect of this document is the minimization of danger and the reframing of recognized side effects. The myoclonic seizures [24] become "muscle spasms or uncontrollable twitching"; the anesthetic coma is "better described as unarousability or deep sedation." Commenting on the sudden falling asleep, the authors find humor in such a response (ignoring the subjects who proceeded to respiratory depression and the women who woke up raped). And the prosexual comments *emphasize* disinhibition as *particularly* marked among women.

Although the initial emphasis in marketing GHB was on its alleged capacity to enhance GH production and muscle building, the real push has centered on its mood-altering and "prosexual" effects. In their book *Better Sex Through Chemistry: A Guide to the New Prosexual Drugs and Nutrients* [19], Morgenthaler and Joy express great enthusiasm for the aphrodisiac effects of GHB.

Nowhere in the Web-available material from their book could we find any serious attention to the possible use of the drug for sexual exploitation of women. This lack of concern is best documented in another Web document, "Dumb on Drugs," linked to the Lycaeum drug archive. The unsigned article in the putative newsletter "Narcolepsy" criticizes the Rape Treatment Center of the Santa Monica-UCLA Medical Center for a brochure warning women against GHB. The article continues [28]:

"We suggest that this information is likely to encourage misuse of GHB. It is an advertising brochure, a shopping list which, in effect, if not intent, encourages potential rapists to try GHB."

The anonymous author does not refute the list of adverse reactions described in the brochure but blames the center for distributing such information. In fact, the Web sites to which "Narcolepsy" was linked offered a detailed "advertising brochure, a shopping list" of the aphrodisiac, disinhibiting, and hypnotic effects of the drug. In our opinion there is a great need to educate the public on the heightened vulnerability of women to this compound. The newest victims may well be young women athletes, who may be offered GHB under the pretext of improving their fitness.

Concluding Remarks: Legal and Ethical Considerations

In summary, a review of the medical usefulness of GHB revealed limited support for the early claims. The highly publicized bodybuilding effect of GHB has proven to be fictitious. Even Duchaine and Morgenthaler admit that the effect is transient if actually present at all [16, 19]. The anesthetic use has been practically abandoned [12]. The literature supporting the effect of GHB in the treatment of alcohol and opioid withdrawal is limited. This can be partly a reflection of the magnification of adverse effects that accompany mixing GHB with ethanol and/or opioids. The likelihood for relapse in addiction is high, particularly during the early phases of recovery. Therefore, the risk from combined use of GHB and alcohol or opioids is quite significant.

The profile of GHB is consistent with its present classification: GHB is now a federal Schedule I controlled substance in the United States. A Schedule I controlled substance is defined as a drug with high potential for abuse and without any currently accepted medical use. Gamma-hydroxybutyric acid is also a controlled substance in several other countries, including Australia, Canada, and Sweden [15].

In response to the vocal defenders and advertisers of GHB (such as Duchaine; Dean; Morgenthaler; Joy; and Fowkes, executive director of the Cognitive Enhancement Research Institute), we do understand that we should be cautious about the legal mandates of government structures and about the economic power behind the scientific facade of pharmaceutical companies [29]. However, the disagreement with specific laws should be expressed in ways different from the ones illustrated in the material we have reviewed. The serious misinformation and the exploitation of the public that characterize the content of these sites have to be condemned.

The characteristics that continue to elicit sustained interest in GHB are the disinhibiting prosexual (aphrodisiac) effects and the mood-enhancing (or mood altering) effects. In other words, GHB's only use is as a recreational drug, one rich in abuse potential, withdrawal phenomena, and serious toxicity.

In our opinion, since the Web has established itself as a very effective marketplace, sellers and buyers alike should be treated no differently from those who operate outside of the virtual market. The person who sells GHB in the Web marketplace is legally as much a drug dealer as the person who conducts the same business on street corners. Legally there is no difference between selling GHB and selling heroin. The transactions on the Web are real, and therefore the legal consequences should be equally real.

We insist on this point because the history of GHB indicates the significant risk implicit in the mass availability of the Web as a place for commerce. Such massive advertisement of GHB as a performance-enhancing, prosexual, disinhibitory, mood-expanding agent (compounded by gross misinformation) endangers the health of athletes and others and offers encouragement and reassurance to thousands of "potential rapists" [28].

References

1. Mandel P, Maitre M, Vayer P, et al. Function of gammahydroxybutyrate: A putative neurotransmitter. J Biochem Soc Transact 15: 215-217, 1987.

2. Kaufman E, Nelson T, Goochee C, et al. Purification and characterization of an NADP-linked alcohol oxido-reductase which catalyzes the interconversion of gammahydroxybutyrate and succinic semialdehyde. J Neurochem 32: 699-712, 1979.

3. Cash CD. Gamma-hydroxybutyrate: An overview of the pros and cons for it being a neurotransmitter and/or a useful therapeutic agent. Neurosci Behav Rev 18(2): 291-304, 1994.

4. Baumann KW, Kassell NF, Olin J, Yamada T. The effects of gammahydroxybutyric acid on canine cerebral blood flow and metabolism. J Neurosurg 57(2): 197-202, August 1982.

5. Gessa GL, Crabat F, Vargiu L, et al. Selective increase of brain dopamine induced by gamma-hydroxybutyrate: Study of the mechanism of action. J Neurochem 15: 377-381, 1968.

6. Galimberti L, Gentile N, Cibin M, Fadda F, Canton G, Ferri M, Ferrara SD, Gessa GL. Gamma-hydroxybutyric acid for treatment of alcohol withdrawal syndrome. Lancet: 787-789, 30 September 1989.

7. Galimberti L, Cibin M, Pagnin P, et al. Gamma-hydrobutyric acid for treatment of opiate withdrawal syndrome. Neuropsychopharmacology 9: 77-81, 1993.

8. Laborit H. Sodium-4-hydroxybutyrate. Int J Neuropharmacol 3: 433-452, 1964.

9. Vickers MD. Gamma-hydroxybutyric acid. Int Anesthes Clin 7: 75-89, 1969.

10. Kam PC, Yoong FF. Gamma-hydroxybutyric acid: An emerging recreational drug. Anaesthesia 53(12): 1195-1198, 1998.

11. Takahara J, Yunoki S, Yakushijiw, et al. Stimulatory effects of gamma-hydroxybutyric acid on growth hormone and prolactin release in humans. J Clin Endocrinol Metab 44: 1014-1016, 1977.

12. Lapierre O, Montplaisir J, Lamarre M, et al. The effect of gammahydroxybutyrate on nocturnal and diurnal sleep of normal subjects: Further considerations on REM sleep-triggering mechanisms. Sleep 12: 24-40, 1990.

13. Scharf MB, Hauck M, Stover R, McDannold M, Berkowitz D. Effect of Gamma-hydroxybutyrate on pain, fatigue, and the alfa sleep anomaly in patients with fibromyalgia. J Rheumatol 25(10): 1986-1990, 1998.

14. Morgenthaler J, Joy D. GHB (gamma-hydroxybutyrate)—Frequently Asked Questions. **www.lycaeum.org/drugs/GHB/ghbfaq.html**. Accessed September 2000.

15. GHB legal status by Erowid. **www.erowid.org/chemical/ghb_law.shtml**.

16. Duchaine D. Underground steroid handbook (II) update. Marina Del Rey, CA: Power Distributors, 1992.

17. **http://www.lycaeum.org/drugs/GHB/ghbfaq.html**.

18. Volpi R, Chiodera P, Caffarra P, Scaglioni A, Malvezzi L, Saginario A, Coiro V. Muscarinic cholinergic mediation of Gh response to gamma-hydroxybutyric acid: Neuro-endocrine evidence in normal and parkinsonian subjects. Psychoneuroendocrinology 25(2): 179-185, 2000.

19. Morgenthaler J, Joy D. Better sex through chemistry: A guide to the new prosexual drugs and nutrients. Petaluma, CA: Smart, 1995.

20. In defense against GHB. By a team of physicians and pharmacists at the University of Florida. **www.lycaeum.org/drug/GHB/okun.html**.

21. Chin M, Kreutzer RA, Dyer JE. Acute poisoning from gamma-hydrobutyrate in California. West J Med 156: 380-384, 1992.

22. Dean W, Morgenthaler J, Fowkes SW. GHB: The natural mood enhancer. Petaluma, CA: Smart, 1997.

23. Li J, Stokes SA, Woeckener A. A tale of novel intoxication: A review of the effects of gamma-hydroxybutyric acid with recommendations for management. Ann Emer Med 31(6): 729-736, 1998.

24. Galloway GP, Frederick SL, Staggers FE Jr., Gonzales M, Stalcup SA, Smith DE. Gamma-hydroxybutyrate: An emerging drug of abuse that causes physical dependence. Addiction 92(1): 89-96, 1997.

25. Sanguineti VR, Angelo A, Frank M. GHB: A home brew. Am J Drug Alc Abuse 23(4): 637-642, 1997.

26. Ola P, D'Aulaire E. Dancing with death. Reader's Digest, June, 2000.

27. Laborit H. Correlations between protein and serotonin synthesis during various activities of the central nervous system (slow and desynchronized sleep, learning and

memory, sexual activity, morphine tolerance, aggressiveness) and pharmacological action of sodium gamma-hydroxybutyrate. Res Comm Chem Path Pharmacol 3(1), 1972.

28. Narcol Sleep Dis 2(4), 1998. As reported in **www.lycaeum.org/drugs/GHB/dumb.pdf**.

29. Valenstein ES. Blaming the brain: The truth about drugs and mental health. New York: Free Press, 1998.

26

Future and Designer Drugs: Emerging Science and Technologies

Gary I. Wadler, MD, FACP, FACSM, FACPM, FCP

The use, misuse, and abuse of drugs have long shaken the foundations of both amateur and professional sport. Competition, at its most basic level, appears to drive athletes to do whatever it takes to win. The problem is not new. Since the beginning of recorded history, athletes have sought a competitive advantage by using various substances we call ergogenic aids. Doping in sport, like the rest of technology, has grown in scientific and ethical complexity. Indeed, so complex is this issue that we cannot even agree on precisely what constitutes doping.

In 1968, the introduction of the banned substances list by the International Olympic Committee (IOC) Medical Commission was coincident with the development of new technologies in the laboratory, and this confluence set the stage for an ongoing contest between those determined to gain an unfair athletic advantage by using drugs and the forensic detectives of the laboratory. It's a struggle between the manipulators and the investigators, and each side's armaments grow more advanced each day. And as science marches on, abuse is never far behind.

British biochemist Guy C. Brown (2000) has noted that athletes' performances have steadily improved since 1900, but emphasized that humans may be soon reaching the limits of their natural physiologic potential.

> What keeps athletes from throwing farther or swimming faster? Where within the body are performance limits set? And why does performance decline when athletes become fatigued? Those questions have intrigued biologists and medical scientists ever since the secrets of anatomy and physiology began to be revealed in the seventeenth century and they have haunted athletes even longer. (p. 32)

Brown postulated that future limits to athletic performance will be determined less by innate physiology of the athlete than by technological advances and evolving judgment about where to draw the line between what is "natural" and what is artificially enhanced. This chapter explores an array of new and emerging technologies that are in the forefront of medical therapeutics, as well as their potential for abuse by athletes determined to gain an unfair athletic advantage. These technologies include gene transfer therapy, stem cell transplantation and

bioregenerative medicine, growth factors, muscle fiber phenotype transformation, red blood cell substitutes including modified hemoglobins and perfluorochemicals, and new drug delivery systems. The chapter examines the scientific underpinnings of these new and emerging technologies, as they are critical to initiatives of prevention including education and ethics, as well as to the detection of abuse. Finally, the history of doping illustrates that invariably, doping agents surface that were not anticipated; and the scientific bases for some of the more notable examples—bromantan, Actovegin, RSR 13, and hydroxyethyl starch (HES)—are discussed.

The Human Genome Project

At the start of the 20th century, a spectacular century of genetic discovery, the seminal work of the monk Gregor Mendel and his pea plants led to the first insights into heredity. Fifty years later, in 1953, Watson and Crick in the journal *Nature* elucidated the structure of DNA, the bearer of the genetic code and the chemical basis for heredity. Some 30 years have passed since the first recombinant DNA molecules were constructed at Stanford University. The techniques of altering the DNA of cells in order to change or produce biologicals have given rise to recombinant human growth hormone and also to erythropoietin, to name but two examples.

Understanding the relationship between disease and genes fascinated scientists throughout the 20th century, whether the disease be sickle cell anemia, Marfan's disease, adrenogenital syndrome, Tay-Sachs disease, adult polycystic kidney disease, or countless others. As the legendary geneticist Victor McKusick noted (1997), "In the case of many Mendelian disorders, however, the nature of the biochemical defect was a mystery until the introduction of the mapping approach to identifying the basic derangement." The first of the diseases to be linked to DNA markers was Huntington's disease. The stunning success in 1983 of mapping the Huntington's disease gene (chromosome four), together with the advances and the ingenuity involved in mapping and sequencing technology, ultimately led the scientific community to call for an organized, systematic effort to map and sequence the entire human genome.

In response, the $3 billion U.S. Human Genome Project was launched in 1990 by the U.S. Department of Energy and the National Institutes of Health (NIH) with the assistance of other countries, including England, France, Germany, Japan, China, and Canada. The objectives were to

- identify all of the approximately 50,000 genes in human DNA;

- determine the sequences of the 3 to 4 billion chemical bases that make up human DNA;

- store this information in databases;

- develop faster, more efficient sequencing technologies;

- develop tools for data analysis;

- address the ethical, legal, and social issues that may arise from the project; and

- compare the human genome to other genomes.

The project was so complex that it literally required millions of times the computing power needed to land a man on the moon. The stunning success of the project at the dawn of the new millennium has the potential for ushering in unimagined new knowledge and technologies that will forever change the diagnostic, therapeutic, and preventive landscapes but also will present challenges to the sport community that heretofore were inconceivable.

A genome is the entire complement of DNA within an organism. Genes are the ordered string of DNA nucleotides that are inherited from one's parents. Human DNA, a double-stranded helix composed of nucleotides, carries the instructions for making every cell in the body including its proteins. Nucleotides are composed of a nitrogen base (either a purine or a pyrimidine), a five-carbon sugar (deoxyribose), and a phosphate group. DNA nucleotides contain two purine bases, adenine (A) and guanine (G); and two pyrimidine bases, thymine (T) and cytosine (C). Adenine on one strand of DNA always binds with thymine on the other strand, and similarly, guanine always binds with cytosine. The order of these bases (A,G,T,C) underlies all of life's diversity and is responsible for the development of a human being from a single cell to an adult. It has been estimated that there are between 3 and 4 billion base pairs in the DNA of the human cell. Astonishingly, in 2000 and 2001, the Human Genome Project laboratories uploaded nearly 20 million bases of the human genetic sequence every night.

On June 26, 2000, the Human Genome Project announced to the world the completion of a working draft reference DNA sequence of the human genome, providing a virtual road map to an estimated 95% of all genes. Recognizing the enormous potential of this new information, President Clinton and Prime Minister Blair proclaimed: "To realize the full promise of this research, raw, fundamental data on the human genome, including the human DNA sequence and its variations, should be made freely available to scientists everywhere."

By February 2001, the publicly funded Anglo-U.S. Human Genome Project and the privately funded Maryland-based Celera Genomics Corporation—the two separate organizations involved with the first analyses of the human gene set—published an array of historical genome breakthroughs in *Nature* and *Science,* respectively. Among the numerous observations was the surprise that humans possess only approximately 30,000 to 35,000 genes—far fewer than the 100,000 previously thought—and only twice as many genes as a worm or a fruit fly. Despite seeming so different from one another, humans are 99.9% genetically identical, though men are twice as likely as women to produce mutations and to subsequently pass them on.

When a gene is isolated, understanding precisely how it works and how sequencing errors can result in a disease may take considerable time. There are thousands of genes that are believed to be directly or indirectly related to the development of human diseases. By the end of 2001, the project was expected to have discovered and catalogued the exact location of more than 1 million genetic markers called single nucleotide polymorphisms (SNPs). These SNPs are places where the genomes of individuals differ by a single genetic letter. Although there may be as many as 10 million such SNPs, the overwhelming majority may do nothing. Analyzing SNPs is not only invaluable from a medical perspective; it will be of great value in shoring up our knowledge of evolution.

Although it was long thought that each gene within the 23 pairs of chromosomes directed the production of a single protein product, that has been known not to be the case for many years. A closer look at gene structure provides some insight into why. Human genes are divided into various segments, and these segments are used in different combinations to make different proteins. The protein-coding segments of DNA are known as exons, and the noncoding segments in between the exons are known as introns. Up to 97% of the noncoding DNA has a largely unknown function and has been referred to as "junk" DNA. While the role of junk DNA is not entirely clear and this DNA may be found to have some message function, it does represent substantial clues to our evolutionary past.

For human cells to make proteins, information from the DNA has to be abstracted from the cell's nucleus. The DNA's exons and the introns, in a copying process known as transcription, are transcribed onto an RNA molecule referred to as messenger RNA (mRNA). However, in a process called alternative splicing, introns are stripped out of the mRNA as the cell produces a mature mRNA. This process of alternative splicing enables exons to be joined together to form specific mRNAs that give rise to specific proteins. For reasons that remain unclear, perhaps related to signals being sent from the introns, certain exons may be skipped and consequently different proteins may be produced. This process enables many proteins to be derived from a single gene.

Once mRNA is formed, it leaves the nucleus into the cytoplasm where it binds with a cell component called a ribosome. Within the ribosome, a protein is assembled by the successive formation of peptide bonds between amino acids that are brought into proper position by transfer RNA (tRNA), cytoplasmic molecules that recognize the base sequence of the mRNA. In effect, the tRNA is an agent of mRNA, reading its code and then bringing amino acids into place one at a time, a process called translation that has been likened to stringing a necklace one bead at a time. Thus, the actual protein factory is within the cell's ribosome. The human body is composed of 100 trillion cells.

Paralleling the strategies that have been utilized to understand DNA (the genome), efforts are under way to better understand the enormous number of proteins produced by a particular genome (proteome), including characterizing their three-dimensional structures, quantity, post-translational modifications, and interactions (proteomics). Unlike some other species, which produce 1 protein per gene, humans average between 3 and 12 proteins per gene. It has been estimated that when compared to the human genome, proteomics involves 1000 times more data. Viewed differently, it has been estimated that there are between 500,000 and one million human proteins, of which the first databases are being unveiled.

It is now believed that the approximately 30,000 human genes direct the production of these numerous proteins, including a complex network of enzymes. And while each cell contains an entire set of genes, different genes are activated in different cells, creating specific proteins, including membrane transporters—proteins that act as cellular gatekeepers, determining whether or not a drug will be taken up by a specific cell. By early 2001, Large Scale Biology Corporation was able to identify 115,963 distinct proteins from healthy tissue. Less than 1.5% of the human genome seems to code for proteins; this is about half the number people thought it would be before the genome map neared completion. And as the Human Genome Project enters its final stages, it is likely that attention will be directed toward a better understanding of the proteins to which the genes give rise. Human proteins are capable of more interactions, including those with other proteins and cellular components, and of doing more things than proteins of other species, and appear to account for much of human complexity.

Implications of the Human Genome Project

While the Human Genome Project holds promise for understanding the hereditary contribution to and molecular bases for nearly all diseases, as well as novel ways to diagnose diseases (before birth and even before conception), it has as goals the prevention of disease, the development of specifically targeted therapies, and the development of designer drugs that are free of side effects, heretofore not possible with any other approach.

In the years and decades ahead, genetic testing will identify at-risk individuals for a variety of diseases, and there is even the possibility that embryos could be selected that are free of genetic diseases. There also exists the potential to manipulate traits such as appearance, intelligence, and athletic attributes.

All this taken to its logical conclusion, the frightening possibility exists that an era of high-tech eugenics could emerge in which individuals are discriminated against because of their genetic profile and/or because of their inability to financially afford genetic enhancements. These issues raise serious ethical, legal, and social challenges, for example job discrimination, insurance discrimination, and privacy issues. So concerned was the NIH that it earmarked 3% to 5% of the Human Genome Project's budget for studies of the ethical, legal, and social implications.

While the Human Genome Project has opened horizons unimaginable just a few years back, what does genetic manipulation mean to the world of sport? The complete sequencing of the human genome will provide vast opportunities for exploring the relationships and interplay between previously unknown genes and the physiologic determinants of performance. And while Congress may have had a broad array of concerns in mind when it mandated that the Human Genome Project address the panoply of ethical, legal, and social issues associated with the project, genetic enhancement to improve athletic ability is not likely to have been in the foreground of those concerns.

Gene Transfer Therapy

The dissection of the human genetic code not only opened a Pandora's box of diagnostic tools and methods; it has significantly paved the way for an array of therapeutic interventions never conceived of before and has spawned the field of pharmacogenetics, which explores how genetic variation influences the way individuals react to medicines and other drugs. In the not-too-distant future, it is likely that drugs will be tailored to meet an individual's specific genetic profile, and methods such as somatic gene transfer therapy and stem cell transplantation will be devised so as to alter one's genetic makeup.

Gene transfer therapy has been defined as the genetic modification of a cell to produce a therapeutic effect. It entails the transferring of new DNA or an entire gene into an individual, usually with the goal of adding new genetic information to compensate for the individual's damaged or missing gene and thus of partially or completely restoring its intended function. Unlike conventional small-molecule therapeutics, gene transfer therapy requires the use of a carrier system to deliver the active agent directly into the target cell population. There are a variety of delivery systems capable of accomplishing this task. Viruses, which have the ability to gain access to cells efficiently, are the most common gene transfer therapy vectors. However, nonviral DNA delivery methods are becoming more popular for a variety of reasons—for example, plasmids are not potentially infectious agents and do not integrate into the host's genome.

For more than a decade, scientists have been developing a vast body of knowledge regarding transgenic animals. Transgenic animals have been genetically modified so as to contain a gene from a different species. The transgenic condition can be achieved through the injection of a foreign gene into a fertilized egg or into embryonic cells. The injected gene then becomes part of the host's DNA and is passed onto all the cells produced during embryonic development. It is thus present in all the cells of the resulting adult organism and is inherited by all its descendants. The transgenic condition can also be achieved through utilization of an unfertilized egg, as demonstrated by scientists at the Oregon Regional Primate Research Center in 2000. Using a retrovirus vector, they were able to produce the first genetically modified monkey by splicing a jellyfish gene, responsible for the jellyfish's green fluorescent protein, into the DNA of unfertilized monkey eggs. Following fertilization, the resulting embryos were placed in the womb of surrogate mother monkeys. One monkey who survived the process was given the name ANDi and actually contained the jellyfish genes.

There can be little question that in the future, gene transfer therapy will be used in the management of sport injuries particularly as it relates to the healing process. Various growth factors and other cytokines (proteins that enable communication between cells) have been identified as important mediators of the healing process. Although currently there are no clinically useful methods of delivery, gene transfer therapy may represent an opportunity to deliver genes to synovia, chondrocytes, tenocytes, and ligamental fibroblasts and may provide a

mechanism to specifically and aggressively target the inflammatory process.

One such cytokine is the protein, transforming growth factor (TGF)-beta, which acts to keep white blood cells from overpopulating tissue in response to inflammation. Injecting the muscles of laboratory rats with genes that encode for TGF-beta protein can reduce inflammation and laboratory-induced arthritis in the rodent's joints. In addition, gene transfer of insulin-like growth factor-1 (IGF-1) has been shown to stimulate production of proteoglycan (a component of joint cartilage) into rabbits with laboratory-induced arthritis of their knee joints, suggesting that such an approach may be possible in individuals with osteoarthritis.

About gene transfer therapy, the renowned Swedish exercise physiologist Bengt Saltin noted, "There is no doubt the medical technology is in place. Certain problems exist but they will be overcome. There are already possibilities for sportsmen." Saltin anticipates, although many in the gene transfer therapy community have a different view, that "commercial" gene transfer therapy will be available within five years.

Genes and Erythropoietin

The introduction of recombinant DNA technology in the 1970s made it possible to obtain pure preparations of a particular DNA segment. This historic breakthrough represented a new approach to therapeutic interventions. Erythropoietin is a case in point. Prior to the development of recombinant DNA technology, the treatment of refractory anemia—for example, the anemia associated with chronic renal failure—was limited to frequent blood transfusions. Sadly, it did not take very long for recombinant human erythropoietin (rhEPO) to fall into the hands of ethically challenged or amoral athletes seeking to artificially enhance their aerobic performance. Not only has this unleveled the playing field; the abuse has also been associated with an alarming number of fatalities of world-class athletes.

It has taken years for the forensic experts in doping to develop a scheme to detect rhEPO abuse. For the 2000 Sydney Olympics, two blood test models were developed by Australian researchers, an "On" model to detect very recent usage and an "Off" model to detect more remote usage. The "On" model measured an array of hematologic parameters while concurrently measuring erythropoietin levels (half-life of 18 hr) in the blood; it can be useful as an out-of-competition test. In addition to the testing of blood, a urine test for the detection of recombinant erythropoietin was developed by French investigators. However, the half-life of rhEPO in the urine is sufficiently short that detection in the urine requires it to have been injected just days prior to the urine test. For the purposes of sanctions in Sydney, a positive "On" blood test as well as a positive urine test was required in order for an athlete to be considered to have doped with erythropoietin. There were no such combined positives at the Games. The "Off" model was not utilized for the purpose of sanctions at the Sydney Olympic Games. Since the desired effect of rhEPO—increased hematocrit—lasts long after the injection, it is likely that athletes learned when to stop rhEPO so as to obtain aerobic enhancement (effective half-life of 14 days) while escaping detection. To date, there has been no opportunity to subject these various testing protocols to the inevitable legal challenges.

Gene transfer therapy likely portends a whole new use and abuse dynamic for erythropoietin, as it is one of the first genes for which a delivery system is being developed. In fact, stable long-term gene expression resulting in sustained increases in circulating red blood cells has been demonstrated in mouse and monkey studies, using techniques akin to those approved for clinical studies for diseases such as hemophilia.

Turning on and off genes is an essential component of gene transfer therapy. Public companies such as Valentis, Inc. have developed a proprietary technology named GeneSwitch that "provides precise control over the level and duration of gene expression when introduced via gene therapy." For example, genes may be turned on or induced by the administration of a pill that in turn determines the level of the therapeutic protein expressed. Similarly, the gene regulation system includes the ability to completely turn off the expression of potent therapeutic genes. This technology is applicable to both viral and plasmid-based gene transfer therapy.

Following the administration of a therapeutic gene into a muscle, for example, a transmembrane electric field pulse to induce microscopic pores in a membrane can be applied to the injection site. This process, called electroporation, is a way of delivering drugs, genetic material (e.g., DNA), or other molecules into cells. The process increases the uptake of a specific gene by the muscle cells and increases protein production by more than 100-fold. By then incorporating a GeneSwitch, one can turn gene expression on by administering an oral bioavailable drug in a dose-dependent fashion.

Using mice, Valentis, Inc. researchers were able to administer plasmids encoding erythropoietin together with a GeneSwitch. Upon oral administration of a small-molecule inducer (mifepristone), a dose-dependent increase in erythropoietin was detected in the blood with a concomitant increase in hematocrit levels. Clinical testing of this specific delivery system is anticipated in 2001.

But this is not the only approach being investigated to address the erythropoietin requirements of patients with chronic anemia. As discussed later in this chapter, new drug delivery systems are being developed to release precise amounts of drugs such as erythropoietin over time. For example, Switzerland's Modex Therapeutics is employing encapsulated cell technology to develop implantable microbioreactors containing encapsulated genetically engineered human fibroblasts that are protected from detection by the host's immune system and that deliver a continuous supply of the therapeutic protein, erythropoietin, over an extended duration. The surgical procedure to insert the product subcutaneously takes less than 10 min. This technology provides a continuous low dose of protein, eliminating the need for frequent injections as is the case with rhEPO.

While such technologies represent major advances in medicine's ever growing therapeutic armamentarium, their potential for abuse by athletes is evident and presents complex new challenges for doping laboratories. Whether as a result of gene transfer therapy or the implanting of encapsulated human cells, the goal is to avoid surges in erythropoietin levels in blood and urine. Erythropoietin produced as a result of these technologies will no longer be "foreign." It will be erythropoietin manufactured within the athlete's own body. This will, for example, invalidate the basis for the urine test for erythropoietin that is predicated on the difference between glycosylation of rhEPO and glycosylation of naturally occurring erythropoietin. In fact, the entire pharmacokinetic and pharmacodynamic profiles of these erythropoietin delivery systems may be entirely different from that associated with rhEPO injected three times per week, as is currently the clinical practice.

Muscle and Growth Factors

Understanding human muscle, its structure and function, has long intrigued scientists—physiologists, anatomists, biochemists, pharmacologists, and more recently, geneticists. Human muscles, like nerve cells, do not replicate throughout life. Accordingly, the human body is endowed with the capacities to induce local muscle repair and to prevent cell death. Skeletal muscle fibers do not have the ability to divide or to form complete new fibers. With age, muscle fibers die, never to be replaced by new ones.

Whether the individual is young or old, muscle bulk can be increased only through the hypertrophy of existing individual fibers that result from the creation of new myofibrils. Myofibrils, the smallest functional unit of muscle, are composed of repeating units of thin (actin, troponin, tropomyosin) and thick (myosin) protein filaments. These very fine contractile fibers extend in parallel along the entire length of the muscle fibers. The interaction between actin and myosin is responsible for the contraction of muscle.

Stress on muscle, for example resistive exercise, triggers signaling proteins to activate genes that cause an increase in muscle bulk (increased myofibrils) by augmenting the production of the contractile proteins, actin and myosin. Like muscle itself, muscle nuclei are incapable of replicating themselves in order to make more myofibrils. To meet the demand for more nuclei to produce more myofibrils, satellite cells—which normally lie dormant adjacent to muscle fibers until some stress or microinjury activates them—replicate and produce more protein and thus more myofibrils. Some of these satellite nuclei become indistinguishable from the muscle cell's nuclei while others remain as satellite cells on the surface of the muscle fiber.

Muscle fibers are basically of two types, slow-twitch and fast-twitch, with the heavy chain myosin determining the functional characteristics of the muscle. The three isoforms of the myosin and the fibers that contain them are known as type I, type IIa, and type IIx. The contractile velocity of a type I fiber is about one-tenth that of a type IIx fiber, with type IIa somewhere in between. The fatigability of these fiber types appears to be inversely related to their contraction times.

Type I slow-twitch fibers tend to have long twitch times and low peak forces and to be highly resistant to fatigue. These fibers are high in oxidative enzymes, but low in glycolytic and adenosinetriphosphatase (ATPase) activity. Type IIa fibers also tend to be fatigue resistant, maintaining their force production even after a large number of contractions. They tend to be high in both oxidative and glycolytic enzymes as well as ATPase activity. The last fiber type, IIx, tends to be the fastest but the most fatigable. Type IIx fibers are high in glycolytic enzyme content and ATPase activity but low in oxidative enzymes. In addition to these fiber types, there are hybrid fibers whose behavior is most like that of the fiber's dominant myosin.

The dominant fiber type, whether I or II, varies from individual to individual; but in general, most individuals have approximately equal amounts of type I and type II fibers. As would be expected, individuals with a preponderance of type I fibers are more likely to excel in endurance events, and individuals with a preponderance of fast-twitch fibers are more likely to excel in short-duration, explosive events.

There has been continuing intense interest in the ability of muscle fibers to convert from slow-twitch to fast-twitch and vice versa. Weight training demonstrates some of the dynamics involved in the distribution of fiber types within an exercised muscle. Specifically, weight training diminishes the number of the fastest (IIx) fibers, converting them to IIa fibers as a consequence of the nuclei in the affected fibers stopping their expression of the IIx gene and replacing it with expression of the IIa gene.

Within the course of one month of weight training, essentially all the IIx fibers transform to IIa fibers, with a concomitant increase in the protein content and thickness of the muscle fibers. After weight training ceases, the type IIa fibers revert to what has been referred to as the default setting of type II fibers, namely, type IIx. However, this does not happen in a linear fashion. Rather, there is an overshoot by approximately a factor of two in the relative amount of type IIx fibers, which lasts for months— a phenomenon that could be advantageous to sprinters if properly timed to coincide with competition.

In addition to increasing the number of IIa fibers from the conversion of IIx fibers into IIa fibers, the number of IIa fibers can also be increased through the conversion of type I fibers into type IIa fibers. Consequently, vigorous weight training combined with other forms of anaerobic exercise converts both type I and type IIx fibers to type IIa fibers, increasing the cross-sectional area of type II fibers twice as much as that of type I fibers.

Given the fact that fiber type and its myosin have a genetic foundation, it follows that the conversion of one fiber type to another, or of one myosin isoform to another, is quite likely to be accomplished by genetic manipulation in the not-too-distant future.

In this regard, a biochemical signaling mechanism has been elucidated that controls muscle fiber gene expression (i.e., the contractile properties of the muscle fiber). Three proteins—calcineurin, NFAT (nuclear factor of activated T cells), and MEF2 (myocyte enhancer factor 2)—participate in a pathway that activates a specific set of genes controlling the abundance of proteins found in type I fibers. It has been established that as a consequence of more frequent motor neuron stimulation (e.g., regular jogging), slow fibers maintain higher levels of intracellular free calcium than fast fibers. When calcium levels remain too high in the muscle cell's cytoplasm, calcineurin is turned on. This in turn causes NFAT to move into the cell's nucleus, where it partners with MEF2 and other proteins to turn on or up-regulate genes specific for type I slow-oxidative fibers. Conversely, inhibition of calcineurin activity by administration of cyclosporin A to intact animals inhibits slow fiber gene expression. In transgenic mice (mice containing a gene from a different species) that expressed activated calcineurin, researchers demonstrated an increase in type I fibers but without evidence of skeletal muscle hypertrophy.

In yet another example of muscle fiber manipulation, Professor Bengt Saltin has noted that the removal, modification, and subsequent reinsertion of a gene can increase the strength of a fly's flight muscles by as much as 300%.

Genes and Growth Factors

There exists a link between mechanical stimulation of various cells of the body and gene expression. As noted previously, skeletal muscle is responsive to changes in functional demands; for example, hypertrophy results from pronounced overloading. During periods of increased loading, myofibers up-regulate the expression and secretion of the growth factor IGF-1 (insulin-like growth factor-1). Growth factors are proteins that bind to receptors on the cell surface, activating cellular proliferation and/or differentiation.

Virtually every tissue type is capable of the autocrine production of insulin-like growth factors. Since, as with neuronal cells, muscle cells do not replicate during life, a mechanism exists to induce local repair and to prevent muscle cell death (apoptosis); and IGF-1 appears to be integral to those mechanisms.

Goldspink has helped elucidate two *local* growth factors involved in the determination of muscle mass, L.IGF-1 and MGF (mechano growth factor). Though produced locally in muscle, L.IGF-1 is similar to liver-type IGF-1 and contributes significantly to the level of circulating IGF-1 when muscle is exercised. The actions of MGF, on the other hand, appear to be quite local, and MGF does not enter the circulation. Mechano growth factor appears to serve a dual function, muscle repair in response to injury and muscle hypertrophy in response to overload.

It appears that IGF-1-induced muscle hypertrophy results from a combination of satellite cell activation and proliferation, as well as increased protein synthesis (actin and myosin) in differentiated myofibers. As previously noted, the up-regulation of genes consequent to muscle stretching and overload alters the muscle fiber's isoform (myosin), and thus its phenotype.

Barton-Davis et al., utilizing viral-mediated gene transfer of IGF-1 (MGF) injected directly into mouse muscle, demonstrated a 15% increase in the mass and a 14% increase in strength of the injected muscle in young adult mice. This method also prevented age-related muscle loss and resulted in a 27% increase in strength as compared with that in uninjected old muscles. Mechano growth factor is significantly more potent and rapid acting than liver-type IGF-1 in effecting an increase in muscle mass.

These observations have enormous therapeutic implications. For example, patients with an array of muscle-wasting diseases can hold out hope that their muscle function and strength can be restored, and that, for example, the incidence of hip fractures in elderly persons coincident with falls secondary to age-related muscle atrophy can be substantially diminished.

However, advances in understanding the interplay of gene transfer technology, growth factors, and muscle physiology raise serious concerns regarding the potential for abuse. In yet another study, IGF-1-producing genes have been successfully introduced into mouse embryos. Is it a stretch to believe that with the new technologies of genetic interventions we are arming parents with the tools to create designer offspring? The illicit systemic use of IGF-1 by elite athletes is already alleged to be a reality. In view of its newness to the marketplace, very little is known about the abuse patterns, availability, and cost, although it has been estimated that the cost on the black market is about $3000 per month. To date, there is no way to detect such abuse.

In the United Sates, IGF-1 is approved for the treatment of Larontype dwarfism and type A insulin resistance syndrome. Like human growth hormone, systemic IGF-1 may predispose an individual to acromegaly. Side effects of its systemic use include headache, adenoidal hyperplasia, jaw pain, and swelling of the hands and feet. Hypoglycemia is common and may have contributed to the death of a German weightlifter.

It should be emphasized that not all growth factors promote growth. The recent discovery of myostatin suggests that negative regulation of tissue growth may also be an important mechanism for controlling skeletal muscle mass. Myostatin, a cytokine, is a member of the TGF-beta superfamily of growth modulators thought to play a role in numerous developmental processes, including the growth and differentiation of skeletal muscle. Myostatin is a potent inhibitor of myoblast differentiation and proliferation and as such is a negative regulator or "brake" on muscle growth. Mice lacking the myostatin gene exhibit significant increases in muscle mass as a result of increased muscle fiber number and size. Similarly, the increase in muscle mass of certain breeds of cattle lacking myostatin has been attributed to marked increases in the number of muscle fibers. Transgenic mice bearing mutated myostatin have exhibited significant (20-35%) increases in muscle mass from myofiber hypertrophy. This certainly brings into play the possibility of altering human muscle size and function by genetic manipulation of myostatin function.

With the application of gene transfer technology to muscle physiology and pathology, it is only a matter of time before abuse of this technology finds its way into the world of competitive athletics. It is not too hard to imagine the day when muscles can be selectively enlarged and/or contoured and isoforms can be selected that best match some athletic objective. The marathoner can acquire a plethora of slow-twitch fibers while the sprinter amasses IIx fibers. Just imagine the consequences of a kinesiologist isolating specific muscles and selectively injecting designer genes into those muscles to maximize their function.

Stem Cells

It was only two years ago that Dr. James Thomson of the University of Wisconsin achieved one of the most coveted goals in biology, isolating from human embryos a primitive cell called a totipotent stem cell. Human totipotent stem cells have an unlimited capacity for replication and an ability to turn into virtually any cell or tissue in the body including muscle, bone, and even brain. Unlike amphibians, whose adult cells have the capacity to "dedifferentiate" into stem cells that can then regenerate into specialized tissues of many types, humans are incapable of regenerating lost organs.

It should be emphasized that not all human stem cells are the same. In addition to the totipotent stem cell, there are progenitor stem cells whose terminal-differentiated progeny consists of a single cell type, and there are multipotent stem cells that give rise to several terminally differentiated cell types constituting a specific tissue or organ. In fact, many mature organs, including the bone marrow and skin, maintain a pool of undifferentiated stem cells that are capable of self-renewal and of differentiation into at least one or more mature cell types. Recently it has been demonstrated that stem cells exist in muscle and brain. Such cells derived from brain can be cultured and transplanted into locations in recipients where they will differentiate into mature neurons. Similarly, skeletal muscle stem cells can be cultured and transplanted into recipient muscle where they will differentiate into myotubes and fuse with endogenous muscle fibers.

Another quality of stem cells that has become increasingly appreciated is their plasticity, or the ability of stem cells of one tissue type to differentiate into cells of another tissue; this raises the possibility of using stem cells from bone marrow, for example, to treat disorders of the nervous system or muscle. The most famous example of cell plasticity was demonstrated in 1997 when a sheep mammary gland cell nucleus was transferred into a sheep oocyte whose own nucleus had been removed, producing the first cloned mammal, the sheep named Dolly. Since then, other mammals have been cloned with use of similar nuclear transfer techniques. However, even Ian Wilmut, the Scottish researcher who brought Dolly into the world, warned that enormous hurdles must be overcome before cloning becomes practical. Out of some 100 attempts to clone an animal, only between 2% and 3% live offspring result. Of the animals that are born, a significant fraction die shortly after birth, while others have serious developmental abnormalities.

Human embryonic totipotent stem cells are derived from the inner cell mass of in vitro-fertilized human blastocysts. Harvesting such stem cells from the embryos has raised serious ethical concerns because retrieving them requires the destruction of the embryo. Only recently did Congress loosen laws restricting federal funds for research involving embryos. Whether or not federally financed funds are available for stem cell research, it is likely that research in the United States in this field will be privately financed. And undoubtedly, stem cell research will continue to move forward in other parts of the world. Such research holds out promise in diseases such as diabetes mellitus, Parkinson's disease, Huntington's disease, and amyotrophic lateral sclerosis. Umbilical cord blood has been identified as another source rich in stem cells, and efforts are under way to capture or harvest these totipotent stem cells before they divide and begin the process of differentiating into tissues such as skin, blood, or nerves.

Stem cell technology holds enormous promise for the future. Some potential advances include the following:

- Providing insights into normal human development and into what goes awry to cause birth defects and diseases such as cancer
- Providing a vehicle in lieu of animal models for developing and testing new drugs
- Generating cells that could be used as replacement cells and tissues to treat conditions such as spinal cord injury, neurodegenerative diseases, heart disease, and various forms of arthritis

Research efforts exploring the potential of the totipotent stem cell are extensive. For example, researchers are examining the interplay between these cells and a host of growth factors, as well as the ways in which such interplay influences the differentiation of these cells into various tissues.

While stem cell therapy and gene transfer therapy hold promise for the treatment of a variety of diseases, the combination of the two may be even more significant. As Kaji and Leiden have pointed out, "implantation of skeletal muscle stem cells that have been modified genetically with vectors that program the expression and secretion of therapeutic proteins, such as erythropoietin and growth hormone, results in the stable delivery of recombinant proteins to the systemic circulation."

From a sports medicine perspective, the potential for the legitimate use of such therapeutic approaches opens up opportunity for "bioregenerative medicine"—which uses the complex interplay between stem cells, growth factors, matrix and cell adhesion molecules, and gene transfer technologies—to construct functional tissues outside the body for implantation to augment or replace damaged tissues and organs within the body. In 2001, researchers at Duke University Medical Center reported the first steps toward creating functional cartilage, not from stem cells, but rather from fat cells derived from liposuction, and specifically from adipose-derived stromal cells.

As initial efforts of bioregenerative medicine have begun to address nervous system disorders such as stroke, Parkinson's disease, and Alzheimer's disease, disorders of tissues such as skin, bone, and muscle cannot be far behind. Already stem cells have been used to grow human heart muscle cells that beat in unison in a petri dish, as well as nerve cells, bone, cartilage and skeletal muscle. To ensure that stem cell research is conducted in an ethically sound manner, a special working group was formed at the NIH to develop research guidelines.

While technologies such as stem cell transplantation and gene transfer hold enormous promise for the future, ethicists remain rightly concerned about their abuse and about consequent genetic discrimination. Is it too far-fetched to imagine a bioengineered 8 ft 6 in. basketball player or a sprinter faster than a thoroughbred horse or a marathoner with a $\dot{V}O_2$max that is off the charts? Is it a stretch to think that with the new technologies of genetic engineering we are arming parents with the tools to create designer offspring? Further, concern has been voiced about the alteration of the genetic composition of germ cells, potentially resulting in germ line transmission of altered genes to the progeny of the treated individual and thus perpetuating designer traits from one generation to the next.

Red Blood Cell Substitutes ("Artificial Blood")

Endurance athletes have long sought to enhance the delivery of oxygen to their working muscles. Reports of blood doping in a controlled scientific setting first appeared in 1947, and by 1966 Ekblom elegantly demonstrated that blood doping indeed improved aerobic capacity. By the 1976 Olympic Games, reports began to surface suggesting that the transfusion procedures were being used by athletes as an ergogenic aid; and by 1984, U.S. cyclists admitted to blood doping for the Los Angeles Olympics. In the late 1980s, recombinant erythropoietin became available, and before long its abuse replaced blood doping. The perception persists that rhEPO is widely abused. During the 2000 Sydney Olympics, the first comprehensive tests for rhEPO abuse were introduced, but the standard for a positive was demanding, and as indicated earlier, there were no reported positives.

With the advances in the development of red blood substitutes, it is likely that athletes will similarly abuse them in the not-too-distant future provided that their use is opaque to the doping laboratory. By the late 1990s, the international cycling federation had issued warnings regarding the abuse of perfluorochemicals. To what extent these red blood substitutes will be readily detectable in blood or urine remains to be seen. Because of the relatively short half-life of these substances, their use is likely to be limited to the time of competition, as contrasted with the out-of-competition abuse of rhEPO.

The increasing demand for blood (the blood industry worldwide is estimated at $2 billion) together with a decreasing blood supply remains a concern, particularly in the developing world. It has been estimated that by the year 2030, there will be an annual shortage of 4 million units of safe blood. Research on blood substitutes began during World War II because of the need for blood to treat war casualties. However, the task was extremely difficult, and attention was soon directed at the development of cell-free oxygen delivery systems.

Normally, oxygen is transported from the lungs to other tissues bound to hemoglobin, an iron-protein compound present in intact red blood cells. In the circulation, red blood cells survive for about 120 days. They are able to withstand severe metabolic and mechanical stresses; for instance, they can deform in order to pass through capillaries with diameters half their own. These cells must also maintain an internal environment that protects the hemoglobin from oxidation and maintains optimum concentrations of 2,3-diphosphoglycerate (2,3-DPG), which is needed for proper hemoglobin function and oxygen delivery.

Normal adult red blood cells contain three forms of hemoglobin, with hemoglobin A being the predominant type. Normal hemoglobin A is a tetramer composed of two α chains and two β chains coded by four genes on chromosome 16. Each globin chain contains a small heme group with an iron atom in the center. Hemoglobin not only gives blood its red color; it transports oxygen, carbon dioxide, and nitric oxide, the latter controlling blood flow through the small blood vessels.

The search for a practical replacement for the red blood cells that would permit stable storage, provide adequate oxygen delivery, and be free of significant toxicity has been long and replete with substantial obstacles. Two major approaches that have shown promise are modified hemoglobins and perfluorochemicals.

Modified Hemoglobins

One approach for producing red blood cell substitutes is to use hemoglobin extracted from red blood cells by removing the cell membrane. However, when free hemoglobin per se is introduced into the circulation, the four-globin tetramer of hemoglobin is broken down into a two-unit dimer that not only does not transport oxygen but also is toxic to the kidneys. Additionally, once the hemoglobin is outside the cell, it no longer has the 2,3-DPG that is required for hemoglobin to readily release oxygen to the tissues. There have been two approaches to modifying hemoglobin so that it may be infused:

• **Microencapsulation of hemoglobin (artificial red blood cells).** Technologic advances, including nanotechnology, have enabled the encapsulation of intact hemoglobin molecules. Unlike normal red blood cell membranes, microencapsulated hemoglobin does not have blood group antigens on its surface and thus does not aggregate in the presence of blood group antibodies. The half-life of these lipid (liposome) membrane-encapsulated artificial cells is in the range of 50 hr as contrasted with the approximately 120 days of normal red blood cells. One advantage of this technique is that the process stabilizes the hemoglobin molecule, enabling its sterilization to eliminate the risk of HIV, hepatitis, and other infectious diseases. Recent efforts have been directed at encapsulating hemoglobin together with its protective enzymes that, for example, prevent the oxidation of hemoglobin to methemoglobin, in 0.15-micron-diameter biodegradable polylactic acid membrane nanocapsules.

- **Cross-linked hemoglobin.** Various methods have been employed to prevent the formation of dimers when free hemoglobin has been used as a red blood cell substitute. One such approach has been cross-linking, that is, connecting or linking amino acids on the surface of the hemoglobin molecule so that they do not break down into nonfunctional, toxic dimers.

One methodology, referred to as intramolecular cross-linking, prevents dimer formation by linking two α or two β chains within a given hemoglobin molecule. Another methodology, polyhemoglobin cross-linking, can link four or five hemoglobin molecules together; 2,3-DPG can then be added to the polyhemoglobin to enhance its oxygen transport function. A variation of this technique cross-links hemoglobin to polymers. Utilizing recombinant DNA technology applied to *Escherichia coli,* a variant of hemoglobin has been formed that retains its tetrameric configuration when it is introduced into the circulation. A newer version of recombinant hemoglobin blocks the nitric oxide receptor site, preventing vasoconstriction when injected into experimental animals and thereby increasing tissue perfusion. All these modifications have a greater ability to release oxygen to the tissues than do intact red blood cells. Recombinant human hemoglobin continues to be tested in clinical trials.

The half-life of recent formulations of polyhemoglobin is 25 to 30 hr, and conjugated hemoglobin lasts even longer. These durations are a function of both dose and species, but nonetheless are orders of magnitude different from the half-life of normal red blood cells. Unlike donor blood that can be refrigerated for no more than one month before being transfused, these blood substitutes can be stored for more than a year and do not require type and cross matching. Because of their short half-life, red blood cell substitutes such as polyhemoglobin are most likely to be used in the setting of acute blood loss, such

as surgery and trauma. In some clinical trials, patients have received as much as 20 units of polyhemoglobin.

Cross-linked hemoglobin is likely to be the first modified hemoglobin ready for clinical use. Clinical trials, including phase III (large-scale efficacy studies), are being conducted by a variety of commercial entities. Such products include Polyheme (human hemoglobin), Hemopure (bovine hemoglobin), and Hemolink (human hemoglobin). In mid-2000, claims were made, though not substantiated, that Hemopure was being used in the track and field community to circumvent the introduction of erythropoietin testing. In response to IOC-accredited laboratories, Biopure Corporation, manufacturer of Hemopure, made available a laboratory test to detect the presence of Hemopure in blood.

Detectable or not, all this is not without risk. For example, an unexpectedly high number of deaths among patients with trauma led to the termination of clinical trials and the withdrawal of two formulations of hemoglobin-based oxygen carriers from further development.

Perfluorochemicals

Perfluorochemicals such as perfluorocarbon (PFC) are inexpensive, synthetic, inert molecules with an enormous capacity to dissolve a variety of gases, including oxygen. They can dissolve as much as 50 times the amount of oxygen that plasma does. However, because of their oxygen-loading characteristics, individuals who use them must inspire concentrations of oxygen as high as 70% to 100%. These chemicals require refrigeration and have a short half-life. Because they are hydrophobic, they must be combined with lipids to enable them to stay in solution in the plasma. Their use has been associated with medical complications including a flulike syndrome, complement activation, cytokine release and suppression of the reticuloendothelial system, and platelet dysfunction. Newer formulations have enabled higher concentrations of PFCs to be used with diminished side effects. Presently, PFCs are not approved for clinical use in the United States.

Rumors of PFC use among athletes first surfaced in early 1998 from the Winter Olympics in Nagano, where cross-country skiers and speed skaters were alleged to have used it. That same year the International Cycling Union issued a warning to its national federations about riders using PFC emulsions. There were rumors that PFC, for example, was also being used by canoeists and was even administered to racehorses.

Drug Delivery Systems

The therapeutic efficacy of certain drugs can be dramatically influenced by the way they are delivered in the body. This has created tremendous interest in the development of innovative drug delivery systems. Historically, there has been an emphasis on maintaining a constant blood level of drugs, eliminating the peaks and troughs of drug concentrations, and for many drugs that is still the objective. Controlled-release systems first appeared in the 1960s and 1970s, and since then the number and variety of controlled-release systems have increased dramatically, enabling less frequent dosing. A more recent trend has been a move toward delivery systems that allow the release rate of a drug to be varied over time and to target the local delivery of certain drugs. Such an approach optimizes the therapeutic properties of the drug while minimizing its adverse or side effects. For other drugs, particularly those that serve as replacement drugs for deficiency states, the objective of a drug delivery system is to mirror the physiologic variations of the naturally occurring substance, for example, the polypeptide hormones. Technologies to accomplish these objectives include biodegradable and nonbiodegradable implants and implantable pump systems. Recent advances in the field of microfabrication and nanotechnology have created the possibility that tiny programmable devices with sensors will be developed that can potentially be integrated into microelectronics enabling the storage and release of drugs on demand. Such smart drug delivery systems will enable the release of exact amounts of medication to meet physiological or therapeutic demands.

Since much of doping forensics depends on the detection of elevated urine and, more recently, elevated blood levels of performance-enhancing drugs, the application of these new technologies is certain to add new confounding variables. As a result of the altered pharmacokinetics and pharmacodynamics associated with new drug delivery systems, those determined to gain unfair athletic advantage will have a window of opportunity for evading detection.

Once again, advances in our knowledge about erythropoietin therapy serve to underscore the challenges that await the doping laboratories. The recent introduction of a hyperglycosylated analog of rhEPO, novel erythropoiesis-stimulating protein (ARANESP), with increased terminal half-life enables patients being treated for anemia will need to dose only every one to two weeks as contrasted with three or more times per week as is the practice with rhEPO. But how might its availability impact the hematologic marker studies done by the Australians or the French urine test that was implemented at the Sydney Olympic Games?

The Always Unexpected and Unknown

Any list of banned drugs should be based on a generally recognized body of science, including laboratory science; and where such science does not exist, the list should be based on a clear, reasoned rationale. Typically, banned lists vary depending on the philosophy, goal, and objectives of the sport's governing body, or in the case of professional sport on the basis of the collective bargaining process. Some lists are quite long and inclusive. Others are relatively short. Then there is always the unexpected and unknown.

Bromantan

No matter what the list, it is likely that there will be drugs that are utilized by athletes that cannot be readily anticipated and therefore will escape specific enumeration on a banned list. Some have suggested that these drugs account for as many as 90% of estimated doping cases. One such drug that captured the headlines during the 1996 Atlanta Olympic Games was bromantan. During the Games, five athletes (Russians and Lithuanians), including two medalists, tested positive for this drug; and it was suspected that its use might have been fairly widespread. The Russian Olympic Committee president had indicated that the drug had been developed by the military as an immune system stimulant for its space program. The Russian literature reported that bromantan boosted the immune system, reduced the perception of fatigue, and enabled the body to better tolerate high temperatures. But the Russian literature had also clearly identified bromantan as a psychostimulant. Nonetheless, it was not specifically enumerated on the banned list.

Although the IOC sanctioned athletes in Atlanta for testing positive for bromantan under the belief that the phrase at the end of the stimulant section "and related substances" encompassed bromantan, the Court of Arbitration in Sport disagreed and lifted the sanctions. According to the IOC Anti-Doping Medical Code in place at the time, the term "related substances" referred to drugs that are related to the class by their pharmacological actions and/or chemical structure. The Court of Arbitration in Sport concluded: "The surrounding circumstances while suspicious do not form a basis for concluding, in light of the scientific evidence, that bromantan is a stimulant." However, the court also concluded, "in view of the probability that bromantan can be indeed classified as a stimulant, its use should be discontinued forthwith."

RSR 13

Hemoglobin's affinity for oxygen can be altered by pH, temperature, and high altitude so as to make oxygen more readily available to the tissues. RSR 13 is a small-molecule drug that binds to hemoglobin causing a dose-dependent, rightward shift of the oxygen dissociation curve and thereby facilitating the release of oxygen from hemoglobin to the body's tissues. The molecule mimics the body's physiologic response to hypoxia, or oxygen deprivation. However, it also significantly impairs oxygen uptake by the lungs. To compensate for this effect on oxygen pulmonary loading, when RSR 13 is used, supplemental oxygen must be administered with an inspired oxygen concentration of 30% as contrasted with the normal atmospheric 21%. RSR 13, an analog of clofibrate, is under investigation as a drug that may improve radiation therapy for cancer patients (a radiation enhancer), since effective radiation requires the presence of oxygen. Radiation excites oxygen molecules, leading to the formation of free radicals that promote cell death, and tumors often have oxygen-depressed areas causing them to be resistant to radiation. RSR 13 may also be useful in the treatment of cardiovascular disease, in bypass surgery, and in treatment of stroke where tissue oxygenation is compromised, as well as in the treatment of inoperable lung cancer. Because of its promising results, the Food and Drug Administration has granted RSR 13 fast tracking status, and it may become commercially available by 2004. It is being tested in Canada, Europe, Australia, and the Middle East.

Even though RSR 13 is years away from clinical use, reports of RSR 13 abuse were rumored in the 2001 Giro d'Italia cycling race. The manufacturer of RSR 13 (Allos Therapeutics, Denver, CO) has always been concerned that the drug's ability to enhance the delivery of oxygen to tissues, including muscle, would potentially be of interest to endurance athletes. Accordingly, Allos has worked with the IOC to deter abuse by athletes and has been working with the IOC-accredited laboratory (UCLA) to develop a urine test for RSR 13. However, even if athletes were able to obtain RSR 13, it is a very difficult drug to abuse. It must be administered intravenously in large volumes; its effects last only 4 to 6 hr; and it must be used with supplemental oxygen. Theoretically, to boost performance, an athlete would have to administer the drug immediately before a competition, and its effects would last only for a limited time. The side effects of RSR 13 include nausea, vomiting, and headaches, and it may interfere with kidney function.

Actovegin

Oxygen delivery is also a function of blood flow. In disease states such as chronic peripheral vascular disease, the inadequate delivery of oxygen to working muscle during walking is manifest by the symptom of intermittent claudication or cramping. Various agents have been utilized either to increase blood flow in disease states or to alter the tissue metabolism in response to hypoxia. In the United States, pentoxifylline (Trental) appears to lower the viscosity of the blood, thereby increasing blood flow into the microcirculation and enhancing tissue oxygenation. In other countries, a substance called Actovegin has been utilized. Actovegin, a dried, deproteinized extract of calf blood, has been reported to work on mitochondrial respiration and energy metabolism. It has been studied at least since the late 1970s and has been used in cases of chronic peripheral arterial vascular insufficiency, cerebrovascular insufficiency, and brain hypoxia. One study suggested that it exerts its effect by improving the transport and utilization of oxygen and glucose. In the 2000 Tour de France, Actovegin (manufactured by the Norwegian company Nycomed) became the center of a controversy when its use was suspected. In December 2000, the IOC became sufficiently concerned that Actovegin was being abused in cycling and placed Actovegin on its banned list. However, in early 2001, Actovegin was removed from the IOC list pending further research on whether it is actually performance enhancing or harmful to the health of athletes.

Hydroxyethyl Starch

At the 2001 Fédération Internationale de Ski (International Ski Federation) Nordic World Ski Championships, the detection of partially methylated alditol acetates— metabolites of a substance barely known to the sport community, hydroxyethyl starch (HES)—led to sanctions against a Finnish skier. The IOC Prohibited Classes of Substances and Prohibited Methods, as enumerated in appendix A of the prevailing Olympic Movement Anti-Doping Code, specifically banned in the "Prohibited Methods" section not only "artificial oxygen carriers" but also "plasma expanders." Normal saline and lactated Ringer's solution are the most commonly used volume expanders. Noncrystalloid volume expanders currently available in the United States include albumin, hydroxyethyl starch, dextrans, and purified protein fractions. While these colloid volume expanders are effective volume substitutes, they do not enhance the oxygen-carrying capacity of blood.

Volume expanders are widely used in resuscitation, intensive care, and operating room settings, in part because they are cheaper than albumin and because they present no risk of transmitting infectious diseases. The use of noncrystalloid volume expanders has been associated with coagulation abnormalities and generalized and anaphylactic reactions, including hypotension, cardiovascular collapse, and death. Use has been associated with severe skin itching. Hydroxyethyl starch is probably the best tolerated of the noncrystalloid volume expanders because it is very similar to glycogen. Hydroxyethyl starch (there are a variety of types) is synthesized from amylopectin, a waxy starch derived from maize, through attachment of hydroxyethyl groups to the starch molecule. Antibodies have been found directed not against the starch molecule but rather against the hydroxyethyl group. The main route of excretion of HES is through the kidney. Ostensibly HES has been used by athletes to dilute their blood in order to mask or obscure self-induced increases in red cell mass.

Conclusion

The number, type, and complexity of new drugs that have come to market since the introduction of doping control in the Olympic movement in 1960s are staggering. It is perhaps ironic that the very science that brings out the best in man in sport has been used to bring out the worst. With the enormous technologic strides of the past few years—the Human Genome Project, gene transfer therapy, genetic engineering, stem cell research, germ line research, cloning, "artificial blood," and new drug delivery systems—we are on the brink of a brave new world of therapeutic opportunities. But we are also left with the daunting possibility that we are about to usher in an alarming grave new world of doping. Stated differently, in the world of doping, milestones too often have become millstones.

In the game of cat and mouse of doping and doping detection, the scientists of the forensic laboratory are forever vigilant in developing new technologies to detect new drugs of abuse. However, ensuring fair play is not as simple as developing new technologies or detecting new drugs.

In Atlanta, for example, it was predicted that performance-enhancing drugs would meet their match in high-resolution mass spectrometry. Yet, it was inevitable that such expectations were to be tempered by legal considerations, as they were when a number of positive steroid cases were not prosecuted because the methodology was so new as to raise legitimate concern that the results could not withstand legal challenges. And good forensic toxicology doesn't necessarily equate with just outcomes. That's why the 1996 Atlanta Games were clouded by the "new" stimulant drug, bromantan, and why political machinations resulted in five athletes being cleared of a doping offense by the on-site Court of Arbitration in Sport.

Now, as we enter the burgeoning world of genetics, the issues become far more complex and the ethical, moral, and biological debate transcends sport. As George Wald, the Nobel Prize-winning biologist and Harvard professor, once said, "Recombinant DNA technology (genetic engineering) faces our society with problems unprecedented not only in the history of science, but of life on earth. It places in human hands the capacity to redesign living organisms, the products of some three billion years of evolution."

We stand at the brink of an uncertain future. The unpredictability and the velocity of change are not an excuse for reserving judgment about some profound distinctions that should fundamentally govern our perspective on the role of sport in our social fabric.

About this, the columnist George Will elegantly opined, "A society's recreation is charged with moral significance. Sport—and a society that takes it seriously—would be debased if it did not strictly forbid things that blur the distinction between the triumph of character and the triumph of the chemistry" (Wadler and Hainline, p. 67).

Tempting as it is to become consumed by the intricacies of anabolic steroids, erythropoietin, or human growth hormone, it is necessary to think expansively and inclusively, to keep the big picture in mind, and to maintain an aerial view, for these drugs are only specific examples that stretch along the continuum from strychnine to genetic enhancement. Only in that way will it be possible to forge a consensus—a unified, expert-wide point of view that will help put the details and the subtleties in proportion. Stay tuned.

References

Abate, T. (February 11, 2001). Genome discovery shocks scientists. *The San Francisco Chronicle.* A1.

Adams, G.R. (1998). Role of insulin-like growth factor-I in the regulation of skeletal muscle adaptation to increased loading. *Exercise and Sports Sciences Reviews.* Vol. 26, 31-60.

Andersen, J.L., Schjerling, P., and Saltin, B. (September 2000). Muscle, genes and athletic performance. *Scientific American.* 48-55.

Aoki, N. (September 15, 2000). Biopure to release test to detect drug misuse by Olympic athletes. *The Boston Globe.* C10.

Aoki, N. (September 27, 2000). Drug makers battle bad sports athletes who abuse new medicines put firms in spotlight—and on defensive. *The Boston Globe.* E1.

Aschwanden, C. (January 15, 2000). Gene cheats. *New Scientist.* 24.

Austin, M. (July 1, 2001). Scandal may aid Denver biotech. Experimental drug lands in spotlight. *The Denver Post.* Business. K-01.

Baltimore, D. (February 15, 2001). Our genome unveiled. *Nature.* Vol. 291, 814.

Barton-Davis, E.R., Shoturma, D.I., Musaro, A., Rosenthal, N., and Sweeney, H.L. (December 22, 1998). Viral-mediated expression of insulin-like growth factor I blocks the aging-related loss of skeletal muscle function. *Proceedings of the National Academy of Sciences.* Vol. 95, No. 25, 15603-15607.

Barton-Davis, E.R., Shoturma, D.I., and Sweeney, H.L. (December 1999). Contribution of satellite cells to IGF-1 induced hypertrophy of skeletal muscle. *Acta Physiologica Scandinavica.* Vol. 167, No. 4, 301-305.

Bass, J., Oldham, J., Sharma, M., and Kambadur, R. (October 1999). Growth factors controlling muscle development. *Domestic Animal Endocrinology.* Vol. 17, No. 2-3, 191-197.

Beauchamp, J.R., Morgan, J.E., Pagel, C.N., and Partridge, T.A. (March 22, 1999). Dynamics of myoblast transplantation reveal a discrete minority of precursors with stem cell-like properties as the myogenic source. *Journal of Cell Biology*. Vol. 6, 1113-1122.

Begley, S., Check, E., and Rogers, A. (February 19, 2001). Solving the next genome puzzle. *Newsweek*. 52.

Biotechnology: Experts point up ethical aspects of human stem cell research. (November 22, 2000). *European Report*.

Brooks, J.R. (June 16, 2001). Experimental drug a lure for athletes, unapproved cancer medication still being tested is in the midst of sports scandal; drug may be new and unapproved, but athletes are after it. *The Salt Lake Tribune*. A1.

Brown, G.C. (October 2000). Speed limits: Will some Olympic records last forever? *The Sciences*. Vol. 40, No. 5, 32-37.

Buffery, S. (August 12, 2000). Doping dilemma. New drug to circumvent EPO tests? *Toronto Sun*.

Chakravarti, A. (February 15, 2001). Single nucleotide polymorphisms . . . to a future of genetic medicine. *Nature*. Vol. 291, 822-823.

Chan, A.W.S., Chong, K.Y., Martinovich, C., Simerly, C., and Schatten, G. (January 12, 2001). Transgenic monkeys produced by retroviral gene transfer into mature oocytes. *Science*. Vol. 291, No. 5502, 309-311.

Chang, T.M. (2000). Future developments in modified hemoglobin as red blood cell substitutes. **http://www.physio.mcgill.ca/artcell/recent.htm**.

Chang, T.M. (December 2000). Red blood cell substitutes. *Bailliere's Best Practice and Research, Clinical Haematology*. Vol. 13, No. 4, 651-667.

Chang, T.M. (2001). Blood substitutes. **http://www.physio.mcgill.ca/artcell/bloodsub.htm#1**.

Chin, E.R., Olson, E.N., Richardson, J.A., Yang, Q., Humphries, C., Shelton, J.M., Wu, H., Zhu, W., Bassel-Duby, R., and Williams, R.S. (August 15, 1998). A calcineurin-dependent transcriptional pathway controls skeletal muscle fiber type. *Genes and Development*. Vol. 12, No. 16, 2499-2509.

Cohen, P. and Concar, D. (May 19, 2001). This week: Cloning special report. *New Scientist*. 14.

Collins, F.S. (July 1, 1999). Shattuck Lecture—Medical and societal consequences of the Human Genome Project. *New England Journal of Medicine*. Vol. 341, No. 1, 28-37.

Collins, F.S. and McKusick, V.A. (February 7, 2001). Implications of the Human Genome Project for medical science. *Journal of the American Medical Association*. Vol. 285, No. 5, 540-544.

Creteur, J., Sibbald, W., and Vincent, J.L. (August 2000). Hemoglobin solutions—not just red blood cell substitutes. *Critical Care Medicine*. Vol. 28, No. 8, 3025-3034.

Dash, A.K. and Cudworth, G.C. 2nd. (July 1998). Therapeutic applications of implantable drug delivery systems. *Journal of Pharmacological and Toxicological Methods*. Vol. 40, No. 1, 1-12.

Davis, J. (February 20, 2001). Doping affair twists and turns at World Nordic Ski Championships. Agence France Presse. Sports.

Egan, M.E. (December 11, 2000). Cell makers. *Forbes*. 220.

Eichelbronner, O., Sielenkamper, A., D'Almeida, M., Ellis, C.G., Sibbald, W.J., and Chin-Yee, I.H. (July 1999). Effects of FI(O(2)) on hemodynamic responses and O(2) transport during RSR13-induced reduction in P(50). *American Journal of Physiology*. Vol. 277, No. 1, Part 2, H290-H298.

Ekblom, B. (1987). Blood-doping, oxygen breathing, and altitude training. In Strauss R.H. (ed.) *Drugs and Performance in Sport*. WB Saunders: Philadelphia, 53.

Evans, C.H., Ghivizzani, S.C., and Robbins, P.D. (May 2000). Potential applications of gene therapy in sports medicine. *Physical Medicine and Rehabilitation Clinics of North America*. Vol. 11, No. 2, 405-416.

Fields, S. (February 16, 2001). Proteomics in genomeland. *Science*. Vol. 291, No. 5507, 1221-1224.

Fresh claims of Australian athletes' drug use erupt. (March 19, 2000). Xinhua News Agency. Sports.

Fretia, R.A. Jr. (July 1998). Exploratory design in medical nanotechnology: A mechanical artificial red cell. *Artificial Cells, Blood Substitutes, and Immobilization Biotechnology*. Vol. 26, No. 4, 411-430.

Friedmann, T. (October 1992). A brief history of gene therapy. *Nature Genetics*. Vol. 2, No. 2, 93-98.

Friedmann, T. and Koss, J.O. (June 2001). Gene transfer and athletics—an impending problem. *Molecular Therapy*. Vol. 3, No. 6, 819-820.

Genetically altered athletes may be next. (November 20, 2000). *Toronto Star*. Edition 1.

Goldspink, G. (April 1999). Changes in muscle mass and phenotype and the expression of autocrine and systemic growth factors by muscle in response to stretch and overload. *Journal of Anatomy*. Vol. 193, Part 3, 323-334.

Goldspink, G. (2000). Cloning of local growth factors involved in the determination of muscle mass. *British Journal of Medicine*. Vol. 34, 159-161.

Growth factor gene transfer in rabbit model stimulates new cartilage production in knee joints. (January 11, 2001). *Gene Therapy Weekly*.

Gussoni, E., Soneoka, Y., Strickland, C.D., Buzney, E.A., Khan, M.K., Flint, A.F., Kunkel, L.M., and Mulligan, R.C. (September 23, 1999). Dystrophin expression in the Mdx mouse restored by stem cell transplantation. *Nature*. Vol. 401, 390-394.

Hagberg, J.M., Moore, G.E., and Ferrell, R.E. (January 2001). Specific genetic markers of endurance performance and VO_2max. *Exercise and Sport Sciences Reviews*. Vol. 29, No. 1, 15-19.

Halliburton, S. (February 1, 2001). Controversial actovegin not banned until more study. *Austin American-Statesman*. C1.

Haney, C.R., Buehler, P.W., and Gulatti, A. (February 28, 2000). Purification and chemical modification of hemoglobin in developing hemoglobin based oxygen carriers. *Advanced Drug Delivery Reviews.* Vol. 40, No. 3, 153-169.

Hextend (6% hetastarch in lactated electrolyte injection) package insert. Final draft. (April 8, 1999). **http://www.fda.gov/cber/ndalabel/hexbio033199LB.pdf**.

Hughes, S.M. (December 3, 1998). Muscle development: Electrical control of gene development. *Current Biology.* Vol. 8, No. 24, R892-R894.

Human genome, the: science genome map. (February 16, 2001). *Science.* Vol. 291, No. 5507, 1218.

Human Genome Project information. (January 2001). **http://www.ornl.gov/hgmis**.

Huuhtanen, M. (March 1, 2001). Finns fear image damaged by sports doping scandal. Associated Press. Sports News.

Initial sequencing and analysis of the human genome. (February 15, 2001). *Nature.* Vol. 409, 860-921.

Kaji, E.H. and Leiden, J.M. (February 7, 2001). Gene and stem cell therapies. *Journal of the American Medical Association.* Vol. 285, No. 5, 545-550.

Kannan, S. (December 14, 1999). Anaphylactic reactions to synthetic colloid plasma substitutes. **http://www.medicinaintensiva-online.org/opexpertos/optoxic/kannan/toxicstarch.html**.

Kanowski, S., Kinzler, E., Lehmann, E., Schweitzer, A., and Kunz, G. (July 1995). Confirmed clinical efficacy of actovegin in elderly patients with organic brain syndrome. *Pharmacopsychiatry.* Vol. 28, No. 4, 125-133.

Kavanagh, B.D., Khandelwal, S.R., Schmidt-Ullrich, R.K., Roberts, J.D., Shaw, E.G., Pearlman, A.D., Venitz, J., Dusenbery, K.E., Abraham, D.J., and Gerber, M.J. (March 2001). A Phase I study of RSR 13, a radiation enhancing hemoglobin modifier: Tolerance of repeated intravenous doses and correlation of pharmacokinetics with pharmacodynamics. *International Journal of Radiation Oncology, Biology, Physics.* Vol. 15, No. 49(4), 1133-1139.

Klein, H.G. (June 1, 2000). The prospects for red-cell substitutes. Editorial. *New England Journal of Medicine.* Vol. 342, No. 22, 1666-1667.

Lamsan, C., Fu, F.H., Robbins, P.D., and Evans, C.H. (2000). Gene therapy in sports medicine. *Sports Medicine.* Vol. 25, No. 2, 73-77.

Lee, S.J. and McPherron, A.C. (October 1999). Myostatin and the control of skeletal muscle mass. *Current Opinions in Genetics and Development.* Vol. 9, No. 5, 604-607.

Lemonick, M.D. (December 25, 2000). Gene mapper: The bad boy of science has jump-started a biological revolution. *Time.* Vol. 156, 110.

Lemonick, M.D. (January 2001). The future of drugs. *Time.* Vol. 157, No. 2, 57-69.

Longman, J. (May 11, 2001). Pushing the limits—a special report; someday soon, athletic edge may be from altered genes. *The New York Times.* A1.

Lowe, K.C. (September 1999). Perfluorinated blood substitutes and artificial oxygen carriers. *Blood Reviews.* Vol. 13, No. 3, 171-184.

MacColl, G.S., Goldspink, G., and Bouloux, P.M. (July 1999). Using skeletal muscle as an artificial endocrine tissue. *Journal of Endocrinology.* Vol. 162, No. 1, 1-9.

MacDougall, I.C. (July 2000). Novel erythropoiesis stimulating protein. *Seminars in Nephrology.* Vol. 20, No. 4, 375-381.

MacDougall, I.C., Gray, S.J., Elston, O., Breen, C., Jenkins, B., Browne, B., and Egrie, J. (November 1999). Pharmacokinetics of novel erythropoiesis stimulating protein compared with epoietin alfa in dialysis patients. *Journal of the American Society of Nephrology.* Vol. 10, No. 11.

Maher, J. and Halliburton, S. (January 12, 2000). Actovegin: Drug of debate; banned substance at center of Tour de France. *Austin American-Statesman.* C1.

McGloughlin, T.M., Fontana, J.L., Alving, B., Mongan, P.D., and Bunger, R. (1996). Profound normovolemic hemodilution: Hemostatic effects in patients and in a porcine model. *Anesthesia and Analgesia.* Vol. 83, No. 3, 459-465.

McKoy, G., Ashley, W., Mander, J., Yang, S.Y., Williams, N., Russell, B., and Goldspink, G. (April 1999). Expression of insulin growth factor-1 splice variants and structural genes in rabbit skeletal muscle induced by stretch and stimulation. *Journal of Physiology (London).* Vol. 516, Part 2, 583-592.

McKusick, V.A. (1997). History of medical genetics. In Emery and Rimon's *Principles of medical genetics.* 3rd ed. Vol. 1, 20, 40.

Modex forges ahead with novel business strategy in cell-based therapies. (November 6, 2000). *2000 Marketletter Publication Ltd.*

Moore, S. and Copetas, A.C. (September 16, 2000). Gene doping's Olympic threat. *The Wall Street Journal.* A6.

Mullon, J., Ciacope, G., Clagett, C., McCune, D., and Dillard, T. (June 1, 2000). Brief report: Transfusions of polymerized bovine hemoglobin in a patient with severe autoimmune hemolytic anemia. *New England Journal of Medicine.* Vol. 342, No. 22, 1638-1643.

Naya, F.J., Mercer, B., Shelton, J., Richardson, J.A., Williams, R.S., and Olson, E.N. (February 18, 2000). Stimulation of slow skeletal muscle fiber gene expression by calcineurin in vivo. *Journal of Biological Chemistry.* Vol. 275, No. 7, 4545-4548.

Nestler, E.J. and Landsman, D. (February 15, 2001). Learning about addiction from the genome. *Nature.* Vol. 291, 834-835.

Odelberg, S.J., Kollhoff, A., and Keating, M.T. (2000). Dedifferentiation of mammalian myotubes induced by msx1. *Cell.* Vol. 103, 1099-1109.

Oligino, T.J., Yao, Q., Ghivizzani, S.C., and Robbins, P. (October 2000). Vector systems for gene transfer to joints. *Clinical Orthopedics.* Vol. 379, Suppl, S17-S30.

Olson, E.N. and Williams, R.S. (June 2000). Remodeling muscles with calcineurin. *Bioessays 2000*. Vol. 22, No. 5, 510-519.

Pace, N., et al. (1947). The increase in hypoxia tolerance of normal men accompanying the polycethemia-induced transition by erythropoietin. *American Journal of Physiology*. 148:152.

Parrish, P. (June 14, 2001). Italian cycling scandal might have Denver tie: Media outlets reporting experimental drug made by small company was one of many confiscated. *Rocky Mountain News*. 1C.

Pennisi, E. (December 22, 2000). Genomics comes of age. *Science*. Vol. 290, No. 5500, 2220-2221.

Pennisi, E. (March 30, 2001). Ribosome's inner workings come into sharper view. *Science*. Vol. 291, No. 5513, 2526-2527.

Pennisi, E. and Vogel, G. (June 9, 2000). Clones: A hard act to follow; cloning research. *Science*. Vol. 288, No. 5472, 1722-1727.

Pollard, T.D. (February 15, 2001). Genomics, the cytoskeleton and motility. *Nature*. Vol. 291, 842-843.

Researchers turn fat cells into cartilage. (March 15, 2000). *Blood Weekly*. 1065-6073.

Robertson, L. (December 14, 2000). Armstrong needs to explain latest accusations. *The Miami Herald*. Sports.

Rusnak, J.M., Kisabeth, R.M., Herbert, D.P., and McNeil, D.M. (March 2001). Pharmacogenomics: A clinician's primer on emerging technologies for improved patient care. *Mayo Clinic Proceedings*. Vol. 76, 299-309.

Saltus, R. (December 22, 2000). Study sees organ growth potential. *The Boston Globe*. A8.

Santini, J.T. Jr., Richards, A.C., Scheidt, R.A., Cima, M.J., and Langer, R.S. (September 2000). Microchip technology in drug delivery. *Annals of Medicine*. Vol. 32, No. 6, 377-379.

Schuldiner, M., Yanuka, O., Itskovitz-Elder, J., Melton, D.A., and Benvenisty, N. (October 10, 2000). Effects of eight growth factors on the differentiation of cells derived from embryonic stem cells. *Proceedings of the National Academy of Sciences*. Vol. 97, No. 21, 11307-11312.

Schultz, O., Sittinger, M., Haeupl, T., and Burmeister, G.R. (2000). Emerging strategies of bone and joint repair. *Arthritis Research*. Vol. 2, No. 6, 433-436.

Scores take up the banner of regrowth: The mission of an increasing number of biotech companies is to overcome the body's constraints to repairing tissue and organs. (November 15, 2000). *Financial Times (London)*. Survey-Biotechnology, 2.

Seppa, N. (July 11, 1998). Gene therapy for arthritis works in rats. *Science News*. Vol. 154, No. 2, 31.

Smith, G. (September 18, 2000). Gotta catch 'em all. *Sports Illustrated*. 84-96.

Standl, T. (May 2000). Artificial oxygen carriers as red blood cell substitutes—perfluorocarbons and cell-free hemoglobin. *Infusionstherapie and Transfusionsmedizin*. Vol. 27, No. 3, 128-137.

Stoneking, M. (February 15, 2001). Single nucleotide polymorphisms: From the evolutionary past. *Nature*. Vol. 291, 821.

Strauss, R.G., Stansfield, C., Heriksen, R.A., and Villhauer, P.J. (May-June 1988). Pentastarch may cause fewer effects on coagulation than Hetastarch. *Transfusion*. Vol. 28, No. 3, 257-260.

Strikeman, A. (January 1, 2001). Drug delivery with muscle; technology information. *Technology Review*. Vol. 104, No. 1, 36.

Swift, E.M. and Yaeger, D. (May 14, 2001). Unnatural selection. *Sports Illustrated*. Vol. 94, No. 20, 86-94.

Urquhart, J. (November 2000). Internal medicine in the 21st century: Controlled drug delivery: Therapeutic and pharmacological aspects. *Journal of Internal Medicine*. Vol. 248, No. 5, 357-376.

U.S. Department of Health and Human Services fact sheet on stem cell research. (February 1, 1999). M2 Presswire.

Valentis announces improved GeneSwitch(TM) gene regulation system. (November 15, 2000). PR Newswire.

Vandegriff, K.D. (September 2000). Haemoglobin-based oxygen carriers. *Expert Opinion on Investigational Drugs*. Vol. 9, No. 9, 1967-1984.

Vermeulen, L.C., Ratco, T.A., Erstad, B.L., Brecher, M.E., and Matuszewski, K.A. (February 1995). A paradigm for consensus. The University Hospital Consortium guidelines for the use of albumin, nonprotein colloid, and crystalloid solutions. *Archives of Internal Medicine*. Vol. 155, No. 4, 373-379.

Verrengia, J.B. (September 27, 2000). Scientists study athletic limits. AP Online.

Vogel, G. (June 8, 2001). Can adult stem cells suffice? *Science*. Vol. 292, No. 5523, 1820-1822.

Wadler, G.I. (1999). Doping in sport: From strychnine to genetic enhancement, it's a moving target! The Duke Conference on Doping. The Duke University School of Law in conjunction with its Center for Sports Law and Policy. Raleigh, North Carolina. **http://www.law.duke.edu./sportscenter/conference.html**.

Wadler, G.I. and Hainline, B. (1989). *Drugs and the athlete*. Philadelphia: F.A. Davis.

Wadler, G.I. (March 1994). Drug abuse update. In The office practice of sports medicine. *Medical Clinics of North America*. Vol. 78, No. 2, 439-455.

Wahr, J.A., Gerber, M., Venitz, J., and Baglia, N. (March 2001). Allosteric modification of oxygen delivery by hemoglobin. *Anesthesia and Analgesia*. Vol. 92, No. 3, 615-620.

Walsh, D. (February 6, 2000). Building the perfect champion. *Sunday Times (London)*. Sport.

Walsh, D. (November 19, 2000). Race against time. *Sunday Times (London)*. Sport.

Walsh, D. (December 7, 2000). Next up...doping from hell. *Calgary Herald*. E1.

Warren, B.B. and Durieux, M.E. (January 1997). Hydroxyethyl starch: Safe or not? *Anesthesia and Analgesia.* Vol. 84, No. 1, 206-212.

Weiss, R. (May 23, 2000). For DNA, a defining moment; with code revealed, challenge will be to find its meaning and uses. *The Washington Post.* A1.

Weiss, R. (January 12, 2001). Scientists create first genetically altered monkey. *The Washington Post.* A1.

Wilmut, I. (December 1998). Cloning for medicine. *Scientific American.*

Wilson, S. (January 25, 2001). Olympics looks into gene therapy. AP Online.

Wilson, S. (February 13, 2001). IOC reviews position on banned drug. AP Online. Sports.

Winslow, R.M. (1999). New transfusion strategies: red cell substitutes. *Annual Review of Medicine.* Vol. 50, 337-353.

Yang, J. and Wu, C.L. (March-April 2001). Gene therapy for pain. *American Scientist.* Vol. 89, No. 2, 126-135.

Yuki, W. (April 9, 2000). New doping problems surface to plague Games. *The Daily Yomiuri (Tokyo).* 21.

Zhu, X., Hadhazy, M., Wehling, M., Tidball, J.G., and McNally, E.M. (May 26, 2000). Dominant negative myostatin produces hypertrophy without hyperplasia in muscle. *Federation of European Biochemical Societies Letter.* Vol. 474, No. 1, 71-75.

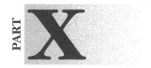
Drug Testing

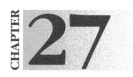
Drug Testing in Sport and Exercise

R. Craig Kammerer, PhD

Small portions of this chapter have appeared in Kammerer, R.C. (2000), Drug testing and anabolic steroids, in *Anabolic Steroids in Sport and Exercise,* C.E. Yesalis (ed.), 2nd ed. (Human Kinetics, Champaign, IL), pp. 415-459; and Kammerer, R.C. (2001), What is doping and how is it detected? in *Doping in Elite Sport,* W. Wilson and E. Derse (eds.) (Human Kinetics, Champaign, IL (pp. 1-28).

The number of therapeutic agents in clinical use today is quite large, with a significant fraction of them requiring some type of drug test in order for their use in therapy to be monitored. An effective drug-testing program designed to combat abuse of a therapeutic agent involves consideration of the concepts listed in figure 27.1. It is important to keep in mind the goals of an "effective" drug test in the program being designed. Clinically, a laboratory test is often effective with a confidence level of about 80%, for several reasons. A clinical test is most often taken in context with other results: a physical exam, presentation of symptoms, discussion of medical history with the attending clinician, or other evaluations to elucidate the problem. In a nonclinical drug-testing program there is usually only one test, along with a corresponding confirmation test; and if the results are not 100% accurate, without any false positives and minimal false negatives, the entire career and livelihood of the person tested are at risk. Drug use still appears to be substantial (Meilman et al. 1995) despite testing programs and technological advances. Along with the ethics and moral issues of a false-positive test, the legal ramifications for the drug-testing organization are often substantial.

Sample collection

Regulatory considerations

Chain of custody

Laboratory analysis

   A. Screening

   B. Confirmation/"B sample"

Pharmacokinetics

Drug metabolism

Drug interactions

Therapy/Drug quantity considerations

Reports/Results

Figure 27.1 Components of effective drug testing.

History of Drug Testing in Sport

Significant drug testing of humans began in the late 1950s, when evidence of drug use was observed following several European cycling and track races. In the 1960 Rome Olympic Games, a cyclist died after apparent amphetamine usage. In 1965, Beckett, Tucker, and Moffat (1967) developed procedures capable of detecting a number of different stimulants that were then used to test participants in the Tour of Britain cycle races. In the 1967 Tour de France, another cyclist died, and amphetamines were found both on his person and in his body. Professor Beckett was a member of the newly formed International

Olympic Committee (IOC) Medical Commission, and his procedures were evaluated on a preliminary basis in the 1968 Mexico City/Grenoble Olympic Games, without testing for anabolic steroids because of the lack of assay procedures. The first "formal" testing (without steroids) occurred at the 1972 Munich/Sapporo Olympic Games (Donike and Stratmann, 1974). The development of complex radioimmunoassay (RIA) screening procedures (Brooks et al., 1979), as well as gas chromatography–mass spectrometry (GC-MS) techniques, led to the introduction of tests for anabolic steroids (AS) at the 1976 Montreal Olympic Games (Bertrand, Masse, and Dugal, 1978). However, only 275 of the 1800 total samples were analyzed for steroids because of the time required for analysis.

During both the 1976 Montreal/Innsbruck Olympics and the 1980 Moscow/Lake Placid Olympics, RIA screening procedures (Brooks, Firth, and Sumner, 1975; Rogozkin, Morozov, and Tchaikovsky, 1979) were used to analyze samples for the presence of AS, and GC-MS analysis was used to confirm positive screening results. Both because of the inherent lack of specificity in RIA screening assays for the steroid metabolites (whose detection was necessary to demonstrate the presence of an AS) and because endogenous testosterone was added to the list of banned drugs, GC-MS was adopted at the 1984 Olympic Games as both the screening and confirmatory method for analysis of AS (Catlin et.al., 1987). The method of assessing whether or not the testosterone arises from illegal usage by the athlete was developed by Donike et al. (1983) based on an earlier study (Baba, Shinohara, and Kasuya, 1980). The test consisted of measuring both testosterone (T) and its epimeric form (a geometric isomer called epitestosterone [E]) in the same sample. Since E is not converted to T in the body to any appreciable extent and since the normal ratio of the quantity of T to the quantity of E is approximately in the range of 1:1 for both males and females, administration of T raises this ratio. A ratio of over 6:1 was considered evidence of having administered T in 1982; and as natural exceptions to this threshold of guilt (discussed later) have appeared, the "informal" guidelines now often used are over 6:1, suspicious; over 10:1, probably guilty. Additional refinement in these guidelines may be forthcoming in the near future.

Drug testing at the 1988 Seoul Summer Olympics was summarized by Chung et al. (1990) and Park et al. (1990). In the 1992 Barcelona Summer Olympic Games, the IOC laboratory reported the detection of several banned drugs in the participating athletes: three cases of stimulant medications (strychnine, norephedrine, and Mesocarb), two clenbuterol positives, and three T/E ratios over 6:1 and between 6 and 10:1 (Segura et al., 1995). Samples containing the stimulant drugs and clenbuterol were formally reported for punitive action, while the three T/E ratios were referred for further study without action against the athletes. In the 1996 Atlanta Olympic Games, most drug positives were disallowed for lack of documentation. Specifically, either the analysis technique (high-resolution mass spectrometry; Horning and Schaenzer 1997[a,b]; Horning, Schaenzer, and Sample, 1998) or the drug (bromantan) was too new for the results to be accepted as valid support of the drug positive.

Testing Matrix: Blood or Urine

Clinically, blood is used for most drug tests. The reason is that the blood level of a drug more reliably correlates with drug action and any therapeutic decision to be made than does a urinary level. A urinary drug level is subject to too many unpredictable variables, like urinary output and fluid intake, to allow therapeutic decision making based on the result. Although a few athletic federations have assessed blood testing outside Olympic competition and some experimental blood testing was performed at the 1994 Lillehammer Winter Olympic Games, urine has been the only permitted testing fluid in most drug programs. Therefore the use of urine requires drug metabolites (or final excretion products) as the molecules that must be detected in order to prove drug use. There are several reasons for limiting testing to the urine matrix. First, the athletes as well as athletic federations feel that obtaining a blood sample is an unnecessary trauma to the athlete. Second, giving a urine sample does not involve needles or any invasive procedure that introduces the possible transmission of disease as well as legal and religious considerations. Other advantages of utilizing urine, rather than blood, include the fact that drug/metabolite concentrations are often higher in urine than in blood and that detection is usually possible for a longer time in urine. Although the possibility of using blood for drug testing is not a new idea (Donike, 1976), in recent years the use of blood has again attracted interest because of the addition of more natural or endogenous compounds, such as human growth hormone (hGH), human chorionic gonadotropin (hCG), and erythropoietin (EPO) to the banned lists. The litigious nature of society today (Jacobs and Samuels, 1995) should slow the introduction of any blood-based drug testing on a wide scale.

A valuable application of the use of blood as the drug-testing matrix has been reported (De la Torre, Segura, and Polettini, 1995; De la Torre et al., 1995). Through use of a blood test, intact T esters have been found in the blood of people who have taken T. Testosterone is usually supplied as an ester of some type in pharmaceutical preparations. Since no T esters are produced naturally (although T is) and since when the ester forms of T are consumed they are *not* excreted intact into the urine, the detection of an intact ester in the blood proves unequivocally that synthetic T was consumed. Since no T ester survives metabolism and excretion into the urine, a urine test per se could not prove usage of T. Thus, the use of blood testing for the verification of T abuse removes any doubt whether exogenous supplementation of natural T occurred. Theoretically, however, the use of T skin patches, gels, or creams would still circumvent this test, as intact esters either would not be used or would not survive passage through the skin intact to the bloodstream. The use of a blood sample to detect T abuse may be of even greater theoretical interest since data demonstrating an actual benefit of T usage for performance in sport have appeared (Bhasin et al., 1996). Also of interest is the work that has been published on the detection of various hormones in blood after T administration (e.g., luteinizing hormone, follicle-stimulating hormone, 17-hydroxyprogesterone, T), as well as the use of the ketoconazole suppression test, all of which are being investigated to verify the recent abuse of T (see Carlstroem et al., 1992; Cowan et al., 1991; Kicman et al., 1990; Oftebro et al., 1994; Palonek et al., 1995).

Figure 27.2 presents the various classes of banned drugs and methods as currently listed by the IOC (2001). Table 27.1 summarizes examples of each class, and table 27.2 lists the maximum allowable concentrations of some classes. Each list details many of the commonly found agents, but these lists are not intended to be complete.

Classes

1. Stimulants
2. Narcotics
3. Anabolic steroids and β_2-agonists
4. Diuretics
5. Peptide hormones

Classes prohibited under certain circumstances

1. Alcohol
2. Cannabinoids
3. Local anaesthetics
4. Glucocorticosteroids
5. Beta-blockers

Methods

1. Blood doping
2. Manipulation (chemical, physical, or pharmacological)
3. Administering artificial oxygen carriers and plasma expanders
4. Aromatase inhibitors: males only

Figure 27.2 Classes of drugs and methods banned by IOC.

Screening Methods

Many standard screening methods are used for the wide variety of drugs to be controlled in sport competition, including GC, high-performance liquid chromatography, GC-MS, immunoassays of various types, and enzyme-linked immunosorbent assay methods. It is beyond the scope of this chapter to summarize the huge number of screening methods, which have been treated elsewhere (Catlin et al. 1987; Hemmersbach et al., 1996; Stenman et al., 1997; Kerrigan and Phillips, 2001).

Confirmation Methods

Fast and efficient screening methods are utilized to decrease the total number of drug samples to be analyzed, so that the slower and more expensive confirmation methods may be used on far fewer samples while still identifying the positive samples correctly. These confirmation methods are thus directed toward fewer possible drug candidates so that much more information may be obtained in a reasonable time frame to assure certainty about the results.

Gas Chromatography–Mass Spectrometry

During gas chromatographic analysis, a solvent extract of a urine sample is injected into a heated long tube (called a column) that interacts with the various components of the sample, retarding some components more than others. Unless the drug/metabolites from the sample extract can be successfully transformed into the gaseous state without destruction of the molecule, gas chromatographic analysis may not be used for such a drug. The time that a substance takes (called the retention time) to pass through a particular column under a specified set of conditions is peculiar to that substance and helps identify it. A mass spectrometer attached to the end of the GC column detects substances passed into it by bombarding the molecules with a beam of electrons that fragments the molecules into ionic pieces; these data constitute an ion fragment fingerprint of that particular substance. That spectrum (collection) of fragment ions, along with the retention time (time spent in the GC column before detection), constitutes information unique to each substance; thus, identification without any doubt is confirmed when these data are the same as those collected when an authentic reference substance (or an extract of a sample taken from someone who has taken the drug) is analyzed under the same conditions. One may obtain this spectrum of ions under full-scan conditions (all possible ions are collected at the same time, without much time spent in defining the signal intensity for any particular ion) or under SIM conditions (selected ion monitoring, in which specific selected ions

Table 27.1 Examples of Banned Drug Classes

Stimulants	Narcotics**	Anabolic steroids/ β₂-agonists/anabolic agents	Diuretics	Peptide hormones, mimetics, and analogues	Beta blockers	Masking agents
Amineptine	Buprenorphine	Androstenediol	Acetazolamide	Corticotrophins (ACTH)	Acebutolol	Bromantan
Amiphenazole	Dextromoramide	Androstenedione	Bendroflumethiazide (Naturetin)	EPO (erythropoietin)	Alprenolol (Sinalol)	Epitestosterone
Amphetamines	Diamorphine (heroin)	Bolasterone	Bumetanide	HCG (human chorionic gonadotrophin) [pro-hibited in males only]	Atenolol (Tenormin)	Probenecid
Bromantan	Methadone	Boldenone (dehydrotestosterone; Vet.)	Chlorthalidone	HGH (human growth hormone; somatotro-phin)	Betaxolol	
Bupropion	Morphine	Clenbuterol (a β₂-agonist)	Canrenone	Insulin [permitted only with certified insulin-dependent diabetes]	Esmolol	
Caffeine*	Pentazocine	Clostebol (Steranabol)	Ethacrynic Acid (Edecrin)	Insulin-like growth factor (IGF-I)	Labetalol	
Cocaine*	Pethidine (meperidine—demerol)	Danazol	Furosemide (Lasix)	Pituitary and synthetic gonadotrophins (lu-teinizing hormone) [prohibited in males only]	Metoprolol (Lopressor)	
Ephedrines*		Dehydrochlormethyltestosterone (Oral-Turinabol; Chlorodianabol)	Hydrochlorothiazide (Esidrix)	Clomiphene [prohibited in males only]	Nadolol (Corgard)	
Fencamfamine		Dehydroepiandrosterone (DHEA)	Spironolactone	Cyclofenil [prohibited in males only]	Oxprenolol	
Mesocarb		Dihydrotestosterone (DHT)	Triamterene	Tamoxifen [prohibited in males only]	Propranolol (Inderal)	
Methylphenidate (Ritalin)		Drostanolone			Sotalol	
Pentetrazol		Ethyllestrenol				
Pipradrol		Formebolone				
Salbutamol		Fluoxymesterone (Halotestin)				
Terbutaline		Furazabol				
Strychnine		Mesterolone (Proviron)				
		Metandienone (Dianabol)				
		Methandriol				
		Methyltestosterone (Metandren)				
		Mibolerone				
		Nandrolone (nortestosterone)				
		19-Norandrostenediol				
		19-Norandrostenedione				
		Norethandrolone (Nilevar)				
		Oxandrolone (Anavar)				
		Oxymesterone (Oranabol)				
		Oxymetholone (Anadrol)				
		Stanozolol (Winstrol)				
		Stenbolone				
		Testosterone^				
		Trenbolone				

*See table 27.2.

**Codeine, dextromethorphan, dextropropoxyphene, dihydrocodeine, diphenoxylate, ethylmorphine, pholcodine, propoxyphene, and tramadol are allowed.

^The presence of a urinary testosterone-to-epitestosterone ratio greater than 6:1 unless there is evidence that this ratio is due to a physiological or pathological condition.

Table 27.2 Summary of Urinary Concentrations Above Which IOC-Accredited Laboratories Must Report Findings for Specific Substances

Substance	Urinary concentrations
Caffeine	>12 µg/ml
Carboxy-THC	>15 ng/ml
Cathine	>5 µg/ml
Ephedrine	>10 µg/ml
Epitestosterone	>200 ng/ml
Methylephedrine	>10 µg/ml
Morphine	>1 µg/ml
19-Norandrosterone	>2 ng/ml in males
19-Norandrosterone	>5 ng/ml in females
Phenylpropanolamine	>25 µg/ml
Pseudoephedrine	>25 µg/ml
Salbutamol	>100 ng/ml as stimulant
Salbutamol	>1000 ng/ml as anabolic agent
T/E ratio	>6

are monitored for a much longer time to define signal intensity). Note that frequently an SIM collection may be virtually as specific as the scan collection when a full scan has only a limited number of ions that is similar to the number monitored under SIM mode

Liquid Chromatography–Mass Spectrometry

Liquid chromatography–mass spectrometry (LC-MS) in principle is a type of analysis similar to GC-MS. The sample is passed through the separation column in the liquid state rather than in the gas phase; and a liquid-solvent carrier medium is used that does not chemically modify the substrate, which moves the sample through the separation column.

LC-MS is already rapidly entering the drug-testing laboratory because of several advantages over the traditional GC-MS techniques. An LC analysis usually proceeds at room temperature, and the solvent moves the substances to be analyzed through the separation column under mild conditions, whereas GC analysis requires the drug to be heated/vaporized into the gaseous state in order to move through the separation column. In the future, LC-MS will gain increasingly major importance in the drug-testing lab because of its ability to confirm

the presence of more drugs besides GC-MS, including the large molecular weight natural hormones (hCG, hGH, EPO, etc.).

High-Resolution Mass Spectrometry

Until recently, high-resolution mass spectrometry (HRMS) would not have been an advantage in drug testing, because sensitivity would have been sacrificed for specificity. In addition, the instruments have been extremely expensive (approximately $300,000 up per instrument). However, costs of these instruments, as with LC-MS instrumentation, have been declining recently, so these instruments may soon be within major lab budget requirements. Because of the improvement in several different electronic and instrumental aspects of HRMS analysis, the technique now possesses increased sensitivity for some drugs. However, background signal (also called experimental noise) is also increased with increased sensitivity; thus the technique may not be of greater value for all substances, since endogenous interferences (background signal) vary with the metabolite being analyzed (Horning and Schaenzer, 1997a,b; Thieme et al., 1996). High-resolution mass spectrometry analysis was introduced in the 1996 Summer Atlanta Olympic Games testing program; but the positive results obtained with the technique were not formally reported, presumably due to anticipated legal problems (Horning, Schaenzer, and Sample, 1998). Only after sufficient results are published addressing detection limits, any false-negative and false-positive issues, and statistics showing the validity of results, will the newer HRMS technique be acceptable both scientifically and legally.

Isotope Ratio Mass Spectrometry

Isotope ratio mass spectrometry (IRMS) is a new technique being evaluated for verification of T positives that could be explained by means other than drug taking. It is based on the claim that the percentage of ^{13}C (a naturally occurring stable nonradioactive isotope of carbon) found in endogenous T, which is made in the body from dietary components whose carbon sources are plants and animals, is different from the percentage of ^{13}C present in the synthetic T from a drug preparation. Isotope ratio mass spectrometry analysis can determine the ratio of $^{13}C:^{12}C$ in the sample, and thus whether the source is a synthetic drug or diet (Aguilera et al., 1996a,b). Even though AS are an old class of drugs (Hoberman and Yesalis, 1995) and the ban on athletic abuse use of T occurred only in 1983, it is has been reported recently that several different situations (figure 27.3) will raise the T/E ratio into the "illegal" >6:1 range without the athlete ever having taken T! If enough data are published that confirm the veracity of the IRMS technique and

- Alcohol use prior to drug test
- Bacteria growth in sample and/or high urinary pH
- Deconjugation conditions used during sample preparation
- Low epitestosterone concentration; need to measure absolute levels of testosterone and epitestosterone
- Female: monthly cycle fluctuations in testosterone/epitestosterone
- Female: birth control pill usage effects on testosterone/epitestosterone
- Endocrine disease
- Genetic enzymatic variations

Figure 27.3 Possible reasons for high testosterone/epitestosterone ratios without drug abuse.

show that it can corroborate whether or not an athlete has taken T, the technique will be utilized despite its expense, time, and special equipment requirements. A recent study of 73 control male athletes and six others whose T/E ratios were over 6:1 evaluated urinary diol metabolites and ^{13}C incorporation (Aguilera et al., 2001) for evidence of T abuse. Considerably more data may be required before the carbon isotope method is validated for proving T abuse.

An IRMS can be used only for isotope ratio analyses and not for other routine assays (such as steroid screening or confirmation tests), so acquisition of the equipment, with its current cost of about $100,000 per instrument, may be difficult for some labs. Isotope ratio mass spectrometry may be of value in resolving the "problems" associated with the documented increase in T/E ratios after alcohol use (Falk, Palonek, and Bjoerkhem, 1988; Karila et al., 1996), a fluctuation in the ratio in women apparently caused by many factors (Engelke, Geyer, and Donike, 1995; Engelke, Flenker, and Donike, 1996), an increased T/E ratio resulting from experimental conditions during sample preparation (Geyer et al., 1996), the possible use of dehydroepiandrosterone (DHEA) (Haning et al., 1991, 1993), or even simultaneous usage of both T and E (Dehennin, 1994). However, because of both the complexity and possible sex differences in the metabolism of DHEA (Haning et al., 1991, 1993), it is not yet clear whether IRMS may be able to distinguish between the use of pharmaceutical and "dietary" DHEA. The use of this technique will increase dramatically in the future. The technique will add considerable costs to the operation of a laboratory since the required instrument

will be useful primarily for the smaller numbers of samples in which T abuse is suspected.

Problem Areas of Testing

This section will focus on the areas of drug testing that are the most difficult to conduct, both legally and scientifically.

Testosterone Use

Testosterone is not converted to its geometric form or 17-epimer, epitestosterone (E), in man or woman. Testosterone exists in amounts approximately equal to that of E in both males and females, but the absolute quantities in females are at least fivefold lower than in males. Thus, theoretically, the T/E ratio should not vary much over 1:1 in "normal" humans. After analysis of thousands of T/E ratios in both athletes and "other" populations, a ratio of 6:1 was chosen as the threshold indicator of illegal supplementation, with the presumption that it would account for ratio variations that might be found for a variety of natural reasons (Donike et al., 1983).

Since 1983, when T abuse was banned in sport by the IOC Medical Commission, a number of other explanations have been found for "high" T/E ratios. Since that time, many of these cases have required long periods of investigation, prompting test challenges, lawsuits, and so on. These other explanations include those summarized in figure 27.3.

An athlete is considered guilty of using T if the testosterone/epitestosterone (T/E) ratio exceeds 6:1, although in actual practice many organizations will not pursue a "positive" unless it is over 9-10:1 because a small number of cases of T/E ratios over 6:1 have been shown not to have arisen from T abuse (Oftebro, 1992; Raynaud et al., 1992, 1993; Garle et al., 1996; Karila et al., 1996). Simultaneous consumption of E and T to keep the ratio of the two substances close to the "normal" ratio of 1:1 should not prevent the identification of exogenous T use (Dehennin, 1994), because the laboratories can calculate the ratios of T, as well as the ratios of E, to other endogenous steroids measured during the drug screening process. These abnormal ratios will be interpreted as atypical by scientists evaluating the data (Dehennin and Matsumoto, 1993; Dehennin, 1994; Norli et al., 1995; Palonek et al., 1995; Geyer et al., 1996). Laboratories have indeed set reference range values for many endogenous steroid levels and ratios (Donike et al., 1995); but the published data to date are rare, and ratios are not uniformly applied by different IOC laboratories. This fact suggests considerable legal problems whenever a positive drug case for the use of any endogenous compound is made public.

Even the published scientific data on the validity of the 6:1 T/E ratio as a means to substantiate T abuse are sparse, at least when evaluating specific natural conditions that may lead to naturally elevated T/E ratios. This situation confers advantages to abusers and their lawyers, because the peer-reviewed data for the test are not available in quantity sufficient to withstand legal challenge. More specifically, information to rigorously define any variations in T/E ratios due to sex, age, diet, common drugs taken (cold medications, alcohol, nicotine-tobacco usage, caffeine, H_2-receptor antagonists [used for ulcer treatment], birth control pills, etc.) is needed. Data for the evaluation of any dependence on T levels at the time of the menstrual cycle, bacteria count in the sample, variation in the pH of the sample, and even the use of other common "permitted" drugs must be available. The T/E data should be on a sufficiently large sample for each category or variable (>10,000) that there is little chance that a false positive would occur in the population of athletes who would normally attend an Olympic Games (usually approximately 10,000+ for a Summer Games). Thus, control of any naturally occurring substance requires the establishment of the "normal" endogenous level in the population and subsequent statistical determination of what constitutes an "abnormal" or abuse level of drug. An excellent recent paper summarizes the T testing "problems" and suggests some possible solutions (Catlin, Hatton, and Starcevic, 1997).

To this author's knowledge, there have been few, if any, reported cases of T abuse attributable to the use of both E and T. Possible reasons are the astute use of both T and E so that urinary levels are not high enough to be conclusive, and/or the anticipated legal issues involved in proving such dual usage. The use of moderate amounts of both T and E will not only not raise the T/E ratio over 6:1, but also will not raise any ratios to other endogenous steroids sufficiently to indicate drug abuse. This situation is analogous to the use of moderate amounts of T only, which raises the T/E ratio, but not over 6:1. Thus, some positive results may not be reported because of the obvious need to protect individuals whose T/E ratios or ratios to other endogenous steroids vary for "natural" reasons and not because of drug use. In either case, use of both T and E constitutes a problem in AS testing, because they are both endogenous substances, and illegal levels must be shown to be due to the illegal use of those substances and not to normal variations in natural hormones (Dehennin, 1994).

Another method for abusing T is the use of the available skin patches (gels) for the application of controlled-release T. A controlled-release preparation delivers the drug into the body on a more consistent basis over time, as opposed to a larger, more sudden dose that is delivered soon after parenteral administration. Thus, controlled release means an even dosing over a longer time period—usually 8 to 12 hr—resulting in a lower peak plasma level than a regular dose, but also a level that varies less and lasts longer. So, relative to parenteral administration, the use of a sustained-release T preparation will yield a more stable blood level of drug with fewer high fluctuations, thereby making drug use "safer" than parenteral administration and resulting in less chance of exceeding the 6:1 T/E ratio (Meikle et al., 1992, 1996). Furthermore, skin (particularly scrotal skin) contains high levels of reductase activity, so that T applied to the skin is quickly converted to dihydrotestosterone (DHT). Thus, DHT levels could be raised by either use of a T skin patch or actual consumption of DHT.

A number of Chinese female swimmers were found positive for DHT (Donike et al., 1995) at the World Swimming Championships in 1994. Their positives were determined by careful comparison of the amount of DHT found in the samples with the amounts of several other endogenous steroids (steroid profile analysis), and were reported in the scientific literature (Southan et al., 1992; Kicman et al., 1995; Donike et al., 1995; Coutts et al., 1997). It was clear that those athletes thought that DHT would not be found during testing, as it was an endogenous compound that had not been controlled before and thus usage would probably go undetected.

Illegal usage of T by female athletes is more difficult to prove than in male athletes because absolute levels are much lower in females; additionally, both the levels of T and E and the T/E ratios fluctuate greatly (Karila et al., 1996; Engelke, Geyer, and Donike, 1995; Engelke, Flenker, and Donike, 1996). There may also be a hormonal cycle-dependent T/E ratio fluctuation (Engelke, Geyer, and Donike, 1995) and a relatively large increase in T/E ratio after alcohol consumption (Falk, Palonek, and Bjoerkhem, 1988; Karila et al., 1996).

Therefore, if the dose of T is carefully chosen and/or combined with sustained-release dosing, significant drug may be utilized both during training and relatively close to competition time, with a very low risk of reaching an illegal T/E ratio. The illegal ratio of T/E was chosen such that some drug abuse would be tolerated in order to protect all innocent athletes.

If future experiments prove that the use of IRMS analysis (discussed earlier) does indeed distinguish between endogenous and exogenous T, or if collection of competition blood specimens is allowed such that the nonendogenous intact T esters may be found when T has been taken (at least after parenteral administration), then many of the lab problems in proving T abuse will disappear.

Circumventing Positive Test Results

The following categories of PES constitute the primary classes of agents that drug takers utilize to escape detection.

Designer Drugs

It is possible but unlikely that an athlete could prevent a positive drug-test result by using a substance containing appropriate interfering or masking ion fragments (figure 27.4). The reason is that laboratories use both the chromatographic retention time (RT) and the mass spectrometric fragment ion pattern for declaring a positive, and the chances of an interfering substance possessing the same RT and ion spectrum as the drug in question are extremely low.

However, designer steroids can and are being made (Bamberger and Yaeger, 1997; Franke and Berendonk, 1997) that may lead to long-term drug abuse without detection. More specifically, a designer or "new" steroid has been chemically produced (synthesized in the laboratory) that retains the anabolic properties desired for such a drug. At the same time the molecular structure (skeleton) is chemically altered so that the currently used steroid screening test (a SIM GC-MS analysis) will not "find" the ions produced by the fragmentation of this new structure. In addition, when such a drug is initially discovered by the laboratory network, the agent must be banned by the various sport federations, the athletes and

Androstenediol

Androstenedione

Bromantan

Cafedrine

DHEA (dehydroepiandrosterone)

DHT (dihydrotestosterone)

Epitestosterone

Polypeptide hormones: erythropoietin, human chorionic gonadotropin, human growth hormone, etc.

Mesocarb/Sydnocarb

Norandrostenediol

Norandrostenedione

Oral-Turinabol metabolite (Chlorodianabol metabolite)

Probenecid

Theodrenaline

Figure 27.4 Some drugs used by athletes to escape detection.

members must be apprised of such bans, and relevant sanctions must be listed so that all athletes, coaches, trainers, physicians, and other appropriate people are notified. The IOC and federations usually require evidence that the prohibition of use of an agent is indicated (that it confers performance enhancement) before issuing the ban. However, the IOC ban of the use of THC (cannabinoids) in 1998 would argue against this rationale, as few would agree that THC confers performance enhancement.

The previously unknown drug bromantan was found in nine athletes in the 1996 Atlanta Olympic Games, and the positive cases reported were disallowed by the World Court of Arbitration for Sport because the drug was too new. The scanty data, scientific knowledge, and literature at the time (from 1967 through July, 1996) were insufficient to enforce the ban. Bromantan was developed in Russia for thermoprotective and stimulant effects, reportedly to be used in army troops. The only published articles described the compound as a psychostimulant. Its chemical structure was unlike that of any other known drug (although one might construe it to be a distant cousin of amantadine, an antiviral drug currently on the market). There was no known metabolic information available in the public scientific literature from 1967 through July 1996. However, some data on the metabolism/detection of the drug has appeared since the 1996 Olympic Games (Sizoi, Bolotov, and Semenov, 1998). Rumors had been circulating that a new drug had been abused in the 1992 Barcelona Olympic Games. Then the IOC labs began to look at competition samples for a new unknown peak during screening, which was identified by mass spectrometry as bromantan, prior to the 1996 Olympic Games.

Natural Hormones Other Than Testosterone

Several polypeptide hormones including hGH, hCG, gonadotropin-releasing hormone (GnRH), insulin, and EPO are being abused in competition. The hGH, GnRH, and hCG all have anabolic effects in their own right and/or stimulate the release of T or other natural anabolic agents (Bradley and Sodeman, 1990; Papadakis et al., 1996; Conn and Crowley, 1994; Laidler et al., 1995). Erythropoietin increases the production of red blood cells, increasing the body's oxygen-carrying capacity. It was widely rumored that EPO was abused at the 1996 Atlanta Olympic Games and 2000 Sydney Games, but no confirmatory lab test was available to enforce a ban or verify any potential reported positives (Bamberger and Yaeger, 1997).

Testing for the many polypeptide hormones is difficult because the confirmatory assays for these compounds by MS are not currently developed and validated and thus not available to laboratories yet (hCG—Laidler et al., 1995; Liu and Bowers, 1995, 1996, 1997; Stenman et al., 1997; EPO—Wide et al., 1995; Ekblom, 1996). Aside from the fact that the presence of polypeptide hormones is difficult to confirm by a specific assay, all of these compounds are naturally present in all healthy people. Thus, doping control programs must establish what levels of polypeptide hormones are abnormal or indicative of abuse and what levels are normal. A considerable database is needed to confirm what concentration ranges for each of these natural components are normal and what variations occur for a variety of "natural" causes. Endogenous hCG levels are minute, in men, except in certain cases of malignancy. Consequently, an athlete accused of hCG abuse can counter with contentions of illness. Levels of hCG are higher in women; shortly after conception, the levels become huge because this compound is a placental hormone (and is the basis of a commonly used pregnancy test). A ban has not been announced for hCG use in women because of insurmountable difficulties in proving abuse.

Athletes take many other endogenous natural agents for a variety of effects, such as release of endogenous growth hormone, enhanced fat burning, and enhanced normal T levels and synthesis (Conn and Crowley, 1994; Laidler et al., 1995). It is important that the athlete take due care in using new or experimental drugs or dosages that significantly exceed therapeutic levels. Although no scientific proof has appeared, recent deaths that were presumably due to the abuse of EPO emphasize this point (Leith, 1991).

Use of Other Substances

Many other substances have become popular for their purported anabolic effects, their effects on endogenous anabolic substances, or stimulant effects. Examples include the following:

- clenbuterol
- Deprenyl
- creatine
- bicarbonate
- Mesocarb/Sydnocarb
- Zeranol

Clenbuterol, a β_2-receptor agonist commonly used to treat asthma in Europe but not approved for medical use in the United States as of this writing, has been shown in animal studies to increase skeletal muscle mass and reduce body fat (Maltin et al., 1987; Satchell, 1996). Widespread abuse of this drug by athletes, including reported positives in the 1992 Barcelona Olympic Games

(Segura et al., 1995), has kept it on most banned lists. A mass spectroscopic method for the detection of clenbuterol and analogs, which also can be used as a confirmation assay, has appeared (Doerge et al., 1995). The labs can detect usage of the drug, but since it is used at very low dosage, and during training prior to competition, it is not known whether usage of the drug has been totally deterred.

The monoamine oxidase inhibitor Deprenyl was approved for use in the United States for Parkinson's disease in 1990 and is abused by athletes for its stimulation effects. However, this drug is converted to methamphetamine and amphetamine in humans, so an athlete taking this drug could be convicted of methamphetamine/amphetamine use (Heinonen, 1994) or for use of the parent drug, which has also been banned by name (Selegiline; IOC, 2001).

Creatine supplementation is claimed to be effective for enhancing the energy supply to muscles and for the recovery of muscle action (Volek and Kraemer, 1996). Creatine is a simple nitrogenous compound that is found in most meat at about 0.5% by weight, and is also made in the body. Creatine is directly involved in maintaining the supply of energy, is rapidly depleted during strenuous exercise, and is involved in energy output/maintenance in muscle tissue. Potential control of abuse is fraught with difficulties because of the normal endogenous level variations. Creatine does not currently appear on any banned list, and so may be used without any risk of penalty as of this date.

Sodium bicarbonate has been used for enhancement of training and prolonging exercise levels (Webster et al., 1993). The mechanism of action is probably neutralization of excess lactate in muscle tissue as exercise and strenuous activity are continued. There is no hope of ever controlling bicarbonate abuse, because large amounts exist in both the diet and the body. An analytical method that would isolate bicarbonate from myriad other inorganic ions naturally present in the body would be difficult at best. Sodium bicarbonate is not currently a banned drug in any sport federation.

Sydnocarb (Mesocarb) is a polar derivative of amphetamine and is classed as a psychostimulant (Breidbach, Sigmund, and Donike, 1995). Its use would confer an advantage in sports in which short-term stimulation would be useful. Because of its polar structure as well as its instability under some conditions of laboratory analysis, Mesocarb is poorly detected by some screening procedures. Recent papers demonstrate how to detect the drug by standard methods in order to enforce a ban on its usage by athletes (Thieme et al., 1995; DeBoer, Ooijen, and Maes, 1995).

Zeranol is a nonsteroid but potent anabolic agent commonly used to fatten cattle (Roche and Davis, 1972).

The USOC has banned Zeranol because of its anabolic activity. When an athlete consumes beef that contains Zeranol, low levels of the drug could be detected. Because Zeranol has no structural similarity to any other AS and is not chemically a steroid, the legal issues of a positive case are unclear.

Consumption of Animals Treated With Banned Drugs

The drugs listed in figure 27.5 have been found in urine samples taken from people who have consumed meat from animals treated with those same drugs. Thus, it is possible to have a "false-positive" drug test in these situations when the individual did not take a drug to enhance performance, but only consumed a meal; in fact, the person did not even know that he had been exposed to the drug at all!

Use of Contaminated Food Supplements

There has been a flurry of recent positive cases of the "use" of the anabolic steroid nandrolone (Masse et al. 1985). It is widely known among athletes that use of nandrolone is not wise, given that the drug is very easy to detect and is not eliminated from the body for a very long time. A logical explanation for this large increase in nandrolone positives is that some immediate precursor(s) to nandrolone is/are being consumed unknowingly via some common over-the-counter agents. A large number of studies have appeared to substantiate the possible source(s) of the rise in nandrolone positives, and possibly define what procedures to use to address the phenomenon (Ciardi et al., 1999; Eendo et al., 1999; Mareck et al., 1999; Lebizek et al., 2000). Evidence that this is the probable explanation has appeared in studies showing that ingestion of norandrostenedione can yield a nandrolone-positive test (Uralets and Gillette, 1999, 2000). In addition, work has appeared showing that commercial androstenedione frequently contains trace levels of a compound that yields a nandrolone-positive drug test (Catlin et al., 2000).

Miscellaneous Drugs

Some drugs may often be used in sport either on purpose or inadvertently. The following are some examples:

Caffeine

Androstenedione

Norandrostenedione

DHEA

Plasma expanders

Caffeine is present in coffee, tea, chocolate, many sodas, and other drinks and is therefore controlled only above a high urinary level, which is very difficult to reach. The valid rationale is that only large levels obviously taken for the stimulation side effects should be punished, not any inadvertent use of one of the most common agents in the world's diets. A recent review of the use of caffeine in sport has treated the subject in depth (Sinclair and Geiger, 2000). It is quite rare that a caffeine positive is reported, so use of the drug does not appear to be a large problem in athletics.

The use of androstenedione increased worldwide after the announcement that the baseball athlete Mark McGwire had use the drug (legal in baseball) while breaking the world's home run record. Work has recently appeared to show that androstenedione consumption may increase T levels (Uralets and Gillette, 1999, 2000; Leder et al., 2000), and, as mentioned earlier, that it has the potential of producing a nandrolone positive due to contamination (Catlin et al., 2000).

The use of DHEA, a steroid, has been increasing in recent years because of its heavily promoted anti-aging effects. Evidence has begun to appear that use of this steroid may increase T levels in either men (Bosy, Moore, and Poklis, 1998; Bowers, 1999) or women (Garde et al., 2000). It also was reported that DHEA usage affects the steroid profile data obtained in the AS screening test (Dehennin et al., 1998). It is becoming quite clear that an athlete must exercise considerable care in determining what he consumes.

In order to potentially increase the oxygen-carrying capacity of the blood, athletes have recently resorted to ingesting plasma expanders, compounds intended to enlarge their oxygen transport. Reports of the abuse of certain perfluorocarbon mixtures (Freons, or PFCs) and hydroxyethyl starch (HES) have resulted in media reports of in-progress test development in order to catch abuse in the future (PFC—see Mathurin et al., 2000; HES—see Thevis, Opfermann, and Schaenzer, 2000). No criteria of abuse or conviction criteria have as yet appeared.

Clenbuterol

Clostebol

Methenolone

Nandrolone

Trenbolone

Zeranol

Figure 27.5 Banned drugs used in animals raised for food.

Future Directions in Drug Testing

Improvements in current tests and new method development will direct much of the laboratory's research efforts.

• **New developments in drug testing may make the process cheaper, faster, and more reliable.** On the other hand, it's also likely that new drugs will be developed that escape detection. The introduction of (a) high-resolution MS-MS analysis (Thieme et al., 1998), (b) LC-MS-MS assays for unstable compounds and polypeptide hormones (Thieme et al., 1998), and (c) isotope ratio combustion MS analysis for use in the T/E assay (Aguilera et al., 2001) will make the testing process more expensive, slower, and more difficult. These instruments and associated assays are considerably more complicated than those used now and will require more staff, further training, and greatly increased overhead costs in a testing lab. In addition, use of other more expensive MS techniques may be examined, but costs will be prohibitive for some time to come (Choi et al., 2001).

• **Confirmation assays are under development for hCG (Laidler et al., 1995), GnRH, hGH, EPO, and other abusable natural products. In addition, there have been press reports that a test for EPO is at hand.** Some federations have used the hemocrit as an indicator of EPO abuse; for example, above 50%, the athlete is simply prohibited from competing, without any punitive action taken. The use of an indirect test such as the hemocrit for "proof" of drug use would not appear to be legally sound, at least in the United States. Recent press has had a flurry of reports of EPO abuse, test development, and captured drug supplies at border crossings between countries. Although a combination test for EPO was reported to be in place for the 2000 Sydney Summer Olympic Games, derived from the combination of a dual serum-based test developed in Australia (Parisotto et al., 2000, 2001) and a urine-based test developed in France (Lasne and Ceaurriz, 2000), no positives were reported for the 2000 Games. Recent articles have reported evaluation of many test methods for EPO (Bialag, Bredbach, and Schaenzer, 2000; Bonfichi, et al., 2000; Breymann, 2000; Ekblom, 2000), and comments from all may be summarized as follows: no good method exists, the methods are unreliable, and there are false positives. Regardless of the current state of the art, frequent press reports state that the IOC will shortly announce a validated test and/or that a test is now ready. Validation of any complicated analytical lab assay, especially for an endogenous hormone, does not consist of holding a meeting claiming validity and announcing same. Even claims of the existence of significant data

proving the validity of such a test do not constitute validation. Publication of such data, replication in other laboratories that can prove their agreement with the previously reported analytical criteria, and substantiation of what constitutes illegal supplementation versus normal variation are all mandatory *before* any acceptance of such claims of validity, no matter *who* is claiming it! Although the mass spectrometric technology clearly exists for the assay and detection of these natural polypeptide products today, there is another major component to the valid detection of abuse of these products: namely, what levels constitute abuse and what levels simply reflect "normal" fluctuation of these compounds that are present in all athletes. Thus, the moral, legal, and ethical issues of calling a drug positive for any of these agents are extremely complex and not easy to define. Under current guidelines and sound scientific rationale, MS should be used for all confirmatory procedures, yet only RIA or other immunoassay methods currently are available for these peptide hormones.

• **Athletic federations may allow blood samples to be used for testing purposes.** Although in some cases, blood (plasma) may contain higher concentrations of a drug than urine does, only limited amounts of blood may be taken; much larger amounts of urine are more easily obtainable. This may minimize the potential benefit of blood as the testing matrix. When esters of T are abused, however, they cannot be detected intact in urine but can be detected in plasma or in hair; this will constitute proof of T abuse. This is an important observation; because T esters are not endogenous (produced in the body), detection of an intact T ester constitutes proof of exogenous T supplementation. Thus, the controversy over the use of the T/E ratio will be avoided and the interpretation of the test result will become obvious (the first scientific proof that this technique is feasible has appeared in De la Torre, Segura, and Polettini, 1995; De la Torre et al., 1995; Kintz, Cirimele, and Ludes, 2000). The use of blood or hair as a testing matrix is still questionable, however, as it must receive approval from the international athletic federations of the relevant sports.

• **Hair analysis may be used.** The hair of a drug user does contain many of the drugs taken by that individual, and analysis of older sections of the hair can reliably indicate chronic use. A report has delineated the mechanism of drug incorporation into human hair (Cone, 1996). Recent reviews of clinical analysis of hair samples (Gaillard and Pepin, 1997; Gleixner and Meyer, 1997) show that T and clenbuterol may be found in human hair (Machnik et al., 1999), and stanozolol has been found in the hair of rats treated with stanozolol (Hold et al., 1996). Henderson et al. (1996)) has proven that cocaine and metabolites are excreted into human hair, and it is also reported that the steroids T and DHEA are excreted into hair (Thieme et al., 1999; Kintz et al., 1999; Kintz, Cirimele, and Ludes, 1999; Kintz et al., 2000). Data have been reported showing that intact T esters were excreted into hair (Kintz et al., 1999), demonstrating that hair, like plasma, could be a useful matrix for proving T supplementation without any doubt. A very recent study (Kintz, Cirimele, and Ludes, 2000) has presented data to show that 19-norsteroids are excreted into human hair, including intact nandrolone. Intact nandrolone is not detectable in urine after 24 hr, so the use of hair as the testing matrix may help verify nandrolone usage. A consensus on guidelines for the use of the hair matrix in doping tests was the result of a recent meeting (Sachs and Kintz, 2000). Thus, it appears that research is progressing on what drugs are excreted into hair, as well as on whether hair is a valid sample for athletic drug-testing programs. Many additional data need to be validated on hair as a testing matrix, including such obvious data sets as the effects of certain dye and shampoo treatments on the drug concentrations over time, bleach or other chemical treatments, and so on.

Conclusion

In order for drug testing to become more effective as a deterrent, protect the athlete's health, and also promote fairness in competition, it must become more widespread and must include more unannounced (out of competition) testing. If athletes know that no one will escape detection for drug abuse with all competitors facing the same uniformly enforced sanctions for use of drugs, most abuse will cease. Athletes are afraid of being at a disadvantage by not using certain performance-enhancing agents because they believe that a majority of their competitors do use performance-enhancing agents.

Sanctions against athletes must be more fairly and uniformly applied. This means that athletes should not be automatically punished in all cases in which their sample shows the presence of a drug, as there are circumstances in which reasons other than drug abuse explain the presence of the drug. In other words, it does matter how the agent got into the athlete's body! Circumstances of drug abuse conviction must always be based on scientific facts, and not on politics, quotas, or other irrelevant criteria. Besides the actual test results, which are almost never in error, at least in IOC labs, scientific facts that should decide a positive drug case include, but are not limited to, any evidence of sabotage, fluctuation of T/E levels as happens due to female hormonal cycle variance (Engelke, Geyer, and Donike, 1995; Engelke, Flenker, and Donike, 1996), genetic evidence of endocrine disease, sample history, conditions

during preparation for testing, and chain of custody. In addition, any positive case showing very low levels of a drug coupled with a normal steroid profile, which indicates no chronic drug use, should not be called positive, since it has been shown that nandrolone metabolites may be generated from the use of some birth control medications (Reznik et al., 1987); boldenone and metabolites have been found in totally naive people who have never taken either boldenone or any steroid (Schaenzer et al., 1995); and several AS metabolites have been found in people who have consumed animals that were treated with the steroids as fattening agents during the raising of the animal (Debruyckere, deSagher, and Peteghem, 1992, 1995; Kicman et al., 1994; Hemmersbach et al., 1995). In addition, pretest consumption of alcohol, incorrect storage of the urine sample, or use of certain specific deconjugation enzymes during sample preparation (Geyer et al., 1996) can artificially raise a T/E ratio and create a false-positive T sample. It should be remembered that a publicly announced positive drug test will ruin the athlete's career, so that when there is *any* doubt about a result, or its interpretation, such a "positive test result" should be considered negative!

The monetary implications and political overtones associated with a drug positive found in an elite or famous athlete are too great to predict anything other than controversy and protracted legal challenges in many cases. Unannounced out-of-competition testing may improve any drug control program's effectiveness, but universal application of such an approach will be difficult to implement worldwide.

References

Aguilera, R., Becchi, M., Grenot, C., Casabianca, H., and Hatton, C.K. (1996a). Detection of testosterone misuse: comparison of two chromatographic sample preparation methods for gas chromatographic-combustion/isotope ratio mass spectrometric analysis. Journal of Chromatography Biomedical Applications, 687(1): 53-54.

Aguilera, R., Becchi, M., Grenot, C., Casabianca, H., Hatton, C.K., Catlin, D.H., Starcevic, B., and Pope, H.G. (1996b). Improved method of detection of testosterone abuse by gas chromatography/combustion/isotope ratio mass spectrometry analysis of urinary steroids. Journal of Mass Spectrometry, 31: 169-176.

Aguilera, R., Chapman, T.E., Starcevic, B., Hatton, C.K., and Catlin, D.H. (2001). Performance characteristics of a carbon isotope ratio method for detecting doping with testosterone based on urine diols: controls and athletes with elevated testosterone/epitestosterone ratios. Clinical Chemistry, 47: 292-300.

Baba, S., Shinohara, Y., and Kasuya, Y. (1980). Differentiation between endogenous and exogenous testosterone in human plasma and urine after oral administration of deuterium-labeled testosterone by mass fragmentography. Journal of Clinical Endocrinology and Metabolism, 50(5): 889-894.

Bamberger, M., and Yaeger, D. (1997). Bigger, stronger, faster. Sports Illustrated, 14 April, 62-70.

Beckett, A.H., Tucker, G.T., and Moffat, A.C. (1967). Routine detection and identification in urine of stimulants and other drugs, some of which may be used to modify performance in sport. Journal of Pharmacy and Pharmacology, 19: 273-294.

Bertrand, M., Masse, R., and Dugal, R. (1978). GC-MS: approach for the detection and characterization of anabolic steroids and their metabolites in biological fluids at major international sporting events. Farmaceutische Tijdschrift Voor Belgie, 55(3): 85-101.

Bhasin, S., Storer, T.W., Berman, N., Callegari, C., Clevenger, B., Phillips, J., Bunnell, N., Tricker, R., Shirazi, A., and Casaburi, R. (1996). The effects of supraphysiologic doses of testosterone on muscle size and strength in normal men. New England Journal of Medicine, 335(1): 1-7.

Bialag, B., Bredbach, A., and Schaenzer, W. (2000). Indicated reference ranges for serum EPO, part II. In Schaenzer, W., Geyer, H., Gotzmann, A., and Engelke, U., eds., Recent Advances in Doping Analysis 7: Proceedings of the 17th Cologne Workshop on Dope Analysis, pp. 301-310, Sport and Buch Strauss, Cologne.

Bonfichi, M., Baldwin, A., Arcaini, L., Lorenzi, A., Marseglia, C., Malcozati, L., Bernardi, L., Passino, C., Spadacini, G., Feil, P., Keyl, C., Schneider, A., Bolardi, A., Bandinelli, G., Greene, R.E., and Beanasconi, C. (2000). Haematological modifications after acute exposure to high altitude; possible implications for detection of recombinant EPO misuse. British Journal of Haematology, 109: 895-896.

Bosy, T.Z., Moore, K.A., and Poklis, A. (1998). The effect of oral dehydroepiandrosterone (DHEA) on the urine testosterone/epitestosterone (T/E) ratio in human male volunteers. Journal of Analytical Toxicology, 22: 455-459.

Bowers, L.D. (1999). Oral dehydroepiandrosterone supplementation can increase the testosterone/ epitestosterone ratio. Clinical Chemistry, 45: 295-297.

Bradley, C.A., and Sodeman, T.M. (1990). Human growth hormone; its use and abuse. Clinics in Laboratory Medicine, 10(3): 473-477.

Breymann, C. (2000). EPO test methods. Bailliere's Clinical Endocrinology and Metabolism, 14(1): 135-145.

Breidbach, A., Sigmund, G., and Donike, M. (1995). Combination of screening procedures—mesocarb detection as an example. In Donike, M., Geyer, H., Gotzmann, A., and Mareck-Engelke, U., eds., Recent Advances in Doping Analysis 2: Proceedings of the 12th Cologne Workshop on Dope Analysis, pp. 301-304, Sport and Buch Strauss, Cologne.

Brooks, R.V., Firth, R.G., and Sumner, N.A. (1975). Detection of anabolic steroids by radioimmunoassay. British Journal of Sports Medicine, 9: 89-92.

Brooks, R.V., Jeremiah, G., Webb, W.A., and Wheeler, M. (1979). Detection of anabolic administration to athletes. Journal of Steroid Biochemistry, 11: 913-917.

Carlstroem, K., Palonek, E., Garle, M., Oftebro, H., Stanghelle, J., and Bjoerkhem, I. (1992). Detection of testosterone administration by increased ratio between serum concentrations of testosterone and 17α-hydroxyprogesterone. Clinical Chemistry, 36: 1779-1784.

Catlin, D.H., Hatton, C.K., and Starcevic, S.H. (1997). Issues in detecting abuse of xenobiotic anabolic steroids and testosterone by analysis of athletes' urine. Clinical Chemistry, 43: 1280-1288.

Catlin, D.H., Kammerer, R.C., Hatton, C.K., Sekera, M.H., and Merdink, J.L. (1987). Analytical chemistry at the games of the XXIIIrd Olympiad in Los Angeles, 1984. Clinical Chemistry, 33(2): 319-327.

Catlin, D.H., Leder, B.Z., Ahrens, B., Starcevic, B., Hatton, C.K., Green, G.A., and Finkelstein, J.S. (2000). Trace contamination of over-the-counter androstenedione and positive urine test results for a nandrolone metabolite. Journal of the American Medical Association, 284: 2618-2621.

Choi, B.K., Hercules, D.M., Zhang, T., and Gusev, A.I. (2001). Comparison of quadrupole, time-of-flight and Fourier transform mass analyzers, for LC-MS applications. LC-GC, 19(3): 514-524.

Ciardi, M., Ciccoli, R., Barbarulo, M.V., and Nicoletti, R. (1999). Presence of norandrosterone in "normal" urine samples. In Schaenzer, W., Geyer, H., Gotzmann, A., and Mareck-Engelke, U., eds., Recent Advances in Doping Analysis 6: Proceedings of the 16th Cologne Workshop on Dope Analysis, pp. 97-104, Sport and Buch Strauss, Cologne.

Chung, B.C., Choo, H.Y.P., Kim, J.W., Eom, K.D., Kwon, O.S., Suh, J., Yang, J.S., and Park, J.S. (1990). Analysis of anabolic steroids using GC/MS with selected ion monitoring. Journal of Analytical Toxicology, 14: 91-95.

Cone, E.J. (1996). Mechanisms of drug incorporation into hair. Therapeutic Drug Monitoring, 18: 438-443.

Conn, P.M., and Crowley, W.F. (1994). Gonadotropin-releasing hormone and its analogs. Annual Reviews of Medicine, 45: 391-405.

Coutts, S.B., Kicman, A.T., Hurst, DT., and Cowan, D.A. (1997). Intramuscular administration of 5α-dihydrotestosterone heptanoate: changes in urinary hormone profile. Clinical Chemistry, 43(11): 2091-2098.

Cowan, D.A., Kicman, A.T., Walker, C.J., and Wheeler, M.J. (1991). Effect of administration of human chorionic gonadotrophin on criteria used to assess testosterone administration in athletes. Journal of Endocrinology, 131: 147-154.

DeBoer, D., Ooijen, R.D.V., and Maes, R.A.A. (1995). Thermostable derivatives of mesocarb and its p-hydroxy-metabolite. In Donike, M., Geyer, H., Gotzmann, A., and Mareck-Engelke, U., eds., Recent Advances in Doping Analysis 2: Proceedings of the 12th Cologne Workshop on Dope Analysis, pp. 305-316, Sport and Buch Strauss, Cologne.

Debruyckere, G., deSagher, R., and Peteghem, C.V. (1992). Clostebol positive urine after consumption of contaminated meat. Clinical Chemistry, 38: 1869-1873.

Debruyckere, G., deSagher, R., and Peteghem, C.V. (1995). Detection of interferences in urinary anabolic steroid analysis. In Donike, M., Geyer, H., Gotzmann, A., and Mareck-Engelke, U., eds., Recent Advances in Doping Analysis 2: Proceedings of the 12th Cologne Workshop on Dope Analysis, pp. 173-184, Sport and Buch Strauss, Cologne.

Dehennin, L. (1994). Detection of simultaneous self-administration of testosterone and epitestosterone in healthy men. Clinical Chemistry, 40: 106-109.

Dehennin, L., Ferry, M., Lafarge, P., Peres, G., and Lafarge, J.P. (1998). Oral administration of dehydroepiandrosterone to healthy men: alteration of the urinary androgen profile and consequences for the detection of abuse in sport by gas chromatography-mass spectrometry. Steroids, 63: 80-87.

Dehennin, L., and Matsumoto, A.M. (1993). Long-term administration of testosterone enanthate to normal men: alterations of the urinary profile of androgen metabolites potentially useful for detection of testosterone misuse in sport. Journal of Steroid Biochemistry and Molecular Biology, 44: 179-189.

De la Torre, R., Segura, J., and Polettini, A. (1995). Detection of testosterone esters in human plasma by GC/MS and GC/MS/MS. In Donike, M., Geyer, H., Gotzmann, A., and Mareck-Engelke, U., eds., Proceedings of the 12th Cologne Workshop on Dope Analysis, pp. 59-80, Sport and Buch Strauss, Cologne.

De la Torre, R., Segura, J., Polettini, A., and Montagna, M. (1995). Detection of testosterone esters in human plasma. Journal of Mass Spectrometry, 30: 1393-1404.

Doerge, D.R., Bajic, S., Blankenship, L.R., Preece, S.W., and Churchwell, M.I. (1995). Determination of β-agonist residues in human plasma using liquid chromatography/atmospheric pressure chemical ionization mass spectrometry and tandem mass spectrometry. Journal of Mass Spectrometry, 30, 911-916.

Donike, M. (1976). The detection of doping agents in blood. British Journal of Sports Medicine, 10(3): 147-154.

Donike, M., Bärwald, K.R., Kostermann, K., Schaenzer, W., and Zimmermann, J. (1983). The detection of exogenous testosterone. In H. Heck, W. Hollmann, H. Liesen, and R. Rost. eds., Sport: Leistung und Gesundheit, pp. 293-298. Cologne: Deutscher Arzte-Verlag.

Donike, M., and Stratmann, D. (1974). Temperature programmed gas-chromatographic analysis of nitrogen containing drugs. Reproducibility of retention times and sample sizes by automatic injection (II). The screening procedure for volatile drugs at the 20th Olympic Games, Munich, 1972. Chromatographia, 7(4): 182-189.

Donike, M., Ueki, M., Koroda, Y., Geyer, H., Nolteemsting, E., and Rauth, S. (1995). Detection of dihydrotestosterone (DHT) doping: alterations in the steroid profile and reference ranges for DHT and its 5α-metabolites. Journal of Sports Medicine and Physical Fitness, 35: 235-250.

Eendo, P.V., Delbeke, F.T., Dejong, F.H., and Debacker, P. (1999). Urinary metabolism of endogenous nandrolone in women. A case study. In Schaenzer, W., Geyer, H., Gotzmann, A., and Mareck-Engelke, U., eds., Recent Advances in Doping Analysis 6: Proceedings of the 16th Cologne Workshop on Dope Analysis, pp. 105-118, Sport and Buch Strauss, Cologne.

Ekblom, B. (1996). Blood doping and erythropoietin. American Journal of Sports Medicine, 24(6): S40-S42.

Ekblom, B.T. (2000). Blood boosting and sport. Bailliere's Clinical Endocrinology and Metabolism, 14(1): 89-98.

Engelke, U.M., Flenker, U., and Donike, M. (1996). Stability of steroid profiles (5): the annual rhythm of urinary ratios and excretion rates of endogenous steroids in female and its menstrual dependency. In Donike, M., Geyer, H., Gotzmann, A., and Mareck-Engelke, U., eds., Proceedings of the 13th Cologne Workshop on Dope Analysis, pp. 177-190, Sport and Buch Strauss, Cologne.

Engelke, U.M., Geyer, H. and Donike, M. (1995). Stability of steroid profiles (4): ratios and excretion rates of endogenous steroids in female urine collected four times over 24 hours. In Donike, M., Geyer, H., Gotzmann, A., and Mareck-Engelke, U., eds., Proceedings of the 12th Cologne Workshop on Dope Analysis, pp. 135-156, Sport and Buch Strauss, Cologne.

Falk, O., Palonek, E., and Bjoerkhem, I. (1988). Effect of ethanol on the ratio between testosterone and epitestosterone in urine. Clinical Chemistry, 32: 1462-1464.

Franke, W.W., and Berendonk, B. (1997). Hormonal doping and androgenization of athletes: a secret program of the German Democratic Republic government. Clinical Chemistry, 43: 1262-1279.

Gaillard, Y., and Pepin, G. (1997). Hair testing for pharmaceuticals and drugs of abuse: forensic and clinical applications. American Clinical Laboratory, October, pp. 18-22.

Garde, A.H., Hansen, A.M., Skovgaard, L.T., and Christensen, J.M. (2000). Seasonal and biological variation of blood concentrations of total cholesterol, dehydroepiandrosterone sulfate, hemoglobin A_{1c}, IgA, prolactin, and free testosterone in healthy women. Clinical Chemistry, 46: 551-559.

Garle, M., Ocka, R., Palonek, E., and Bjoerkhem, I. (1996). Increased urinary testosterone/epitestosterone ratios found in Swedish athletes in connection with a national control program. Evaluation of 28 cases. Journal of Chromatography Biomedical Applications, 687(1): 55-60.

Gleixner, A., and Meyer, H.H.D. (1997). Methods to detect anabolics in hair: use for food hygiene and doping control. American Laboratory, December, 44-47.

Geyer, H., Schaenzer, W., Mareck-Engelke, U., and Donike, M. (1996). Factors influencing the steroid profile. In Donike, M., Geyer, H., Gotzmann, A., and Mareck-Engelke, U., eds., Proceedings of the 13th Cologne Workshop on Dope Analysis, pp. 95-114, Sport and Buch Strauss, Cologne.

Haning, R.V. Jr., Flood, C.A., Hackett, R.J., Loughlin, J.S., McClure, N., and Longcope, C. (1991). Metabolic clearance rate of dehydroepiandrosterone sulfate, its metabolism to testosterone, and its intrafollicular metabolism to dehydroepiandrosterone, androstenedione, testosterone, and dihydrotestosterone in vivo. Journal of Clinical Endocrinology and Metabolism, 72(5): 1088-1095.

Haning, R.V. Jr., Hackett, R.J., Flood, C.A., Loughlin, J.S., Zhao, Q.Y., and Longcope, C. (1993). Plasma dehydroepiandrosterone sulfate serves as a prehormone for 48% of follicular fluid testosterone during treatment with mentropins. Journal of Clinical Endocrinology and Metabolism, 76(5): 1301-1307.

Heinonen, E.H. (1994). Pharmacokinetic aspects of l-deprenyl (selegiline) and its metabolites. Clinical Pharmacology and Therapeutics, 56: 742-749.

Hemmersbach, P., Tomten, S., Nilsson, S., Oftebro, H., Havrevoll, O., Oen, B., and Birkeland, K. (1995). Illegal use of anabolic agents in animal fattening-consequences for doping analysis. In Donike, M., Geyer, H., Gotzmann, A., and Mareck-Engelke, U., eds., Proceedings of the 12th Cologne Workshop on Dope Analysis, pp. 185-192, Sport and Buch Strauss, Cologne.

Henderson, G.L., Harkey, M.L., Zhou, C.H., Jones, R.T., and Jacob, P. (1996). Incorporation of isotopically labeled cocaine and metabolites into human hair. 1. Dose-response relationships. Journal of Analytical Toxicology, 20: 1-12.

Hoberman, J.M., and Yesalis, C.E. (1995). The history of synthetic testosterone. Scientific American, February, 60-65.

Hold, K.M., Wilkins, D.G., Crouch, D.J., Rollins, D.E., and Maes, R.A. (1996). Detection of stanozolol in hair by negative ion chemical ionization mass spectrometry. Journal of Analytical Toxicology, 20(10): 345-349.

Horning, S., and Schaenzer, W. (1997a). Basics of high resolution mass spectrometry (HRMS). In Schaenzer, W., Geyer, H., Gotzmann, A., and Mareck-Engelke, U., eds., Recent Advances in Doping Analysis 4: Proceedings of the 14th Cologne Workshop on Dope Analysis, pp. 253-260, Sport and Buch Strauss, Cologne.

Horning, S., and Schaenzer, W. (1997b). Steroid screening using GC/HRMS. In Schaenzer, W., Geyer, H., Gotzmann, A., and Mareck-Engelke, U., eds., Recent Advances in Doping Analysis 4: Proceedings of the 14th Cologne Workshop on Dope Analysis, pp. 261-270, Sport and Buch Strauss, Cologne.

Horning, S., Schaenzer, W., and Sample, B. (1998). HRMS analysis performed at the 1996 Summer Olympic Games. In Schaenzer, W., Geyer, H., Gotzmann, A., and Mareck-Engelke, U., eds., Recent Advances in Doping Analysis 5: Proceedings of the 15th Cologne Workshop on Dope Analysis, pp. 329-337, Sport and Buch Strauss, Cologne.

IOC (International Olympic Committee). (2001). Prohibited classes of substances and methods, Lausanne, Switzerland, 1 September.

Jacobs, J.B., and Samuels, B. (1995). The drug testing project in international sports: dilemmas in an expanding regulatory regime. Hastings International and Comparative Law Review, 18(3): 557-589.

Karila, T., Kosunen, V., Leinonen, A., Taehtelae, R., and Seppaelae, T. (1996). High doses of alcohol increase testosterone-to-epitestosterone ratio in females. Journal of Chromatography Biomedical Applications, 687(1): 109-116.

Kerrigan, S., and Phillips, W.H. (2001). Comparison of ELISAs for opiates, methamphetamine, cocaine metabolite, benzodiazepines, phencyclidine and cannabinoids in whole blood and urine. Clinical Chemistry, 47: 540-547.

Kicman, A.T., Brooks, R.V., Collyer, S.C., Cowan, D.A., Nanjee, M.N., Southan, G.J., and Wheeler, M.J. (1990). Criteria to indicate testosterone administration. British Journal of Sports Medicine, 24: 253-264.

Kicman, A.T., Coutts, S.B., Walker, C.J., and Cowan, D.A. (1995). Proposed confirmatory procedure for detecting 5α-dihydrotestosterone doping in male athletes. Clinical Chemistry, 41(11): 1617-1627.

Kicman, A.T., Cowan, D.A., Myhre, L., Nilsson, S., Oftebro, H., Havrevoll, O., Oen, B., and Birkeland, K. (1994). Effect on sports drug tests of ingesting meat from steroid (methenolone)-treated livestock. Clinical Chemistry, 40: 2084-2087.

Kintz, P., Cirimele, V., Deveaux, M., and Ludes, B. (2000). Dehydroepiandrosterone (DHEA) and testerone concentrations in human hair after chronic DHEA supplementation. Clinical Chemistry, 46: 414-415.

Kintz, P., Cirimele, V., Jeanneau, T., and Ludes, B. (1999). Identification of testosterone and testosterone esters in human hair. Journal of Analytical Toxicology, 23: 352-356.

Kintz, P., Cirimele, V., and Ludes, B. (1999). Physiological concentrations of DHEA in human hair. Journal of Analytical Toxicology, 23: 424-428.

Kintz, P., Cirimele, V., and Ludes, B. (2000). Discrimination of the nature of doping with 19-norsteroids through hair analysis. Clinical Chemistry, 46: 2020-2022.

Laidler, P., Cowan, D.A., Hider, R.C., Keane, A., and Kicman, A.T. (1995). Tryptic mapping of human chorionic gonadotropin by matrix-assisted laser desorption/ionization mass spectrometry. Rapid Communications in Mass Spectrometry, 9: 1021-1026.

Lasne, L., and Ceaurriz, J. (2000). EPO testing. Nature, 405: 635.

Lebizec, C., Gaudin, I., Pohu, A., Monteau, F., and Andre, F. (2000). Identification of endogenous 19-norandrosterone in human urine. In Schaenzer, W., Geyer, H., Gotzmann, A., and Engelke, U., eds., Recent Advances in Doping Analysis 7: Proceedings of the 17th Cologne Workshop on Dope Analysis, pp. 109-122, Sport and Buch Strauss, Cologne.

Leder, B.Z., Longcope, C., Catlin, D.H., Ahrens, B., Schoenfeld, D.A., and Finkelstein, J.S. (2000). Oral androstenedione administration and serum testosterone concentrations in young men. Journal of the American Medical Association, 283: 779-782.

Leith, W. (1991). Cyclists don't die like this. The Independent on Sunday, 14 July, 3-4.

Liu, C., and Bowers, L.D. (1995). Studies towards confirmation of HCG using HPLC/MS. In Donike, M., Geyer, H., Gotzmann, A., and Mareck-Engelke, U., eds., Recent Advances in Doping Analysis 2: Proceedings of the 12th Cologne Workshop on Dope Analysis, pp. 235-242, Sport and Buch Strauss, Cologne.

Liu, C., and Bowers, L.D. (1996). Immunoaffinity trapping of urinary human chorionic gonadotropin and its high-performance liquid chromatographic-mass spectrometric confirmation. Journal of Chromatography Biomedical Applications, 687(1): 213-220.

Liu, C., and Bowers, L.D. (1997). Mass spectrometric characterization of the β-subunit of human chorionic gonadotropin. Journal of Mass Spectrometry, 32: 33-42.

Machnik, M., Geyer, H., Horning, S., Breidbach, A., Delahaut, P., and Schaenzer, W. (1999). Long term detection of clenbuterol in human scalp hair. In Schaenzer, W., Geyer, H., Gotzmann, A., and Mareck-Engelke, U., eds., Recent Advances in Doping Analysis 6: Proceedings of the 16th Cologne Workshop on Dope Analysis, pp. 31-37, Sport and Buch Strauss, Cologne.

Maltin, C., Delday, M., Hay, S., Smith, F., Lobley, G., and Reeds, P. (1987). The effect of the anabolic agent, clenbuterol, on the overloaded rat skeletal muscle. Bioscience Reports, 7: 143-148.

Mareck-Engelke, U., Geyer, H., and Schaenzer, W. (1999). 19-Norandrosterone: criteria for the decision making process. In Schaenzer, W., Geyer, H., Gotzmann, A., and Mareck-Engelke, U., eds., Recent Advances in Doping Analysis 6: Proceedings of the 16th Cologne Workshop on Dope Analysis, pp. 119-130, Sport and Buch Strauss, Cologne.

Masse, R., Laliberte, C., Tremblay, L., and Dugal, R. (1985). Gas chromatographic/mass spectrometric analysis of 19-nortestosterone urinary metabolites in man. Biomedical Mass Spectrometry, 12(3): 115.

Mathurin, J.C., Ceaurriz, J.D., Sicant, M.T., Marion, B., Audran, M., and Krafft, M.P. (2000). Development of an analytical strategy for detection of PFC's for anti-doping control: analysis of breath and blood samples after IV injection of PFC emulsions in rats. In Schaenzer, W., Geyer, H., Gotzmann, A., and Engelke, U., eds., Recent Advances in Doping Analysis 7: Proceedings of the 17th Cologne Workshop on Dope Analysis, pp. 21-30, Sport and Buch Strauss, Cologne.

Meikle, A.W., Arver, S., Dobs, A.S., Sanders, S.W., Rajaram, L., and Mazar, N.A. (1996). Pharmacokinetics and metabolism of a permeation-enhanced testosterone transdermal system in hypogonadal men: influence of application site—a clinical research center study. Journal of Clinical Endocrinology and Metabolism, 81: 1832-1840.

Meikle, A.W., Mazer, N.A., Moellmer, J.F., Stringham, J.D., Tolman, K.G., Sanders, S.W., and Odell, W.D. (1992). Enhanced transdermal delivery of testosterone across nonscrotal skin produces physiological concentrations of testosterone and its metabolites in hypogonadal men. Journal of Clinical Endocrinology and Metabolism, 74(3): 623-628.

Meilman, P.W., Crace, R.K., Presley, C.A., and Lyerla, R. (1995). Beyond performance enhancement; polypharmacy among collegiate users of steroids. Journal of the American College of Health, 44: 98-104.

Norli, H., Esbensen, K., Westad, F., Birkeland, K.I., and Hemmersbach, P. (1995). Chemometric evaluation of urinary steroid profiles in doping control. Journal of Steroid Biochemistry and Molecular Biology, 54(1-2): 83-88.

Oftebro, H. (1992). Evaluating an abnormal urinary steroid profile. Lancet, 359: 941-942.

Oftebro, H., Jensen, J., Mowinckel, P., and Norli, H.R. (1994). Establishing a ketoconazole suppression test for verifying testosterone administration in the doping control of athletes. Journal of Clinical Endocrinology and Metabolism, 78: 973-977.

Palonek, E., Gottlieb, C., Garle, M., Bjoerkhem, I., and Carlstroem, K. (1995). Serum and urinary markers of exogenous testosterone administration. Journal of Steroid Biochemistry and Molecular Biology, 55(1): 121-127.

Papadakis, M.A., Grady, D., Black, D., Tierney, M.J., Gooding, G.A.W., Schambelan, M., and Grunfeld, C. (1996). Growth hormone replacement in healthy older men improves body composition but not functional ability. Annals of Internal Medicine, 124: 708-716.

Parisotto, R., Gore, C.J., Hahn, A.G., Ashenden, M.J., Olds, T.S., Martin, D.T., Pyne, D.B., Gawthorn, K., and Brugnara, C. (2000). Reticulocyte parameters as potential discriminators of recombinant human erythropoietin abuse in elite athletes. International Journal of Sports Medicine, 21: 471-479.

Parisotto, R., Wu, M., Ashenden, M.J., Emslie, K.R., Gore, C.J., Howe, C., Kazlauskas, R., Sharpe, K., Trout, G.J., Xie, M., and Hahn, A.G. (2001). Detection of recombinant human EPO abuse in athletes utilizing monitors of altered erythropoiesis. Haematologica, 86: 128-137.

Park, J.S., Park, S., Lho, D.S., Choo, H.P., Chung, B., Yoon, C., Min, H., and Choi, M.J. (1990). Drug testing at the 10th Asian Games and 24th Seoul Olympic Games. Journal of Analytical Toxicology, 14: 66-72.

Raynaud, E., Audran, M., Brun, J.F., Fedou, C., Chanal, J.L., and Orsetti, A. (1992). False-positive cases in detection of testosterone doping. Lancet, 340: 1468-1469.

Raynaud, E., Audran, M., Pages, J. Ch., Fedou, C., Brun, J.F., Chanal, J.L., and Orsetti, A. (1993). Determination of urinary testosterone and epitestosterone during pubertal development: a cross-sectional study in 141 normal male subjects. Clinical Endocrinology, 38: 353-359.

Reznik, Y., Herrou, M., Dehennin, L., Lemaire, M., and Leymarie, P. (1987). Rising plasma levels of 19-nortestosterone throughout pregnancy: determination by radioimmunoassay and validation by gas chromatography-mass spectrometry. Journal of Clinical Endocrinology and Metabolism, 64(5): 1086-1088.

Roche, T., and Davis, W. (1972). Evaluating growth promoters for beef cattle. Farm and Food Research, 7: 146-148.

Rogozkin, V.A., Morozov, V.I., and Tchaikovsky, V.S. (1979). Rapid radioimmunoassay for anabolic steroids in urine. Schweizerische Zeitschrift für Sport Medizin, 27(4): 169-173.

Sachs, H., and Kintz, P. (2000). Consensus of the Society of Hair Testing on hair testing for doping agents. Forensic Science International, 107: 3.

Satchell, M. (1996). Raising "boxcars" out in the barn. U.S. News and World Report, 18 March, 40-41.

Schaenzer, W., Geyer, H., Gotzmann, A., Horning, S., Mareck-Engelke, U., Nitschke, R., Nolteemsting, E., and Donike, M. (1995). Endogenous production and excretion of boldenone (17β-hydroxyandrosta-1,4-dien-3-one), an androgenic anabolic steroid. In Donike, M., Geyer, H., Gotzmann, A., and Mareck-Engelke, U., eds., Proceedings of the 12th Cologne Workshop on Dope Analysis, pp. 211-212, Sport and Buch Strauss, Cologne.

Segura, J., de la Torre, R., Pascual, J.A., Ventura, R., Farre, M., Ewin, R.R., and Cami, J. (1995). Antidoping control laboratory at the games of the XXV Olympiad Barcelona '92. In Donike, M., Geyer, H., Gotzmann, A., and Mareck-Engelke, U., eds., Recent Advances in Doping Analysis 2: Proceedings of the 12th Cologne Workshop on Dope Analysis, pp. 413-430, Sport and Buch Strauss, Cologne.

Sinclair, C.J.D., and Geiger, J.D. (2000). Caffeine use in sports. Journal of Sports Medicine and Physical Fitness, 40: 71-79.

Sizoi, V.F., Bolotov, S.L., and Semenov, V.A. (1998). Studies of Bromantan metabolites structure. In Schaenzer, W., Geyer, H., Gotzmann, A., and Mareck-Engelke, U., eds., Recent Advances in Doping Analysis 5: Proceedings of the 15th Cologne Workshop on Dope Analysis, pp. 287-300, Sport and Buch Strauss, Cologne.

Southan, G.J., Brooks, R.V., Cowan, D.A., Kicman, A.T., Unnadkat, N., and Walker, C.J. (1992). Possible indices for the detection of the administration of dihydrotestosterone to athletes. Journal of Steroid Biochemistry and Molecular Biology, 42(1): 87-94.

Stenman, U.H., Kallio, L.U., Korhonen, J., and Alfthan, H. (1997). Immunoprocedures for detecting human chorionic gonadotropin: clinical aspects and doping control. Clinical Chemistry, 43(7): 1293-1298.

Thevis, M., Opfermann, G., and Schaenzer, W. (2000). GC-MS detection of HES in human urine In Schaenzer, W., Geyer, H., Gotzmann, A., and Engelke, U., eds., Recent Advances in Doping Analysis 7: Proceedings of the 17th Cologne Workshop on Dope Analysis, pp. 31-40, Sport and Buch Strauss, Cologne.

Thieme, D., Grosse, J., Lang, L., and Mueller, R.K. (1995). Detection of mesocarb metabolite by LC-TS/MS. In Donike, M., Geyer, H., Gotzmann, A., and Mareck-Engelke, U., eds., Recent Advances in Doping Analysis 2: Proceedings of the 12th Cologne Workshop on Dope Analysis, pp. 275-284, Sport and Buch Strauss, Cologne.

Thieme, D.J., Grosse, R., Lang, R., Mueller, R.K., and Wahl, A. (1998). Interpretation of high-resolution and tandem-MS data: two relevant cases of steroid metabolites at pg level in blood and urine. In Schaenzer, W., Geyer, H., Gotzmann, A., and Mareck-Engelke, U., eds., Recent Advances in Doping Analysis 5: Proceedings of the 15th Cologne Workshop on Dope Analysis, pp. 157-168, Sport and Buch Strauss, Cologne.

Thieme, D.J., Grosse, R., and Mueller, R.K. (1996). Application of high-resolution and tandem-MS to the identification of anabolic agents. In Donike, M., Geyer, H., Gotzmann, A., and Mareck-Engelke, U., eds., Proceedings of the 13th Cologne Workshop on Dope Analysis, pp. 285-297, Sport and Buch Strauss, Cologne.

Thieme, D., Grosse, T., Sachs, H., and Mueller, R.K. (1999). Detection of several anabolic steroids of abuse in human hair. In Schaenzer, W., Geyer, H., Gotzmann, A., and Mareck-Engelke, U., eds., Recent Advances in Doping Analysis 6: Proceedings of the 16th Cologne Workshop on Dope Analysis, pp. 9-30, Sport and Buch Strauss, Cologne.

Uralets, V., and Gillette, P.A. (1999). Over-the-counter anabolic steroids. 4-Androsten-3,17-dione; 4-androsten-3β, 17β-diol; and 19-nor-4-androsten-3,17-dione; excretion studies in men. Journal of Analytical Toxicology, 23: 357-366.

Uralets, V., and Gilette, P.A. (2000). Over-the-counter Δ^5 anabolic steroids 5-androsten-3,17-dione; 5-androsten-3β,17β-diol; dehydroepiandrosterone; and 19-nor-5-androsten-3,17-dione excretion studies in men. Journal of Analytical Toxicology, 24: 188-193.

Ventura, R., and Segura, J. (1996). Detection of diuretic agents in doping control. Journal of Chromatography B(1), 687: 127-144.

Volek, J.S., and Kraemer, W.J. (1996). Creatine supplementation: its effect on human muscular performance and body composition. Journal of Strength and Conditioning Research, 10(3): 200-210.

Webster, M.J., Webster, M.N., Crawford, R.E., and Gladden, L.B. (1993). Effect of sodium bicarbonate ingestion on exhaustive resistance exercise performance. Medicine and Science in Sports and Exercise, 25(8): 960-965.

Wide, L., Bengtsson, C., Berglund, B., and Ekblom, B. (1995). Detection in blood and urine of recombinant erythropoietin administered to healthy men. Medicine and Science in Sports and Exercise, 27(11): 1569-1576.

CHAPTER 28

Form Over Substances: The Legal Context of Performance-Enhancing Substances

Charles E. Petit, JD

"[T]o be a great athlete today you need a great coach, a great chemist and a great lawyer."

Bamberger & Yeager, 1997:64

The other chapters in this book discuss many aspects of performance-enhancing substances (PES). The discussion would remain incomplete without consideration of the legal context of PES. The law interacts—as we shall see, often in a self-defeating manner—with the scientific and ethical aspects of PES use.

It would be pleasant to report that one must understand only one set of legal principles, statutes, and results to comprehend the legal context of PES. It would also be untrue. The existing patchwork of inconsistent—and all too often contradictory—treaties, statutes, regulations, and case law creates so many exceptions to general rules one might draw concerning PES regulation that the exceptions swallow the rules. Much of the legal context remains completely speculative, as there is little legal authority on PES abuse other than anabolic steroids. The Sydney Olympics will profoundly affect how the PES "culture" treats, and is treated by, the various legal systems. However, the scope of this effect is difficult to predict and will take years to become clear. Whether *any* existing legal system can handle the issues presented by PES without substantial legislation is in question; whether the legal system *should* do so is even more uncertain. The law is a heavy hammer, but this job may require a saw or screwdriver.

The legal context of PES will continue to change. Government treatment of PES will continue to change, as will the legal response of the international athletic community. Most importantly, the science (and hopefully reliability) of PES testing will continue to advance; simultaneously, new PES or combinations will emerge. Because PES other than steroids have been either rarely used or rarely testable, most of the PES-related law that has been tested concerns anabolic steroids, their precursors, and their metabolites. Anabolic steroids leave direct, known biochemical evidence of their use. At present, testing regimes cannot directly detect other popular PES like erythropoietin (EPO) and human growth hormone (hGH), but must infer their presence through elevated levels of other, marker biochemicals and

functions. This further muddies the already murky waters of PES testing policy and its legal implementation, because it is entirely possible that successful athletes naturally have somewhat elevated levels of some of these supposed markers (Williams, 1998; Jacobs & Samuels, 1995; *cf.* Walsh & Fallain, 2000). This last may well prove a chicken-and-egg issue that undermines any attempt at regulation. Unlike chromosomal "anomalies" in "female" athletes (Senn, 1999), an individual's precise chemical makeup is not accurately testable or evaluable in current or foreseeable medical contexts.

This chapter begins with a short examination of U.S. regulation of PES outside of athletic competition, considering both the privacy issues surrounding drug testing and potential defenses to criminal charges based on intoxication or other diminished capacity due to PES use. Next, the chapter takes a short look at international regulation of PES outside of athletic competition, primarily relating to drug trafficking. This background leads into the most publicized aspect of PES: the consequences of positive test results. Unlike scientific knowledge, legal reasoning must be more consistent with individual circumstances than with abstract principles of "fair play" or "good science," because the legal system necessarily takes a step beyond knowledge and policy to remedy (Deason, 1999, 1998; Benson, 1991). This section examines a few actual examples of legal application of PES policies to see what these trees reveal about the forest of legal PES policy concerning competitive athletes. The last section steps from these retail examples to the wholesale issue of the sources and rationale of legal authority for regulating PES in competition. One major issue that this chapter does *not* cover, except as it provides context for the remainder of the discussion, is the application of the law to PES use and abuse outside the context of competitive athletics. This is an intractable area of law (e.g., Kleinman & Petit, 2000), and excessive consideration of noncompetitive PES use and abuse will mask some of the important issues involved in competitive use. Further, such regulation will necessarily be even more chaotic than in the competitive arena, as there is no organization with the will or authority to impose uniform standards, let alone uniform conduct.

United States Regulation of Performance-Enhancing Substances

Athletes are most immediately, if at all, concerned about the direct consequences to them of PES—that is, getting caught (e.g., Voet, 1999; Francis & Coplon, 1990). The most highly publicized aspect of U.S. law is the struggle over the allowable scope of individualized, suspicionless drug testing. Generally, drug testing in the United States must pass muster under the Fourth Amendment's proscription against unreasonable searches and seizures:

> The right of the people to be secure in their persons, houses, papers, and effects, against unreasonable searches and seizures, shall not be violated, and no Warrants shall issue, but upon probable cause, supported by Oath or affirmation, and particularly describing the place to be searched, and the persons or things to be seized. (U.S. Const. Amd. IV)

These words have created nearly as much U.S. law since 1914 as the remainder of the Constitution combined. Most importantly, contrary to the general perception, the Fourth Amendment is not limited to actions by the police, or to a criminal context (e.g., *Acton,* 1995). In practice, there appears to be a "drug-testing exception" to the Fourth Amendment. Looking closely at the context of the relevant cases, however, indicates that the exception is not quite so clear (see also Kleinman & Petit, 2000).

Drug Testing

The clearest PES-related decision from the Supreme Court of the United States is *Vernonia School District 47J v. Acton,* which directly concerns scholastic and collegiate athletics (*Acton,* 1995). The Supreme Court ruled that a school district's random drug testing of its athletes was constitutional under the Fourth Amendment. As in *Von Raab* and *Skinner,* the Court found that government-compelled urinalysis implicated an individual's privacy interests (*Von Raab,* 1989; *Skinner,* 1989). The Court relied on its earlier decision in *New Jersey v. T.L.O.,* which held that because the urinalysis was conducted in the public school setting, probable cause did not apply: "Fourth Amendment rights are different in public schools than elsewhere; the 'reasonableness' inquiry cannot disregard the schools' custodial and tutelary responsibility for children" (*T.L.O.,* 1985). The continual regulation of public school children—for example, required student vaccinations and physical exams—diminishes their expectations of privacy. The Court found that students, in particular athletes, have diminished expectations of privacy because they subject themselves to a more regulated life, and they voluntarily expose themselves to the revealing circumstances of the locker room (*Acton,* 1995).

Although the Supreme Court held that the privacy interests were diminished, they were not completely eliminated. Thus, the court turned to considering the intrusiveness of urinalysis, which intrudes on a bodily function traditionally accorded great privacy, aside from any Constitutional protections. The Court held that the seriousness of the intrusion turns upon how the testing is monitored, and concluded that the Vernonia School District's policy was not significantly intrusive because the male athletes remained fully clothed and were monitored, if at all, from behind, and the female athletes provided urine samples in enclosed stalls.

The Court dismissed the drug-testing program as a required disclosure of private medical records because the test screened only for illicit drugs. In addition, the kind of drugs tested for did not vary from individual to individual, and the results were available only to a limited group of school personnel. Prevention of false-positive results due to prescription medication—a defense, one must note, not available to athletes competing internationally (Bamberger & Yeager, 1997; see also the following discussion of Andreea Raducan)—was dismissed as a significant difficulty, because the school policy did not prohibit a student from providing the relevant data directly to the testing facility. Although this rationale remains the law in the United States, it simply removes the intrusion one additional step, to a party unknown to (and unanswerable to) the student or her parents, and requires breaking the district's policy of withholding the identity of the individuals who provide particular samples (*Acton,* 1994). A student who both takes prescription medication and values the privacy of her medical records, then, is caught in an insoluble dilemma: She must either reveal data from her medical records to a testing laboratory, and thus identify to a third party which sample is hers, or risk discipline for a false-positive test result. The difficulty is further underscored by the allegedly foolproof chain of custody (*Acton,* 1995, 1994). One can argue that, when relying on such chains of custody, no set of procedures can prevent substantial and distressingly common difficulties caused by human failures—accidental or otherwise. This is consistent with the author's personal experience.

This weakness of the *Acton* rationale, however, pales next to the problems caused by the procedural posture and standard of review. The Supreme Court is not a fact-finding body; instead, it accepts cases for appellate review, and must establish its view of the facts of a case based only on material in the record of proceedings in the trial court, supplemented by the appellate record (*Acton,* 1992, 1994). The district court made a very close finding that the school district did, in fact, have reasonable suspicion that there was a significant problem with illicit drugs (cocaine, marijuana, and amphetamines) among student-athletes (*Acton,* 1992). This factual finding was not reviewed in the later decisions, although it forms a critical part of the Fourth Amendment analysis (*Acton,* 1995, 1994). Thus, one cannot be certain that a truly suspicionless testing program for PES among student-athletes, such as a blanket requirement that seventh-grade football players be tested for anabolic steroid or EPO use, could withstand Fourth Amendment scrutiny (*cf. Todd,* 1998). On the other hand, a statutory requirement for either random or universal testing based on a legislative finding of fact would provide a legally sufficient factual basis, even though the test subjects had no opportunity to refute the legislative analysis (*cf. Hill,* 1994; Meloch, 1987; Locke & Jennings, 1986).

A more interesting, and as yet untested, question concerns the Fourth Amendment rights of adults who undergo suspicionless testing for substances that may be prescribed by physicians in good faith. *Acton* turns on the limitations imposed on students' Fourth Amendment rights by *T.L.O.* The rationales presented in *Von Raab* and *Skinner* do not help much, as both of those cases involved testing individuals whose performance clearly impacts public safety and welfare. Conversely, the Supreme Court has rejected suspicionless testing in contexts in which drug use would not clearly impact public safety and welfare (*Chandler,* 1997). The major sport leagues have gotten around the Fourth Amendment problem by including detailed testing requirements in their collective bargaining agreements ([Unattributed], 2000; Williams, 1998; see also Yesalis, Courson, & Wright, 2000). What, then, about "amateur" athletic competition, or other contexts in which there is no labor agreement between a controlling league authority and the competitors, such as tennis or golf? These competitors vastly outnumber the major leaguers; for example, four times as many runners entered the Chicago Marathon in 2000 as are on the combined rosters of all NFL teams. The closest fact-pattern thus far considered in the federal appeals system is Butch Reynolds's dispute with the International Amateur Athletics Federation (IAAF), the international governor of track and field (*Reynolds,* 1994). However, the actual decision in *Reynolds* concerns whether U.S. courts can assert jurisdiction to review decisions of the IAAF, not the validity of Reynolds's test results. United States courts have successfully evaded this issue, except as it concerns students (*Hill,* 1994).

The only way out of this dilemma, absent a comprehensive regulation scheme that applies to competitions held under auspices other than those of the established sport federations and other participants in the Court for Arbitration of Sport (CAS), is a contractual agreement between the individual athletes and the competition's organizers. Such a contract might be similar to that required of competitors in the 1996 Atlanta Olympics, which prohibited athletes from making court challenges to doping decisions absent gross violation of due process, fundamental rights, or public order (Downes, 1998). This solution has its own serious problems. The CAS system appears, on its face, to violate American notions of due process (Kleinman & Petit, 2000; *Hooters,* 1998). It is unlikely that a smaller organization could establish an arbitration or other process that would both be binding and respect the individual rights of the athletes.

Conversely, these regimes must overcome significant legislation and case law that protect workers' general privacy and employment rights and that restrict arbitrary and capricious action against individual workers in support of an employer's or organization's broader policy concerns (*cf. Bosman,* 1995; *Barnes,* 1993). The *Bosman* case provides an excellent example of how general employment law can affect athletic competition. Traditionally, football (soccer) has relied on sale of player contracts between clubs for a "transfer fee," rather than the American tradition of trading a player for other players or draft choices. Jean-Marc Bosman reached the end of his contract with Standard Liege, one of the leading Belgian clubs. He did not sign a new contract, but wished to try his luck on the open employment market. Standard Liege, however, refused to release his official registration, even though he was out of contract. This should sound a lot like the now-abrogated "reserve clause" that prevented free agency in American baseball (*Flood,* 1972). The European Court of Justice held, however, that athletic tradition and efficiency could not overcome the general freedom enjoyed by European workers to move between jobs (*Bosman,* 1995). The Treaty of Rome, which functions somewhat as does the U.S. Constitution for European Union issues, was held to supercede both the international federation's rules and the Belgian statute relied on by Standard Liege. *Bosman* demonstrates that arbitrary or discretionary determinations that a particular policy or practice is "good for sport" may not hold under general law, thus counseling caution. Michelle Smith de Bruin, whose circumstances are discussed further on, is at this writing attempting to use the *Bosman* rationale in a challenge to her "conviction" for steroid misuse.

"Roid Rage" and Other Behavioral Consequences

Many PES have dangerous behavioral side effects; some of the intended effects, such as heightened aggression resulting from amphetamine use, are equally problematic. Statistically, some athletes (and others) who use PES on a regular basis are likely to commit crimes, possibly under the influence of the PES. In such a case, is the athlete liable for or guilty of the underlying offense? If not, what theory provides a valid defense? Unfortunately, the answer to this question is even more difficult than developing a legal method to control international drug trafficking.

Leaving philosophical and ethical considerations of responsibility aside, U.S. law—and that of other common-law countries—offers three potential defenses based on drug use:

- Voluntary intoxication, an incomplete defense (i.e., it reduces the gravity of the charge or the penalty, but does not result in acquittal)

- Involuntary intoxication, which may be a complete defense in some circumstances but is usually an incomplete defense

- Legal insanity, which is normally a complete defense but is occasionally treated as an incomplete defense

Drunk driving—abuse of a performance-*inhibiting* substance—provides an excellent test example. In an ordinary homicide, the charge is based on the general culpability of the defendant, and can range from involuntary manslaughter to murder (Lafave & Scott, 1986). Intoxication usually acts to reduce the charge from murder, and virtually always eliminates the death penalty as a potential consequence. One typical statute reads as follows:

> In cases involving reckless homicide, being under the influence of alcohol or any other drug or drugs at the time of the alleged violation shall be presumed to be evidence of a reckless act unless disproved by evidence to the contrary. (720 ILCS 5/9-3(b))

The major difficulty for defendants is proving that the PES they were taking did, in fact, create a level of intoxication or insanity. Research concerning these questions often results in contradictory or borderline findings (Kleinman & Petit, 2000; Bahrke, Yesalis, & Wright, 1996). The defense of "roid rage"—an assertion more akin to legal insanity than to simple intoxication—has had, at best, mixed results (Kleinman & Petit, 2000; Nack, Yeager, & Clive, 1998; Bidwill & Katz, 1989; *cf. Williams,* 1986).

Civil liability is another area for concern. These three defenses have much less force in a civil proceeding, resulting in substantially greater risk of a finding of liability for acts "instigated" by steroids, or amphetamines, or barbiturates (Lafave & Scott, 1986). In addition, the burden of proof is much lower in civil matters than criminal ones. In the United States, the difference is between "beyond a reasonable doubt" and "preponderance of the evidence." There are similar differences in burdens of proof in most Western nations (Boyle, 1988). A finding of civil liability for wrongfully causing a death can, in some circumstances, result in more severe consequences than a criminal conviction for involuntary manslaughter.

International Regulation of Performance-Enhancing Substances

Most international regulation of PES concerns trafficking in controlled substances. This is intertwined with efforts to control other illicit drugs (Bahrke, 1994). Possession of PES is typically treated the same as possession of illicit drugs like cocaine, at least in the relevant statutes (Anabolic Steroids Control Act of 1990; *cf.* Yesalis et al., 1997). In the United States, this is typically treated as a relatively minor state-law offense (Taylor, 1991, 1987). Although possession of a controlled substance without prescription is in fact a federal offense (Anti-Drug Abuse Act of 1988), in practice federal prosecutors will not prosecute for mere possession; instead, the federal authorities concentrate on trafficking and leave possession issues to the states, unless possession is somehow intertwined with another, more serious, offense (Bertram et al., 1996).

The effectiveness of antitrafficking efforts to date is not open to question—it is largely a story of occasional "drug busts" that do little to stem the supply of PES.

> Swiss star Armin Meier was one of a handful of competitors who admitted to police they had used a performance-enhancing substance known as EPO [erythropoietin] to counter their exhaustion during the gruelling 3,877-km race. "Yes, I said that I had taken EPO, how I took it and why I took it," Meier said, adding this: "I'm just a victim of the system." (Deacon, 1998)

The prosecution of Willy Voet is an excellent example of the difficulties with stopping PES trafficking (Voet, 1999; Walsh, 2000). Voet was caught with several hundred vials of EPO as a result of a fairly routine traffic stop at the border between Belgium and France prior to the 1998 Tour de France. Initially, Voet was castigated by the cycling community as a traitor and liar; he never denied that the Festina team had a coordinated, physician-supervised program of administering PES, particularly EPO, to its athletes. The wall of silence has since crumbled. During Voet's trial for trafficking in France, other participants have started to admit that PES usage in cycling is at least as widespread as Voet has claimed publicly (Walsh, 2000), and other sports are also under serious investigation (Walsh & Fallain, 2000). A French court in Lille fined Voet 30,000 francs and imposed a suspended prison sentence of 10 months. The court fined

Bruno Roussell, the former head of Festina (the cycling team for which Voet had been working), 50,000 francs and imposed a suspended prison sentence of one year, but acquitted rider Richard Verenque. Conversely, there has been little publicized response to the Australian discovery of human growth hormone in a Chinese swimmer's luggage, aside from expulsion of the swimmer from the competition and the country (Lord, 2000). The Dutchman's finger is in the dike, but the rest of the dike leaks like a sieve (Kleinman & Petit, 2000; Ryan, 1988; Bertram, et al., 1996).

Legal Procedure and Individual Misuse

Unfortunately, as in U.S. law concerning illegal searches and seizures, virtually our only reported glimpses of the procedures actually used in confronting individual instances of PES misuse by athletes result from instances in which there has been a positive test for a PES. To the present, this has virtually always meant anabolic steroids, as testing regimes for other PES seldom have been sufficiently sophisticated and reliable for use in regulating competition.

> Without a reliable test, officials are at a loss even to say how widely abused [EPO and hGH] are. Scattered evidence suggests troubling pervasiveness, at least in some sports or among certain teams. "If this were a basketball game, we'd be behind about 98 to 2," remarks a former official of the U.S. Olympic Committee (USOC) who asked not to be identified. (Zorpette, 2000:20)

Michelle Smith de Bruin: When in Geneva, Do As the Genevans Do

Michelle Smith de Bruin won the first-ever Irish swimming medal at the 1996 Atlanta Olympics. In the two years preceding the Games, she had shattered her own personal records by several seconds. This led to far-from-circumspect accusations (whether true or not) of steroid use from both inside and outside the international swimming community. In early 1998, Smith de Bruin was selected to give an out-of-competition urine sample for analysis. The sample was contaminated with ethanol at several times the lethal dose, apparently straight from a whiskey bottle. Ironically, the contamination failed to mask anabolic steroid metabolites found in the sample by the testing laboratory in Spain (Lord, 1999, 1998a, 1998b).

The subsequent legal odyssey points out many of the difficulties with human factors in any drug-testing regime, and particularly with observation of sample provision and the chain of custody. Whether one believes Smith's story (that the sample was contaminated with both the steroidal metabolites and the alcohol after she provided it to the testing authority's representative) or the representative's (that he smelled a strong odor of whiskey from the sample as Smith de Bruin gave it to him), the procedure followed to obtain and process the sample was clearly unsatisfactory (Lord, 1999, 1998a). At her various hearings, Smith de Bruin's counsel raised credible objections both to the method of obtaining and safeguarding the sample itself and to internal procedures at the testing laboratory (Lord, 1998b). Left unstated were questions concerning the "random selection" of Smith de Bruin for testing.

Regardless of Smith de Bruin's substantive guilt, the public proceedings were little short of a circus. Lawyers on both sides tried the case in front of both the media and the arbitral tribunal (Lord, 1999). Yet an athlete who provides an allegedly positive sample during competition would envy Smith de Bruin's opportunity to consult experts, attorneys, and publicists; to avoid immediate public humiliation; to reflect on his situation. In-competition test results are dealt with quickly and harshly. The speed of resolution works to the severe disadvantage of competitors, as it prevents any meaningful investigation into particular circumstances and allows surprise theories of guilt to go unopposed, as allegedly occurred in the Ben Johnson incident in Seoul (Francis & Coplon, 1990).

Andreea Raducan: The Cold Hard Facts

The reaction of the International Olympic Committee (IOC) to a positive test for pseudoephedrine (a common over-the-counter cold medication) at the Sydney Olympics demonstrates many of the difficulties with the current PES control regime. The afternoon before the individual all-around final in women's gymnastics, Andreea Raducan, of the Romanian team, complained to the team doctor of a stuffy head. The team doctor prescribed a single dose of a common cold medication to relieve the stuffiness. The following afternoon, Raducan won the gold medal in the individual all-around. Shortly thereafter, she tested positive for pseudoephedrine, which is prohibited as a PES by the international federations. Under the zero-tolerance policies in place at the Sydney Olympics, Raducan was stripped of her gold medal. Not surprisingly, test results for the team all-around (which preceded the individual all-around) and for the competitions on individual apparatus (which followed the individual all-around) did not detect pseudoephedrine or any other banned substance, because the drug exits the system quickly (Chaudhary, 2000b; Williams, 1998).

This particular incident demonstrates the hypocrisy of the current PES control system. One must initially question whether pseudoephedrine is a PES at all *for gymnasts*. Pseudoephedrine's physiological effects allegedly include mild stimulation coupled with somewhat heightened aggressiveness (figure 28.1) (Williams, 1998). These defects have made pseudo-ephedrine, available as an over-the-counter drug in North America as Sudafed and in Europe as Nurofen, popular with professional hockey players. Stimulation, aggressiveness, and clearance of the sinus passages are obvious benefits in a team contact sport played on ice. Gymnastics, however, requires not stimulation and aggression, but concentration and control. Also unlike hockey players, gymnasts typically have significant rest periods between individual exercises. This makes the performance-enhancing effect of pseudoephedrine questionable for a gymnast, except insofar as promoting normal sinus function would be considered "performance enhancing." The IOC and CAS admitted that pseudoephedrine would not have enhanced a gymnast's performance (Chaudhary, 2000b, 2000a). One must therefore question whether the rationale for this particular ban is concern for the integrity of competition or something more self-interested. The recent decision concerning Casey Martin's use of a golf cart demonstrates other difficulties with assuming a rationale based on the integrity of competition (*Martin*, 2001).

The IOC's reaction in itself was also quite troubling. Under its own rules, any athlete who tests positive at any time for any banned PES is to be excluded from the Games from that point and must forfeit all medals won at that Games (Olympic Movement Anti-Doping Code,

1999). All records set by that athlete during those Games are also to be stricken. The IOC, however, did not do this. Raducan was allowed to keep her gold medal from the team all-around competition and her individual silver medal on the vault (Chaudhary, 2000a). This inconsistency is only the beginning of the arbitrary and capricious reaction of the IOC to this incident. A review by a truly disinterested authority, such as is available to parties after "arbitration" in the United States, would have seriously questioned this arbitrary, inconsistent, and capricious result (FAA, § 4; Gorman, 1995; see Kleinman & Petit, 2000).

From a legal perspective, then, the IOC's reaction was unsatisfactory. The incident demonstrates that "zero-tolerance" systems simply do not work to control individual behavior concerning PES. A zero-tolerance system may be of some value for controlling organizational behavior (e.g., Boyle, 1988); it may be of some value in controlling trafficking in a prohibited substance. Raducan's apparently innocent mistake in this incident, however, was not so much taking pseudoephedrine as trusting the team doctor. The IOC's treatment of a teenaged Romanian gymnast can only encourage self-medication—which is, in all probability, far more dangerous than trusting even a negligent team physician. This leads to the most troubling aspect of this particular positive test result: The team physician's stated (and based on the situation obvious) motivation was to ensure the health of the athlete. Conversely, concern for the athletes' health is

PES	Pseudoephedrine
Available as	Nonprescription decongestant, including brands such as Sudafed, Triaminic, Dimetapp, Drixoral, Chlor-Trimeton, Myfedrine, and Benylin
	Nonprescription cold remedies, including brands such as Tylenol Sinus, Nyquil, Dayquil
Dosage	As ergogenic: >120 mg not more than two hours prior to performance
	As decongestant: 60 mg every 4-6 hours (120 mg every 12 hours for "long-acting" formulas), not exceeding 240 mg in 24 hours
Positive test result	Urine concentration > 25 g/ml
Classification	Stimulant (purported; ergogenic effectiveness contested)
Effectiveness	Unproven in clinical trials (Williams, 1998; Gillies, 1997)
Banned by	All international federations who follow the World Antidoping Agency
Prominent cases	Andreea Raducan (see discussion in text); Rick DeMont (1972 Olympics, swimming; prescription asthma medication)

Figure 28.1 Profile of pseudoephedrine as a PES, as of 2001.

Sources: Consumer Reports, 2001; World Antidoping Agency, 2001; Williams, 1998; Gillies et al., 1997; Anti-Doping Convention, 1989

the most common value-neutral justification for blanket banning of specific substances as PES.

So what, then, *is* the actual justification for blanket bans that disdain medical advice tailored to the particular athlete's health, situation, and circumstances? What, given the actual justification, is the appropriate legal response? Although there is little direct testimony from decision makers, the actual justification appears to be the reputation and economic well-being of the major sponsoring organizations, particularly the IOC (Zorpette, 2000). If the organizations truly wished to prevent cheating, they would emphasize unannounced out-of-competition testing of a relatively large proportion of athletes—which would cost a significant amount of money (Deacon, 1998; Kleinman & Petit, 2000). That Smith de Bruin's test was an unannounced out-of-competition test in itself points out the need to rely on such testing. Continued reliance on in-competition testing to control PES use smacks of both selective prosecution, which risks legal challenges (Lafave & Scott, 1986), and misuse of legal mechanisms for inappropriate ends (*cf.* Farber & Frickey, 1991).

Regulating Performance-Enhancing Substances: A Question of Authority

Lurking beneath these questions of individual rights and proper procedure is a more subtle issue: What is the source of an international federation's authority to regulate or punish doping? The facile answer is the agreement of the athletes to compete. This is neither complete nor, in itself, satisfactory. In the Western democracies, we are fond of saying that "government governs only with the consent of the governed." One must remember, however, that international athletic federations are anything but democracies (Senn, 1999).

One might also argue that international athletic federations obtain their authority from the sovereign states that are members of the federations. This argument is, at best, circular. The international athletic federations base their policies and structures on perceived value to the sport, not on the interests of any of the nations that contribute to those federations. Although the federations have on occasion been pressured by individual nations or groups of nations, international sporting bodies tend to be much more obstinate (Senn, 1999). Looking at the history of relations between the nations and the athletic federations dispassionately, this structure resembles the relations between the American states of the old South and the American national government during the first half of the 19th century. This implies that the international federations—and, in particular, the IOC—act as virtual sovereigns within the area of athletics. The IOC's recent efforts to establish a "Court for Arbitration of Sport"

only reinforce this conclusion (Senn, 1999). The one structural responsibility remaining to the modern nation-state is the provision of a system for resolving disputes between its citizens (Moynihan, 1992; de Groot, 1983).

If the international athletic federations talk like sovereigns and behave with the self-assurance of sovereigns, should they not be treated as sovereigns? If so, are there other legal principles that regulate the exercise of the federation's assumed authority? International and human rights law was not an invention of the victors of World War II. De Groot (1983) long ago theorized about abstract principles of law that regulate the conduct of nations; the Hague and Geneva conventions of the early 20th century regulate the treatment of both combatants and noncombatants (Boyle, 1988). Comparison of the actions and policies of the international athletic federations to third-world regimes generally agreed on as human rights violators, however, is disquieting. There seems little doubt that a nation-state whose legal system behaved and was structured like that of the federations would earn substantial criticism from human rights organizations. The only possible distinction is the assertion that competing in athletics is not a right, but a privilege. This, however, smacks of the controversy over "professionalism" that has dogged the modern Olympics for its entire history, based more on prejudice, tradition, and class preconceptions than on any real benefit to competition (Senn, 1999; *cf. Martin,* 2001).

The differences between scientific and legal knowledge further obscure the appropriate legal response to misuse of PES. One can say with a scientific degree of certainty that a given sample, whether of urine or blood, has tested positive for a given substance (Kammerer, 2000). Leaving aside the possibility of chemical false positives, this scientific conclusion is *not* necessarily congruent with the legal conclusion that the individual to whom the sample is attributed misused the given PES (Deason, 1999, 1998). Some factors that complicate this congruence—all of which appear to have occurred in at least one publicly disclosed testing incident—include the following:

- Unknowing, one-time introduction of a banned substance to the competitor, such as apparently happened to Andreea Raducan

- Misattribution of the result, either through misidentification of the sample itself or mistaken correlation of the sample with the test subject, as claimed by Mary Decker Slaney (Downes, 1998)

- Contamination of the sample at the source, as alleged in the Smith de Bruin test (Lord, 1999, 1998a, 1998b)

- Contamination or other difficulties during transmission of the sample from the test subject to the laboratory (Lord, 1998b)

This list of systemic failures does not take into account the possibility of purposeful alteration of a sample or results (*cf.* Lord, 1998b). Although the author is not aware of a provable instance of such corruption, other widespread corruption of the international athletics community and the economic incentives to remove one's competitors create a nontrivial risk that the present system does little to control, or even consider (Francis & Coplon, 1990; Senn, 1999; see Ferstle, 2000).

Mistaken certainty of physiological origin provides yet another reason that the legal response to PES should remain cautious. The recent spate of positive tests for nandrolone—a substance that has been banned since the early 1970s and that resulted in exclusion of seven competitors from the 1984 Los Angeles Olympics (Senn, 1999; Goldman, Bush, & Klatz, 1984)—is instructive. Some research indicates that contemporary nutritional supplements may be providing a false-positive result (Goodbody, 2000). Logically, this makes sense, as nandrolone is no longer a "preferred" anabolic steroid; it is neither as effective as some newer synthetics nor as short-lived in the body (Masse et al., 1985; Masse & Goudreault, 1992). Identification of nandrolone metabolites in urine is fairly well established (Hampl & Stárka, 1991; Kammerer, 2000; see Goldman, Bush, & Klatz, 1984), and athletes know this. It is difficult to understand the wide variety of athletes suddenly using nandrolone in light of the public crackdown on PES (see Kammerer, 2000). "To be caught is not easy; it only happens," says Emil Vrijman, director of the Netherlands' doping control center, "when an athlete is either incredibly sloppy, incredibly stupid[,] or both" (Bamberger & Yeager, 1997:63).

Conclusion

Improper and uninformed use of PES is a serious problem. Leaving aside the question of the integrity of athletic competition, many PES can be extraordinarily dangerous, either through toxicity or side effects. Long before modern drug-testing protocols, marathon runners used strychnine during the early years of the Olympics as a supposed PES, with easily imaginable consequences (Senn, 1999). Despite the draconian reaction of some contemporary sport regulating bodies, other PES are so common that it may be difficult to find competitors in some events who are *not* using banned substances (Zorpette, 2000; Hughes, 2000).

[A]longside the stirring spectacle of Olympic competition in Sydney, there will be another struggle so complex that the average viewer will probably have a hard time grasping the rules, let alone getting excited about it. Unfortunately, the loser will be fair competition. (Zorpette, 2000:20)

Recognizing the problem, however, is only the initial step. Effective and appropriate responses are as important in a social or legal context as they are in medicine, while ineffective and inappropriate responses are as counterproductive. There is little reason to believe that imposing prohibition on PES, even with better technology, has been or will be any more effective than the American experience of the 1920s with alcohol; quite the opposite (Ryan, 1998; Currie, 1993). Law provides an effective and appropriate means to control the behavior of individuals whose behavior is controlled by scruples. Absent those scruples, though, whether through ignorance, disagreement with underlying values, or sheer apathy, law is neither an effective nor an appropriate response.

Law can, in some circumstances, correct behavior; it can occasionally deter behavior (Lafave & Scott, 1986). It cannot do so, however, when working at cross-purposes with other factors motivating athletes, both economic and (un)ethical (Bamberger & Yeager, 1997). Further, a legal system can provide effective behavior modification only when it is widely believed to impose accurate, even-handed results. As long as economic sponsorship makes winning the only thing, draconian legal responses to misuse of PES will remain not just ineffective, but counterproductive.

References

720 ILCS 5/9-3(b) [Illinois]. Offenses Against the Person: Homicide: Involuntary Manslaughter and Reckless Homicide.

Anabolic Steroids Control Act of 1990. Title XIX of Pub. L. No. 101-647, 104 Stat. 4851 (codified at 21 U.S.C. § 333(e)).

Anti-Drug Abuse Act of 1988. Pub. L. No. 100-690, § 2403, 102 Stat. 4230 (codified at 21 U.S.C. § 333).

Acton, Vernonia Sch. Dist. No. 47J v., 515 U.S. 646 (1995).

Acton v. Vernonia Sch. Dist. No. 47J, 23 F.3d 1514 (9th Cir. 1994).

Acton v. Vernonia Sch. Dist. No. 47J, 796 F. Supp. 1354 (D. Ore. 1992).

Bahrke, M.S. (1994). International conference on abuse and trafficking of anabolic steroids. *International Journal of Drug Policy,* 5(1):23-26.

———, Yesalis, C.E., & Wright, J.E. (1996). Psychological and behavioural effects of endogenous testosterone levels and anabolic-androgenic steroids among males, a review. *Sports Medicine,* 10(5): 303-337.

Bamberger, M., & Yeager, D. (1997, 14 Apr.). Over the edge. *Sports Illustrated:* 60-70.

Barnes v. International Amateur Athletic Federation, 862 F. Supp. 1537 (D.W. Va. 1993).

Benson, P. (1991). The priority of abstract right and constructivism in Hegel's legal philosophy. In Cornell, D.,

Rosenfeld, M., & Carlson, D.G., eds., *Hegel and Legal Theory.* New York: Routledge, Chapman, & Hall.

Bertram, E., Sharpe, K., & Andreas, P. (1996). *Drug War Politics: The Price of Denial.* Berkeley: University of California Press.

Bidwill, M.J., & Katz, D.L. (1989). Injecting new life into an old defense: Anabolic steroid-induced psychosis as a paradigm of involuntary intoxication. *University of Miami Entertainment and Sports Law Review,* 7(1):19-21.

Bosman, Union Royale Belge des Sociétés de Football Association ASBL v. (1995). 1995 E.C.R. I-5040 *et seq.,* no. C-415/93.

Boyle, F.A. (1988). *Defending Civil Resistance Under International Law.* Salem, OR: Center for Energy Research.

Chandler v. Miller, 520 U.S. 305 (1997).

Chaudhary, V. (2000a, 28 Sep.). A tale of two citings: Drug sympathy for Raducan, none for fellow Romanian Melinte. *Guardian* (UK).

———. (2000b, 29 Sep.). Bitter pill as tiny gymnast loses gold: Tiriac quits over "innocent" victim of war against drugs. *Guardian* (UK).

Currie, E. (1993). *Reckoning: Drugs, the Cities, and the American Future.* New York: Hill & Wang.

Deacon, J. (1998, 10 Aug.). The Tour de shame: The sports world reels from new drug scandals. *Macleans:* 43.

Deason, E.E. (1999). Incompatible versions of authority in law and science. *Social Epistemology,* 13(2): 147-164.

Deason, E.E. (1998). Court-appointed expert witnesses: Scientific positivism meets bias and deference. *University of Oregon Law Review,* 77(1): 59-156.

De Groot ("Grotius"), H. (trans. van Holk, L.E., & Rölofsen, C.G.). (1983). *Grotius Reader: A Reader for Students of International Law and Legal History.* The Hague: T.M.C. Asser Instituut.

Downes, S. (1998, 29 Nov.). Drug charges haunt Slaney. *The Times* (London).

Farber, D.A., & Frickey, P.F. (1991). *Law and Public Choice.* Chicago: University of Chicago Press.

Federal Arbitration Act (1998). 9 U.S.C. §§ 1-16.

Ferstle, J. (2000). Evolution and politics of drug testing. In Yesalis, C.E., ed., *Anabolic Steroids in Sport and Exercise.* Champaign, IL: Human Kinetics, 363-413.

Flood v. Kuhn, 407 U.S. 258 (1972).

Francis, C., & Coplon, J. (1990). *Speed Trap: A Track Coach's Explosive Account of How the World's Greatest Athletes Win—With Drugs.* New York: St. Martin's.

Goldman, B., Bush, P., & Klatz, R. (1984). *Death in the Locker Room: Steroids and Sports.* South Bend, IN: Icarus Press.

Goodbody, J. (2000, 22 Aug.). Tainted Christie loses out in the long run. *The Times* (London).

Gorman, R. (1995). The *Gilmer* decision and the private arbitration of public-law disputes. *University of Illinois Law Review,* 1995(3):635-681.

Hampl, R., & Stárka, L. (1991). Endocrine effects and immunoassay procedures of anabolics. In Shipe, J.R., & Savory, J., *Drugs in competitive athletics: Proceedings of the first international symposium held on the Islands of Brioni, Yugoslavia 29 May-2 June 1988.* Oxford: Blackwell Scientific.

Hill v. National Collegiate Athletic Ass'n, 865 P.2d 633, 7 Cal.4th 1, 26 Cal. Rptr.2d 834 (1994).

Hooters of America v. Phillips, 1998 U.S. Dist. LEXIS 3962 (D.S.C. Mar. 12, 1998).

Hughes, R. (2000, 29 Oct.). Finally, mask of deceit torn from laboratory on wheels. *The Times* (London).

Jacobs, J.B., & Samuels, B. (1995). The drug testing project in international sports: Dilemmas in an expanding regulatory regime. *Hastings International and Comparative Law Review,* 18(3):557-589.

Kammerer, R.C. (2000). Drug testing and anabolic steroids. In Yesalis, C.E., ed. *Anabolic Steroids in Sport and Exercise.* Champaign, IL: Human Kinetics, 415-459.

Kleinman, C.C., & Petit, C.E. (2000). Legal aspects of anabolic steroid use and abuse. In Yesalis, C.E., ed., *Anabolic Steroids in Sport and Exercise.* Champaign, IL: Human Kinetics, 333-359.

Lafave, W.R., & Scott, A. (1986). *Criminal Law* (2d ed.). St. Paul: West.

Locke, E., & Jennings, M. (1986). The constitutionality of student-athlete mandatory drug testing programs: The bounds of privacy. *University of Florida Law Review,* 38:581-613.

Lord, C. (2000, 12 Sep.). Chinese pledge has empty sound. *The Times* (London).

———. (1999, 4 May). Smith defiant in face of accusers. *The Times* (London).

———. (1998a, 5 June). IOC finds flaws in one of Smith's lines of defence. *The Times* (London).

———. (1998b, 16 Oct.). Smith takes on issue of right to test. *The Times* (London).

Martin v. P.G.A. Tour, Inc., 121 S. Ct.1879 (2001).

Masse, R., & Goudreault, D. (1992). Studies on anabolic steroids XI. 18-hydroxylated metabolites of mesterolone, methenolone, and stenbolone: New steroids isolated from human urine. *Journal of Steroid Biochemistry and Molecular Biology,* 43:399-410.

Masse, R., Laliberte, C., Tremblay, L., & Dugal, R. (1985). Gas chromatographic/mass spectrometric analysis of 19-nortestosterone urinary metabolites in man. *Biomedical Mass Spectrometry,* 12(3): 115-121.

Meloch, S.L. (1987). An analysis of public college athlete drug testing programs through the unconstitutional condition doctrine and the fourth amendment. *Southern California Law Review,* 60:815-850.

Moynihan, P.D. (1992). *On the Law of Nations.* New York: Harvard University Press.

Nack, W., Yeager, D., & Clive, T. (1998, 18 May). The muscle murders. *Sports Illustrated:* 96-106.

Olympic Movement Anti-Doping Code. 1999. Reproduced at **http://www.gnoc.com/code.htm** (current version).

Only 12 test positive for drugs in NBA's new screening. (2000, 7 Feb.). *New York Times.*

Reynolds v. International Amateur Athletic Fed., 23 F.3d 1110 (6th Cir.), *cert. denied,* 115 S. Ct. 423 (1994).

Ryan, K.F. (1998). Clinging to failure: The rise and continued life of U.S. drug policy. *Law and Society Review,* 32(1):221-242.

Senn, A.E. (1999). *Power, Politics, and the Olympic Games.* Champaign, IL: Human Kinetics.

Skinner v. Railway Labor Executives Ass'n, 489 U.S. 602 (1989).

Taylor, W.N. (1991). *Macho Medicine: A History of the Anabolic Steroid Epidemic.* Jefferson, NC: McFarland.

————. (1987). Synthetic anabolic-androgenic steroids: A plea for controlled substance status. *Physician and Sportsmedicine,* 15(5):145.

T.L.O., New Jersey v., 469 U.S. 325 (1985).

Todd v. Rush Cty. Schools, et al., 139 F.3d 571 (7th Cir. 1998) (Ripple and Rovner, *JJ.,* dissenting).

Voet, Willy. (1999). *Massacre á la Chaîne: Révélations sur 30 ans de tricheries* [Chain Massacre: Revelations of 30 Years of Deception]. Paris: Calmann-Lévy.

Von Raab, National Treasury Employees Union v., 489 U.S. 656 (1989).

Walsh, D. (2000, 29 Oct.). When the lying had to stop. *The Times* (London).

————, & Fallain, J. (2000, 29 Jan.). Poison in the heart of sport. *The Times* (London).

Williams, State v. No. C-5630/5631/5634 (Cir. Ct. St. Mary's Cty., Md., Apr. 3, 1986).

Williams, M.H. (1998). *The Ergogenics Edge: Pushing the Limits of Sports Performance.* Champaign, IL: Human Kinetics.

Yesalis, C.E., Bahrke, M.S., & Wright, J.E. (2000). Societal alternatives. In Yesalis, C.E., ed., *Anabolic Steroids in Sport and Exercise.* Champaign, IL: Human Kinetics, 461-474.

Yesalis, C.E., Courson, S.P., & Wright, J.E. (2000). History of anabolic steroid use in sport and exercise. In Yesalis, C.E., ed., *Anabolic Steroids in Sport and Exercise.* Champaign, IL: Human Kinetics, 51-71.

Yesalis, C.E., Barsukiewicz, C.K., Kopstein, A.N., & Bahrke, M.S. (1997). Trends in anabolic-androgenic steroid use among adolescents. *Archive of Pediatric and Adolescent Medicine,* 151:1197-1206

Zorpette, G. (2000, May). All doped up—and going for the gold. *Scientific American:* 20, 22.

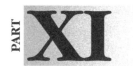
Conclusion

Issues, Concerns, and the Future of Performance-Enhancing Substances in Sport and Exercise

Michael S. Bahrke, PhD

Charles E. Yesalis, MPH, ScD

It's clear—athletes have used a myriad of performance-enhancing substances since ancient times. And it is no secret that today's athletes continue to use a wide range of performance-enhancing substances, from anabolic agents (anabolic steroids, prohormones, and β-2 agonists) to stimulants (ephedrines, amphetamines, caffeine, bromantan, and mesocarb). Athletes also use relatively simple medical techniques to improve performance, such as blood doping, and scientists may be inadvertently making it easier for them by creating new delivery modalities to administer "old" drugs, such as testosterone, via nasal mists, skin patches, and gels, which are then co-opted by athletes, coaches, and their scientific advisors for performance-enhancement use.

The sport pharmacy of today includes substances such as cyproterone acetate, a "brake drug" used by young female gymnasts to delay development of the hips and breasts associated with onset of puberty. In addition, recent advances in science are providing athletes with even more substances and methods to enhance performance and appearance. As scientists are attempting to develop valid doping tests for erythropoietin (EPO), athletes and their scientific advisors have already turned to other leading edge replacements such as perfluorocarbon (PFC), which has the ability to dissolve a variety of gasses including oxygen, and Actovegin, a derivative of calf blood serum that has several medical uses including the treatment of open wounds, but is believed to be used by athletes to increase the oxygen-carrying capacity of the blood. Another new substance is hydroxyethyl starch (HES), a plasma volume expander or drug that dilutes the concentration of hemoglobin and oxygen-carrying red blood cells. It is taken intravenously, and was recently discovered being used by Finnish cross-country skiers. Moreover, new psychotropic drugs will undoubtedly enable athletes from such diverse sports as wrestling, ice hockey, and diving to suppress pain, summon aggression, and eliminate anxiety. So, it comes as no surprise that a recent survey of athletes competing in the Sydney Olympic Games revealed athletes using an average of 6 to 7 types of performance-enhancing substances, includ-ing one competitor who was using 29 substances!

Performance-Enhancing Substance Users

The National Institute on Drug Abuse estimates that more than one million adults have abused anabolic steroids, and a recent government study of adolescent drug use shows an alarming increase in anabolic steroid use among middle school youths from 1998-1999, with an estimated 2.7% of eighth graders saying they have used the drugs. Researchers at the Mayo Clinic in Rochester, Minnesota recently found more than 8% of high school athletes in their region have used creatine and, in a larger survey conducted by Blue Cross and Blue Shield, it is estimated that one million U.S. children between the ages of 12 and 17 years old may have taken performance-enhancing substances, including creatine. This may be one of the reasons why, in the year following slugger Mark McGwire's use of androstenedione (andro) while breaking professional baseball's home run record, sales of androstenedione surged more than 1000 percent to more than $50 million, as industry figures show. Perhaps of even more concern, especially to the parents of adolescent athletes, is that more "hard core" substances such as the new testosterone gel, AndroGel, might soon become available over the Internet.

While estimates of performance-enhancing substance use among elite athletes range widely, from 10% to 99%, and researchers say it is impossible to know exactly how many athletes are doping, most experts believe the use of performance-enhancing substances by athletes is epidemic. Results of anti-doping tests taken during the 2000 Tour de France revealed the presence of doping products in the urine of 45% of the competitors participating in the testing.

In professional sports, San Diego Padres general manager Kevin Towers commented on the prevalence of anabolic steroids among professional baseball players, "I think the stuff is more prevalent in major league clubhouses than alcohol, tobacco, or any other drug, but the attitude seems to be, 'Let's not worry about it until someone dies.'" On the other hand, we would never know the level of steroid use among major league baseball players because Major League Baseball does not have a program for the random or regular drug testing of players.

Even law enforcement personnel are using substances such as anabolic steroids to improve their performance and appearance. Officers say they do it because their job can be physical at times and they feel as though having big muscles gives them "a little edge."

Health Effects of Performance-Enhancing Substances

As documented in the preceding chapters, while we know some of the short-term adverse effects for several performance-enhancing substances, we know very little about others. For example, we know one of the adverse effects of erythropoietin (EPO) includes increased viscosity of the blood, thereby putting users at greater risk for cardiovascular accidents, and EPO has been suspected (but not proven) as the cause of death for about 20 European cyclists since the late 1980s. Among the side effects of ephedrine are hypertension, paranoia, insomnia, nervousness, and neurological and cardiovascular incidents such as seizures, myocardial infarctions, and cerebral hemorrhages. Since 1994, products containing ephedrine have been linked to at least 80 deaths and more

than 1400 complaints by consumers reporting adverse effects. Conversely, we know less about the short-term adverse effects of supplementation with other performance-enhancing substances such as the testosterone precursors, dehydroepiandrosterone (DHEA) and androstenedione (andro).

While we have some information on the acute effects of a number of the drugs used by athletes, much of this information comes as a result of clinical studies. Unfortunately, the subjects in many of these studies were infirm and the studies employed dosing regimens that are often quite different than those used by athletes. Thus the applicability of this clinical information to the health of athletes is problematic. Other information on adverse drug affects is derived from case studies, clinical anecdotes, or accounts in the lay press, the conclusions from which potentially suffer from significant threats to internal and external validity. Episodic use of doping agents also presents a methodological problem. For example, we know what happens when the body produces excessive growth hormone over long periods of time (i.e., acromegally). However, will an athlete using recombinant human growth hormone (rhGH) in an episodic fashion—two 8-week cycles in a year—develop acromegally?

Even when acute effects have been well documented, as with the long-established masculinizing effects of AAS, the information is often ignored. An example is the East German physicians who from 1974 to 1989 administered large doses of anabolic steroids to female athletes. Many of the women are now infertile, have deepened voices and no breasts, have given birth to deformed children, and, in one woman's case she took so many steroids and developed so many male characteristics she underwent a sex-change operation to become a man.

Of greater importance is the dearth of knowledge of the long-term health effects of most performance-enhancing drugs. Again, anabolic steroids serve as a good example. These drugs have been part of the medical armamentarium for more than 65 years and they have been used as doping agents for almost that long. However, we have yet to perform a comprehensive, epidemiological investigation of the long-term health effects of anabolic steroids, similar to those studies conducted for tobacco, alcohol, marijuana, and other substances. Even for a supplement as ubiquitous as creatine, we have yet to determine the health consequences of high-dose use 10 years or more down the road. Furthermore, to conduct such sophisticated longitudinal investigations would take large amounts of time and money. To date, neither government agencies nor sport federations have been willing to devote substantial resources to such endeavors.

Another potential confounder in epidemiologic investigations of the health effects of doping is that athletes come in all sizes, shapes, and colors. In particular, there has been well-deserved criticism that many of the epidemiologic studies of doping agents have tended to focus on white males. In addition, athletes, even within the same sport, can differ greatly regarding their training regimens and diets. These differences can also serve as potential confounders in studies on doping.

The Real Performance Effects of Performance-Enhancing Substances

What do we really know (scientifically) about the effects of performance-enhancing substances? Based on the research presented in this volume, it is apparent that some substances are effective in enhancing performance and/or appearance. For other substances, additional research will be needed before we can confirm their efficacy as performance-enhancers. Also, it is apparent that there are some substances that have been evaluated for which there is little or no scientifically sound evidence demonstrating performance-enhancement, but some athletes continue to use those substances in hopes of improving their performance and/or appearance. Clearly the motivational aspects of the psychological phenomena of the "placebo effect," the "self-fulfilling prophecy," "group affiliation," and "herd behavior" are alive and well in the area of performance-enhancing substances—phenomena some unscrupulous nutrition supplement manufacturers use to full advantage in the marketing and sales of their products.

The Blur Between "Drugs" and "Supplements"

More than 100 million Americans consume some type of nutritional supplement each day—everything from vitamin-fortified drinks to various powders, pills, and bars containing an assortment of amino acids and other nutrients, and consumers are paying more than $14 billion annually for these products. Even mainstream food companies such as Snapple and Ben & Jerry's are adding ginseng, ginkgo biloba, and other herbs to trendy foods and drinks.

The range of supplements available to athletes has increased dramatically over the past few years with the loosening of regulations regarding their sale. The 1994 Dietary Supplement Health and Education Act (DSHEA) substantially reduced the control of the United States Food and Drug Administration (FDA) over supplements and permitted the introduction of new supplements as long as they occurred naturally in food. In other words, if a substance occurs naturally—and as long as manufacturers do not claim it has medical benefits—the FDA can not monitor it. As a result, the DSHEA allows the sale of some steroid hormones such as androstenedione

(andro) and dehydroepiandrosterone (DHEA) as over-the-counter dietary supplements. Consequently, for the consumer, the distinction between what is a drug and what is a supplement is often blurred.

Exacerbating the drug vs. supplement problem is the confusion surrounding what exactly is a prohibited substance. For example, most elite sport governing bodies have already declared androstenedione (andro) a banned substance. The International Olympic Committee, the National Collegiate Athletic Association, and the National Football League have banned androstenedione use among players, and recently the National Basketball Association included androstenedione on a list of nine newly prohibited substances. However, the NBA Players Association has been fighting the androstenedione ban. The NBA Players Association only recently agreed to add marijuana to the NBA list of banned substances. Major League Baseball does not ban androstenedione. To add to this confusion, there is scant research to support the notion that androstenedione enhances performance, while there are a number of studies that support the performance effects of creatine—a supplement that is not on any banned list.

A related issue is whether athletes are using medication for treating or cheating. Asthma products and other medicines were used by hundreds of athletes during the recent Sydney Olympic Games where 607 athletes (about 6% of the total of 10,600 athletes who competed at Sydney) produced waivers for asthma medication, compared with about 1% of the general population. As the World Anti-Doping Agency (WADA) Chairman Dick Pound remarked, "It's surprising how many of them are taking medications. You look at it and say how can all of the finest athletes on the face of the earth be so sick?"

Contamination and improper labeling are other problems associated with food supplements. Up to 20% of 200 different food supplements purchased randomly from store shelves in a recent International Olympic Committee-sponsored investigation showed traces of banned substances such as anabolic steroids. Hundreds of athletes throughout the world have tested positive for nandrolone, the muscle-building anabolic steroid, over the past two years. Almost 350 nandrolone cases across all sports were reported in 1999 alone. These positive tests add to the increasing speculation that many of these positive results for nandrolone are the result of athletes inadvertently taking mislabeled or contaminated nutritional supplements.

On the college level, a recent National Collegiate Athletic Association survey found 42% of college athletes use nutritional supplements that are unregulated and may contain banned substances such as ephedrine. The same survey showed the use of amphetamines, anabolic steroids, and ephedrine, while still low, had increased slightly over the past four years. Almost 60% of those using supplements acquired them from retail stores, according to the survey. Unfortunately, athletes frequently are unaware that substances such as ephedrine are contained in some supplements. They do not recognize the risk because they purchase the products, such as Ripped Fuel, Xenadrine, and Hydroxycut, at nutritional stores throughout the country. However, the rules of most sport governing bodies state that athletes are responsible for whatever substances they put into their bodies.

While many feel the DSHEA needs to be revised, the United States Food and Drug Administration and DHEA are working to classify several over-the-counter dietary supplements, such as andro and DHEA, as controlled substances making them more difficult to get and easier to regulate.

The Rapidly Growing List of Performance-Enhancing Substances

As the booming biotechnology and pharmaceutical industries discover new ways to fight disease, scientists and athletes are also discovering ingenious new ways to subvert those substances and methods to enhance performance and appearance. Some greedy scientists attend academic meetings and perch like vultures waiting to figure out how substances can be tweaked for athletic use. Then, a few months later, the new substances are being sold as nutritional supplements, or we learn about athletes who are experimenting with them. However, many believe the current use of anabolic steroids and the injection of synthetic hormones and blood substitutes will soon be passé because athletes will be injecting genes to enhance performance and appearance. Within the next 8-10 years or less (some predict this may occur as early as 2004), it is quite possible that genetic engineering will profoundly change the course of competitive sport by allowing scientists to create the "perfect" athlete. Genetic engineering has already been achieved in animals, and it is only a matter of time before athletes do it. Researchers have shown in rodents that they can inject a gene directly into a target muscle and increase its performance by 25%.

In the attempt to deter genetic therapy, the International Olympic Committee's Medical Commission is developing high-tech anti-abuse tests that analyze blood and saliva for antibodies produced as a result of taking gene medications, and it's working on the creation of gene footprints by looking at gene proteins. However, given previous attempts by the International Olympic Committee to reduce and eliminate doping in sport, the prospects of halting the genetic engineering of athletes are slim to none.

The Track Record of Dope Testing

As documented in this volume, performance-enhancing substance use in Olympic sport has remained unchanged for years, as has the blind eye Olympic officials have cast toward the problem. However, what has changed over the years are the substances of choice and the methods athletes have used to thwart drug tests. In the past, enforcement has fallen upon a patchwork of groups, including sports federations that test before and during national and international competitions. Unfortunately, some organizations would test for certain substances and some for others. Also, prior to the 1990s, tests were performed only at competitions, so cheaters doped before and after.

The International Olympic Committee has a history of testing halfheartedly and in some cases, covering up positive results to avoid embarrassment. Since a list of banned drugs was introduced at the 1968 Olympic Games in Mexico City, 11,053 tests have been conducted at the Games. Only 48 or 0.43% have been positive. In Sydney, 11 (0.001%) of the nearly 11,000 athletes who competed tested positive for banned drugs. Dr. Wade Exum, former Director of Drug Control Administration for the United States Olympic Committee, claims that half of United States athletes who tested positive for banned substances went unpunished in recent years.

Even with new tests on the way, researchers say, there remains a panoply of performance-enhancing substances that they cannot detect. And, while blood and urine EPO testing is finally being instituted (athletes can still resort to autologous blood doping), there are no reliable tests for recombinant human growth hormone (rhGH) and other performance boosters such as insulin-like growth factor-1 (IGF-1). To combat the continuing doping war, late in 1999 the International Olympic Committee created the World Anti-Doping Agency (WADA), an independent body that coordinates anti-doping enforcement for the Olympics and other international competitions. However, as former International Olympic Committee President Juan Antonio Samaranch was quoted as saying upon relinquishing his position, "In doping, the war is never won."

A Brief View Into the Crystal Ball: The Future of Performance-Enhancing Substances in Sport and Exercise

It would be wonderful if athletes did not use performance-enhancing substances, but they do and they are not going to stop. As one writer observed, the genie is out of the bottle (and perhaps it has been out for hundreds or even thousands of years?) and there is no returning it. With so many athletes using performance-enhancing substances, should these substances be legalized, at least in professional sports, thus leveling the playing field? Athletes would be free to use whatever substances they wished. Performance-enhancing substances could be regulated and administered under the guidance of the team physician. Consuming optimal dosages could minimize adverse effects.

Perhaps we should have two Olympic Games: one drug-free and the other drugged? Athletes participating in the Dope Olympics could use any substance they wished to enhance performance and appearance. Athletes competing in the dope-free Games testing positive for a performance-enhancing substance would be banned for life.

Perhaps the list of banned substances should be reduced to a more manageable level. Near the end of his tenure as International Olympic Committee President, Juan Antonio Samaranch recommended lowering the number of banned substances, contending the list was not realistic.

Perhaps the heart of the problem is social: do we overemphasize the importance of winning? Winners become heroes, so society creates a culture of worshiping winners. And, while some believe all athletes are winners just by competing, the fact is, in athletic competition there is only one first place finisher—*the* winner. Not every athlete who competes wins, and for those lacking natural talent, performance-enhancing substances offer the means by which they may become "winners." Unfortunately, for some athletes, the temptations and rewards of winning in sports are too great and they succumb to doping. The use of various substances by athletes to enhance performance and appearance will never be completely eliminated. There is too much fame and fortune to be gained by being a winner in sports. If sport fans around the world were polled and asked: "Are you upset by doping?" "Are you against doping?" virtually everyone would say, "Yes." However, a far more relevant question is: "Are you upset enough about the doping to turn off your television set and not watch sports events?" Judging by the continuing profitability and popularity of both amateur and professional sports, most would answer, "No."

Appendix

Web Sites for Selected Sports Governing and Sports Medicine Organizations

Doping Policies

World Anti-Doping Agency
http://www.wada-ama.org/asiakas/003/WADA_HomePage.nsf/start?readform

United States Anti-Doping Agency
http://www.usantidoping.org

Position Stands/Papers

American Academy of Pediatrics
http://www.aap.org/family/steroids.htm

American College of Sports Medicine
http://www.acsm-msse.org/

Drug Regulations and Programs

Amateur Athletic Union
http://www.aausports.org/mytp/home/index.jsp

Federation Internationale de Football Association
http://www.fifa.com/

International Association of Athletics Federations
http://www.iaaf.org/

International Olympic Committee Prohibited Classes of Substances and Prohibited Methods
http://www.nodoping.olympic.org/pos_anti_dop_code_e.html

International Tennis Federation Schedule of Prohibited Substances
http://www.itftennis.com/html/rule/frameset.html

Major League Baseball Drug Policy and Prevention Program
http://sports.findlaw.com/drugs/policy/baseball/

Major League Soccer Drug Policy
http://sports.findlaw.com/drugs/policy/soccer/

National Basketball Association/National Basketball Players Association/Women's National Basketball Association Anti-Drug Program
http://sports.findlaw.com/drugs/policy/basketball/index.html

2001-2002 National Collegiate Athletic Association Banned-Drug Classes
http://www.ncaa.org/sports_sciences/drugtesting/

National Football League Policy and Program for Substances of Abuse
http://sports.findlaw.com/drugs/policy/football/index.html

National Hockey League Drug Policy
http://sports.findlaw.com/drugs/policy/hockey/index.html

Union Cycliste Internationale
http://www.uci.ch/english/about/rules/ch14_dopage.pdf

United States Olympic Committee
http://www.usoc.org/

USA Powerlifting Drug Testing/Doping Control Program Overview
http://www.adfpa.com/drug_testing/index.shtml

United States Soccer Federation
http://www.ussoccer.com/home/default.sps

USA Track and Field
http://www.usatf.org/

White House Drug Policy and National Youth Anti-Doping Media Campaign
http://www.playclean.org/

World Boxing Council Rule 4 Medical and Antidoping Regulations
http://www.wbcboxing.com/home/home.html

Index

Note: The italicized *f* and *t* following page numbers refer to figures and tables, respectively.

About the Editors

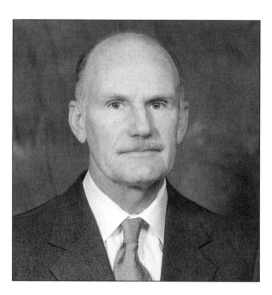

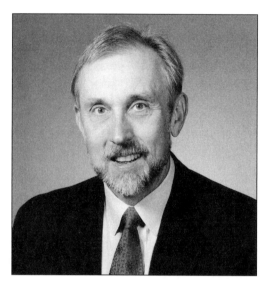

Michael S. Bahrke, PhD, received his MS in exercise physiology and his PhD in sport psychology from the University of Wisconsin at Madison. Dr. Bahrke has been an assistant professor at the University of Kansas, director of research for the U.S. Army Physical Fitness School, fitness area coordinator at the University of Wisconsin, and project director for a National Institute on Drug Abuse-funded anabolic steroids research grant in the School of Public Health, Division of Epidemiology and Biostatistics, at the University of Illinois in Chicago. This research project was designed to investigate the use of performance-enhancing substances in the Chicago area and is one of the largest research projects ever funded by the NIDA. Dr. Bahrke has authored, or co-authored, more than 50 scientific articles and chapters and made presentations at numerous scientific meetings including the International Conference on the Abuse and Trafficking of Anabolic Steroids, sponsored by the U.S. Drug Enforcement Administration. He is a fellow of the American College of Sports Medicine and is currently an acquisitions editor in the Scientific, Technical, and Medical Division of Human Kinetics.

Charles E. Yesalis, MPH, ScD, received his BS and MPH degrees from the University of Michigan, and he was awarded his doctoral degree by the Johns Hopkins School of Hygiene and Public Health in 1975. He then joined the faculty at Johns Hopkins for one year. Dr. Yesalis was a member of the department of preventive medicine and environmental health at the University of Iowa, College of Medicine, from 1976-1986. Currently, he is professor of health policy and administration and exercise and sport science at Pennsylvania State University. For the past 23 years, much of Dr. Yesalis' research has been devoted to the non-medical use of anabolic-androgenic steroids (AAS) and other performance-enhancing drugs. In 1993 he edited, *Anabolic Steroids in Sport and Exercise.* The second edition of *Anabolic Steroids in Sport and Exercise* was released in August, 2000. His other book, *The Steroids Game* (1998), focuses on prevention, education, and intervention regarding AAS use by adolescents. Dr. Yesalis has been a consultant to, among others, the U.S. Senate Judiciary Committee, the Drug Enforcement Administration, the Centers for Disease Control and Prevention, the Food and Drug Administration, the NFL Players Association, the U.S. Olympic Committee, the National Collegiate Athletic Association, and the National Strength and Conditioning Association.

About the Contributors

Hervé J. Allain, MD, obtained his neurology degree in 1977 from the University of Rennes, Rennes, France. He was trained in pharmacology in Paris, then in Rochester, New York on behalf of Pr Lasagna in 1979. He has been the head of the department of experimental and clinical pharmacology at Rennes Medical School, University of Rennes since 1992. Most of his research concerns the use of central nervous system drugs in humans.

Louis C. Almekinders, MD received his medical degree from Erasmus University in Rotterdam, The Netherlands. After completing an orthopaedic residency at the University of North Carolina and a fellowship at Duke University, he joined the faculty of the department of orthopaedic surgery at the University of North Carolina at Chapel Hill. He is currently an associate professor working in orthopaedic sports medicine and soft tissue injury research.

Lawrence E. Armstrong, PhD, FACSM, is an associate professor of exercise science at the Human Performance Laboratory, University of Connecticut. His research specialties include physiological responses to exercise, dietary intervention (e.g., low salt diets, glucose-electrolyte solutions), heat tolerance, and pharmacologic influences on thermoregulation and acclimatization to heat as they apply to athletic and military populations. Professor Armstrong's field studies have focused on heat exhaustion in military units (Panama), heat stress monitors (Australia), heat illness (Texas), casualty rates at the Boston Marathon (Massachusetts), fluid-electrolyte balance in tennis players (Florida), and cooling of heatstroke patients after a summer road race (Falmouth, Massachusetts). He is the author of *Performing in Extreme Environments* (Human Kinetics, 2000).

Danièle Bentué-Ferrer, PhD, was trained in biology at the University of Lyon, France and obtained her pharmacology degree at the University of Paris and the University of Rennes. She is in charge of the unit of kinetics and metabolism in the department of pharmacology at Rennes. Most of her research concerns the impact of drugs on neurotransmitters and the deciphering of the mechanism of action of new psychotropics.

Michel Bourin, MD, PharmD, was trained as a pharmacist at Tours University in 1970 and received his medical degree there in 1979. He also was trained in pharmacology in Paris, France. He has held the position of head of psychopharmacology research since 1981 at the University of Nantes. He is currently professor of pharmacology at the University of Nantes and associate professor in the department of psychiatry at the University of Alberta in Edmonton, Canada. He is treasurer of the European College of Neuropsycho-pharmacology.

J. David Branch, PhD, FACSM received his PhD from the University of South Carolina at Columbia. In 1994 he joined the faculty at Old Dominion University in Norfolk, Virginia where he is the coordinator of the undergraduate exercise science program. He is a fellow in the American College of Sports Medicine.

Priscilla M. Clarkson, PhD, is a professor of exercise science and associate dean for the school of public health and health sciences (SPHHS) at the University of Massachusetts at Amherst. She is a fellow in the American College of Sports Medicine, and she has served as a member of the board of trustees. Currently president of the national ACSM, she also has served as its vice-president and as president of the New England regional ACSM chapter. She is the 1997 recipient of the ACSM Citation Award and the 1999 recipient of the New England ACSM Honor Award. Professor Clarkson has published more than 100 scientific articles and has given numerous national and international scientific presentations. The major focus of her research is on exercise-induced muscle soreness and damage. She has also published in the area of sport nutrition, especially nutritional supplements for weight loss and weight gain. Currently the editor for the *International Journal of Sport Nutrition,* Professor Clarkson serves on the Research Review Board of the Gatorade Sports Science Institute and as a scientific advisor to the International Life Sciences Institute (ILSI). She has served as a member of the Science Working Group at NASA to develop laboratories for Space Station, as scientific advisor to the National Space Biomedical Research Institute and as a member of the NCAA Competitive and Medical Safeguards Committee.

Rachelle Jansevics Cohen, PhD, is a licensed clinical psychologist specializing in addiction treatment. She received her BS in psychology from the University of Washington and her PhD from the University of Georgia. She has been a staff psychologist in the Substance Abuse Treatment Program at the Birmingham VA Medical Center and a coordinator in a similar treatment program at the Atlanta VA Medical Center. In addition, she has served as adjunct faculty at the University of Alabama at Birmingham and Emory University. Most recently, Dr. Jansevics Cohen has been employed as an instructor at Washington State University.

Ellen Coleman, RD, MA, MPH, received a BS degree in home economics from Cal Poly San Luis Obispo in 1975, a MPH in nutrition from Loma Linda University in 1977, and a MA degree in physical education from the University of California at Davis in 1981. She is the nutrition consultant for *The Sport Clinic* in Riverside, California and coauthor of *Ultimate Sports Nutrition* (Bull Publishing 1999). Ellen has completed the Hawaii Ironman triathlon twice. .

Robert K. Conlee, PhD, received his BS and MS degrees from Brigham Young University in physical education and his PhD in exercise physiology from the University of Iowa in 1975 under Charles Tipton. After completing his postdoctoral work at Washington University School of Medicine with John Holloszy, he joined the faculty at Brigham Young University in 1977. He currently is a professor of exercise physiology and dean of the college of health and human performance at Brigham Young University and a fellow of the American College of Sports Medicine.

Dean F. Connors, MD, PhD, received his BS and MS degrees in secondary education from Baylor University in 1976 and 1977 respectively. He received his PhD in exercise physiology from Purdue University in 1984. He was on the staff of the U.S. Army Physical Fitness School from 1983 to 1985. Dr. Connors earned his MD from Michigan State University in 1990 and completed his training in anesthesiology at the Cleveland Clinic Foundation in 1998. Dr. Connors is currently an associate professor of clinical anesthesiology on the faculty of the St. Louis University School of Medicine.

Björn T. Ekblom, MD, received his PhD and MD at the Karolinska Institute, Stockholm, Sweden, in 1969 and 1970, respectively, and since 1977 has been a full professor in physiology at the same institute. In 1973-1974 he was visiting professor in physiology for 9 months at Harvard Medical School at Boston. He currently is a board member of the National Institute of Public Health in Sweden, the Science Academy and the Election Commission for the IOC Prize of the International Olympic Committee, and the Swedish National Center for Research in Sports, and is Chairman of the Medical Commission of the Swedish Football Association. He frequently serves as the science research expert for several national delegations concerned with public health and sport.

Marion Rudin Frank, EdD, is a licensed psychologist with more than 25 years experience in private practice in Philadelphia. She is board certified in medical psychotherapy, group psychotherapy, and clinical hypnotherapy. Dr. Frank serves as president of Professional Psychology Services, PC, a company she founded to address the psychological needs of the business community. She has had several book chapters and numerous articles published, ranging in topics from groups and relationship issues to psychosocial aspects of illness. She is systems-, cognitive-, feminist-, and Jungian-oriented. Formerly, Dr. Frank was a clinical instructor at the Medical College of Pennsylvania, on staff at Temple and Jefferson Universities, and a founding member of the Philadelphia Women's Network. She received her doctorate from Temple University and a master's degree from Columbia.

Duncan N. French, MS, obtained his BS and qualified teacher status in exercise physiology from the University of Northumbria, United Kingdom. He received his MS degree (with distinction) from Leeds Metropolitan University in the United Kingdom, where his major field of study was sport and exercise physiology. Following completion of his masters program, Mr. French was a physical education teacher at a high school in the north east of England for a short period. Presently, Mr. French is a doctoral fellow in the department of kinesiology at the University of Connecticut where he has research interests in the neuromuscular and neuroendocrine responses to resistance training and high intensity exercise.

Stephen J. Heishman, PhD, received his BA in psychology from Vanderbilt University and his PhD in experimental psychology from the University of Louisville. From 1982 to 1986, he was on the psychology faculty at St. Anselm College, Manchester, New Hampshire. After completing a postdoctoral fellowship at Johns Hopkins School of Medicine in 1988, Dr. Heishman joined the intramural research program of the National Institute on Drug Abuse (NIDA), where currently he is a senior investigator in the Clinical Pharmacology and Therapeutics Branch. He is also associate director for Education and Training at NIDA.

R. Craig Kammerer, PhD, is a senior research scientist, consultant, and medical writer in the pharmaceutical industry in New Jersey. Dr. Kammerer obtained his PhD in chemistry from UCLA and then did considerable postdoctoral work in biological chemistry-psychiatry, medicinal chemistry, and pharmacology, before becoming assistant professor of pharmacology at the UCLA School of Medicine in 1978. He was chosen as the founding associate director and technical head of the UCLA-Paul Ziffren Olympic Analytical Laboratory at its inception in 1982, and was one of two faculty that oversaw the development of the 1984 Olympic Games laboratory in Los Angeles. In 1987, he left UCLA for the pharmaceutical industry, and has done research since that time in drug metabolism, analytical pharmacology, toxicology, drug testing, and medical device development.

Steven B. Karch, MD, received his undergraduate degree from Brown University in Providence, Rhode Island, and attended graduate school in anatomy and cell biology at Stanford University. He received his MD degree from Tulane University School of Medicine in New Orleans, did postgraduate training in neuropathology at the Royal London Hospital, and in cardiac pathology at Stanford University at Palo Alto. He is currently assistant medical examiner in San Francisco. He is the author of nearly 100 papers and book chapters, most having to do with the effects of drug abuse on the heart. He has published four books (*The Pathology of Drug Abuse,* 1st and 2nd editions, *Drug Abuse Handbook*, *A Brief History of Cocaine,* and *The Consumer's Guide to Herbal Medicine).* Dr. Karch is a fellow of the American Academy of Forensic Sciences, and a member of the Society of Forensic Toxicologists (SOFT) and the National Association of Medical Examiners (NAME). He is also a fellow of the Royal Society of Medicine in London and The Forensic Science Society (UK).

William J. Kraemer, PhD, is currently a full professor in the department of kinesiology and the human performance laboratory as well as the director of research in the dean's office of the Neag School of Education at the University of Connecticut. Prior to his current position, he held the John and Janice Fisher Endowed Chair in Exercise Physiology and from 1998 until June of 2001 was director of the human performance laboratory and a full professor at Ball State University in Muncie, Indiana. In addition, Dr. Kraemer was an adjunct professor of physiology and biophysics at the Indiana University School of Medicine. Prior to his 1998 appointment at Ball State University, he was a full professor of applied physiology at the Pennsylvania State University. At Penn State he had served as director of the laboratory for sports medicine, was director of research for the center for sports medicine on the University Park campus, and held an appointment in the department of orthopedics in the College of Medicine at Penn State's Milton S. Hershey Medical Center, Hershey, Pennsylvania. He also served as the associate director for the center for cell research at

Penn State and held appointments in the inter-college program in physiology, the department of kinesiology, and in the gerontology center. His research has focused on the endocrine responses and target cell adaptations to exercise and resistance training.

Gordon S. Lynch, PhD, is an assistant professor in the department of physiology at the University of Melbourne. He received his BSc with honors from La Trobe University in 1987 and his PhD from the University of Melbourne in 1992. He was awarded a C.J. Martin Research Fellowship from the National Health and Medical Research Council (NHMRC) of Australia for postdoctoral study at the University of Michigan, where he worked for two-and-a-half years with his mentor, Professor John A. Faulkner. In 1995 he was awarded the A.K. McIntyre Medal from the Australian Physiological and Pharmacological Society for contributions to physiology during his predoctoral and early postdoctoral years. On return to Australia, he was awarded a R. Douglas Wright Fellowship (NHMRC) and a fellowship from the Australian Research Council, and then took up a lectureship at the University of Melbourne in 1999. Dr. Lynch also holds the Certified Strength and Conditioning Specialist qualification from the National Strength and Conditioning Association.

Michael R. McGuigan, PhD, completed his doctorate in exercise physiology at Southern Cross University in Australia. He then completed a postdoctoral research fellowship at in the Human Performance Laboratory at Ball State University. He is currently an assistant professor in the department of exercise and sport science at the University of Wisconsin at La Crosse.

Kurt A. Mossberg, PT, PhD, received a BS degree in biological sciences from Illinois State University, a MS degree in physical therapy from Texas Woman's University, and a PhD degree in physiology/metabolism from the University of Texas Health Science Center at Houston. He is currently associate professor and chair of the physical therapy program at the University of Texas Medical Branch at Galveston. His research focuses on the cardiorespiratory adaptations of individuals with acquired brain and spinal cord pathology.

Bradley C. Nindl, PhD, received his doctoral degree in physiology from the Pennsylvania State University. He is currently a research physiologist and principal investigator in the Military Performance Division at the U.S. Army Research Institute of Environmental Medicine in Natick, Massachusetts, where his lines of research focus on somatotrophic hormonal influences and optimization of soldier physical performance. Dr. Nindl is a fellow in the American College of Sports Medicine (ACSM) and is on the executive committee of the New

England chapter of ACSM. His other professional affiliations include the American Physiological Society, the Endocrine Society, and the National Strength and Conditioning Association. He is a regular reviewer for *Medicine and Science in Sports and Exercise* and the *Journal of Applied Physiology*. He is an author/coauthor of more than 60 publications, chapters, and technical reports on endocrinological, body compositional, and physical performance responses to exercise and military operational stress.

Claire Peel, PhD, PT, received a BS degree in biology from Southwestern University, a MS degree in physical therapy from the University of Southern California, and a PhD degree in physical education from the University of Iowa. She is currently associate professor in the division of physical therapy and assistant dean for academic affairs in the school of health related professions at the University of Alabama at Birmingham. Her research focuses on the role of physical activity in preventing functional decline in older adults.

Charles E. Petit, JD, received his ABs in English and chemistry from Washington University (St. Louis) and his JD magna cum laude from the University of Illinois, where he was articles editor for the University of Illinois Law Review. He became interested in the legal aspects of drug testing as a commanding officer in the U.S. Air Force while handling the aftermath of more than 20 positive drug tests, including two for steroids. He is currently in private practice in Urbana, Illinois.

Eric S. Rawson, PhD, received his PhD from the department of exercise science at the University of Massachusetts at Amherst. He is currently in preventive and behavioral medicine at the University of Massachusetts Medical School in Worcester, Massachusetts. He is a member of the American College of Sports Medicine and has presented research both regionally and nationally. A major focus of his research is the effects of nutritional supplements on exercise performance and weight gain. Dr. Rawson has received funding for this research from the American Federation for Aging Research, the American College of Sports Medicine, and the National Strength and Conditioning Association.

Stan Reents, PharmD, is currently the editor-in-chief of the on-line drug reference "Clinical Pharmacology." Prior to this, he was a clinical specialist with the Adult Internal Medicine service at Shands Hospital at the University of Florida and was also a certified personal trainer. He received his PharmD from the University of the Pacific and completed his residency at the University of Illinois. He recently published *Sport and Exercise Pharmacology,* a text summarizing drug-exercise issues

Pierre Rochcongar, MD, is head of the unit of biology of sport and leads research into the epidemiology of prevention and physiology of physical exercise. He is a member of the executive committee of Société Française de Médecine du Sport as well as Société Française de Traumatologie of Sport, and was physician to the French soccer team from 1988 to 1993.

Martyn R. Rubin, MS, received a BS in kinesiology from Indiana University and a MS in exercise and sport science from the University of Memphis. He is currently a doctoral candidate in the department of kinesiology at the University of Connecticut. His primary research interests are in the areas of exercise endocrinology and nutritional endocrinology with particular emphasis on growth hormone.

Vincenzo R. Sanguineti, MD, is associate professor of psychiatry at Jefferson Medical College in Philadelphia. He was born and raised in Eritrea, completed medical school at the Universita' Degli Studi of Milan, conducted studies in anthropology in the Eritrean western downlands and published field research in tropical medicine in Northern Nigeria, where he also directed a missionary hospital. He came to the United States in 1970, completed his training in psychiatry at Yale and was a member of its faculty until he moved to Philadelphia in 1989. He has published in several leading journals on severe psychopathology and co-morbidity from substance abuse. His latest book *Landscapes in my Mind* addresses the largely unresearched field of subjectivity. He is presently in private practice in Philadelphia.

Lawrence L. Spriet, PhD, received his BSc in kinesiology from the University of Waterloo, MSc in exercise physiology from York University and PhD in medical sciences from McMaster University. After a postdoctoral fellowship at Huddinge University Hospital in Sweden, he joined the department of human biology and nutritional sciences, where he is currently a professor of exercise physiology. Dr. Spriet's teaching and research focuses on the effects of exercise and nutrition on the regulation of energy metabolism in human skeletal muscle and the effects of ergogenic aids on athletic performance. He is also a member of the Gatorade Sports Medicine Review Board.

Robert D. Stainback, PhD, is a licensed clinical psychologist and a private practice consultant in sport psychology. Previously, he directed the Substance Abuse Treatment Program at the Birmingham Department of Veterans Affairs Medical Center in Birmingham, Alabama and served as an assistant professor in psychology and psychiatry at the University of Alabama at Birmingham. He has more than 20 years of experience in the substance abuse treatment field. Dr. Stainback received his PhD and MBA from the University of Alabama.

Suzanne Nelson Steen, DSc, RD, is the sports nutritionist for the University of Washington Huskies athletic teams and is a faculty member in the graduate nutritional sciences program, department of epidemiology, University of Washington. Prior to joining the Husky staff, Dr. Steen was an assistant professor and chair of the graduate nutrition education department at Immaculata College in Pennsylvania. She has also served as clinical director of the weight and eating disorders center at the University of Pennsylvania School of Medicine, department of psychiatry. Dr. Steen was a consulting nutritionist to USA Wrestling and a member of the nutrition advisory committee for US Swimming. Throughout her career, Dr. Steen has worked with many different athletic teams and counseled both recreational and elite athletes. She has given presentations across the country on various topics in sports nutrition and exercise science to coaches, athletes, and health professionals. Dr. Steen's work with athletes has been published in numerous journal articles, book chapters, and books. Her most recent books include *The Ultimate Sports Nutrition Handbook, Nutrition for Sport and Exercise,* and *Play Hard Eat Right: A Parents' Guide to Sports Nutrition for Children.* Steen earned her BS in psychology at Ursinus College, a MS in clinical nutrition at Drexel University, and a PhD in nutritional science at Boston University. She is a registered dietitian of the American Dietetic Association, and a member of the American College of Sports Medicine. Dr. Steen serves on the Gatorade Sports Nutrition Advisory Board, on the editorial board of the *International Journal of Sport Nutrition,* and is a past member of the Gatorade Board of Advisors for Science and Education–North America.

John Sudkamp, MD, received his AS in radiological technology from George Washington University, Washington, DC, while on active duty in the US Navy. After discharge from active duty he received his BS in health sciences from the Medical University of South Carolina in Charleston, South Carolina and his MD from the University of Illinois College of Medicine, Rockford, Illinois. He completed two years of surgical residency in Syracuse, New York prior to joining the St. Louis University anesthesia residency where he is currently serving as chief resident.

Gary I. Wadler, MD, FACP, FACSM, FACPM, FCP, received his medical degree from Cornell University Medical College and completed his residency in internal medicine at the New York Hospital. From 1980 to 1991, he served as the tournament physician at the US Open Tennis Championships. He was the lead author of the seminal text, *Drugs and the Athlete.* In 1993, he was the recipient of the IOC President's Prize for his work in the field of doping. He has served as a trustee of the American College of Sports Medicine and the Women's Sports Foundation where he is currently on the Board of Stewards. Dr. Wadler has served as a steroid expert for the Department of Justice in a number of criminal prosecutions and has represented the United States at WHO international conferences on the prevention of doping. He served as a member of the Technical Advisory Group of the CASA National Commission on Sports and Substance Abuse and was a consultant in the preparation of its report, *Winning at Any Cost: Doping in Olympic Sports.* Dr. Wadler serves as the medical advisor to the White House Office of National Drug Control Policy where he participated in the preparation of its position document, *Enhancing U.S. International Efforts to Combat Drug Use and Doping in Sport,* and he was a participant in the White House Task Force on Drug Use in Sports. He is a U.S. member of the World Anti-Doping Agency's Health, Medicine and Research Committee and is the Substance Abuse Advisor to the National Basketball Association. Dr. Wadler is the chairman of the Nassau County Sports Commission in New York and is a member of the board of directors of OATH (Olympic Advocates Together Honorably). He is an associate professor of clinical medicine at the NYU School of Medicine and a senior attending physician at North Shore University Hospital in Manhasset, New York, where he is in the private practice of internal medicine and sport medicine.

Michael J. Webster, PhD, received a BS degree from Oregon State University in 1985, a MS degree from the University of Northern Iowa in 1987, and a PhD degree from Auburn University in 1992. He served on the faculty at Western Illinois University from 1992-1997. In 1997 he joined the faculty at the University of Southern Mississippi where he is presently an associate professor of exercise physiology and director of the laboratory of applied physiology in the school of human performance and recreation. His research focus has been nutritional supplementation and muscle fatigue. Michael and his wife Miriam have four boys.

Melvin H. Williams, PhD, FACSM, received his PhD from the University of Maryland in 1968 and immediately joined the faculty at Old Dominion University in Norfolk, Virginia. He established the Human Performance Laboratory whose research focus for 30 years involved the effect of various pharmacological, physiological, and nutritional ergogenic aids on human exercise and sport performance, culminating in several authored and edited books on performance-enhancing substances. Dr. Williams is also the founding editor of the *International Journal of Sport Nutrition and Exercise Metabolism.* Currently he is an eminent scholar emeritus at Old Dominion University.

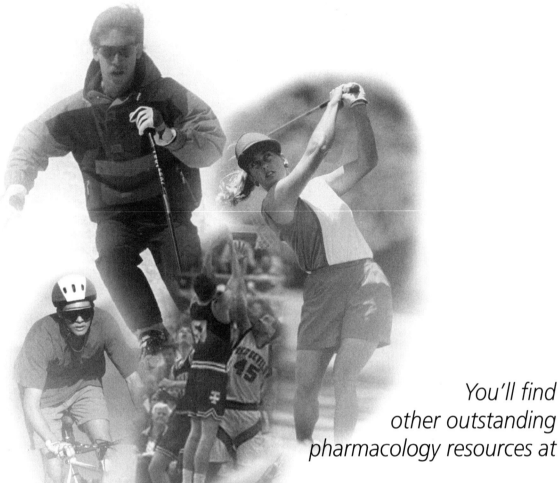